PHARMACY & FEDERAL DRUG LAW REVIEW

A PATIENT PROFILE APPROACH

PHARMACY & FEDERAL DRUG LAW REVIEW
A PATIENT PROFILE APPROACH

EDITORS

DAVID C. KOSEGARTEN, PhD, RPh

Emeritus Professor of Pharmacology and Toxicology
Massachusetts College of Pharmacy and Health Sciences
Boston, Massachusetts

DOUGLAS J. PISANO, PhD, RPh

Associate Provost for Pharmacy Education
Dean, School of Pharmacy–Boston
Massachusetts College of Pharmacy and Health Sciences
Boston, Massachusetts

McGRAW-HILL
MEDICAL PUBLISHING DIVISION

New York / Chicago / San Francisco / Lisbon / London / Madrid / Mexico City
Milan / New Delhi / San Juan / Seoul / Singapore / Sydney / Toronto

Pharmacy & Federal Drug Law Review
A Patient Profile Approach

3 4 5 6 7 8 9 0   QPD/QPD   0 9

Set ISBN: 0-07-144560-9
Book ISBN: 0-07-146809-9
CD-ROM ISBN: 0-07-146810-2

This book was set in Souvenir by TechBooks.
The editors were Michael Brown, Christie Naglieri, and Patrick Carr.
The production supervisor was Catherine H. Saggese.
The cover designer was Pehrsson Design.
Quebecor World was the printer and binder.

This book is printed on acid-free paper.

Tell the authors and publisher what you think about this book by sending your comments to pharmacy@mcgraw-hill.com. Please put the author and title in the subject line.

Library of Congress Cataloging-in-Publication Data

Kosegarten, David C.
    Pharmacy & federal drug law review : a patient profile approach /
David C. Kosegarten, Douglas J. Pisano.— Ist ed.
        p. cm.
    Includes bibliographyical references and index.
    ISBN 0-07-144560-9 (softcover)
    1. Pharmacy. 2. Pharmacy—Law and legislation—United States.
I. Title: Pharmacy and federal drug law review. II. Pisano, Douglas J.
III. Title.

RS92.K67 2006
615'.1—dc22
                                                            2005050527

*To the hard working faculty for their tireless efforts to publish
a case study book that is truly reflective of present day
pharmacy practice, and thus an important review
for student success.*

CONTRIBUTORS

Michael Angelini, MA, PharmD, BCPP

Assistant Professor of Clinical Pharmacy
Massachusetts College of Pharmacy and Health Sciences, School of
  Pharmacy–Boston
Pharmacotherapist
Veterans Affairs, Boston Healthcare System, Outpatient Clinic
[Patient Profiles # 18, 38, 55, 62, 74, 95, 111, 122, 131, 150,
  168, 179, 188, 222, and 248]

Paul Belliveau, PharmD, RPh

Associate Professor of Pharmacy Practice
Massachusetts College of Pharmacy and Health Sciences, School of
  Pharmacy–Worcester
[Patient Profiles # 67, 126, 183, 224, and 250]

Dawn Chandler-Toufieli, PharmD, RPh

Assistant Professor of Pharmacy Practice
Massachusetts College of Pharmacy and Health Sciences, School of
  Pharmacy–Boston
[Patient Profiles # 198, 200, 202, 206, 209, 212, and 215]

Maryann R. Cooper, PharmD, BCPS

Assistant Professor of Pharmacy Practice
Massachusetts College of Pharmacy and Health Sciences, School of
  Pharmacy–Boston
[Patient Profiles # 19, 86, 142, 199, and 232]

Ronald J. DeBellis, PharmD, RPh

Chair and Associate Professor, Department of Pharmacy
  Practice
Massachusetts College of Pharmacy and Health Sciences, School of
  Pharmacy–Worcester
[Patient Profiles # 7, 10, 15, 23, 30, 33, 46, 50, 64, 69, 79, 87,
  98, 103, 123, 143, 155, 158, 160, 180, 207, and 236]

Claire DiFrancesco, RPh

Instructor of Pharmacy Practice
Massachusetts College of Pharmacy and Health Sciences, School of
  Pharmacy–Worcester
[Patient Profiles # 54, 114, 171, 218, and 244]

Kaelen Dunican, RPh

Instructor of Pharmacy Practice
Massachusetts College of Pharmacy and Health Sciences, School of
  Pharmacy–Worcester
[Patient Profiles # 58, 118, 175, 220, and 246]

Trisha Ford-LaPointe, PharmD, BCPS

Assistant Professor of Pharmacy Practice
Massachusetts College of Pharmacy and Health Sciences, School of
  Pharmacy–Boston
Pharmacist Faculty
Massachusetts General Hospital
[Patient Profiles # 25, 91, 148, 203, and 234]

James M. Gagnon, PharmD

Assistant Professor of Pharmacy Practice
Massachusetts College of Pharmacy and Health Sciences, School of
  Pharmacy–Boston
Clinical Pharmacist
Brooks Pharmacy
[Patient Profiles # 41, 104, 161, 211, and 239]

Nancy Huff, PharmD

Assistant Professor of Pharmacy
Massachusetts College of Pharmacy and Health Sciences, School of
  Pharmacy–Boston
[Patient Profiles # 14, 34, 51, 70, 93, 107, 127, 149, 164, and 184]

Courtney I. Jarvis, PharmD

Assistant Professor of Pharmacy Practice
Massachusetts College of Pharmacy and Health Sciences, School of
  Pharmacy–Worcester
[Patient Profiles # 56, 116, 173, 219, and 245]

David C. Kosegarten, PhD, RPh

Professor of Pharmacology and Toxicology, Emeritus
Massachusetts College of Pharmacy and Health Sciences, School of
  Pharmacy–Boston

Susan Krikorian, MS, RPh

Associate Professor of Pharmacy Practice
Massachusetts College of Pharmacy and Health Sciences, School of
  Pharmacy–Boston
[Patient Profiles # 20, 27, 31, 39, 57, 76, 92, 96, 113, 133, 145,
  153, 170, and 205]

Karen W. Lee, PharmD, BS Chem, CDM

Assistant Professor of Pharmacy Practice
Massachusetts College of Pharmacy and Health Sciences, School of
  Pharmacy–Boston
[Patient Profile # 21, 88, 144, 201, and 233]

Matthew R. Machado, PharmD

Assistant Professor of Pharmacy Practice
Massachusetts College of Pharmacy and Health Sciences, School of
  Pharmacy–Boston
[Patient Profiles # 13, 83, 138, 195, and 230]

Eric J. Mack, PhD, RPh

Assistant Professor of Pharmaceutics
Loma Linda University, School of Pharmacy
[Patient Profiles # 8, 28, 47, 66, 84, 101, 121, 141, and 178]

Michael J. Malloy, PharmD

Dean and Professor
Massachusetts College of Pharmacy and Health Sciences, School of
  Pharmacy–Worcester/Manchester
[Patient Profiles # 48, 110, 167, 216, and 242]

Michele Matthews, PharmD

Assistant Professor of Pharmacy Practice
Massachusetts College of Pharmacy and Health Sciences, School of
Pharmacy–Worcester
Clinical Pharmacist, Hahnemann Family Health Center/UMass
Memorial Healthcare
[Patient Profiles # 3, 73, 128, 185, and 225]

William W. McCloskey, PharmD, RPh

Associate Professor of Pharmacy Practice
Massachusetts College of Pharmacy and Health Sciences, School of
Pharmacy–Boston
[Patient Profiles # 6, 17, 26, 44, 63, 82, 85, 99, 119, 139, 140,
156, 176, 194, 197, and 231]

Lisa McDevitt, PharmD, BCPS

Assistant Professor of Pharmacy Practice
Clinical Specialist in Organ Transplantation
Massachusetts College of Pharmacy and Health Sciences, School of
Pharmacy–Boston
[Patient Profiles # 9, 77, 134, 191, and 228]

Ahmed S. Mehanna, PhD

Associate Professor of Medicinal Chemistry
Massachusetts College of Pharmacy and Health Sciences, School of
Pharmacy–Boston
[Patient Profiles # 16, 29, 36, 53, 72, 89, 94, 109, 129, 147,
151, 166, 186, 204, and 235]

Anna K. Morin, PharmD

Assistant Professor of Pharmacy Practice
Massachusetts College of Pharmacy and Health Sciences, School of
Pharmacy–Worcester
[Patient Profiles # 45, 108, 165, 214, and 241]

S. Mimi Mukherjee, PharmD, BCPS, CDE

Assistant Professor
Massachusetts College of Pharmacy and Health Sciences, School of
Pharmacy–Boston
Primary Care Pharmacist
Boston Veterans Administration Health Care System
[Patient Profiles # 11, 81, 136, 193, and 229]

Nicole M. Nolan, PharmD, RPh

Assistant Professor of Pharmacy Practice
Massachusetts College of Pharmacy and Health Sciences, School of
Pharmacy–Worcester
[Patient Profiles # 4, 24, 42, 52, 61, 80, 112, 117, 137, 154,
169, 174, 192, 217, and 243]

Marie Normand, PharmD

Assistant Professor of Pharmacy Practice
Massachusetts College of Pharmacy and Health Sciences, School of
Pharmacy–Boston
[Patient Profiles # 5, 75, 132, 189, and 227]

Douglas J. Pisano, PhD, RPh

Dean, School of Pharmacy–Boston
Associate Professor of Pharmacy Administration
Massachusetts College of Pharmacy and Health Sciences, School of
Pharmacy–Boston
[Law Section: Patient Profiles # 1, 2, 3, 4, 5, 6, 7, 8, 9, 10, 11,
12, 13, 14, and 15]

Dorothea Rudorf, PharmD, MS(G), RPh

Associate Professor of Pharmacy Practice
Clinical Pharmacy Specialist in Infectious Diseases
Massachusetts College of Pharmacy and Health Sciences, School of
Pharmacy–Boston
[Patient Profiles # 35, 100, 157, 208, and 237]

Sheila Seed, RPh, MPH, BS Pharm

Assistant Instructor of Pharmacy Practice
Massachusetts College of Pharmacy and Health Sciences, School of
Pharmacy–Worcester
[Patient Profiles # 60, 120, 177, 221, and 247]

Matthew A. Silva, PharmD, RPh

Assistant Professor of Pharmacy Practice
Massachusetts College of Pharmacy and Health Sciences, School of
Pharmacy–Worcester
Adjunct Assistant Professor, Department of Family Medicine
University of Massachusetts Medical School & Family Health Center
of Worcester
[Patient Profiles # 65, 124, 181, 223, and 249]

Blaine T. Smith, RPh, PhD

Assistant Professor of Pharmacy Practice
Massachusetts College of Pharmacy and Health Sciences, School of
Pharmacy–Worcester
[Patient Profile # 43, 106, 163, 213, and 240]

Karyn M. Sullivan, RPh, MPH

Assistant Professor of Pharmacy Practice
Massachusetts College of Pharmacy and Health Sciences, School of
Pharmacy–Worcester
[Patient Profiles # 1, 71, 128, 185, and 225]

Tobias C. Trujillo, PharmD, RPh

Assistant Professor of Clinical Pharmacy
Massachusetts College of Pharmacy and Health Sciences, School of
Pharmacy–Boston
[Patient Profiles # 2, 22, 40, 59, 78, 97, 115, 135, 152, 172,
190, and 196]

Caroline S. Zeind, PharmD, RPh

Chair and Associate Professor, Department of Pharmacy Practice
Massachusetts College of Pharmacy and Health Sciences, School of
Pharmacy–Boston
[Patient Profiles # 12, 32, 37, 49, 68, 90, 102, 105, 125, 146,
159, 162, 182, 210, and 238]

CONTENTS

PART II:

LAW / 315

PATIENT PROFILES:

PART III:

ANSWERS WITH EXPLANATIONS AND REFERENCES / 345

PART III

PREFACE

Pharmacy students become pharmacy practitioners only after successfully passing the national licensure examination as well as state and federal law examinations. These exams are the North American Pharmacist Licensure Examination (NABPLEX) and the Multi-State Pharmacy Jurisprudence Exam (MJPE). Overall, the pass rate for these examinations is quite good, the majority of students passing these exams and obtaining state pharmacy practice licenses on the first attempt. While this is statistically admirable, it does not speak to the preparation needed to accomplish this very difficult task. The purpose of this review book is to help with that task by offering more than 200 real life case study reviews of disease states, pharmacotherapeutics, pharmaceutic, pharmacologic and other basic science refreshers as well as an overview of federal pharmacy law.

The authors, either current or former members of faculty of the Massachusetts College of Pharmacy and Health Sciences, School of Pharmacy Boston–Worcester, who have prepared cases for this book have taken great care to develop relevant and meaningful exercises. In addition, each case has a number of thought provoking questions to accompany it, several hundred in fact, with detailed answers and citations to better explain the concepts. Great pains were taken to incorporate the criteria as described by the National Association of Boards of Registration in Pharmacy (NABP) who administer these exams. On behalf of the Editors and faculty authors, we wish you the very best success in your future and rewarding careers as pharmacy professionals.

David C. Kosegarten, PhD, RPh
Douglas J. Pisano, PhD, RPh

PART I

PATIENT PROFILES:
CASE PRESENTATIONS,
QUESTIONS, AND ANSWERS

OVER-THE-COUNTER PRODUCTS

PRESENTATION

CC: "How am I going to keep track of all these pills?"

HPI: WM is a 55-year-old Caucasian man who is being released from the hospital today after having a heart attack while cutting his lawn 3 weeks ago.

PMH: Hypertension, hyperlipidemia, gout, status post myocardial infarction

MH: Lisinopril 20 mg PO qd, atorvastatin 20 mg PO qd, allopurinol 300 mg PO qd, enteric-coated aspirin 325 mg PO qd, nitroglycerin 0.4-mg tablets SL PRN

Allergies: PCN (urticaria)

FH: Father died at age 78 owing to unknown causes. Mother died at age 82 with Alzheimer's disease. WM has two brothers, ages 64 and 59, who both have a history of hypertension.

SH: WM has been married for 30 years. He works as a chemical engineer for a large company. He occasionally works 14-hour days and considers his job to be extremely stressful. WM does not exercise and has poor eating habits owing to his long workdays. He denies the use of alcohol, tobacco, and illicit drugs. He usually drinks about 8 cups of coffee per day.

PHYSICAL EXAMINATION

Gen: Overweight Caucasian male who is nervous about going home on his new medications

VS: Blood pressure: 135/95 mm Hg; pulse: 96 beats per minute; respiratory rate: 20 respirations per minute; temperature: 98.9°F; height: 5 ft, 7 in; weight: 105 kg

HEENT: PERRLA; fundi clear; ears clear

CV: Normal S_1, S_2 heart sounds; no m/r/g

Pulm: Clear to A&P

Abd: Soft, nontender; bowel sounds present in all four quadrants.

Neuro: A&O × 3; reflexes are symmetric and active.

Ext: Normal skin turgor; no joint tenderness or swelling

LABORATORY VALUES

Sodium: 141 mEq/L

Potassium: 4.6 mEq/L

Chloride: 105 mEq/L

CO_2 content: 26 mEq/L

Blood urea nitrogen (BUN): 15 mg/dL

Serum creatinine: 1.1 mg/dL

Glucose: 105 mg/dL

Albumin: 4 mg/dL

Hemoglobin: 17 g/dL

Hematocrit: 50%

Platelets: 200 K/mm³

White blood cell (WBC) count: 6000/mm³

Total cholesterol: 320 mg/dL

Triglycerides: 390 mg/dL

High-density lipoprotein (HDL) cholesterol: 58 mg/dL

Low-density lipoprotein (LDL) cholesterol: 184 mg/dL

QUESTIONS

1. Which of the following should be added to WM's list of discharge medications?

   A. Digoxin
   B. Doxazosin
   C. Atenolol
   D. Amlodipine
   E. Candesartan

2. What is the maximum daily dosage of aspirin?

   A. 4 g
   B. 2.4 g
   C. 3.2 g
   D. 1.5 g
   E. 600 mg

3. Which of the following is *not true* regarding the addition of niacin to WM's therapy?

   A. Niacin is associated with cutaneous flushing and itching.
   B. Aspirin administration prior to niacin ingestion can reduce the prostaglandin-mediated response that commonly occurs.
   C. Nicotinamide is an effective agent used to reduce cholesterol and triglyceride levels.
   D. Niaspan is a sustained-release form of niacin that is associated with fewer dermatologic reactions.
   E. WM's gout may be exacerbated by niacin because it can cause hyperuricemia.

4. WM comes to the pharmacy to find out which over-the-counter product he should take for his headache. He holds up a bottle of acetaminophen and a bottle of ibuprofen. Which therapy would be the best choice for WM, taking his current medication list into account?

   A. Ibuprofen and acetaminophen are both acceptable options for WM.
   B. Acetaminophen; the antihypertensive effects of angiotensin-converting enzyme (ACE) inhibitors may be antagonized with concurrent

ibuprofen administration if used more than several days.

C. Ibuprofen; the antihypertensive effects of ACE inhibitors may be antagonized with concurrent acetaminophen administration if used more than several days.

D. Ibuprofen; ibuprofen has a higher maximum daily dosage than acetaminophen.

E. Neither acetaminophen nor ibuprofen is a good alternative for WM because they both inhibit platelet aggregation, and this may interfere with his aspirin therapy.

5. Which of the following is(are) *true* regarding aspirin administration in cardiac patients?

   I. Clopidogrel is a useful alternative in patients with a true aspirin sensitivity.
   II. Aspirin should be given indefinitely to patients who have experienced ST-segment or non-ST-segment elevation myocardial infarction (MI).
   III. According to current guidelines, patients with a suspected MI should immediately chew and swallow 160 to 325 mg non-enteric-coated aspirin.

   A. I only
   B. III only
   C. I and II only
   D. II and III only
   E. I, II, and III

6. WM returns to his doctor for a checkup and complains of a nonproductive cough that does not seem to go away. Which of WM's medications could be responsible for this reaction?

   A. Allopurinol
   B. Aspirin
   C. Nitroglycerin
   D. Lisinopril
   E. Atorvastatin

7. Which statement *most accurately* identifies the mechanism of action of aspirin regarding its effect on platelets?

   A. Aspirin decreases prostaglandin E_2 (PGE_2) synthesis.
   B. Aspirin irreversibly acetylates cyclooxygenase, which reduces thromboxane A_2 (TXA_2).
   C. Aspirin increases prostaglandin synthesis in the central nervous system (CNS).
   D. Aspirin traps free radicals and stabilizes lysosomal membranes.
   E. Aspirin increases arachidonic acid release.

8. Aspirin in usual doses may be associated with all the following *except*

   A. Metabolic alkalosis
   B. Urticaria
   C. Bronchoconstriction
   D. Prolonged bleeding time
   E. Reye's syndrome

9. Acetaminophen can produce which of the following effects?

   I. Analgesic
   II. Antipyretic
   III. Antiplatelet

   A. I only
   B. III only
   C. I and II only
   D. II and III only
   E. I, II, and III

10. Which nonprescription medication should be *avoided* in WM unless he is under medical supervision?

    A. Senna
    B. Guaifenesin
    C. Docusate
    D. Chlorpheniramine
    E. Pseudoephedrine

PATIENT PROFILE 2

CORONARY ARTERY DISEASE

PRESENTATION

RT is a 52-year-old man brought into the ED with complaints of chest pain, shortness of breath, and palpitations.

RT was at home this morning reading the paper after breakfast when he experienced chest pain of sudden onset in the sternal area that radiated to the left arm and jaw. He describes his chest pain as pressure, 8 out of 10, not associated with any type of exertion. RT immediately took SL nitroglycerin 0.4 mg every 5 minutes × 3 with no relief. RT's wife then called 911. During the ambulance ride the paramedics administered SL nitroglycerin 0.4 mg, and this provided some relief for RT (chest pain now 5/10). On his arrival in the ER, RT was still complaining of 5/10 chest pain, palpitations, dizziness, and shortness of breath.

Past medical history includes CAD for 4 years, no prior acute myocardial infarction, hypertension for 10 years, hyperlipidemia for 10 years, gout, and previous treatment for *Helicobacter pylori* infection.

Current medications are aspirin 325 mg po qd, nifedipine XL 60 mg po qd, lovastatin 20 mg po qd, and allopurinol 200 mg po qd.

RT's father died of AMI at 49. His mother died of breast cancer at 54. RT's social history includes occasional use of alcohol. He stopped smoking 6 months ago and denies use of illicit drugs.

PHYSICAL EXAMINATION

BP: 100/65, HR: 140, RR: 24, T: afebrile
GEN: Middle-aged man in moderate respiratory distress
HEENT: Unremarkable
NECK: No JVD
CHEST: Rales heard at the bases
COR: Tachycardia; SI, S2, and S3 heard
ABD: Unremarkable
EXT: No edema
Neuro: Unremarkable
EKG: ST-segment depression in V4-V6

LABS

Na: 139	K: 3.4
Cl: 100	CO_2: 24
BUN: 118	GLU: 105
SCr: 1.2	Hgb: 13.4
Total chol: 210	WBC: 5.6 K
LDL chol: 145	Hct: 41.5
HDL chol: 30	Plts: 230,000
Trig: 175	

QUESTIONS

1. Which of the following is not a risk factor for the development of CAD?

   A. Smoking
   B. Hypertension
   C. Hyperlipidemia
   D. Family history
   E. Gout

2. RT is diagnosed with unstable angina. Which of the following should be immediately administered to RT?

   A. Diltiazem 30 mg
   B. Isosorbide dinitrate 10 mg
   C. Amiodarone 200 mg
   D. Aspirin 325 mg
   E. Ticlopidine 250 mg

3. RT is transferred to the coronary care unit. Which of the following would not be appropriate to initiate in RT at this time?

   A. IV unfractionated heparin
   B. Nifedipine 30 mg po q4h
   C. IV nitroglycerin
   D. Metoprolol 25 mg po bid
   E. Aspirin 325 mg po qd

4. Which of the following would be appropriate in treating RT for chronic CAD?

   A. Increase nifedipine to 120 mg po qd
   B. Increase lovastatin to 40 mg po qd
   C. Decrease lovastatin to 10 mg po qd
   D. Discontinue aspirin; start ticlopidine 250 mg po bid
   E. Decrease nifedipine to 30 mg po qd

5. Which of the following is not true regarding patient education with sublingual nitroglycerin?

   A. SL nitroglycerin should be replaced every 6 months.
   B. SL nitroglycerin should be stored in a cool, dry place.
   C. After opening a new bottle, the patient should leave the cotton in the bottle to maintain the potency of the medication.
   D. Do not keep in the bathroom medicine cabinet.
   E. Before administering SL nitroglycerin, the patient should sit down.

ATTENTION-DEFICIT/HYPERACTIVITY DISORDER (ADHD)

NC is a 6-year-old boy who presents with his mother to his primary care physician for routine health care maintenance. During his physical examination, NC's mother begins to discuss certain behavioral changes that NC has displayed over the past 7 months. She has brought with her a letter written by his first grade teacher that states that he "blurts out answers in class, constantly leaves his seat, is significantly louder than the other children, uses inappropriate language, does not listen when spoken to, consistently interrupts lessons, does not complete assignments, and has become aggressive with his classmates." His mother states that she has also noticed that NC has become increasingly agitated and "cannot sit still." She explains that he has an 11-year-old brother who has "ADD," and she thinks that NC has similar but worse symptoms. She does not want NC to see a psychiatrist but would like this physician to treat his symptoms.

NC's past medical history includes chronic ceruminosis that is treated with Debrox. His mother gives him acetaminophen for fevers. She states that he has no allergies to medications. NC lives at home with his parents and two older brothers. When questioned about life at home, he says that his parents "yell at each other a lot." His family history is significant for an 11-year-old brother with ADHD (currently taking Adderall XR 20 mg every morning). NC is 35 in tall and weighs 25 kg. Vital signs are within normal limits, and his physical and neurologic examinations are unremarkable. NC has undergone IQ testing in the past and has scored within the normal range for his age. Learning and developmental disorders have been ruled out.

The physician believes that NC has ADHD and initiates immediate-release methylphenidate 5 mg PO twice daily. He schedules NC for a return visit in 1 month to assess his response to the methylphenidate.

QUESTIONS

1. Which of the following patient characteristics meets the *Diagnostic and Statistical Manual of Mental Disorders*, fourth edition (DSM-IV), criteria for the diagnosis of ADHD?

    A. The presence of symptoms both at home and at school
    B. The presence of symptoms for 7 months
    C. His age

    D. A and B only
    E. All the above

2. Which of the following has been shown to be an effective adjunctive therapy in the management of ADHD?

    A. Cognitive behavioral therapy
    B. Electrotherapy
    C. Acupuncture
    D. Relaxation techniques

3. Which of the following statements regarding the use of methylphenidate is correct?

    A. Methylphenidate has been associated with a high incidence of hematologic disorders such as thrombocytopenia; complete blood counts should be assessed monthly.
    B. Methylphenidate can be discontinued abruptly without withdrawal symptoms.
    C. Methylphenidate causes appetite suppression; growth parameters and eating habits should be assessed frequently during therapy.
    D. Methylphenidate causes a dose-dependent increase in blood pressure; vital signs should be assessed monthly.

4. Which of the following are contraindications to methylphenidate therapy?

    A. Tourette's syndrome
    B. Anxiety
    C. Monoamine oxidase (MAO) inhibitor use
    D. B and C only
    E. All the above

5. How long after initiating methylphenidate therapy will it take to see an initial clinical response in NC?

    A. 1 day
    B. 2 weeks
    C. 1 month
    D. 6 months

6. NC returns for his 1-month visit. His mother claims that NC has been having "problems" on methylphenidate. Although both she and his teacher have noticed an improvement in his ADHD symptoms,

she is unable to get him to fall asleep at night. She states that she has been following the directions on the prescription bottle and has been giving him the methylphenidate twice a day at 7 AM and 7 PM. Which of the following is the best recommendation that you can make at this time regarding NC's treatment?

A. Administration of the second dose may be too close to NC's bedtime, and he may be experiencing insomnia from the methylphenidate; doses should be administered at 7 AM and 12 noon.
B. Methylphenidate may be causing insomnia, and therapy should be changed to Adderall because it lacks this side effect.
C. Consider the addition of a hypnotic such as zolpidem to alleviate the insomnia caused by methylphenidate.
D. Consider referring NC to a sleep specialist to determine the cause of his insomnia.

7. NC returns again 1 month later, and his mother is quite happy with the changes that were made to his therapy. She has been reading more about ADHD and has heard about this new medication called Strattera. Which of the following statements regarding Strattera is correct?

A. Strattera has only been approved for use in adults with ADHD.
B. Unlike methylphenidate, Strattera is not scheduled as a CII controlled substance.
C. Unlike methylphenidate, Strattera can be used safely in patients taking MAO inhibitors.
D. Strattera is considered a "nonstimulant" and therefore lacks side effects such as anorexia and anxiety.

8. The physician is considering switching NC to Concerta. Which of the following statements correctly represents an important counseling point that should be relayed to NC's mother?

A. Concerta tablets should not be chewed because this could release the medication too quickly and cause severe side effects.
B. Components of the Concerta tablet called *ghosts* may be seen in the stool; this is normal.
C. Concerta should only be given on an empty stomach.
D. A and B only
E. All the above

9. NC is doing well on his ADHD therapy, but his teacher has noted that his aggressiveness with his classmates has not subsided. His mother wants to know if there is any way to treat this. She states that her nephew was treated years ago for ADHD and that he also had aggressive symptoms, but she cannot remember the name of the medication he was given. Which one of the following medications has been used to treat aggressive behaviors in children?

A. Clonazepam
B. Clonidine
C. Imipramine
D. Venlafaxine

10. NC's mother says that the name of the medication that was used to treat her nephew's ADHD was pemoline. Which of the following statements regarding the use of pemoline is correct?

A. It has been associated with fatal hepatotoxicity and is no longer considered a first-line therapy in the management of ADHD.
B. It has been associated with hematologic side effects such as aplastic anemia.
C. It has been associated with ocular side effects such as nystagmus.
D. All the above

PATIENT PROFILE 4

HYPERTENSION

PRESENTATION

LB is a 56-year-old white woman who undergoes a routine examination by her primary care physician. She has a history of asthma, gastroesophageal reflux disease (GERD), type II diabetes mellitus, and peripheral neuropathy. She is post-menopausal. LB has no known drug allergies and currently takes conjugated estrogen 0.625 mg po qd, medroxyprogesterone 5 mg po qd, albuterol MDI 2 puffs qid prn, ranitidine 300 mg po qhs, and glyburide 10 mg po qd. She has smoked 1½ packs of cigarettes per day for the past

20 years. LB's blood pressure at this office visit is recorded in the chart as 158/94.

QUESTIONS

1. You want to determine whether the blood pressure was measured correctly. Which of the following is false regarding the measurement of blood pressure?

   A. Measurement should begin after at least 5 minutes of rest.
   B. Patients should refrain from smoking or ingesting caffeine during the 30 minutes before the measurement.
   C. Two or more readings separated by 2 minutes should be averaged.
   D. The bladder within the cuff should encircle ≥ 80% of the arm.
   E. The first appearance of sound is used to define diastolic blood pressure.

2. LB's blood pressure is above normal at each of two visits after the initial screening. Hypertension is diagnosed. Which of the following medications is the best initial therapy for LB?

   A. Hydrochlorothiazide
   B. Losartan
   C. Clonidine
   D. Propranolol
   E. Enalapril

3. The goal blood pressure for LB is

   A. <140/90 mm Hg.
   B. <140/80 mm Hg.
   C. <120/80 mm Hg.
   D. <130/80 mm Hg.
   E. <110/90 mm Hg.

4. Which of the following are risk factors for the development of cardiovascular disease?

   A. Diabetes mellitus
   B. Smoking
   C. Sex (men and postmenopausal women)
   D. Only A and B
   E. A, B, and C

PATIENT PROFILE 5

DIABETES

PRESENTATION

CC: KE is a 48-year-old man who presents to your pharmacy with a prescription for metformin. This is the first time he will be taking this medication.

HPI: After talking to KE, you discover that he was diagnosed with type 2 diabetes last week after routine blood tests at his regular checkup. He was given a blood glucose monitor and supplies and was told to test his blood sugar two to three times daily, record the results in a log book, and bring it with him to his next appointment in 3 months. KE has brought his laboratory work with him to the pharmacy for you to see.

PMH: Hypertension, dyslipidemia, obesity, osteoarthritis (right knee)

ALL: NKDA

MH: Amlodipine 5 mg PO qd, naproxen 500 mg PO bid, niacin SR 1000 mg PO qd, atorvastatin 10 mg PO qd, MVI 1 PO qam

FH: Mother, 74, alive; 30-year history of type 2 diabetes; right toe amputation. Father, 76, alive; status post myocardial infarction at age 64.

SH: Married, two children, high school math teacher. Denies smoking; admits to occasional alcohol use.

Tried unsuccessfully to lose weight twice in the past year.

VS: BP = 144/92 mm Hg; temperature = 98.7°F; height = 5 ft, 11 in; weight = 248 lb.

Labs: 140 101 16; total cholesterol: 210 mg/dL; low-density lipoprotein (LDL) cholesterol: 150 mg/dL; 134; high-density lipoprotein (HDL) cholesterol: 38 mg/dL; triglycerides: 154 mg/dL; 4.2 27 1.2

VISIT NOTES

KE would like to have a printout for metformin. He likes to read about a new medication before he takes it.

He has a friend who is taking this medication and knows it may upset his stomach. Since he is at school all day, he is particularly worried about this side effect. He also wants to purchase some glucose tablets to bring to school with him.

QUESTIONS

1. Which of the following is *true* regarding KE's blood pressure, according to current guidelines?

A. KE's blood pressure of 144/92 mm Hg is at goal. He should continue his amlodipine regimen.
B. KE is not at goal. He should be started on lisinopril, and the dose should be titrated to reach a goal blood pressure of less than 140/90 mm Hg.
C. KE is not at goal. He should be started on lisinopril, and the dose should be titrated to reach a goal blood pressure of less than 130/80 mm Hg.
D. KE is not at goal. He should be started on lisinopril, and the dose should be titrated to reach a goal blood pressure of less than 125/75 mm Hg.

2. Which of the following is *true* regarding KE's lipid levels, according to current guidelines?

A. KE should start cholestyramine to lower his triglyceride level.
B. KE's lipid levels are at goal. He should continue with his atorvastatin regimen.
C. KE's lipid levels are not at goal. He should be treated to reach a goal LDL of les than 100 mg/dl and HDL of greater than 40 mg/dl.
D. KE should not continue to take his niacin because it may raise his blood sugar. The atorvastatin is sufficient to treat his dyslipidemia.

3. Which of the following is the *most appropriate* recommendation for KE regarding eye examinations?

A. KE should have a full dilated and comprehensive eye examination by an ophthalmologist or an optometrist as soon as possible, and the examination should be repeated annually.
B. KE should have a full dilated and comprehensive eye examination by an ophthalmologist or an optometrist in 5 years, and the examination should be repeated every 5 years if it is normal.
C. KE should have a full dilated and comprehensive eye examination by an ophthalmologist or an optometrist in 3 years, and the examination should be repeated every 5 years if it is normal.
D. KE should have a full dilated and comprehensive eye examination by an ophthalmologist or an optometrist as soon as possible, and the examination should be repeated every 5 years if it is normal.

4. Which of the following is the *most appropriate* recommendation for KE regarding the influenza vaccine?

A. KE should receive his flu shot annually.
B. KE should receive an annual flu shot starting at 65 years of age.
C. KE should only receive a flu shot if there is no national shortage of influenza vaccine.
D. KE should receive one lifetime flu shot and should be revaccinated when he is 65 years of age.

5. Which of the following is the *most appropriate* recommendation for proper foot care in KE?

A. KE should have his first foot examination in 5 years.
B. KE should have a full and comprehensive foot examination every 3 months.
C. KE should have a full and comprehensive foot examination annually, and his feet should be examined visually at every routine visit.
D. KE should be counseled to clip his toenails regularly and to cut away any bunions or blisters that may appear between doctor visits.

6. Which of the following is the *most appropriate* statement regarding the use of metformin in KE?

A. Metformin is not appropriate for KE. It should not be used as monotherapy.
B. Metformin is not appropriate for KE. He should be started on glyburide because it is not associated with weight gain.
C. Metformin is appropriate therapy for KE. He should be counseled regarding the high risk of hypoglycemia associated with its use.
D. Metformin is appropriate therapy for KE. He should be counseled on the risk of nausea and vomiting when starting this medication.

7. Which of the following is a risk factor for diabetic foot infections?

A. Family history of diabetes
B. Diabetes less than 5 years
C. Presence of one or more diabetic complications
D. Family history of amputation due to a foot infection

8. Which of the following may be a contraindication to metformin therapy?

A. Age >65 years
B. Serum creatinine >1.0
C. Circulatory dysfunction
D. Concurrent insulin therapy

9. What is KE's body mass index (BMI)?

A. 27
B. 30
C. 35
D. 40

10. According to current guidelines, does KE have the metabolic syndrome?

A. Yes, KE meets the criteria for diagnosis of the metabolic syndrome.
B. No, KE does not meet the criteria for diagnosis of the metabolic syndrome.

PATIENT PROFILE 6

SEIZURE DISORDERS

PRESENTATION

ZM is a 20-year-old woman receiving 300 mg phenytoin for treatment of a generalized disorder secondary to a motor vehicle accident 1 year ago. Although seizure free for the past 6 months, she now reports being increasingly confused and lethargic. Nystagmus is detected at physical examination. She is taking no other medications, but has been dieting to lose weight before her upcoming wedding. A total phenytoin concentration is obtained and is reported to be 14 mg/L (desired range, 10 to 20 mg/L). Other laboratory results are as follows:

Na: 138 mEq/L (135–145 mEq/L)
BUN: 10 mg/dL (8–20 mg/dL)
Cr: 1.0 mg/dL (0.7–1.5 mg/dL)
Albumin 2.5 g/dL (3.5–5 g/dL)
K: 3.5 mEq/L (3.5–5 mEq/L)
Cl: 98 mEq/L (96–106 mEq/L)
ALT: 8 IU/L (0–35 IU/L)
AST: 10 IU/L (0–40 IU/L)

QUESTIONS

1. What is this patient's primary drug-related problem?

   A. Phenytoin toxicity secondary to impaired hepatic function
   B. Phenytoin toxicity secondary to impaired renal function
   C. Phenytoin toxicity secondary to a decrease in protein binding
   D. Phenytoin toxicity secondary to a decrease in free phenytoin concentration
   E. Phenytoin toxicity secondary to serum electrolyte abnormalities

2. Which of the following side effects of phenytoin therapy is not related to increased serum concentrations?

   A. Ataxia
   B. Sedation
   C. Hirsutism
   D. A and B
   E. A, B, and C

3. After her phenytoin therapy has been optimized, ZM returns to the clinic just before her wedding and requests an oral contraceptive. Which of the following statements regarding oral contraceptives and phenytoin is most correct?

   A. There is no potential drug-drug interaction.
   B. Phenytoin inhibits the metabolism of oral contraceptives and may increase their side effects.
   C. Oral contraceptives inhibit the metabolism of phenytoin and may increase its side effects.
   D. Phenytoin induces the metabolism of oral contraceptives and may decrease their efficacy.
   E. Oral contraceptives induce the metabolism of phenytoin and may decrease its efficacy.

4. ZM returns for a routine follow-up visit in 1 year after the wedding. She is relatively seizure free, and she and her husband are considering starting a family. Which of the following vitamin supplements is recommended for women taking anticonvulsants to reduce the potential for teratogenic effects?

   A. Thiamine
   B. Ascorbic acid
   C. Vitamin K
   D. Folic acid
   E. Vitamin B_{12}

5. During the follow-up visit ZM exhibits moderate gingival hyperplasia and asks about an alternative medication to phenytoin. Which of the following would be the least appropriate alternative for treatment of her type of seizure disorder?

   A. Phenobarbital
   B. Carbamazepine
   C. Valproic acid
   D. Ethosuximide
   E. All of the above

RESPIRATORY TRACT INFECTIONS

PRESENTATION

PJ is a 51-year-old white man who is homeless. He has a fever, cough, and chills that have lasted for 2 days. PJ reports bronchitis for 2 weeks before admission and had a dry cough that resolved without drug treatment. Two days before admission, PJ had an onset of fever, chills, and sweats and was treated at a clinic for the homeless with Tylenol (acetaminophen), which provided some relief.

PJ had pneumonia in May of 1994 and had rheumamtic fever at the age of 4 or 5. He has a resulting heart murmur. PJ has no known durg allergies. PJ is homeless, unemployed, and lives on the street. He is single and has no children. He became homeless 2 years ago after his mother died of a long illness for which he cared for her. He has smoked 1 pack of cigarettes per day for 25 years, uses alcohol occasionally (likes to drink beer), and has gone without a drink for 1 week. PJ is a disheveled-looking 51-year-old man who appears far older than his stated age. He complains of a cough and states that if he can't get a cigarette, he will hold someone hostage until he does.

PHYSICAL EXAMINATION

VS: Blood pressure:: 130/90 mm Hg; hear rate: 108 beats per minute; respiratory rate: 12 breaths per minute; temperature: 39°C; SaO_2: 95%

Chest: Note E to A egophony and fremitus

LABORATORY VALUES

Na: 131	K: 3.5
Cl: 97	CO_2: 20
White blood cell (WBC) count: 16.1	Hgb: 12.9
Platelets: 157	Hct: 38
Blood urea nitrogen (BUN): 18	Neutrphils: 84
Serum Cr: 0.99	Lymphocytes: 4
Glucose: 123	Bands: 5

A/P: PJ is a 51-year-old homeless, unemployed man who has a history of drinking and smoking who presents with a community-acquired pneumonia.

QUESTIONS

1. Which of the following pathogens is *most likely* the organism that caused the pneumonia?

   A. *Streptococus pneumoniae*
   B. *Mycoplasma pneumoniae*
   C. *Pseudomonas aeruginosa*
   D. A and C
   E. A and B

2. According to criteria, PJ can be treated for pneumonia as an outpatient. PJ has enrolled in an indigent care program and is eligible for pharmaceutical samples free of charge. He has shown in the past that he is largely noncompliant. Which of the following antibioitics would be *most appropriate* for PJ to take orally as an outpatient?

   A. Ceftazidime
   B. Amoxicillin and clavulanate
   C. Azithromycin
   D. Erythromycin
   E. Cefaclor

3. The culture and sensitivity report from a sputum sample indicates that pneumococci have grown and are sensitive to penicillin, doxycycline, cefuroxime, and erythromycin. The result of a urine *Legionella* antibody test is positive. Which choice would you consider the best therapeutic decision?

   A. Discontinue the azithromycin because there is a pharmacoeconomic advantage to using penicillin 500 mg PO qid in its place.
   B. Continue azithromycin therapy because this macrolide antibiotic will cover both pneumococci and *Legionella* species.
   C. Consider the addition of gentamicin 300 mg IV q24h to cover the gram-negative organism *Legionella*.
   D. Switch the current therapy to cefuroxime 500 mg PO bid for better pneumococcal coverage.
   E. Add metronidazole to the current therapy for additional gram-positive coverage.

4. PJ returns to the emergency department 10 days later with similar symptoms. He admits to not finishing his prescribed course of azithromycin. The *S. pneumoniae* infection is now thought to be penicillin-resistant at an intermediate level. Knowing that his financial and compliance concerns remain largely the same, select an antibiotic from the following list that would be the *most useful* to PJ.

   A. Trovafloxacin 300 mg Po qd is necessary to treat this patient. Its broad spectrum will ocver both *Pseudomonas aeruginosa* and *Bacteroides fragilis*, which may be causing the pneumonia.

B. Ampicillin 500 mg PO qid would be useful to PJ because of its extended gram-negative spectrum.
C. A switch from azithromycin to clarithromycin 500 mg PO bid should be enough to eradicate the resistant penumococcal infection.
D. Intravenous vancomycin 1 g q12h is deemed necessary for intermediate-resistance *S. pneumoniae*.
E. Levofloxacin 500 mg PO qd should be sufficient to control the penicillin-resistant strain of *S. penumoniae*.

5. PJ becomes noncompliant with the regimen. He returns to the emergency department with pleuritic chest pain. A chest x-ray shows dense bilateral infiltrates, which are worse than those on previous radiographs. PJ is hypoxic and is intubated because of respiratory failure. He is admitted to an intensive care unit with the diagnosis of severe community-acquired pneumonia. PJ has no drug allergies. Which of the following antibiotic regimens would be the best choice to treat PJ?

A. Doxycycline 500 mg IV q12h and metronidazole 500 mg IV q12h
B. Ceftriaxone 1 g IV q24h and azithromycin 500 mg IV q24h
C. Gentamicin 50 mg IV q24h and imipenem 500 mg IV q12h
D. Ampicillin 2 g IV q6h, metronidazole 500 mg IV q8h, and gentamicin 70 mg IV q24h
E. Bactrim (trimethoprim-sulfamethoxazole) 10mg/kg/d IV in three divided doses as the only antibiotic

PATIENT PROFILE 8
BUFFER SOLUTIONS

PRESENTATION

The pH of maximum stability for a new drug in formulation studies is 5.000. An appropriately prepared acetic acid (Ka 1.75×10^{-5}, MW 60) and sodium acetate (MW 82) buffer solution will be used to manufacture a stable parenteral formulation. The total buffer concentration should be 3.75×10^{-2} M.

QUESTIONS

1. Which of the following is a true statement?

    A. The pH of maximum stability is the pH at which the drug degradation rate is at a minimum.
    B. The pH of maximum stability is the minimum in a plot of log k_{obs} versus pH.
    C. The pH of maximum stability is the pH at which optimal solubility occurs.
    D. A and B
    E. All of the above

2. What is the pKa of acetic acid?

    A. -4.757
    B. 0.999
    C. 1.000
    D. 4.757
    E. 5.757

3. What is the molar ratio of salt to acid needed to achieve a pH of 5.000?

    A. 10,000 : 1
    B. 1.75 : 1
    C. 0.571 : 1
    D. 1 : 1.75
    E. 1 : 100,000

4. What are the molar concentrations of salt and acid needed to achieve a pH of 5.000?

    A. 0.0136 M salt and 0.0238 M acid
    B. 0.0214 M salt and 0.0375 M acid
    C. 0.0238 M salt and 0.0136 M acid
    D. 0.0375 M salt and 0.0214 M acid
    E. 1.000 M salt and 1.000 M acid

5. How many milligrams of salt and acid are needed to prepare 0.5 L of buffer solution?

    A. 82 mg salt and 60 mg acid
    B. 558 mg salt and 714 mg acid
    C. 976 mg salt and 408 mg acid
    D. 1116 mg salt and 1428 mg acid
    E. 1952 mg salt and 816 mg acid

PATIENT PROFILE 9

END-STAGE RENAL DISEASE

PRESENTATION

HPI: SG is a 58-year-old woman who arrives to the dialysis center for routine hemodialysis. Her access catheter is noted to be red and erythematous.

PMH: End-stage renal disease secondary to diabetes mellitus type II and hypertension. She receives hemodialysis for 3 hours three times per week. She makes little to no urine.

SH: Married with no children. Used to work as a high school teacher but is currently on disability.

FH: Father died in a motor vehicle accident (MVA) when SG was 10 years old. Mother died 2 years ago from sepsis after a coronary artery bypass graft (CABG).

VS: Temperature: 36.2°C; blood pressure: 133/68 mm Hg; heart rate: 64 beats per minute; respiratory rate: 18 breaths per minute; weight: 165 lb

LABORATORY AND DIAGNOSTIC TESTS

Sodium: 141 mEq/L

Chloride: 105 mEq/L

Blood urea nitrogen (BUN): 133 mg/dL

Glucose: 193 mg/dL

Phosphorus: 6.8 mg/dL

Hemoglobin: 7.8 g/dL

Platelets: 172,000/mm^3

Potassium: 4.2 mEq/L

CO_2: 23 mEq/L

Serum creatinine: 3.8 mg/dL

Calcium: 8 mg/dL

White blood cell (WBC) count: 12,000/mm^3

Hematocrit; 24.6%

CURRENT MEDICATIONS

Allopurinol 100 mg PO qd

Amlodipine 10 mg PO qd

Citalopram 40 mg PO qd

Epoetin alfa 4,000 units SQ after each HD

Insulin aspart sliding scale with meals

Insulin glargine 40 units SQ qhs

Metoprolol 100 mg PO bid

Trazodone 100 mg PO qhs

QUESTIONS

1. What is SG's creatinine clearance?

   A. <10 mg/dL
   B. 10–19 mg/dL
   C. 20–39 mg/dL
   D. 40–59 mg/dL
   E. >60 mg/dL

2. SG's physician wishes to start her on a medication to treat her hyperphosphatemia. Which of the following would be the *most appropriate* recommendation?

   A. Calcium acetate 667 mg tid on an empty stomach
   B. Calcium acetate 667 mg tid with meals
   C. Sevelamer 800 mg tid on an empty stomach
   D. Sevelamer 800 mg tid with meals
   E. No treatment is necessary because dialysis should remove the excess phosphorus.

3. Which of the following *best describes* appropriate monitoring parameters specifically for the use of Phoslo to treat hyperphosphatemia?

   A. Serum phosphorus levels
   B. Serum phosphorus and calcium levels
   C. Serum phosphorus, calcium, and potassium levels
   D. Renal function tests
   E. Serum phosphorus and calcium levels and hepatic function tests

4. Which of the following medications have been associated with renal toxicity?

   A. Vancomycin IV
   B. Tobramycin IV
   C. Amphotericin B IV
   D. A and B
   E. All the above

5. SG's physician wishes to initiate an angiotensin-converting enzyme (ACE) inhibitor. Which of the following statements *most accurately* describes the effect of these agents on the kidney?

   A. ACE inhibitors are useful in all patients with renal insufficiency because they increase renal blood flow by vasodilating the afferent arteriole.
   B. ACE inhibitors are useful in all patients with renal insufficiency because they decrease renal blood flow by vasoconstricting the afferent arterioles.
   C. ACE inhibitors are particularly useful in patients with proteinuria because they decrease glomerular pressure by vasodilating the efferent arterioles.
   D. ACE inhibitors are particularly useful in patients with proteinuria because they increase glomerular pressure by vasoconstricting the efferent arterioles.
   E. ACE inhibitors maintain efficacy in treating hypertension despite renal insufficiency because they enhance the effect of diuretics in the distal tubule.

6. Which of the following adverse effects are associated with ACE inhibitor therapy?

   A. Bradycardia, hyperkalemia, and dry cough
   B. Hyperkalemia, dry cough, and an elevated serum creatinine
   C. Hyperkalemia, hyperphosphatemia, and renal insufficiency
   D. Erythrocytosis, dry cough, and an elevated serum creatinine
   E. Bradycardia, angioedema, and hyperphosphatemia

7. A prescription is written to increase SG's epoetin alfa dose to 8000 units SQ three times per week with hemodialysis. Which of the following products may be used to fill this prescription?

   A. Procrit
   B. Epogen
   C. Aranesp
   D. A or B
   E. B or C

8. When do you expect to see an increase in the hemoglobin and hematocrit as a result of the new epoetin alfa dose?
   (*Note:* The new dose is 8000 units SQ three times weekly with hemodialysis.)

   A. Immediately after the first dose of 8000 units
   B. Shortly after the third dose of 8000 units
   C. Within 2 days
   D. Within 2 to 4 weeks
   E. Within 2 to 4 months

9. Which of the following is the *most accurate* statement regarding iron therapy in this patient?

   A. Epoetin alfa treatment increases iron demand, and patients receiving epoetin alfa commonly will develop iron deficiency.
   B. Because this patient has anemia of chronic renal insufficiency, monitoring for iron deficiency is not necessary.
   C. Iron therapy will antagonize the effectiveness of epoetin alfa.
   D. This patient should be switched from epoetin alfa to intravenous iron therapy to effectively treat the anemia.
   E. This patient will never require iron therapy.

10. Blood cultures drawn today in the dialysis center are positive for *Staphylococcus aureus*. Sensitivities are as follows:

Cefazolin	Sensitive
Ciprofloxacin	Sensitive
Oxacillin	Sensitive
Vancomycin	Sensitive

   Which of the following would be the *most appropriate* treatment for this infection?

   A. Cefazolin IV
   B. Ciprofloxacin PO
   C. Nafcillin IV
   D. Vancomycin PO
   E. Vancomycin IV

PATIENT PROFILE 10
BACTEREMIA AND SEPSIS

PRESENTATION

AV is a 48-year-old Hispanic woman whose boyfriend found her unconscious with shallow respirations and three fentanyl patches on her leg. AV was given naloxone and 50 mL 50% dextrose solution in the field without a response. She was intubated in the field and brought to the emergency department for treatment of an overdose. Her medical history includes depression, migraine headaches, and hypothyroidism. Medications being taken on arrival are fentanyl patches, amitriptyline, and fluoxetine. She has no known allergies. Review of systems reveals that AV is a 90-kg woman who looks younger than her stated age; she is intubated and unconscious. Vital signs are BP 90/45, HR 130, RR 32, T 99.6 degrees. WBC count is

$15/mm^3$ with a left shift. A Swan-Ganz catheter is placed and reveals the following numbers: CVP 12, PA 50/20, PCWP 16, SVR 310, CI 5.5. CXR findings are consistent with bilateral patchy alveolar infiltrates. The diagnosis is septic shock.

QUESTIONS

1. Which of the following scenarios listed best defines sepsis?

   A. The presence of viable bacteria in the blood
   B. The systemic inflammatory response to a variety of severe clinical insults
   C. The systemic response to infection

D. A systolic blood pressure <90 mm Hg or a reduction of >40 mm Hg from baseline in the absence of other causes for hypotension

E. The presence of altered organ function in an acutely ill patient such that homeostasis cannot be maintained without intervention.

2. The types of organisms that most frequently cause gram-negative bacteremia are

A. Enteric gram-negative bacilli
B. Non–lactose-fermenting gram-negative rods
C. *Pseudomonas aeruginosa*
D. *Bacteroides fragilis*
E. Group D streptococci

3. After adequate fluid resuscitation with either 0.9% NaCl or Ringer's lactate and not much of a blood pressure response, a pharmacologic vasopressor should be chosen. Which of the following choices would be considered the best for this patient with septic shock as diagnosed on the basis of Swan-Ganz catheter findings?

A. Low-dose dopamine at 2-3 μg/kg/min for vasoconstriction
B. Norepinephrine titrated for a systolic blood pressure >90 mm Hg

C. Phenylephrine <0.03 μg/kg/min
D. Nitroprusside sodium 0.3 μg/kg/min titrated for a systolic blood pressure >90 mm Hg
E. Esmolol 50 μg/kg/min titrated for a systolic blood pressure >90 mm Hg

4. Which of the following goals of antibiotic therapy for sepsis should be considered when choosing an agent for AV?

A. To cover a broad range of organisms
B. To cover polymicrobial infections
C. To prevent the emergence of resistance from bacterial subpopulations that may be resistant to one of the antibiotic components
D. To provide an additive or synergistic agent
E. All of the above

5. If AV has an intraabdominal source of sepsis, which antibiotic regimen should be chosen?

A. Cefazolin and metronidazole
B. Piperacillin-tazobactam and gentamicin
C. Ceftriaxone and gentamicin
D. Clindamycin and tobramcyin
E. None of the above

PATIENT PROFILE 11

DIABETES MELLITUS

PRESENTATION

MB is a 54-year-old white man seen in pharmacy clinic for poor blood sugar control. His PMH includes type 2 diabetes mellitus, rheumatoid arthritis, hypertension, hyperlipidemia, obesity, and chronic obstructive pulmonary disease. He denies any drug allergies. His current medications are glyburide 10 mg twice daily, atorvastatin 10 mg once daily, methotrexate 7.5 every Tuesday, amlodipine 5 mg once daily, and albuterol metered-dose inhaler (MDI) 2 puffs every 6 hours as needed. He also was placed on prednisone 10 mg once daily for a flare of his rheumatoid arthritis about 2 weeks ago. He states that he does not take any alternative or over-the-counter (OTC) medications other than aspirin EC 325 mg once daily, which he started taking a week ago on the advice of his father. He states that he is adherent with his medication regimen.

MB's father and MB's only brother both have type 2 diabetes mellitus. MB's mother died when he was 8 years old. MB recently met with a dietician and has been trying to decrease his weight and improve his blood sugars. He has

been taking a 15-minute walk almost every day for about a month. He was unable to walk briefly when his rheumatoid arthritis first began to flare up. However, the addition of the prednisone has been very effective for his symptoms. He uses his glucose meter to check a fasting blood sugar every morning, and despite his best attempts to decrease the carbohydrate content of his meals, he has noticed that his blood sugars have been rising over the past couple of weeks. He is very frustrated by his rising blood sugars because he feels that he has been adherent with several of the suggested lifestyle modifications. One month ago his fasting morning blood sugars averaged about 100 mg/dL. Last week his fasting morning blood sugars averaged about 200 mg/dL. MB denies symptoms of increased thirst or increased frequency of urination but states that he has been feeling very tired over the past 2 weeks, which he attributed to the warm and humid weather.

MB smokes about a pack of cigarettes per day and has been smoking since age 20 when he was in college. He has tried to quit on several occasions but was unsuccessful each time. He has a difficult time not smoking when he is stressed. He is a criminal lawyer and is frequently stressed by his job. Over the past 2 weeks he has been smoking a pack and a half per day. As a result, he has needed to use his albuterol MDI more frequently. He occasionally will have a glass of wine with his evening meal but otherwise does not drink alcohol. He has never used illicit drugs. He lives alone and does his own grocery shopping and cooking. MB confirms that he fasted 12 hours before his blood was drawn at the laboratory today.

MB's height is 5 ft, 11 in. MB's weight is 230 lb. MB's vital signs are as follows: blood pressure: 145/90 mm Hg; heart rate: 80 beats per minuite; respiratory rate: 18 breaths per minute; and temperature: 98.6°F. MB's laboratory values today are as follows: A1c: 6.9%; Na: 135 mEq/L; K: 4.0 mEq/L; blood urea nitrogen (BUN): 21 mg/dL; serum creatinine: 0.9 mg/dL; glucose: 230 mg/dL; total cholesterol: 212 mg/dL; low-density lipoprotein (LDL) cholesterol: 130 mg/dL; high-density lipoprotein (HDL) cholesterol: 58 mg/dL, and triglycerides: 120 md/dL. All liver function tests and components of his complete blood count were within normal limits.

You review MB's medical chart and note that at his last visit 3 months ago his vital signs were as follows: blood pressure: 126/78 mm Hg; heart rate: 78 beats per minute; respiratory rate: 18 breaths per minute; and temperature: 98.6°F. His laboratory values 3 months ago were as follows: A1c: 6.5%, total cholesterol: 240 mg/dL, LDL cholesterol: 180 mg/dL, HDL cholesterol: 40 mg/dL, and triglycerides: 100 mg/dL. Both his previous spot urine microalbumin:creatinine ratios were around 200 μg/mg creatinine, which is consistent with microalbuminuria. MB states that the atorvastatin 10 mg once daily had been added to his medication regimen 3 months ago. He denies muscle pain or any other side effects from any of his medications.

QUESTIONS

1. Which of the following is the *most likely* cause of MB's hyperglycemia?

   A. Initiation of aspirin EC 325 mg once daily
   B. Initiation of prednisone 10 mg once daily
   C. Initiation of atorvastatin 10 mg once daily
   D. Increased tobacco use increasing glipizide metabolism
   E. Increased albuterol MDI use

2. Which of the following medication regimen changes would be *most appropriate* to help control MB's blood sugars?

   A. Add repaglinide 1 mg with each meal
   B. Switch glyburide to glipizide 10 mg twice daily
   C. Increase glyburide dose to 20 mg twice daily

   D. Add metformin (Glucophage) 1000 mg twice daily
   E. Add pioglitazone (Actos) 15 mg once daily

3. Which of the following medication regimen changes would be *most appropriate* to help control MB's cholesterol?

   A. No change to MB's medication regimen is necessary. His lipid profile levels are at goal.
   B. Increase atorvastatin to 20 mg once daily
   C. Add gemfibrozil 600 mg twice daily
   D. Switch atorvastatin 10 mg once daily to niacin sustained release (Niaspan) 500 mg at bedtime
   E. Add cholestyramine one 4-g packet twice daily

4. Because MB is taking glyburide and has started to exercise recently, which of the following counseling points is important to mention?

   A. Glyburide can cause dry mouth. Drink plenty of water when exercising.
   B. Glyburide can cause sedation. Use heavy machinery with caution.
   C. Glyburide rarely can cause muscle pain. If you experience this side effect, contact your care provider immediately.
   D. Glyburide can cause a low blood sugar reaction. Make sure that you carry something with 15 g of carbohydrate with you at all time.
   E. Glyburide rarely can cause damage to your lungs. If you experience increased shortness of breath, contact your care provider as soon as possible.

5. MB has microalbuminura. Which of the following medication classes have been shown to prevent progression of diabetic nephropathy?

   A. Angiotensin-converting enzyme (ACE) inhibitors
   B. β-Blockers
   C. α_1-Antagonists
   D. Nondihydropyridine calcium channel blockers
   E. Diuretics

6. If a thiazolidinedione is added to MB's medication regimen, which of the following laboratory parameters is the *most important* to monitor?

   A. Liver function tests
   B. Complete blood count
   C. Sodium
   D. Albumin
   E. Creatinine

7. Which of the following disease states can the addition of a thiazolidinedione exacerbate?

   A. Chronic heart failure
   B. Eczema
   C. Gastroesophageal reflux disease

D. Chronic obstructive pulmonary disease
E. Epilepsy

8. Acarbose (Precose) is added to MB's medication regimen. Which of the following side effects are caused *most commonly* by acarbose?

A. Dizziness
B. Increased flatulence
C. Tremor
D. Photosensitivity
E. Sedation

9. Which of the following is the *most appropriate* way to initiate acarbose (Precose)?

A. Take 50 mg three times daily with first bite of meal

B. Take 200 mg three times daily with first bite of meal
C. Take 50 mg three times daily an hour before each meal
D. Take 200 mg three times daily an hour before each meal

10. MB's blood pressure is currently elevated compared with his blood pressure 3 months ago. Which medication(s), if decreased, could help lower and improve his blood pressure?

A. Atorvastatin
B. Prednisone
C. Glipizide
D. Methotrexate
E. All the above

PATIENT PROFILE 12

HIV, AIDS

PRESENTATION

LR is a 25-year-old-woman with HIV infection that was diagnosed in 1996. She has been taking zidovudine (Retrovir®, AZT) and didanosine (Videx®, ddI) since 1996. She recently went to a clinic for a routine check-up. LR's physician assessed the CD4+ cell count and viral load (Quantiplex™ HIV RNA assay) and is considering adding the protease inhibitor indinavir (Crixivan®) to the current regimen of zidovudine 300 mg bid and didanosine 200 mg bid. LR appears to be a good candidate because of her financial situation and a history of compliance with her current medications. She has no known drug allergies.

QUESTIONS

1. Which statement(s) concerning zidovudine (Retrovir®, AZT) therapy is/are true?

A. LR must be monitored for adverse hematologic effects such as anemia and granulocytopenia.
B. Drugs requiring gastric acidity (e.g., dapsone, ketoconazole, itraconazole, and tetracycline) should be given 2 hours before or 2 hours after zidovudine.
C. Zidovudine and indinavir should be avoided in a regimen because of in vitro antagonism, and you must notify LR's physician.
D. A and B
E. All of the above

2. Which statement(s) concerning indinavir (Crixivan®) therapy is/are true?

A. Because of a problem with nephrolithiasis, LR should be counseled that adequate hydration (six 8-ounce glasses of liquids within the course of 24 hours) is important.
B. Lipodystrophy and other metabolic interferences, such as hyperglycemia, have been reported during postmarketing surveillance of patients with HIV infection undergoing antiretroviral regimens that include indinavir and other protease inhibitors.
C. LR should be counseled that indinavir must be administered with a high-fat meal to increase the bioavailability of this agent.
D. A and B
E. All of the above

3. Which statement(s) concerning didanosine (Videx®, ddI) therapy is/are true?

A. Didanosine should be administered on an empty stomach, 1 hour before or 2 hours after a meal.
B. LR should be monitored for signs and symptoms of peripheral neuropathy and pancreatitis.
C. LR should be counseled that with each dosage she should take two tablets (100 mg each) to prevent gastric acid degradation of didanosine.
D. A and B
E. All of the above

4. Another agent that could be added to LR's current regimen is nevirapine (Viramune®), a non-nucleoside reverse transcriptase inhibitor. LR's physician asks you to provide drug information regarding this agent. Which of the following statement(s) concerning nevirapine (Viramune®) is/are true?

A. Nevirapine is an inducer of the cytochrome P450 oxidative system, and women should avoid concomitant administration with oral contraceptives and use an alternative form of birth control.

B. A lead-in period should be used when initiating therapy with nevirapine to lessen the frequency of rash.

C. Patients should be informed to stop the medication and notify the doctor immediately if a severe rash develops or a rash develops that is accompanied by symptoms such as a fever, blistering, mouth sores, conjunctivitis, and swelling.

D. A and B

E. All of the above

5. The physician asks you to provide drug information regarding the FDA-approved agent, efavirenz (Sustiva™). Which of the following statement(s) concerning efavirenz (Sustiva™) is/are true?

A. Efavirenz is dosed once daily (600 mg daily) which is beneficial for patients who prefer simplified regimens.

B. Information from preclinical trials showed that efavirenz appears to cause birth defects; women should be screened for pregnancy before initiating treatment and should be encouraged to use effective contraception while taking this agent.

C. Adverse effects reported with this agent on initiation of therapy include dizziness, trouble sleeping, drowsiness, trouble concentrating, unusual dreams, or a combination of these effects.

D. A and B

E. All of the above

PATIENT PROFILE 13

HYPERLIPIDEMIA

PRESENTATION

AM is a 55-year-old man brought into the pharmacist-coordinated lipid clinic for evaluation and modification of his risk factors for coronary heart disease. AM was discharged from the hospital 1 year ago, having been admitted to the emergency room with chest pain. It was determined that he had a myocardial infarction (MI). At present, he has no significant complaints. Past medical history includes an MI 1 year ago. He has had a right shoulder replacement following an accident skiing. A current medication list according to the patient reveals the following: atenolol 50 mg PO qd, aspirin 325 mg qd, and lovastatin 20 mg qpm. AM's father died of an acute MI at age 49. His mother died of ovarian cancer at age 67. AM's social history includes occasional use of alcohol. He also currently smokes 1 pack of cigarettes per day.

PHYSICAL EXAMINATION

Blood pressure: 164/92 mm Hg; heart rate: 76 beats per minute; respiratory rate: 18 breaths per minute; temperature: afebrile
GEN: Alert, oriented, and pleasant patient.
Chest: Heart reveals regular rhythm.
ABD: Soft and nontender without masses.
EXT: No edema

LABORATORY VALUES

Na: 140 mEq/L
Cl: 113 mEq/L
Blood urea nitrogen (BUN): 15 mg/dL
Serum Cr: 0.9 mg/dL
Low-density lipoprotein (LDL) cholesterol: 170 mg/dL

K: 3.5 mEq/L
CO_2 content: 28 mEq/L
Glucose: 93 mg/dL

Total cholesterol: 305 mg/dL
High-density lipoprotein (HDL) cholesterol: 32 mg/dL Triglycerides: 525 mg/dL AST: 25 mg/dL ALT: 22 mg/dL HbA1c: 5.9%

Uric acid: 5 mg/dL

QUESTIONS

1. The addition of which of the listed antibiotics could result in a potentially dangerous drug interaction with AM's lipid lowering therapy?

I. Erythromycin
II. Itraconazole
III. Cephalexin

A. I only
B. III only
C. I and II only

D. I and III only
E. I, II, and III

2. Which of the following HMG-CoA reductase inhibitors (statins) is not metabolized through the cytochrome P450 system and thus would avoid interactions with drugs metabolized via that particular system?

   A. Fluvastatin
   B. Fenofibrate
   C. Simvastatin
   D. Ezetimibe
   E. Pravastatin

3. When a patient is brought in for a suspected MI, what laboratory values should be evaluated and within what time frame?

   A. A full lipoprotein profile. This needs to occur within 24 hours of the event.
   B. A full lipoprotein profile. This needs to occur within 48 hours of the event.
   C. HDL cholesterol and total cholesterol. This needs to occur within 24 hours of the event.
   D. HDL cholesterol and total cholesterol. This needs to occur within 36 hours of the event.
   E. HDL cholesterol and total cholesterol. This needs to occur within 48 hours of the event.

4. According to the NCEP ATP III guidelines, what are AM's risk factors that modify LDL cholesterol goals?

   A. Age, cigarette smoking, high HDL
   B. Age, cigarette smoking, low HDL
   C. Alcohol use, hypertension, low HDL
   D. Alcohol use, hypertension, high HDL
   E. Alcohol use, cigarette smoking, high HDL

5. AM's 10-year coronary heart disease risk is 15%. Based on AM's history and profile, what is his LDL cholesterol goal according to the ATP III guidelines?

   A. <200 mg/dL
   B. <190 mg/dL
   C. <160 mg/dL
   D. <130 mg/dL
   E. <100 mg/dL

6. How do HMG-CoA reductase inhibitors exert their lipid-lowering effects?

   I. By blocking lipase
   II. By binding bile acids

III. By inhibiting the rate-limiting step in cholesterol synthesis

   A. I only
   B. III only
   C. I and II
   D. II and III
   E. I, II, and III

7. The addition of which of the following fibrates has been shown to result in a two- to fourfold increase in systemic statin levels for lovastatin?

   A. Fenofibrate
   B. Colesevelam
   C. Gemfibrozil
   D. Clofibrate
   E. Ezetimibe

8. Which of the following are therapeutic lifestyle modifications (TLCs) that could be initiated?

   A. Weight management
   B. Cholesterol intake <200 mg/day
   C. Decreased soluble fiber
   D. A and B
   E. A, B, and C

9. Niacin is mentioned as a potential additive therapy. AM is concerned about the flushing associated with the immediate-release form of niacin. What counseling points can you inform AM of that will help to relieve this side effect?

   I. Eating 30 minutes before taking a dose
   II. Taking aspirin 325 mg 30 minutes before taking the dose
   III. Taking the dose with a cool rather than hot beverage

   A. I only
   B. III only
   C. I and II only
   D. II and III only
   E. I, II, and III

10. While you are counseling AM, he asks about the side effects of statins. Which of the following are side effects seen with statins?

   A. Rash
   B. Headache
   C. Abdominal pain
   D. Muscle pain
   E. All the above

PATIENT PROFILE 14

ONCOLOGY: BREAST CANCER

PRESENTATION

BH is a 52-year-old white woman who goes to her physician's office because she has found a lump in her right breast. The lump had been intermittently palpable by the patient for the past 4 months. The patient's medical history includes mild hypertension and non-insulin-dependent diabetes mellitus. Current medications include glyburide 5 mg bid and captopril 25 mg bid. BH has no known drug allergies. The family history includes a mother with breast cancer. BH is married and has six children. She had her first child at 24 years of age. The social history reveals that BH does not smoke and uses alcohol socially.

Physical examination at the time of presentation revealed a healthy woman in no apparent distress. The findings were as follows:

BP: 140/85, HR: 80, RR: 16, T: 98.6
Ht: 5'1", Wt: 160 lb
HEENT: WNL
COR: No murmurs, rub, or gallops
PULM: + BS, no rales or rhonchi
CHEST: Palpable lump upper, outer quadrant right breast

LABS

Electrolytes: WNL
SCr: 1.1
WBC: 4000
Hgb: 12.9
Hct: 38

Mammogram reveals a highly suspicious area in right breast. BH chose surgical intervention and adjuvant antineoplastic therapy with cyclophosphamide, low-dose methotrexate, and 5-FU. Pathology identified a 2.5-cm tumor, ER+, and 3 of 15 positive lymph nodes.

QUESTIONS

1. On basis of the history presented, what is BH's most important risk factor for breast cancer?

   A. Social alcohol use
   B. Actual body weight greater than ideal body weight
   C. First-degree relative with breast cancer
   D. Birth of first child after age 20
   E. Use of oral hypoglycemic agent

2. What would be the dose-limiting toxicity of the regimen selected by BH and her physician?

   A. Nephrotoxicity
   B. Peripheral neuropathy
   C. Gastrointestinal upset
   D. Bone marrow suppression
   E. Urinary tract infection

3. The primary indication for systemic antineoplastic therapy in BH's case is to

   A. prevent disease spread to the lymph nodes.
   B. target microscopic malignant cells in the circulation.
   C. prevent disease spread to the CNS.
   D. increase cell kill at the tumor site.
   E. prevent disease spread to the bone.

4. After completing her antineoplastic therapy, BH starts therapy with tamoxifen. What is the rationale for this therapy?

   A. Hormonal manipulation has been shown effective in the treatment of ER+ patients.
   B. Progesterone therapy is effective in fighting microscopic malignant disease.
   C. Tamoxifen is the drug of choice for patients younger than 60 years.
   D. Tamoxifen will limit the toxicity of the antineoplastic regimen just completed.
   E. Estrogen therapy has been effective in delaying disease recurrence.

5. Five years later BH has no signs of disease. She reports hot flashes, irritability, and other effects of menopause. She wants your opinion regarding starting hormone replacement therapy (HRT) before discussing it with her physician. What would be your best response to her inquiry?

   A. Recommend against HRT because of her history of breast cancer
   B. Recommend against HRT because of increased cardiovascular risk
   C. Recommend HRT to decrease her risk of ovarian cancer
   D. Recommend HRT at low doses to minimize estrogen effects
   E. Recommend HRT with continual dosing to minimize monthly bleeding

PATIENT PROFILE 15
RESPIRATORY TRACT INFECTIONS

PRESENTATION

MK is a 34-year-old white man who comes to the emergency department because of shortness of breath, pleuritic chest pain, and a 2-day history of diarrhea. He is not bringing up much sputum, but a chest x-ray shows bilateral patchy infiltrates that suggest pneumonia.

QUESTIONS

1. Which would be the *most likely* choice of antibiotics for this hospitalized patient with community-acquired pneumonia?

    A. Ceftazidime and tobramycin
    B. Ceftriaxone and azithromycin
    C. Penicillin and erythromycin
    D. Clindamycin and metronidazole
    E. Trimthoprim-sulfamethoxazole

2. After 1 day of therapy, a rash develops. An alternative single agent that can be used intravenously or orally to manage pathogens that cause community-acquired pneumonia (*Streptococcus pneumoniae* and atypical pathogens) would be which of the following?

    A. Levofloxacin
    B. Clindamycin
    C. Imipenem
    D. Cefixime
    E. Loracarbef

3. A *Legionella* urine antigen assay comes back negative. This can be translated into which of the following clinical manifestations?

    A. Macrolide therapy should be discontinued because this patient does not have *Legionella* infection.
    B. Discontinue the β-lactam therapy and continue the macrolide because the patient most likely does not have pneumococcal pneumonia.
    C. Switch antibiotic therapy primarily to cover anaerobes.
    D. A negative urine antigen test does not confirm that a patient does not have *Legionella* infection, and macrolide therapy should be continued.
    E. Discontinue all antibiotic therapy and follow chest x-rays and fever curve.

4. Erythromycin is likely to be used to manage community-acquired pneumonia, and administration of this antibioitic does not necessitate hospitalization. Which is the most common adverse reaction associated with both IV and oral administration of erythromycin?

    A. Prolonged QT interval leading to torsades de pointes when used with nonsedating antihistamines such as astemizole
    B. Motilin activation in the gastrointestinal (GI) tract that initiates uncoordinated peristalsis resulting in anorexia, nausea, or vomiting
    C. Transient reversible deafness or tinnitus with doses higher than 4 g/day among patients with hepatic or renal dysfunction
    D. Cholestatic hepatitis among adults but not children
    E. Rash

5. Culture shows a highly resistant strain of *S. pneumoniae* with a minimum inhibitory concentration (MIC) >2. Which of the following IV antibiotics will provide coverage against this highly resistant strain?

    A. Vancomycin and rifampin
    B. Vancomycin as a single agent
    C. Cefotaxime
    D. Ceftriaxone
    E. All the above

PATIENT PROFILE 16

MEDICINAL CHEMISTRY

PRESENTATION AND QUESTION

Mr. B, a truck driver who spends most of his day time on the road, has so-called seasonal allergic rhinitis. He stops by the pharmacy where you work and asks your help for a medication that can alleviate his suffering. What would you recommend?

A. Diphenhydramine (structure 16.1) 25-mg capsules
B. Diphenhydramine 50-mg capsules
C. Diphenhydramine elixir (12.5 mg/5 mL)
D. Chlorpheniramine maleate (structure 16.2), 12-mg extended release tablets
E. Fexofenadine (structure 16.3), 60-mg oral capsules

16.1

16.2

16.3

PATIENT PROFILE 17

SEIZURES

PRESENTATION

RT is a 24-year-old woman who has been taking 300 mg phenytoin for treatment of a generalized seizure disorder secondary to a motor vehicle accident over 2 years ago. While she has been seizure-free over the past several months, she now complains of being increasingly lethargic, confused, and uncoordinated. On physical examination, she is noted to have bilateral nystagmus and mild gingival hyperplasia. She has no other significant medical history and takes no medications except acetaminophen for occasional headaches. She does admit to going on a "serious diet" to lose weight for her upcoming wedding. Her laboratory results are reported as follows:

Na: 138 mEq/dl (135–145 mEq/L)

K: 3.5 mEq/L (3.5–5 mEq/L)

Blood urea nitrogen (BUN): 10 mg/dL (8–20 mg/dL)

CL: 98 mEq/L (96–106 mEq/L)

Cr: 1.0 mg/dL (0.7–1.5 mg/dL)

ALT: 8 IU/L (0–35 IU/L)

Albumin: 2.5 g/dL (3.5–5 g/dL)

AST 10 IU/L (0–40 IU/L)

Total phenytoin level: 14 mg/L (10–20 mg/L)

QUESTIONS

1. What might best explain RT's symptoms?

   A. Phenytoin toxicity owing to decreased hepatic metabolism
   B. Phenytoin toxicity owing to decreased renal clearance
   C. Phenytoin toxicity owing to decreased free phenytoin concentrations
   D. Phenytoin toxicity owing to serum electrolyte abnormalities
   E. Phenytoin toxicity owing to decreased protein binding

2. What phenytoin side effect that RT is experiencing is concentration-dependent?

   A. Lethargy
   B. Confusion
   C. Gingival hyperplasia
   D. Nystagmus
   E. All the above

3. After her phenytoin therapy has been optimized, RT returns to clinic prior to her wedding and requests an oral contraceptive. Which of the following statements concerning the combination of an oral contraceptives and phenytoin is *most correct*?

   A. There is no drug interaction.
   B. Phenytoin may induce the metabolism of oral contraceptives and decrease their efficacy.
   C. Phenytoin may inhibit the metabolism of oral contraceptives and increase their side effects.
   D. Oral contraceptives may inhibit the metabolism of phenytoin and increase its side effects.
   E. Oral contraceptives may induce the metabolism of phenytoin and decrease its efficacy.

4. RT returns for a routine follow-up in 1 year. She has been seizure-free for several months, and now RT and her husband are thinking about starting a family. Which of the following is recommended as a supplement for women on antiepileptic agents to reduce possible teratogenic effects?

   A. Thiamine
   B. Ascorbic acid
   C. Vitamin K
   D. Vitamin B_{12}
   E. Folic acid

5. In several months, RT's husband brings her to the emergency room (ER) in a semiconscious state. She has experienced three tonic-clonic seizures over the past 45 minutes without recovering full consciousness between "attacks." He says that he suspects that RT stopped taking her medication since she complained about unacceptable side effects, and she has been having more frequent seizures of late. What is RT most likely experiencing?

   A. Partial complex seizure
   B. Febrile seizure
   C. Status epilepticus
   D. Phenytoin toxicity
   E. Absence seizure

6. Which of the following would be *most appropriate* to administer to RT in the ER?

   A. Oral phenytoin
   B. Intramuscular diazepam
   C. Intravenous phenobarbital
   D. Intravenous lorazepam
   E. Oral carbamazepine

7. After initial therapy, the ER physician wants to initiate intravenous (IV) phenytoin. What is the maximum rate of administration of phenytoin IV?

   A. 5 mg/min
   B. 10 mg/min
   C. 25 mg/min
   D. 50 mg/min
   E. 100 mg/min

8. The ER only stocks fosphenytoin for IV administration. Which of the following statements concerning fosphenytoin is *most correct*?

   A. It is more active than phenytoin.
   B. It is less water soluble than phenytoin.
   C. It may be administered more rapidly than phenytoin.
   D. It is less expensive than phenytoin.
   E. Lack of propylene glycol diluent makes it more likely to cause cardiovascular side effects.

9. Since RT finds side effects of oral phenytoin unacceptable, an alterative therapy for control of her

seizures is being explored. Which of the following agents would *not* be effective for treating her type of seizure disorder?

A.   Ethosuximide
B.   Carbamazepine
C.   Valproate
D.   A and B
E.   A, B, and C

10. RT's physician asks about the possibility of multiple-drug therapy for her. Which of the following statements concerning the use of a combination of agents for the treatment of seizures is *most correct*?

A.   Multiple-drug therapy is generally recommended when possible.
B.   Multiple-drug therapy significantly improves seizure control.
C.   Multiple-drug therapy may increase overall compliance.
D.   Multiple-drug therapy generally is less expensive than monotherapy.
E.   Multiple-drug therapy may increase the risk of side effects.

PATIENT PROFILE 18

PANIC DISORDER

PRESENTATION

RB is a 17-year-old boy who had experienced what he calls a panic attack 4 days ago while watching television. These attacks have occurred twice in the past year, and the patient is fearful that one may occur when he is at school or on a date.

The history of the present illness is that 4 days ago the patient was watching television when he felt his heart racing, became short of breath, and he thought he was going to die. He ran around the house and eventually hid underneath his kitchen table. The symptoms subsided about 10 minutes later. He claims to have had similar symptoms twice in the past 10 to 12 months although not as severe. There appears to be no precipitant to these attacks.

The past medical history is noncontributory. The surgical history is tonsillectomy in 1991. RB is allergic to cefuroxime; he experiences a rash. He is taking no medications.

RB's paternal aunt has diagnosed depression and a generalized anxiety disorder. RB is currently a junior in high school. He works part time as a clerk in a grocery store.

PHYSICAL EXAMINATION

BP sitting R arm: 120/76, HR: 70, RR: 16, T: 99.6°F.

A/P: Patient is a 17-year-old boy who seeks treatment of panic symptoms experienced three times over the last year. His most recent attack was 4 days ago.

QUESTIONS

1. Patients who experience panic attacks have a high likelihood of developing what type of phobia?

A.   Belonophobia
B.   Xenophobia
C.   Pharmacophobia
D.   Agoraphobia
E.   Photophobia

2. What other causes can precipitate a panic attack—like state?

A.   Caffeine
B.   Hyperthyroidism
C.   Cocaine
D.   A and B
E.   A, B, and C

3. Effective treatment strategies for panic disorder include

A.   pharmacotherapy.
B.   relaxation training.
C.   cognitive and behavioral therapy.
D.   A and B
E.   A, B, and C

4. Which of these medications is/are effective in the treatment of patients with panic disorder?

A.   Paroxetine
B.   Brofaromine
C.   Imipramine

D. A and B
E. A, B, and C

5. Because of intolerance of fluoxetine, the patient is being switched to phenelzine. How should the medication change be managed?

A. Start phenelzine the same day as the last dose of fluoxetine.

B. Start phenelzine the day after the last dose of fluoxetine.

C. Start phenelzine 1 week after the last dose of fluoxetine.

D. Start phenelzine 5 weeks after the last dose of fluoxetine.

E. Start phenelzine 6 months after the last dose of fluoxetine.

P A T I E N T   P R O F I L E   1 9

BREAST CANCER

PRESENTATION

CC: CF is a 35-year-old premenopausal African-American woman recently diagnosed with left breast cancer.

HPI: CF had a painless lump discovered in the upper outer quadrant of her left breast by a plastic surgeon during a preoperative examination for breast augmentation surgery. She subsequently received a mammogram, which revealed a suspicious mass in the left breast. A core biopsy of the lesion was positive for infiltrating ductal carcinoma. CT scan, chest x-ray, and bone scan were negative for metastasis. CF received a total mastectomy with axillary lymph node dissection, revealing a 4.2×3.4 cm mass with 4+ ipsilateral axillary lymph nodes involved.

PMH: None

FH: Smoked 1 pack of cigarettes per day for 20 years; quit 5 months ago; no drug use; occasional alcohol use.

SH: Single female; works as a pharmaceutical sales representative; no children; mother died 5 years ago from breast cancer at age 62; father alive with type 2 diabetes mellitus.

ALL: Penicillin → hives

MH: Ortho Tri-Cyclen 1 tab PO qd

ROS: No complaints except for some pain at surgical site

VS: Temperature: 98.8°F; blood pressure: 122/75 mm Hg; heart rate: 58 beats per minute; respiratory rate: 16 breaths per minute; O_2 saturation: 98% RA

Height: 63 in; weight: 152 lb

General: Pleasant overweight woman in NAD

HEENT: PERRLA, EOMI

Neck: Supple, no LAD, no thyromegaly

Lungs: CTA bilaterally

Heart: RRR, no MRG

ABD: Soft, nontender/nondistended, positive bowel sounds

EXT: No C/C/E

Neuro: A&O × 3

CBE: Healed mastectomy scar on the left; no palpable lesions/lymph nodes

LABORATORY DATA

Na: 140 mEq/L	K: 3.5 mEq/L
Cl: 107 mEq/L	CO_2: 28 mEq/L
Blood urea nitrogen (BUN): 8 mEq/L	Serum Cr: 0.6 mg/dL
Glucose: 120 mg/dL	Ca: 9.1 mg/dL
Mg: 2.4 mg/dL	PO_4: 2.6 mg/dL
Total bilirubin: 0.8 mg/dL	ALP 60 IU/mL
Low-density lipoprotein (LDH) cholesterol: 580 IU/mL	Albumin: 4.0 mg/dL
Hgb: 13 g/dL	Hct: 37%
Platelets: 150,000/mm³	White blood cell (WBC) count: 5000/mm³, 60% P, 33% L, 6% M, 1% E

DIAGNOSTIC TESTS

Echocardiogram: LVEF > 60% with normal wall motion

Mastectomy specimen (left breast): 4.2×3.4 cm mass (IDC) with 4+ ipsilateral axillary lymph nodes involved.

Tumor is estrogen/progesterone receptor positive and over expresses HER2/*neu.*

ASSESSMENT/PLAN

CF is a 35 year old African-American woman with stage IIB breast cancer. The treatment plan will include chemotherapy with doxorubicin, cyclophosphamide, and paclitaxel followed by radiation and tamoxifen for 5 years.

QUESTIONS

1. What is the mechanism of action of cyclophosphamide?

    A. Inhibits DNA synthesis by intercalation between base pairs
    B. Prevents cell division by cross-linking DNA strands
    C. Promotes the assembly of microtubules
    D. Competitively binds to estrogen receptors

2. Which of the following is(are) risk factor(s) for the development of breast cancer in this patient?

    A. Smoking history
    B. Oral contraceptive use
    C. Family history
    D. All the above

3. Which of the following is an adverse reaction to paclitaxel?

    A. Hypersensitivity reactions
    B. Cardiomyopathy
    C. Hemorrhagic cystitis
    D. Nephrotoxicity

4. Which of the following chemotherapeutic agents is classified as a vesicant?

    A. Cyclophosphamide
    B. Doxorubicin
    C. Paclitaxel
    D. Tamoxifen

5. Tamoxifen is associated with which of the following adverse events?

    A. Hot flashes
    B. Mood changes
    C. Deep vein thrombosis
    D. All the above

6. Which metabolite of cyclophosphamide is responsible for causing hemorrhagic cystitis?

    A. Acrolein
    B. Chloracetylaldehyde
    C. Hexamethylamine
    D. Hydroxycyclophosphamide

7. Which chemoprotectant can be used to prevent hemorrhagic cystitis from cyclophosphamide?

    A. Amifostine
    B. Dexrazoxane
    C. Mesna
    D. Allopurinol

8. Which of the following adverse reactions is associated with doxorubicin treatment?

    A. Congestive heart failure
    B. Peripheral neuropathy
    C. Constipation
    D. Nephrotoxicity

9. Which one of BF's chemotherapeutic agents is cell-cycle-specific, and which phase of the cell cycle is it specific to?

    A. Doxorubicin, S phase
    B. Paclitaxel, M phase
    C. Cyclophosphamide, G_1 phase
    D. Paclitaxel, S phase

10. BF's oncologist ordered ondansetron and dexamethasone to be given before chemotherapy. What is the role of dexamethasone in this patient?

    A. Antineoplastic
    B. Pain management
    C. Prevent infusi reactions with cyclophosphamide
    D. Antiemetic

RENAL TRANSPLANTATION

PRESENTATION

Institution	Nursing home
Patient	JB
Age	55
Sex	Male
Allergies	NKA
Race	White
Height	5'10"
Wt	159 lb

Diagnosis	Primary	1. s/p cadaveric kidney transplant August 1998
		2. HTN
		3. IDDM
	Secondary	1. Chronic gout
		2. Hypercholesterolemia (controlled with dietary restriction)

	Date	Test		
Lab/diagnostic tests	11/25	BUN 35 mg/dL		
	11/25	SCr 2.8 mg/dL		
	11/25	K 4.9 mEq/mL		
	11/25	Glucose 195 mg/dL		

	Date	Drug and Strength	Route	Sig
Med orders	11/25	Cyclosporine microemulsion (Neoral®) 100 mg	po	bid
	11/25	Mycophenolate mofetil 1500 mg (CellCept®)	po	bid
	11/25	Prednisone 15 mg	po	qam
	11/25	Diltiazem CD 240 mg	po	qd
	11/25	HCTZ 25 mg	po	qd
	11/25	Regular insulin sliding scale (ss)	sc	As dir
Additional orders	11/25	Serum cyclosporine 455 ng/mL		
	11/25	BP 140–150/89–94		
Pharmacist notes	11/25	On 11/05 baseline SCr 1.4 mg/dL and BUN 24 mg/dL, BP WNL		
	11/25	Patient was switched from Sandimmune® to Neoral® on 11/05		
	11/26	Patient's blood glucose controlled with sliding scale regular insulin		

QUESTIONS

1. What is the most significant difference between the cyclosporine formulations, Sandimmune® and Neoral®?

    A. Capsule size
    B. Frequency of administration
    C. Bioavailability
    D. Cost
    E. Availability

2. A serum trough cyclosporine level of 455 ng/mL (normal 50–300 ng/mL) predisposes the patient to

    A. osteoporosis.
    B. nephrotoxicity.
    C. congestive heart failure.
    D. hyperthyroidism.
    E. hepatic failure.

3. One of the clinical signs of dose-related cyclosporine toxicity is

   A. hyperglycemia.
   B. blurred vision.
   C. psychosis.
   D. paresthesia.
   E. tremors.

4. In this case, cyclosporine was temporarily discontinued then restarted at a lower daily dose. What laboratory determinations will aid in monitoring JB's cyclosporine therapy?

   I. Serum creatinine (SCr) and BUN
   II. Cyclosporine blood concentrations
   III. Thyroid panel

   A. I only
   B. III only
   C. I and II only
   D. II and III only
   E. I, II, and III

5. Which of the following drugs is an inhibitor of CYP3A4 and is used concomitantly with cyclosporine to maintain therapeutic drug levels at lower cyclosporine doses?

   A. Mycophenolate mofetil
   B. Prednisone
   C. Azathioprine
   D. Tacrolimus
   E. Diltiazem

PATIENT PROFILE 21

DIABETES MELLITUS: COMPLICATIONS

PRESENTATION

CC: "Recently, I have experienced uncontrollable pain in my feet and hands."

HPI: VB is a 43-year-old woman who was diagnosed with diabetes mellitus type 2 about 10 years ago. VB is non-compliant with her medications and self-monitoring of blood glucose. Therefore, VB has poor blood glucose control. Last year, VB reported symptoms of tingling in her fingers and feet. Based on these reports, VB's primary care physician strongly reiterated his recommendation that VB perform self foot care and visit a podiatrist at least once a year. During VB's last visit to her primary care physician about 3 months ago, she did not show any signs of other diabetes-related complications. VB was sent to a pharmacist-run outpatient clinic for counseling on the importance of compliance with medications and self-monitoring strategies.

Medications: Metformin 500 mg PO qd, repaglinide 2 mg with each meal, aspirin 81 mg PO qd

PMH: Diabetes type 2 diagnosed 10 years ago

PSH: None

FH: Father deceased at age 40 from cardiovascular complications; mother (75 years old) with breast cancer.

SH: Single; drinks alcohol occasionally; denies illicit drug use

ALL: NKDA

PHYSICAL EXAMINATION

General: Overweight Chinese woman; appearance reflects apparent age.

VS: Blood pressure: 160/92 mm Hg; heart rate: 70 beats per minute; respiratory rate: 20 breaths per minute; temperature: 37°C

Height: 5 ft, 2 in; weight: 82 kg

Skin: Normal skin turgor

HEENT: PERRLA; EOM intact; mucous membranes normal.

COR: RRR; no murmur, rubs, or gallops; posterior tibial and dorsalis pedis pulses absent.

Chest: Lungs CTA

ABD: Soft, nontender, normal bowel sounds

GU: Normal output

RECT: Normal anus

EXT: Ulcers on right foot

NEURO: Normal

ECG: Normal

LABORATORY VALUES

Na: 121 mEq/L	K: 5.3 mEq/L
Cl: 98 mEq/L	HCO_3: 5.6 mEq/L
Blood urea nitrogen (BUN): 25 mg/dL	Serum Cr: 1.4 mg/dL
Glucose: pending	Hgb: 14.5 g/dL
Hct: 42.3%	Platelets: $270 \times 10^3/mm^3$
PT: N/A	aPTT: N/A
Triglycerides: 152 mg/dL	Total cholesterol: 212 mg/dL
High-density lipoprotein (HDL) cholesterol: 31 mg/dL	Low-density lipoprotein (LDL) cholesterol: 120 mg/dL

QUESTIONS

1. In order to assess VB's compliance to medication therapy, VB's primary care physician would measure which of the following tests?

   A. Blood pressure
   B. Cholesterol panel
   C. Fasting blood glucose
   D. Glycosylated hemoglobin
   E. Postprandial blood glucose

2. VB's primary care physician may have recommended which of the following self foot care strategies?

   I. Well-fitted walking shoes
   II. Daily visual foot inspection
   III. Self-removal of calluses

   A. I only
   B. II only
   C. I and II
   D. II and III
   E. I, II, and III

3. Which of the following is evaluated during an annual visit to the podiatrist?

   I. Skin integrity
   II. Vascular status
   III. Protective sensation

   A. I only
   B. II only
   C. I and II
   D. II and III
   E. I, II, and III

4. VB's poor blood glucose control may place her at risk for which of the following diabetes-related long-term complication(s)?

   I. Hypoglycemia
   II. Sexual dysfunction
   III. Retinopathy

   A. I only
   B. II only
   C. I and II
   D. II and III
   E. I, II, and III

5. Which of the following should be screened/performed for VB on every routine diabetes visit with her primary care physician?

   A. Lipid panel
   B. Blood pressure
   C. Eye examination
   D. Cardiac stress test
   E. Microalbuminuria

6. Which of the following medications may be initiated in VB based on her family history of coronary vascular disease?

   I. Ibuprofen
   II. Aspirin
   III. Atorvastatin

   A. I only
   B. II only
   C. I and II
   D. II and III
   E. I, II, and III

7. Which of the following medications may be initiated in VB in order to prevent nephropathy?

   I. Verapamil
   II. Lisinopril
   III. Irbesartan

   A. I only
   B. II only
   C. I and II
   D. II and III
   E. I, II, and III

8. Which of the following medications may be initiated in VB to treat her neuropathic pain?

   I. Gabapentin
   II. Amitryptiline
   III. Ibuprofen

   A. I only
   B. II only
   C. I and II
   D. II and III
   E. I, II, and III

9. For what diabetes-related long-term complication may VB be initiated on metoclopramide?

   A. Retinopathy
   B. Neuropathy
   C. Hypertension
   D. Gastroparesis
   E. Orthostatic hypotension

10. Which of the following laboratory data *best* represents one of the recommended lipid panel values for VB?

    A. LDL < 70 mg/dL
    B. LDL < 100 mg/dL
    C. HDL > 35 mg/dL
    D. Triglycerides < 160 mg/dL
    E. Total cholesterol < 250 mg/dL

PATIENT PROFILE 22

ARRHYTHMIAS

PRESENTATION

SB is a 57-year-old woman who arrives in the emergency department stating that she feels light-headed and has palpitations. She states she was going about her normal morning routine of working in her garden when she suddenly felt dizzy and went inside to sit down. After ½ hour the palpitations and dizziness had not gone away, and SB decided to seek medical attention. She denies dizziness or palpitations in the past and currently she is having no chest pain.

PAST MEDICAL HISTORY

Hypertension
CAD: s/p AMI 2 years ago
CHF: EF = 40% 6 months ago
Hyperlipidemia
Asthma
Depression

MEDICATIONS

Enalapril 10 mg po bid
Lasix® (furosemide) 40 mg po qd
KCl 20 mEq po qd
Aspirin 81 mg po qd
Simvastatin 20 mg po qd
Azmacort® (triamcinolone acetonide) 2 puffs qid
Albuterol 2 puffs prn
Sertraline 60 mg po qd

The family history is noncontributory. The patient denies ETOH use, smoking, or substance abuse.

PHYSICAL EXAMINATION

BP: 90/55 (150/90 last visit), HR: 140, RR: 20, T: afebrile
GEN: Middle-aged woman in mild distress
HEENT: Normal
NECK: No JVD
COR: Irregularly irregular S1 and S2, no S3
ABD: Normal
EXT: No edema

LABS

Na: 138	K: 4.0
Cl: 99	CO_2: 26
BUN: 23	SCr: 1.2
Gluc: 145	TSH: 1.3 (0.3-5.0)
INR: 1.0a	WBC: 5.6
Hgb: 12.5	Hct: 38.3
Plts: 219,000	PT: 12.5
PTT: 28.5	

ECG: Atrial fibrillation with a ventricular rate of 140–150 beats/min

QUESTIONS

1. What should be the initial management of atrial fibrillation for SB?

   A. Anticoagulation with IV unfractionated heparin
   B. Give IV amiodarone at 1 mg/min
   C. Give IV diltiazem drip 5 mg/h
   D. Restore normal sinus rhythm with direct current cardioversion
   E. Give digoxin IV 0.25 mg q6h × 24 h

2. Which of the following would not be appropriate to use for long-term control of SB's ventricular rate?

   A. Diltiazem 120 mg po qd
   B. Metoprolol 50 mg po qd
   C. Digoxin 0.125 mg po qd
   D. Verapamil 120 mg po qd
   E. All of the above

3. Which of the following antiarrhythmics would be the most appropriate choice for SB to maintain normal sinus rhythm?

   A. Amiodarone
   B. Quinidine
   C. Lidocaine
   D. Sotalol
   E. Flecainide

4. Which of the following interventions is appropriate to initiate in SB's care at this time?

   A. Increase aspirin to 325 mg po qd
   B. Discontinue aspirin, start ticlopixdine 250 mg po bid

C. Discontinue aspirin, start clopidogrel 75 mg po qd
D. Start warfarin 2.5 mg po qd
E. Start enoxaparin 30 mg sq bid

5. Which of the following medications may result in a drug interaction with amiodarone?

A. Enalapril
B. Digoxin
C. Aspirin
D. Albuterol
E. Azmacort™

RESPIRATORY TRACT INFECTIONS

PRESENTATION

When CM goes to pick up his child at the day-care center, a rambunctious child expectorates onto him. Not thinking too much of this, CM wipes off the goo and proceeds to eat some Cheerios. The following morning, CM finds himself short of breath with a fever of 103°C. He takes some acetaminophen and goes to work. Six hours later the fever returns, and CM coughs up purulent, rust-colored sputum. He also notices that his heart is racing and thinks that it might be a good idea to seek medical attention.

QUESTIONS

1. When CM gets to his primary care physician's office, he is asked to expectorate an induced sputum sample. Complete blood count (CBC) results yield a white blood cell (WBC) count of 15.3 (high), lymphocytes 6 (low), and bands 12 (high). A Gram stain on the sputum sample shows gram-positive cocci in chains. What is the *most likely* organism, assuming that CM has no underlying disease?

A. *Legionella pneumophilia*
B. *Haemophilus influenzae*
C. *Streptococcus pneumoniae*
D. *Acinetobacter calcocoeticus*
E. *Bacteroides fragilis*

2. While waiting for the culture and sensitivities results, you are asked to recommend an antibiotic for empirical treatment. Which of the following antimicrobial agents would be the *best* empirical choice for CM if he is admitted to the hospital?

A. Ceftriaxone
B. Gentamicin
C. Metronidazole
D. Tetracycline
E. Aztreonam

3. While eating his eighth piece of apple pie, CM is found in his room choking. A slice of apple is halfway into his trachea before the nurse places her fingers in CM's mouth and removes the food. Because CM has aspirated the pie, it would be *most prudent* to add which of the following antibiotics to the regimen to improve anaerobic and gram-positive coverage?

A. Vancomycin
B. Ceftazidime
C. Imipenem
D. Clindamycin
E. Metronidazole

4. It is well known that underlying diseases can predispose patients to lower repiratory tract infections. It is also known that among patients with aspiration pneumonia, anaerobic organisms (which commonly cannot be cultured) are responsible in part for the pneumonia. The presence of underlying disease among patients with pneumonia shifts the bacterial flora toward yielding which of the following types of bacteria in addition to typical bacterial pathogens that occur among this patient population?

A. Gram-positive cocci in clusters
B. Gram-positive cocci in chains
C. Lactose-fermenting gram-negative rods
D. Non-lactose-fermenting gram-negative rods
E. Atypical organisms

5. Of the nondrug therapies to augment management of pneumonia, which is designed to loosen mucous a secretions trapped in the lower airways?

A. Pulse oximetry
B. Measuring intake and output
C. Nasotracheal suctioning
D. Postural percussion and draina
E. Nasally applied saline mist

HYPERTENSION

PRESENTATION

TC is a 36-year-old white man with diagnosed hypertension. He has no past medical problems. His baseline blood pressure is 162/96 mm Hg.

ALL: Codeine causes stomach upset
MEDS: Maalox® 30 cc po prn
FH: Father has hypertension and arthritis; mother has COPD
SH: Drinks socially on weekends (2–4 drinks per weekend); does not smoke tobacco or use illicit drugs
PE: Unremarkable

LABS

Na: 140 mEq/L	BUN: 12 mg/dL
K: 4.1 mEq/L	Cr: 0.8 mg/dL
Gluc: 100 mg/dL	

QUESTIONS

1. Atenolol 25 mg po qd is initiated. This is a first-line agent for young, white men with no medical history. What other treatment is considered a first-line therapy for TC? Select the best answer.

   A. Doxazosin
   B. Hydrochlorothiazide
   C. Nifedipine
   D. Captopril
   E. Methyldopa

2. Which of the following describes adverse effects that may occur with atenolol?

   A. Light-headedness
   B. Bradycardia
   C. First-dose syncope
   D. Only A and B
   E. A, B, and C

MENSTRUAL DISORDERS/VAGINAL INFECTION

PRESENTATION

A 26-year-old woman presents with complaints of extremely painful periods. The pain is typically so bad during the first 48 to 72 hours of her period that she is unable to ⬛⬛⬛⬛⬛⬛ that her mood changes significantly ⬛⬛⬛⬛ it where it has interfered ⬛⬛⬛⬛ nd her spouse. Over the ⬛⬛⬛⬛ eme vaginal itching and

⬛⬛⬛⬛ ciency anemia,

⬛⬛⬛⬛ hildren. Drinks occasionally ⬛⬛⬛⬛ ned recently from a ⬛⬛⬛⬛ t by the pool all day. ⬛⬛⬛⬛ good health.

PHYSICAL EXAMINATION

VS: Blood pressure: 120/80 mm Hg; heart rate: 70 beats per minute; respiratory rate: 12 breaths per minute; temperature: 98.6°F
General: Well-appearing 26-year-old
HEENT: PERRLA, EOMI
Heart: Normal
Lungs: CTA
GU: Vagina red, swollen with a white cottage cheese–like discharge
GI: Normal
EXT: Normal

LABORATORY VALUES

135	112	1.2	
3.7	38	20	80

Total cholesterol: 160 mg/dL
Low-density lipoprotein   High-density lipoprotein
  (LDL) cholesterol: (HDL) cholesterol: 60 mg/dL
  100 mg/dL
Triglycerides: 100 mg/dL   AST: 30 IU/L
                           ALT 32 IU/L
Cultures: Vaginal swab: Positive for *Candida*
Pap smear: 6 months ago: Normal
STD panel: Negative

MEDICATIONS

Centrum 1 tablet PO qd
Claritin 10mg PO qd
Flonase 1 puff intranasally bid
Excedrin Migraine 1 tablet q6h PRN for headache
Levaquin 500 mg PO qd × 7 days (stopped 2 days ago)
Ferrous sulfate 325 mg PO tid

QUESTIONS

1. Which of the following symptoms is(are) consistent with dysmenorrhea?

    A. Nausea/vomiting
    B. Breakthrough bleeding
    C. Seizures
    D. Blurry vision

2. Common treatment strategies for the management of dysmenorrhea include

    I. Oral contraceptive
    II. Nonsteroidal anti-inflammatory drugs (NSAIDs)
    III. Ferrous sulfate

    A. I
    B. III
    C. I and II
    D. II and III

3. The patient's physician has decided to manage her dysmenorrhea with naproxen. Which medication should be limited/avoided while being used concurrently naproxen?

    A. Loratidine
    B. Excedrin Migraine
    C. Fluticasone
    D. Ferrous sulfate

4. What is a significant difference between premenstrual syndrome (PMS) and premenstrual dysphoric disorder (PMDD)?

    A. PMDD is considered a psychiatric condition.
    B. PMS is considered psychiatric condition.
    C. PMS requires treatment with a benzodiazepine.
    D. PMDD requires treatment with an Midol.

5. The patient has been diagnosed with PMDD, and her physician has prescribed Sarafem, which is commonly associated with which side effect?

    A. Asthenia
    B. Nausea
    C. Headache
    D. Diarrhea

6. How much elemental iron does ferrous sulfate 325 mg provide?

    A. 325g
    B. 162 mg
    C. 65 mg
    D. 300 mg

7. This patient has been diagnosed with a vaginal *Candida* infection (yeast infection). Which of the following is(are) considered risk factor(s) for developing a yeast infection?

    I. Wearing wet, tight clothing
    II. Recent antibiotic use
    III. Taking ferrous sulfate

    A. I
    B. III
    C. I and II
    D. II and III

8. *Lactobacillus acidophilus* is an active culture that has been associated with preventing/treating vaginal yeast infections. What class of therapy is *Lactobacillus* considered?

    A. Antibiotic
    B. Antifungal
    C. Probiotic
    D. Antidiarrheal

9. Recurrent vaginal yeast infections may be associated with which of the following more serious medical conditions?

    I. Endocarditis
    II. Diabetes
    III. HIV infection

    A. I
    B. III

C. I and II
D. II and III

10. Which of the following is a significant difference between the 1-, 3-, and 7-day vaginal yeast infection over-the-counter therapies?

A. 7-day therapy is more effective than the 3-day therapy.

B. 1-day therapy is more effective than the 3- and 7-day therapy.

C. 1-day therapy is associated with a higher incidence of adverse effects than the 3- and 7-day therapy.

D. 7-day therapy is associated with more adverse effects than the 3-day therapy.

PATIENT PROFILE 26

SEIZURE DISORDER

PRESENTATION

AN is a 25-year-old man who recently started taking carbamazepine for new-on-set complex partial seizures. During his first clinic follow-up visit 2 weeks after beginning therapy, AN informed his physician that he was seizure free and experiencing no ill effects from the medication. His carbamazepine level on this visit was 9 mg/L (8–12 mg/L). Because the seizures were under control, the physician advised AN to come back to the clinic in 3 months. However, 6 weeks later (8 weeks after starting therapy), AN returns to the clinic reporting increasing seizure frequency over the past 10–14 days. A carbamazepine level drawn on this visit is 5.5 mg/L. AN states emphatically that he is taking his medication, and his wife agrees.

QUESTIONS

1. What is the most appropriate assessment of this patient's problem?

A. Carbamazepine is the wrong drug for this patient's seizure and another medication should be prescribed instead.

B. The patient does not have optimal control, and a second medication should be added to the regimen.

C. The regimen should not be altered because the patient is probably not going to achieve any better seizure control without intolerable side effects.

D. The dose of carbamazepine should be increased because autoinduction of carbamazepine metabolism has occurred.

E. The dose of carbamazepine should be decreased because the patient is experiencing drug toxicity.

2. Which of the following side effects may be associated with carbamazepine therapy?

A. Leukopenia
B. Blurred vision
C. SIADH
D. A and B
E. A, B, and C

3. At a 6-month evaluation. AN is still experiencing 1–2 seizures per week despite optimal carbamazepine therapy. AN's physician asks you what medication could be added to the regimen that would be the least likely to interact with carbamazepine. Which of the following is the most appropriate?

A. Phenytoin
B. Phenobarbital
C. Lamotrigine
D. Felbamate
E. Gabapentin

4. AN's physician wants to initiate valproic acid therapy. What baseline tests should be performed before valproic acid therapy is started?

A. Liver function tests
B. Renal function tests
C. Serum electrolytes
D. ECG
E. No baseline testing is necessary

5. Several months later, AN's physician asks about starting lamotrigine therapy. Lamotrigine dosing should be initiated slowly to decrease the incidence of which side effect?

A. Hepatotoxicity
B. Renal toxicity
C. Cardiotoxicity
D. Neutropenia
E. Skin rash

RENAL TRANSPLANTATION

PRESENTATION

CC: A 45-year-old man presents to the emergency room at the local hospital with complaints of fever, tenderness, and mild pain at the incision site.

HPI: Four months ago, the patient received a cadaveric donor kidney transplant (2 of 6 HLA match, PRA >50%). He now has flank pain and graft tenderness and was brought to the hospital by his wife. He states that 2 days ago he began feeling "feverish," and his urine output decreased significantly. His wife claims that he has been compliant with his medications during this recent illness. He is status post acute rejection episode 2 months ago treated with methyl prednisolone (Solu-Medrol) 1000 mg pulse doses IV qd × 3, followed by OKT3 (Orthoclone) 5 mg IV daily × 2 weeks. Oral prednisone taper was instituted the day after the last IV pulse dose of methyl prednisolone.

PMH: Status post renal transplantation 4 months ago, end-stage renal disease (ESRD), type 1 diabetes mellitus (DM) since childhood, hypertension (HTN) × 10 years, grand mal seizures × 2 years, hyperlipidemia × 1 year; good medication adherence

Medications on admission: prednisone (Deltasone) 20 mg qd, mycophenolate mofetil (Cellcept) 1500 mg bid, cyclosporine (CSA) microemulsion (Neoral) 200 mg bid, diltiazem LA (Cardizem LA) 240 mg qd, atorvastatin (Lipitor) 40 mg qd, phenytoin (Dilantin) 300 mg qd, ganciclovir (Cytovene) 500 mg tid, regular insulin sliding scale as directed by his physician

ALL: Captopril (cough)

SH: No tobacco, no illicit drug use, no alcohol; lives with wife and one daughter; employed as a secondary school psychologist

FH: Father deceased (myocardial infarction at 55 years of age); mother in good health; no siblings

Physical examination: Generally, a pleasant, soft-spoken AA male who appears uncomfortable experiencing flank pain (5/10) and tenderness

HEENT: EOMI, PERRLA, MMM

Neck: Soft, supple

COR: RRR

PULM: CTA

ABD: Soft, diffusely tender, nondistended, positive bowel sounds

Back: Paraspinal tenderness

EXT: Positive distal pulses; no edema

NEURO: Cranial nerves (CNs) II–XII intact; no gross deficit

VS: Temperature: 100.1°F; blood pressure: 154/94 mm Hg; heart rate: 80 beats per minute; respiratory rate: 19 breaths per minute

Weight: 80 kg; height: 5 ft, 11 in

LABORATORY VALUES

Na: 140 mEq/L	K: 5.1 mEq/L
Cl: 101	Total CO_2: 22
Blood urea nitrogen (BUN): 70	Serum Cr: 3.8 (baseline 1.0)
BG 201	White blood cell (WBC) count: 7.1
Red blood cell (RBC) count: 3.0	Hct: 39%
Hgb: 13.2	Platelets: 300
Ca: 8.2	PO_4: 5.1
Albumin: 3.4	

Adjusted serum phenytoin concentration: 12 mg/mL
CSA trough level: 90 ng/mL
Estimated creatinine clearance (Cl_{cr}) < 15 mL/min (on admission)
Estimated baseline Cl_{cr}: 96 mL/min
Urine: mod. hyaline casts, RBC 1–2
Urine output: < 10 mL/h

The medical team makes the following assessments:

1. Oliguric acute renal failure (ARF) most likely due to acute allograft rejection episode
2. Hypertension and hyperkalemia most likely due to ARF

QUESTIONS

1. What is the *most significant* difference between cyclosporine formulations Sandimmune and Neoral?

   A. Capsule size
   B. Frequency of administration
   C. Bioavailability
   D. Cost
   E. Short supply

2. What is the *most likely* cause of the second episode of acute allograft rejection after renal transplant in this patient?

   A. Insufficient immunosuppression as a consequence of phenytoin and CSA drug interaction

    B. Insufficient immunosuppression as a consequence of decreased CSA bioavailability

    C. Nephrotoxicity as a consequence of diltiazem and CSA drug interaction

    D. Nephrotoxicity as a result of atorvastatin and CSA drug interaction

    E. Medication nonadherence

3. The medical team is considering either OKT3 or methylprednisolone as treatment for acute allograft rejection and would like your opinion. What is the *most compelling* reason to avoid the administration of a second course of OKT3 in this patient?

    A. Cost burden

    B. Requires prolonged hospitalization of the patient

    C. Lack of efficacy because the drug was administered during the first rejection episode

    D. Possible severe hypersensitivity reaction owing to preformed antibodies from previous drug exposure

    E. All the above

4. In this case, the acute rejection episode is managed successfully with methyl prednisolone treatment followed by prednisone taper to 20 mg qd. The dose of cyclosporine (CSA) is adjusted up to provide optimal immunosuppression, prevent allograft rejection, and avoid drug-induced toxicity. All other drugs and doses remain the same. What laboratory determinations will aid in the monitoring of the patient's CSA therapy?

    I. Serum creatinine and blood urea nitrogen (BUN) concentrations

    II. CSA blood concentration

    III. Blood pressure determinations

    A. I only

    B. III only

    C. I and II only

    D. II and III only

    E. I, II, and III

5. All the following complications are associated with chronic prednisone therapy *except*

    A. Osteonecrosis

    B. Hyperglycemia

    C. Peptic ulcer disease

    D. Chronic allograft rejection

    E. Hypertension

6. Which of the following drugs may be associated with rhabdomyolysis resulting from cytochrome P450 3A/3 enzyme inhibition by CSA?

    A. Atorvastatin

    B. Ganciclovir

    C. Mycophenolate mofetil

    D. Prednisone

    E. Diltiazem

7. Which of the following indications is *correct* in describing the role of ganciclovir in posttransplant patients?

    A. Prophylaxis of *Pneumocystis carinii* (PCP) pneumonia

    B. Prophylaxis of *Mycobacterium avium* complex (MAC)

    C. Prophylaxis of cytomegalovirus (CMV) infection

    D. Prophylaxis of toxoplasmosis

    E. All the above

8. What are two risk factors leading to the development of chronic rejection in this patient?

    A. Prolonged mycophenolate mofetil (MMF) and prednisone use

    B. Prolonged CSA use and prior allograft rejection episodes

    C. OKT3 administration and pulse-dose methyl prednisolone

    D. Cadaveric donor kidney and diltiazem

    E. OKT3 and methyl prednisolone administration

9. One year later, the team now needs your assistance in optimizing immunosuppressive maintenance therapy to avoid the potential of drug-induced chronic rejection and malignancies. What is the *most appropriate* therapeutic strategy to recommend in this patient?

    A. Switch MMF to azathioprine

    B. Switch CSA to sirolimus

    C. Switch CSA to tacrolimus

    D. Discontinue diltiazem

    E. Increase the dose of CSA

10. Which of the following drugs is associated with posttransplant lymphoproliferative disorders (PTLD) and malignancies?

    A. OKT3

    B. Methyl prednisolone

    C. Diltiazem

    D. Ganciclovir

    E. Cyclosporine

PATIENT PROFILE 28
ANTIBIOTIC SUSPENSIONS

PRESENTATION

An *ampicillin for suspension* dosage form when constituted, has a concentration of 250 mg/5 mL. The instructions to the patient read: *1 tsp qid × 10 d.*

QUESTIONS

1. Which size commercial container should be chosen to complete the prescription?

   A. 30 mL
   B. 50 mL
   C. 100 mL
   D. 200 mL
   E. 240 mL

2. Ampicillin is available as a for-suspension dosage form for which of the following reasons?

   A. Ensure drug stability when constituted for the time span of the dosage regimen
   B. Ensure drug stability for the nonconstituted dosage form for the labeled shelf-life product dating
   C. Product line extension
   D. A and B
   E. All of the above

3. Ampicillin is formulated as a for suspension dosage form rather than as a solution for which of the following reasons?

   A. Increase in shelf-life product dating for nonconstituted product

   B. Increase in solubility of ampicillin in water
   C. Increase in stability of ampicillin
   D. A and C
   E. All of the above

4. Regarding the constitution of a for suspension dosage form, which of the following statements is/are true?

   A. Sterile water must be used for constitution.
   B. The amount of water to be added is equivalent to the desired final volume of the dosage form.
   C. The amount of water to be added is less than the desired final volume of the dosage form.
   D. The volume of the powder to be constituted is considered insignificant in regard to the amount of water to be used.
   E. B and D

5. Which of the following is not true regarding the stability of ampicillin for suspension dosage forms?

   A. Exposure of the constituted suspension to extreme heat for prolonged periods would decrease stability.
   B. The expiration dating of the constituted suspension dosage form is longer than that of ampicillin constituted as a solution dosage form.
   C. The stability of the suspension dosage form exceeds that of the solution dosage form.
   D. B and C
   E. All of the above

PATIENT PROFILE 29
DIABETES

PRESENTATION

SL is a 45-year-old woman. SL has noticed recently that her visits to the bathroom have increased dramatically. SL scheduled an appointment with her primary care physician (PCP) to find out what is going on. The doctor performed a quick blood sugar test for SL. The test result revealed that her blood sugar level reads 240 mg/dL.

QUESTIONS

1. What do you think about her blood sugar level?

   A. It is within the normal range.
   B. It is far below the normal range.
   C. It is far above the normal range.

2. What is the normal value for blood glucose levels (in mg/dL)?

   A. 50–80
   B. 80–100
   C. 120–140
   D. 160–200
   E. 200–240

3. Assuming that the PCP concluded that SL is diabetic, can you predict what type of diabetes she might have?

   A. Juvenile
   B. Adult onset
   C. Insulin resistant
   D. Both A and C
   E. Both B and C

4. Why do diabetics have frequent visits to the bathroom?

   A. An elevated blood sugar levels pharmacologically induces bladder contractions.
   B. Diabetes is one of such disease states in which sodium excretion is remarkably increased.
   C. When sugar appears in urine at higher concentrations than normal, it acts as an osmotic diuretic.

5. If SL is confirmed to have type 2 diabetes, which of the following medications is(are) expected to be prescribed for her?

   A. Glipizide (glucotrol, Structure 29.1)
   B. Tolbutamide (orinase, Structure 29.2)
   C. Pioglitazone (Structure 29.3)
   D. A or B
   E. A, B, or C

6. What is the chemical class to which the drugs glucotrol and tolbutamide belong called?

   A. Sulfonylurea
   B. Bigaunide
   C. Thiazolidinedione

7. Considering the acid-base properties of glucotrol, how would concurrent administration of urine alkalinizers such as antacids affect its duration of action?

   A. Make it shorter
   B. Make it longer
   C. No effect

8. What is the *most appropriate* description for the mechanism of the antidiabetic action of sulfonylurea drugs?

   A. They directly stimulate glucose entry into the cell.
   B. They stimulate insulin secretion from pancreatic beta cells.
   C. They stimulate the synthesis of insulin receptors through interaction with DNA.
   D. They directly stimulation glucose conversion into glycogen in the liver.

9. What does insulin-resistant diabetes mean?
   A. Insulin is not formed in the pancreas at all.
   B. Insulin is formed but not released from the beta cell.
   C. Insulin receptors on target cells are defective.

10. If SL's blood sugar does not level off after 2 weeks of therapy with glucotrol 5 mg bid, what would you recommend as an alternative regimen to SL?

   A. Increase the glucotrol dose to 10 mg bid.
   B. Switch to piolglitazone 15 mg once a day.
   C. Add pioglitazone 15 mg once a day to current regimen of glucotrol.
   D. Discontinue glucotrol and switch to orinase 250 mg bid.

CH_3—pyrazine—$CONHCH_2CH_2$—benzene—$SO_2NHCONH$—cyclohexane

29.1

CH_3—benzene—$SO_2NHCONH-C_4H_9$

29.2

pyridine(CH_3)—CH_2CH_2O—benzene—CH_2—thiazolidinedione

29.3

BACTEREMIA AND SEPSIS

PRESENTATION

TN is a 77-year-old 80-kg white man who was admitted to the intensive care unit after resection of colon cancer. Other problems TN is experiencing include atrial fibrillation, *Staphylococcus aureus* pneumonia, GI bleeding, and a question of bowel ischemia. His past medical history includes an MI with an ejection fraction of 25%, ischemic heart disease, an INR >8, atrial fibrillation, benign prostatic hypertrophy, right lower lobectomy, and colon cancer. Laboratory values are consistent with infection. Culture results are as follows:

10/2 Sputum: 1+ *Aspergillus fumigatus*

10/12 Blood: Enterococcus sensitive to ampicillin, gentamicin (in combination with ampicillin), and vancomycin

10/12 Sputum: 4+ *Staphylococcus aureus* sensitive to tetracycline, Bactrim® (trimethoprim and sulfamethoxazole), levofloxacin, cefazolin, clindamycin, erythromycin, oxacillin

10/15 Gallbladder: 3+ enterococci sensitive to ampicillin, gentamicin (in combination with ampicillin), and vancomycin

Active infections are the enterococcal bacteremia, *S. aureus* pneumonia, and enterococcal gallbladder infection.

QUESTIONS

1. Which of the following antibiotic regimens would you consider the best choice to manage TN's gallbladder infection?

   A. Because vancomycin covers all gram-positive infections including enterococcal infection, it should be considered the standard of therapy in all enterococcal infections. Dose at 1g IV q12h.
   B. Metronidazole traditionally is considered to cover infections below the diaphragm. By anatomic design, the gallbladder lies below the diaphragm and should be covered by 500 mg IV q8h.
   C. The culture and sensitivity results can be used to guide your antibiotic therapy. Ampicillin 2 g IV q6h + gentamicin 80 mg IV q12h for synergy against the enterococci should be the therapy of choice.
   D. A second-generation cephalosporin such as cefotetan 1 g IV q12h can be used to manage this enterococcal infection below the diaphragm.
   E. A third-generation cephalosporin such as ceftriaxone, which is eliminated partially through the hepatobiliary tree, can be used to manage this gallbladder infection.

2. Further laboratory reporting of the culture results shows the strain of *Staphylococcus aureus* in TN's sputum to be methicillin resistant. TN has normal renal function. After discontinuing the selected antibiotics, which antibiotic should be used to treat TN for MRSA?

   A. Imipenem 500 mg IV q6h
   B. Vancomycin 1g IV q12h
   C. Imipenem 500 mg IV q12h
   D. Vancomycin 1g IV q6h
   E. Nafcillin 2 g IV q6h

3. TN has severe diarrhea with green, foul-smelling stool. A stool sample for *Clostridium difficile* toxin and fecal leukocytes has been sent to the microbiology laboratory for identification. Which therapy and dose would you select, if any, for empiric management of *C. difficile* colitis?

   A. Two lactobacillus packets mixed in apple sauce before each meal
   B. Vancomycin 1g IV q12h
   C. Yogurt with activated cultures tid
   D. Metronidazole 500 mg po tid
   E. Wait for culture results before beginning treatment

4. Which of the following statements is the most correct regarding vancomycin monitoring for TN?

   A. In general, a peak level between 20 and 50 mg/dL and a trough level less than 10 mg/dL are considered therapeutic.
   B. The sample for the peak vancomycin level should be drawn immediately after the infusion has been completed.
   C. Vancomycin should be infused over 15–30 minutes.
   D. Vancomycin dosing is based on ideal body weight.
   E. All of these statements regarding vancomycin are true.

5. All of the following can be considered toxicities of vancomycin except

   A. red neck syndrome, which can occur with rapid infusion <60 minutes.
   B. trough accumulation over time that may necessitate dose adjustment.
   C. nephrotoxicity when vancomycin is used in the absence of other nephrotoxic drugs.
   D. nephrotoxicity when vancomycin is used in combination with aminoglycosides.
   E. ototoxicity.

PATIENT   PROFILE   3 1

ACUTE RENAL FAILURE

PRESENTATION

CC: Patient was transported from home to the emergency room in a private ambulance.

HPI: The patient is a 67-year-old man who was discharged from the hospital with resolving pneumonia one day PTA. He is accompanied by his son, who claims to have found him unconscious on the bathroom floor. On arrival to the emergency room, the patient remains unconscious and unresponsive to stimuli, with shallow respiratory breathing.

PMH: Type 2 diabetes mellitus (DM) × 15 years, hypertension (HTN) × 10 years, mild chronic renal insufficiency (CRI) × 2 years, congestive heart failure (ACC/AHA stage B) × 1 year, asthma (unknown history), community-acquired pneumonia (recent hospital admission), headaches

Medications on admission: Levofloxacin (Levoquin) 500 mg PO qd × 1 week left, lisinopril (Zestril) 20 mg qd, furosemide (Lasix) 20 mg qd in the morning, carvedilol (Coreg) 25 mg bid, glyburide (Micronase) 5 mg qd, albuterol (Proventil) IH 2 puffs qid PRN, ibuprofen (Advil) 200 mg (2 tablets) PRN for headaches

ALL: NKDA

SH: Widower, lives alone, retired

FH: Noncontributory

PHYSICAL EXAMINATION

General: White male who is semiconscious and ill-appearing with labored breathing.

HEENT: EOMI, PERRLA, MMM

Neck: Soft, supple

COR: RRR, S_1, S_2 gallop

PULM: Rales lower left lobe

ABD: Soft, nontender, nondistended

EXT: Positive distal pulses, positive BL edema

Neuro: Not able to perform tests

VS: Temperature: 98.7°F; blood pressure: 124/84 mm Hg; heart rate: 80 beats per minute; respiratory rate: 15 breaths per minute

Weight: 58 kg; height: 5 ft, 6 in

LABORATORY VALUES

Na: 140 mEq/L
Cl: 99
Blood urea nitrogen (BUN): 101
K: 7.5
Total CO_2: 18
Serum Cr: 6.2 (baseline 1.4)

Glucose: 160
Red blood cell (RBC) count: 4.2
Hgb: 11.4
Ca: 7.9
Albumin: 4.0
White blood cell (WBC) count: 15
Hct: 35%
Platelets: 180
PO_4: 8.2

U/A: No sediment, no protein, Gram's stain (−)
Urine output: <10 mL/h
ECG: Flattened P waves, widened QRS segment

The medical team makes the following assessments:

1. ECG changes consistent with life-threatening hyperkalemia
2. Oliguric acute renal failure probably due prerenal azotemia from volume overload
3. r/o septicemia

QUESTIONS

1. Which of the problems listed below is(are) biochemical and hemodynamic manifestations consistent with acute renal failure (ARF)?

   I.   Metabolic acidosis
   II. Hyperkalemia
   III. Oliguria

   A. I only
   B. III only
   C. I and II only
   D. II and III only
   E. I, II, and III

2. Which of the following diagnostic tools may be used to differentiate drug-induced prerenal azotemia from intrinsic renal failure?

   A. Urine chemistries
   B. Urinalysis
   C. Glycosylated hemoglobin A_{1C}
   D. A and B
   E. A and C

3. Which one of the following drugs may lead to a false-positive FeNa value?

   A. Levofloxacin
   B. Carvedilol
   C. Furosemide

D. Lisinopril
E. Glyburide

4. Identify the agents in this case that may be responsible for suspected drug-induced prerenal azotemia.

A. Lisinopril and furosemide
B. Lisinopril and ibuprofen
C. Ibuprofen and levofloxacin
D. Levofloxacin and carvedilol
E. Carvedilol and glyburide

5. All the following are considered risk factors for ARF-associated mortality *except*

A. advanced age.
B. oliguria.
C. markedly elevated serum creatinine.
D. septicemia.
E. hyperglycemia.

6. What is the *most appropriate* agent for the management of hyperkalemia associated with ARF in this patient?

A. Calcium gluconate IV
B. Sodium bicarbonate IV
C. Furosemide IV
D. Regular insulin IV
E. Sodium polysterene sulfonate PO

7. Which of the following drugs may have exacerbated hyperkalemia in the presence of declining renal function in this patient?

A. Levofloxacin
B. Carvedilol
C. Furosemide
D. Lisinopril
E. Glyburide

8. Which of the following statements is *false* regarding prerenal azotemia?

A. Urine output is between 50 and 400 mL/day.
B. FeNa is <1%.
C. BUN:SCr ratio is >20:1.
D. Nonsteroidal anti-inflammatory drugs (NSAIDs) are safe to use in the presence of prerenal azotemia.
E. Prerenal azotemia is reversible.

9. Choose the diuretic of *first choice* for converting the patient from oliguria to nonoliguria?

A. Spironolactone
B. Furosemide
C. Hydrochlorothiazide
D. Metolazone
E. Mannitol

10. In the ensuing 12-hour stay in the emergency room, the patient's cardiac and renal functions have improved, electrolytes have stabilized, consciousness has been restored, septicemia has been ruled out, and urine output has increased to more than 40 mL/h. The medical team would like to continue the levofloxacin, and they turn to you for dosing recommendations. Which of the following determinations is important to consider before making a recommendation in this patient?

I. WBC count and differential
II. Estimated ClCr
III. Route of administration (IV or PO)

A. I only
B. III only
C. I and II only
D. II and III only
E. I, II, and III

PATIENT PROFILE 32

OPPORTUNISTIC INFECTIONS: HIV, AIDS

PRESENTATION

RT is a 32-year-old, 64-kg, white, homosexual man admitted to the hospital with shortness of breath, fever, and a dry cough of 2 weeks' duration. A chest radiograph reveals bilateral interstitial markings, and arterial blood gas analysis reveals hypoxemia with a Pao_2 of 55 mm Hg, $Paco_2$ of 44 mm Hg, and a pH of 7.3. Hypertonic saline nebulization for sputum induction and subsequent bronchoalveolar lavage were performed. Examination of the specimens revealed intracystic bodies and extracystic trophozoites. RT is given the diagnosis of moderate *Pneumocystis carinii* pneumonia (PCP). He had never been tested for HIV infection, and this episode of PCP is his AIDS-defining illness. He has NKDA. Ibuprofen and acetaminophen on an as needed (prm) basis are the only medications that he has taken in the past.

QUESTIONS

1. The most appropriate treatment regimen for RT is the following:

   A. Initiate trimethoprim-sulfamethoxazole (TMP-SMZ, co-trimoxazole) therapy and corticosteriod therapy for approximately 21 days.

   B. Initiate dapsone therapy with corticosteriod therapy for approximately 21 days.

   C. Initiate trimetrexate therapy and folinic acid along with corticosteriod therapy for approximately 21 days.

   D. Initiate TMP-SMZ therapy for approximately 21 days; corticosteriod therapy is not warranted in the treatment of this patient.

   E. Initiated dapsone therapy for approximately 21 days; corticosteroid therapy is not warranted in the treatment of this patient.

2. RT responds well to 21 days of therapy for PCP. This patient needs secondary prophylaxis. Which is the preferred prophylactic regimen for RT?

   A. TMP-SMZ
   B. Dapsone
   C. Aerosolized pentamidine
   D. Atovaquone
   E. Dapsone, pyrimethamine, and leucovorin

3. Once the acute PCP infection resolved, RT's physician ordered viral load studies and a CD4+ cell count. The results were as follows: viral load 300,000 copies/mL (Quantiplex™ HIV RNA assay) and CD4+ cell count 45/mm^3. The physician wants to initiate antiretroviral therapy with two nucleoside reverse transcriptase inhibitors and one protease inhibitor. He wants to avoid choosing agents that have similar toxicity profiles. Which of the following regimens has at least two agents with similar toxicity profiles and would not be a good initial regimen?

   A. Zidovudine (Retrovir®, AZT), lamivudine (Epivir®, 3TC), and indinavir (Crixivan®)

   B. Didanosine (Videx®, ddI), zalcitabine (Hivid®, ddC), and nelfinavir (Viracept®).

   C. Zidovudine (Retrovir®, AZT), didanosine (Videx®, ddI), and saquinavir (Fortovase®).

   D. Lamivudine (Epivir®, 3TC), abacavir (Ziagen™), and nelfinavir (Viracept®)

   E. Stavudine (Zerit®, d4T), lamivudine (Epivir®, 3TC), and nelfinavir (Viracept®)

4. The physician also must consider issues of patient compliance. He remembers reading about an FDA-approved medication that contains a combination of two nucleoside analogues; this combination agent allows twice daily dosing and reduces the number of pills taken daily. You provide the correct name of the medication, which is Combivir® and tell him that it is a combination of the following agents:

   A. Zidovudine (Retrovir®, AZT) and stavudine (Zerit®, d4T)

   B. Stavudine (Zerit®, d4T) and lamivudine (Epivir®, 3TC)

   C. Didanosine (Videx®, ddI) and zalcitabine (Hivid®, ddC)

   D. Zalcitabine (Hivid®, ddC) and stavudine (Zerit®, d4T)

   E. Zidovudine (Retrovir®, AZT) and lamivudine (Epivir®, 3TC)

5. The physician also wants to initiate *Mycobacterium avium-intracellulare* complex (MAC) prophylaxis because RT's CD4+ count is low. Which of the following is/are appropriate prophylactic therapy for MAC?

   A. Clarithromycin (Biaxin®)
   B. Azithromycin (Zithromax®)
   C. Ciprofloxacin (Cipro™)
   D. A and B
   E. All of the above

BACTEREMIA AND SEPSIS

PRESENTATION

AV is a 48-year-old Hispanic woman whose boyfriend found her unconscious with shallow respirations and three fentanyl patches on her leg. AV was given naloxone and 50 mL 50% dextrose solution in the field without a response. She was intubated in the field and brought to the emergency room for treatment of an overdose. Her medical history includes depression, migraine headaches, and hypothyroidism. Medications being taken on arrival were fentanyl patches, amitriptylene, and fluoxetine. She has no known allergies. Review of systems reveals that AV is a 90-kg female who looks younger than her stated age; she is intubated and unconscious. Vital signs are blood pressure: 90/45 mm Hg; heart rate: 130 beats per minute; respiratory rate: 32 breaths per minute; and temperature: 99.6°F. White blood cell (WBC) count is $15/mm^3$ with a left shift. A Swan-Ganz catheter is placed and reveals the following numbers: CVP: 12; PA: 50/20; pulmonary capillary wedge pressure (PCWP): 16; SVR: 310; and cardiac index (CI): 5.5. Chest x-ray findings are consistent with bilateral patchy alveolar infiltrates. The diagnosis is sepsis shock.

QUESTIONS

1. Which of the following scenarios *best defines* sepsis?

   A. The presence of viable bacteria in the blood
   B. The systemic inflammatory response to a variety of severe clinical insults
   C. The result of an infectious insult that triggers a localized inflammatory reaction that then spills over to cause the systemic inflammatory response syndrome (SIRS)
   D. A systolic blood pressure of less than 90 mm Hg or a reduction of greater than 40 mm Hg from baseline in the absence of other causes for hypotension
   E. Presence of altered organ function in an acutely ill patient such that homeostasis cannot be maintained without intervention

2. What are the types of organisms that *most frequently* cause gram-negative bacteremia?

   A. Enteric gram-negative bacilli
   B. Non-lactose-fermenting gram-negative rods
   C. *Pseudomonas aeruginosa*
   D. *Bacteroides fragilis*
   E. Group D streptococci

3. After adequate fluid resuscitation with either 0.9% NaCl or Ringer's lactate and not much of a blood pressure response, a pharmacologic vasopressor should be chosen. Which of the following choices would be considered the *best* for this patient with septic shock as diagnosed on the basis of Swan-Ganz catheter findings?

   A. Low-dose dopamine at 2 to 3 μg/kg/min for vasoconstriction
   B. Norepinephrine titrated to a systolic blood pressure of greater than 90 mm Hg
   C. Phenylephrine <0.03 μg/kg/min
   D. Nitroprusside sodium 0.3 μg/kg/min titrated for a systolic blood pressure of greater than 90 mm Hg
   E. Esmolol 50 μg/kg/min titrated for a systolic blood pressure of greater than 90 mm Hg

4. Which of the following goals of antibiotic therapy for sepsis should be considered when choosing an agent for AV?

   A. To cover a broad range of organisms.
   B. To cover polymicrobial infections.
   C. To prevent the emergence of resistance from bacterial subpopulations that may be resistant to one of the antibiotic components.
   D. To provide an additive or synergistic agent.
   E. All the above goals should be considered when an antibiotic choice is made in a septic patient.

5. If AV has an intra-abdominal source of sepsis, which antibiotic regimen should be chosen?

   A. Cefazolin + metronidazole
   B. Piperacillin-tazobactam + gentamicin
   C. Ceftriaxone + gentamicin
   D. Clindamycin + tobramcyin
   E. None of the available choices is applicable.

PATIENT PROFILE 34

ONCOLOGY: PROSTATE CANCER

PRESENTATION

DE is a 66-year-old man who sees his physician for his annual physical. His only complaints are occasional headaches treated with ibuprofen 1–2 tablets and nocturia 1–2 episodes each night over the past few months. The medical history is significant for vasectomy at age 34. Current medications include low-dose aspirin 162 mg qd, a daily multivitamin, and the ibuprofen. DE has a documented allergy to cephalexin (hives). He is married with three children all alive and well. DE's father died at age 80 (cardiac event). His mother is age 86, alive and well. DE smokes less than one pack of cigarettes per day and drinks only red wine at social events. He continues to exercise three times per week (exercise bicycle and walking).

PHYSICAL EXAMINATION

BP: 124/78, HR: 80, RR: 14, T: 98.6
Ht: 6'1", Wt: 85 kg
Pulmonary examination shows some rhonchi
Digital rectal examination shows enlarged prostate

LABS

Electrolytes: WNL
SCr: 1.4
PSA: 10

QUESTIONS

1. On the basis of the information obtained, what risk factors for prostate cancer are present?

   A. Smoking history and social alcohol use
   B. Advanced age and previous vasectomy
   C. Intermittent ibuprofen use and increased SCr
   D. Family history and low blood pressure
   E. Enlarged prostate and possible BPH

2. Recommendations for early detection of prostate cancer include the following:

   A. Yearly prostate biopsy after age 70
   B. Yearly digital rectal examination after age 40
   C. Yearly transrectal ultrasonography after age 70
   D. Monthly PSA monitoring after age 40
   E. Monthly testicular examination after age 40

3. DE is found to have prostate cancer and is treated with external radiation. Two years later, a routine PSA is found to be elevated to 50. Hormonal therapy is instituted with leuprolide depot and bicalutamide. What is the primary goal of this combined therapy?

   A. Maximize circulating estrogen levels
   B. Maximize circulating androgen levels
   C. Minimize production of peripheral progesterone
   D. Minimize circulating testosterone
   E. Minimize production of gonadotropin-releasing hormone

4. What drug counseling information must be provided to DE to prepare him for the early effects of the leuprolide depot and bicalutamide regimen?

   A. Increased risk of alopecia
   B. Increased risk of severe nausea and vomiting
   C. Increased risk of worsening symptoms for the first couple weeks
   D. Increased risk of bone marrow suppression after 10 days
   E. Increased risk of secondary malignant disease

5. DE initially responds to therapy then returns to his physician reporting hip and back pain. He has used acetaminophen 650 mg q6h for the past 2 days without adequate pain relief. He states his pain is 4 on a scale of 1 to 10. After the source of the pain has been identified as disease progression to bone, what would be the most appropriate pain control regimen for DE at this time?

   A. Ibuprofen 600 mg q8h
   B. Morphine immediate release 20 mg q4h prn
   C. Transdermal fentanyl 25 μg q72h
   D. Buffered aspirin 1–2 tabs q6h prn
   E. Meperidine PCA

PYELONEPHRITIS

PRESENTATION

LK is an 85-year-old woman who is brought to the emergency room of the local hospital by her daughter, who indicates that her mother experienced nausea, fever, chills, and back pain for the last 24 hours and also has become progressively confused. She states that LK used ice packs on her forehead to relieve the fever and also took several Tylenol® tablets at home.

PMH: Hypertension
 PUD
 Frequent urinary tract infections (UTIs)
 Degenerative joint disease
 Osteoporosis

Medications: Lisinopril 20 mg PO QD
 Ibuprofen 400 mg PO PRN
 Maalox PRN
 Calcium carbonate (Tums® ultra) 1 tablet QD

All: NKDA

SH: Lives alone; daughter takes care of her

Upon examination the following results are recorded:

Temp 37.9°C, BP 95/60 mm Hg, heart rate 90 beats/min

HEENT: Dry mucous membranes

Heart: Sinus tachycardia

Abdomen: Positive CVA tenderness, flank pain

Neuro: Oriented only to person

Selected laboratory data:

WBC 16.5 cells/mm^3 (83% neutrophils, 10% bands, 5% lymphocytes, 2% eosinophils)

Scr 1.1 mg/dL; BUN 25 mg/dL

Na 133 mEq/L; K 3.3 mEq/L; Cl 96 mEq/L

UA: pH 8, cloudy urine, + nitrite, pyuria, hematuria, many bacteria

Gram stain: Gram-negative rods

Urine culture and sensitivity results are pending

A: LK is an elderly woman in slight distress complaining of "feeling sick" with a history of frequent UTIs, hypertension, PUD, and DJD who presents with pyelonephritis.

QUESTIONS

1. Which of LK's findings *most specifically* indicates the presence of an infection?

   A. Her temperature
   B. Her heart rate
   C. Her white blood count (WBC)
   D. Her WBC and differential
   E. Her neutrophil count

2. Which of the following laboratory parameters observed in the patient LK indicates a "shift to the left?"

   A. The percentage of neutrophils
   B. The percentage of bands
   C. The percentage of lymphocytes
   D. The percentage of eosinophils
   E. The total WBC

3. The most likely microorganism(s) causing LK's pyelonephritis is/are:

   A. Staphylococci and Streptococci
   B. Enterococci
   C. *E. coli* or other *Enterobacteriaceae*
   D. *Pseudomonas aeruginosa*
   E. *Bacteroides fragilis*

4. In order to treat LK's pyelonephritis she should be empirically started on:

   A. IV ceftriaxone
   B. PO ciprofloxacin
   C. IV vancomycin
   D. IV metronidazole
   E. PO Bactrim

5. In addition to the antibiotic, the patient needs to receive:

   A. IV hydration with normal saline
   B. IV hydration with normal saline and at least 20 mEq KCl
   C. Sufficient orally administered fluids with potassium supplements
   D. Antipyretics such as acetaminophen to decrease her high fever
   E. Nothing because she is nauseous and may vomit

6. Two days after the start of the antibiotic therapy the urine culture and sensitivity report are available with the following information:
   Microorganism identified: *Klebsiella pneumoniae*
   Resistant to ceftazidime, Bactrim, levofloxacin
   Intermediately sensitive to: ceftriaxone
   Sensitive to: cefazolin, ciprofloxacin, imipenem, piperacillin/tazobactam

Given the newly available information, what is the most appropriate treatment approach for LK?

A. Treat with cefazolin PO for optimal antimicrobial coverage.

B. Treat with ceftriaxone IV because this drug is renally eliminated.

C. Switch patient to imipenem IV for the broadest antimicrobial coverage.

D. Switch the patient to piperacillin/tazobactam IV for broadest antimicrobial coverage.

E. Treat patient with ciprofloxacin IV for optimal outcome.

7. If the pathogen identified had been *Pseudomonas aeruginosa,* which of the following parenteral treatment regimens could have been initiated?

I. Piperacillin-tazobactam
II. Ceftazidime
III. Cefotaxime
IV. Ciprofloxacin
V. Aztreonam

A. I and II only
B. II and III only
C. V only
D. All except III
E. IV and V only

8. Four days after admission LK feels much better and all her previous symptoms have disappeared. She is alert and oriented × 3. Her vital signs are now: Temp 37°C, BP 130/88 mmHg, HR 75 beats/min. Which is the *most appropriate* way to manage LK at this point?

A. Discharge her to home because she has successfully finished the 3-day antibiotic course that is recommended for treatment of UTI.

B. Obtain a urine gram stain to see if her UTI has cleared.

C. Continue the previously initiated treatment (see Question 6) for a total course of 14 to 1 days.

D. Switch her to an oral antibiotic regimen to finish a total course of 14 to 21 days.

E. Assume that her infection has cleared and initiate prophylactic treatment.

9. Upon discharge from the hospital LK is prescribed ciprofloxacin 500 mg PO BID and is instructed to follow up with her primary care physician. Which of the following characteristics applies to this drug?

A. The bioavailability of IV and PO ciprofloxacin is comparable; therefore, the doses are the same.

B. Ciprofloxacin frequently causes convulsions and psychosis; therefore, it should not be administered to elderly patients such as LK.

C. Ciprofloxacin frequently causes cardiotoxicity (increases hypertension); therefore, the patient should be carefully monitored.

D. Ciprofloxacin may interact with antacids and calcium preparations; therefore, the patient should be counseled to space the intake of these drugs at least 2 hours apart.

E. Ciprofloxacin is metabolized in the liver; therefore, a liver profile should be obtained from the patient before initiating the drug. 10. LK may use which of the following options as prophylaxis against UTI?

I. Cranberry juice or cranberry-concentrate tablets
II. Topical estrogen cream
III. Continuous therapy with low-dose Bactrim, trimethoprim, nitrofurantoin, or norfloxacin for 6 months

A. I only
B. II only
C. III only
D. I and II
E. All are suitable options

PATIENT PROFILE 36
MEDICINAL CHEMISTRY

PRESENTATION

An 80-year-old female patient calls you, her trusted pharmacist, in the pharmacy stating that the medication she is taking for chronic arthritis does not relieve the pain. You examine her file and find that she is taking Clinoril® (sulindac, structure 36.1) one 200-mg tablet once a day. You call her physician, who is unaware of the difference between sulindac and other NSAIDs in this class. The physician asks for your recommendation.

QUESTION

1. What would you recommend?

   A. Increase the dosing frequency of sulindac from once to twice a day
   B. Switch from sulindac to nabumetone (structure 36.2)
   C. Switch from sulindac to naproxen (structure 36.3)
   D. Switch to steroid therapy, as with prednisone (structure 36.4)
   E. A or B

36.1

36.2

36.3

36.4

PATIENT PROFILE 37

HIV/AIDS

PRESENTATION

RS is a 25-year-old-woman who has just been diagnosed with HIV infection. She has a past history of trichomoniasis and gonorrhea. The clinician discusses the various combinations of antiretroviral agents for treatment of HIV infection with RS. After discussing the options, the clinician and RS decide on the following regimen: zidovudine + lamivudine (Combivir®) and lopinavir + ritonavir (Kaletra®). She has been adherent to medications in the past. She currently is taking the following medications: one multivitamin daily and ibuprofen as needed. She has no known drug allergies.

QUESTIONS

1. Which statement concerning the antiretroviral agents in RS's regimen is true?

   A. Zidovudine and lamivudine are protease inhibitors.
   B. Zidovudine and lamivudine are fusion inhibitors.
   C. Lopinavir and ritonavir are nucleoside reverse transcriptase inhibitors.
   D. Zidovudine and lamivudine are nucleoside reverse transcriptase inhibitors.
   E. Lopinavir and ritonavir are non-nucleoside reverse transcriptase inhibitors.

2. Which statement about zidovudine is true?

   A. Zidovudine is an inhibitor of cytochrome P450.
   B. Zidovudine is an inducer of cytochrome P450.
   C. RS should be counseled that zidovudine should be taken with a high-fat meal.
   D. RS should be counseled that zidovudine can be taken without regard to meals.
   E. RS should be counseled that if gastrointestinal upset occurs with zidovudine, the dose can be reduced by 50%.

3. Which statement about lamivudine is true?

   A. Lamivudine is an inhibitor of cytochrome P450.
   B. Lamivudine is an inducer of cytochrome P450.
   C. RS should be counseled that lamivudine should be taken with a high fat meal.
   D. RS should be counseled that lamivudine can be taken without regard to meals.
   E. RS should be counseled that if gastrointestinal upset occurs with lamivudine, the dose can be reduced by 50%.

4. Which statement about ritonavir is true?

   A. Ritonavir is an inhibitor of cytochrome P 450.
   B. Ritonavir should be administered on an empty stomach.
   C. Ritonavir is only available as capsules.
   D. Ritonavir causes minimal gastrointestinal upset.
   E. Ritonavir inhibits the final stages of viral entry by binding to a region on the envelope glycoprotein 41 of HIV-1.

5. Which of the following statements about the antiretroviral agents in the coformulation lopinavir and ritonavir is true?

   A. Ritonavir is coformulated with lopinavir in order to achieve adequate plasma concentrations of lopinavir.
   B. Lopinavir is metabolized primarily via the kidneys.
   C. Lopinavir and ritonavir are formulated together because each drug has a different mechanism of action.
   D. The coformulation of ritonavir and lopinavir must be taken on an empty stomach.
   E. RS should be counseled to separate administration of lopinavir/ritonavir (Kaletra®) and zidovudine/lamivudine (Combivir®).

6. Which of the antiretroviral agents below is matched appropriately with the potential adverse effect?

   A. Zidovudine: anemia
   B. Lamivudine: rhabdomyolysis

   C. Ritonavir: nephropathy
   D. Lopinavir: hyperthyroidism
   E. All of the above are matched appropriately.

7. RS asks you for information about efavirenz (Sustiva®), another antiretroviral agent. Which of the following statements is true about this agent?

   A. Efavirenz is a nucleoside reverse transcriptase inhibitor.
   B. Efavirenz should be administered with a high-fat meal.
   C. Efavirenz has been reported to cause central nervous system effects.
   D. Efavirenz is an inhibitor of cytochrome P450.
   E. Patients taking efavirenz should be counseled that they must drink 48 ounces of water daily.

8. RS asks you for information about one of the newer antiretroviral agents, enfuvirtide (Fuzeon®). You correctly reply that:

   A. Enfuvirtide is a protease inhibitor.
   B. Enfuvirtide is a nucleoside reverse transcriptase inhibitor.
   C. Enfuvirtide is a non-nucleoside reverse transcriptase inhibitor.
   D. Enfuvirtide is a fusion inhibitor.
   E. Enfuvirtide is a Tat antagonist.

9. RS asks you for information about administration of enfuvirtide. You correctly reply that:

   A. Enfuvirtide is administered orally.
   B. Enfuvirtide is administered as a subcutaneous injection.
   C. Enfuvirtide is administered intravenously.
   D. Enfuvirtide is administered as an intramuscular injection.
   E. Enfuvirtide is administered intranasally.

10. Which of the antiretroviral agents is matched appropriately with its class and potential adverse effect?

   A. Indinavir (Crixivan®): protease inhibitor, nephrolithiasis
   B. Abacavir (Ziagen®): nucleoside reverse transcriptase inhibitor, oral paresthesias
   C. Tenofovir disoproxil fumarate (Viread®), non-nucleoside reverse transcriptase inhibitor, renal insufficiency
   D. Fosamprenavir (Lexiva®), nucleoside reverse transcriptase inhibitor, peripheral neuropathy
   E. Stavudine (Zerit®), protease inhibitor, cardiotoxicity

GENERALIZED ANXIETY DISORDER

PRESENTATION

OA is a 47-year-old woman who says she always feels nervous and indecisive. She also reports aching joints.

The history of the present illness is that 2 months ago OA started taking sertraline for the management of depression. Although her mood is elevated, she continues to have persistent feelings of nervousness and indecisiveness. These feelings seem to persist throughout the day and do not seem to be related to any specific event.

The past medical history is hypertension for 3 years, GERD for 5 years, and depression diagnosed 2 months ago. There are no known drug allergies. The medication history is lisinopril 10 mg qd, cimetidine 300 mg bid, and sertraline 100 mg qd.

OA's father died of MI at age 61. Her mother is still alive. OA is a receptionist at an insurance office. She has two adult children, denies tobacco use, and drinks an occasional glass of wine.

PHYSICAL EXAMINATION

Well-dressed woman who appears stated age
BP sitting R arm: 136/86, HR: 88, RR: 22, T: 98°F

A/P: The patient has recently diagnosed depression, is being treated with sertraline 100 mg qd, and continues to report symptoms of anxiety.

QUESTIONS

1. Which of the symptom(s) is/are characteristic of generalized anxiety disorder?

   A. Indecisiveness
   B. Nervousness
   C. Aching joints
   D. A and B
   E. A, B, and C

2. Which is a more common adverse effect among users of sertraline?

   A. Blurred vision
   B. Alopecia
   C. Orthostatic hypotension
   D. Sexual dysfunction
   E. Extrapyramidal side effects

3. The patient is to start taking diazepam. What clinically significant drug-drug interactions will exist in OA's profile?

   A. Cimetidine can prolong the elimination half-life of diazepam.
   B. Cimetidine can shorten the elimination half-life of diazepam.
   C. Sertraline can decrease the amount of diazepam absorbed.
   D. Lisinopril can decrease the renal elimination of diazepam.
   E. Lisinopril can increase the renal elimination of diazepam.

4. Lorazepam has fewer pharmacokinetic drug interactions than diazepam because lorazepam is metabolized primarily through which pathway?

   A. Cytochrome P450 1A2
   B. Cytochrome P450 2D6
   C. Cytochrome P450 3A4
   D. Renal elimination
   E. Glucuronidation

5. Patients who have a history of substance abuse but need anxiolytic therapy should be treated with which medication?

   A. Lorazepam
   B. Buspirone
   C. Diazepam
   D. Bupropion
   E. Chlordiazepoxide

RENAL TRANSPLANTATION

PRESENTATION

Institution	Nursing home	
Patient	MEJ	
Age	59	
Sex	Female	
Allergies	Sulfa	
Race	White	
Ht	5'4"	
Wt	112 lb	
Diagnosis	Primary	1. s/p second cadaveric kidney transplant October 1998
		2. NIDDM
		3. HTN
		4. Lupus nephritis
	Secondary	1. DVT (1997)
		2. s/p TAH (1991)

	Date	Test		
Lab/diagnostic tests	10/31	BUN 90 mg/dL, SCr 6.8 mg/dL		
	10/31	WBC 11,100/mm^3		
	10/31	K 5.5 mEq/mL		
	10/31	Na 142 mEq/mL		
	10/31	Daily I&O		
	10/31	Blood C & S		
	10/31	Cyclosporine blood conc.		
	10/31	ABGs		
	10/31	Chest x-ray		
	10/31	Hct 33.2		
	10/31	Hg 10.8		
	10/31	BG (finger sticks 7×/d)		
	11/02	Renal biopsy		

	Date	Name and Strength	Route	Sig
Med orders	10/31	Methyprednisolone 1000 mg	IV bolus	qd × 3
	10/31	Cyclosporine microemulsion (Neoral®) 100 mg	po	bid
	10/31	Mycophenolate mofetil (CellCept®) 1000 mg	po	tid
	10/31	Prednisone 20 mg	po	On hold
	10/31	Glyburide 5 mg	po	On hold
	10/31	Regular insulin	SC	Sliding scale
	10/31	Diltiazem CD 180 mg	po	qd
	10/31	Furosemide 40 mg	po	On hold
	10/31	Furosemide 100 mg	IV	Stat × 1
	10/31	D$_5$NS @50–100 mL/h	IV	Continuous
	11/01	Furosemide 100 mg	IV	One dose
	11/02	OKT3 1 mg	IV	One dose
	11/02	OKT3 5 mg	IV	qd × 14 d

Additional orders	10/31	Maintain hydration with D$_5$NS IV @50–100 mL/h
	11/02	Renal biopsy findings consistent with acute allograft rejection
Pharmacist notes	11/07	SCr and BUN values are steadily decreasing
	11/03	Prednisone po restarted
	11/02	Premeds administered. Patient tolerates OKT3
	11/02	Therapeutic cyclosporine blood concentration

QUESTIONS

1. The pharmacist who receives the October 31 drug order for methylprednisolone should recognize that the dose is

   A. a test dose.
   B. a loading dose.
   C. the therapeutic dose.
   D. the recommended dose for allograft rejection episodes.
   E. not a recommended dose.

2. Which of MEJ's drugs is most likely to cause psychosis?

   A. Neoral® (cyclosporine)
   B. CellCept® (mycophenolate mofetil)
   C. Methylprednisolone
   D. OKT3
   E. Diltiazem

3. The possibility that MEJ has pulmonary edema should be ruled out before she is given

   A. prednisone.
   B. glyburide.
   C. cyclosporine.
   D. OKT3.
   E. furosemide.

4. OKT3 belongs to the following class of drugs:

   A. Polyclonal antibodies
   B. Monoclonal antibodies
   C. Antithymocyte globulins
   D. Antilymphocyte globulins
   E. None of the above

5. The pharmacist who receives the November 2 drug order for OKT3 should recognize that the dose is

   A. a test dose.
   B. a loading dose.
   C. the therapeutic dose.
   D. the recommended dose for patients with renal impairment.
   E. not a recommended dose.

6. The potential effects of cytokine release syndrome by OKT3 therapy necessitate the vigilant monitoring of the following:

   I. Temperature
   II. Pulse
   III. Blood pressure

   A. I only
   B. III only
   C. I and II only
   D. II and III only
   E. I, II, and III

PATIENT PROFILE 40

ARRHYTHMIAS

PRESENTATION

SB is a 62-year-old man who arrives in the emergency department with light-headedness, palpitations, and shortness of breath that have lasted for 2 days.

SB is an active 62-year-old who walks 2 miles daily and rides an exercise bicycle three times a week. He states he has felt palpitations previously but that they were associated with exercise and usually went away with rest. Two days ago while cleaning dishes in the kitchen SB began feeling short of breath and noticed his heart was racing. He hoped that the palpitations would go away as they usually did, but when they continued, SB came to the hospital.

The medical history includes hypertension for 20 years, hyperlipidemia for 5 years, and chronic renal failure for 2 years. SB had rheumatic heart disease (mitral valve) as a child.

SB reports adhering to a step 1 diet for the last 2 years. A review of systems is noncontributory. The medication history includes enalapril 5 mg po bid, furosemide 20 mg po qd, and gemfibrozil 600 mg po qd. SB has no known drug allergies.

PHYSICAL EXAMINATION

GEN: Well-developed man in moderate distress
BP: 120/75, HR: 146, RR: 22, T: 37.2°C, Ht: 177.8 cm, Wt: 80 kg
HEENT: PERRLA, no JVD, mild AV nicking
CHEST: Clear to auscultation
COR: Rate irregularly irregular, no murmurs or gallops
ABD: Soft, nontender, active bowel sounds
GU: Deferred
RECT: WNL
EXT: No edema, normal pulses throughout
NEURO: A/O × 3

LABS

Na: 136

Gluc: 120

K: 4.5

Cl: 97

PO_4: 6.3

CO_2: 22

BUN: 60

Cholesterol: 240 mg/dL

Trig: 180 mg/dL

Hct: 26.0

Hgb: 9.5

Ca: 6.5

Mg: 2.1

SCr: 3.5

WBC: 8.0

Plts: 175,000

HDL: 34 mg/dL

LDL: 170 mg/dL

WBC differential: WNL

PT/INR: 13.0 s/1.1

Urinalysis: No RBC, no WBC, (+) protein, (+) hyaline casts

Chest x-ray: Clear

ECG: Atrial fibrillation, no P waves, variable R-R interval, normal QRS Echocardiogram: Enlarged atria, mild left ventricular hypertrophy, no thrombi

QUESTIONS

1. Which of the following therapeutic interventions is most appropriate at this time?

   A. Start amiodarone 400 mg po tid
   B. Start amiodarone continuous infusion at 1 mg/min
   C. Start diltiazem infusion at 5 mg/h
   D. Restore normal sinus rhythm with direct current cardioversion
   E. Start procainamide continuous infusion at 2 mg/min

2. After controlling SB's ventricular rate, which of the following interventions would be most appropriate at this time?

   A. Start warfarin at 5 mg po qd
   B. Start unfractionated heparin at 5000 units sq bid
   C. Start amiodarone at 200 mg po qd
   D. Start flecainide at 100 mg po qd
   E. Start aspirin at 325 mg po qd

3. A decision is made to try to keep SB in normal sinus rhythm. Which of the following interventions would not be appropriate at this time?

   A. Start amiodarone at 400 mg po tid
   B. Start mexiletine 200 mg po q8h
   C. Start sotalol 80 mg po bid
   D. Start quinidine 324 mg po q8h
   E. Start procainamide 750 mg SR po qid

4. The physician decides to initiate long-term warfarin therapy with SB. Which of the following medications will not interact with warfarin?

   A. Amiodarone
   B. Aspirin
   C. Gemfibrozil
   D. Enalapril
   E. Verapamil

5. Which of the following interventions would be most appropriate in SB's care at this time with regard to cholesterol-lowering therapy?

   A. Increase gemfibrozil to 900 mg po bid
   B. Decrease gemfibrozil to 300 mg po bid
   C. Add lovastatin 20 mg po qd to current therapy
   D. Discontinue gemfibrozil, start lovastatin 20 mg po qd
   E. Add cholestyramine 4 g po bid to current therapy

PATIENT PROFILE 41

DIABETES

PRESENTATION

TB is an obese 49-year-old white woman who complains of not feeling well lately. TB lives alone and currently works as a receptionist in a law firm. She has just moved to the area and has not yet set up an appointment with her new practitioner. Upon discussion with TB it is discovered that she was diagnosed with type II diabetes approximately 5 years ago by her long-time primary care physician. TB only takes glyburide at a dose of 5 mg twice a day for treatment of diabetes. TB states that she occasionally monitors her blood sugar, but does not do it regularly. She states that she is not allergic to any medications that she is aware of but does have a history of seasonal allergies, for which she uses Claritin®. TB also informs you that she takes a daily vitamin, as well as an aspirin once a day. She reports no other herbal or over-the-counter use. TB admits to having a glass of wine occasionally with dinner and states that she does not smoke. TB is an only child. Her father died of a heart attack at the age of 60 and her mother is currently alive with type II diabetes. TB does admit to not feeling well lately and that her random blood glucose readings have been "a little high," but she does not recall the exact number, nor does she keep track of the readings. She does know that her HbA1C is 9%, which increased from 8.5% 6 months ago. Her blood pressure has remained consistent at 135/85 over the past year. TB states a major reason for this consistency in blood pressure results from her compliance with her exercise schedule that was set up by her prior practitioner. She does admit that she has not been as compliant with her assigned diet because of excessive gas and upset stomach.

Medication History:
Claritin® 10 mg by mouth once a day for seasonal allergies
Aspirin 81 mg by mouth once a day
Glyburide 5 mg by mouth twice a day
Lisinopril 10 mg by mouth once a day
Atorvastatin 10 mg by mouth once a day
Medical History:
Type II diabetes diagnosed 5 years ago
Hypertension diagnosed 4 years ago
Dyslipidemia diagnosed 4 years ago
Significant labs:
LDL: 130
HDL: 50
Triglycerides: 200

1. The two fundamental metabolic defects associated with TB's diabetes are which of the following?

   A. Normal insulin secretion and tissue resistance to insulin
   B. Impaired insulin secretion and tissue resistance to insulin
   C. Total loss of insulin secretion and tissue resistance to insulin
   D. Normal insulin secretion and increased hepatic glucose production
   E. Impaired insulin secretion and decreased hepatic glucose production

2. Which of the following is the most important counseling point that should be made to TB concerning her glyburide?

   A. Gastrointestinal upset is common.
   B. A rash is seen in most patients.
   C. Vigorous exercise should be initiated.
   D. Weight gain is associated with this medication.
   E. It is important not to miss a meal while on this medication.

3. Which of the following would not describe TB if she were to become hypoglycemic?

   A. Hunger
   B. Tremor
   C. Sweating
   D. Bradycardia
   E. Palpitations

4. What is the most imperative action for TB to take if she begins to suffer from hypoglycemia?

   A. Eat a sandwich.
   B. Chew a piece of gum.
   C. Drink a glass of water.
   D. Take one to two glucose tablets.
   E. Administer insulin on a sliding scale.

5. Which of the following best describes how glyburide works to treat TB's diabetes?

   A. Glyburide inhibits hepatic glucose production.
   B. Glyburide reduces insulin resistance in the periphery.
   C. Glyburide stimulates insulin release from the pancreas.
   D. Glyburide slows intestinal absorption of carbohydrates in the intestine.
   E. All of the above

6. Which of the following medications could interact with TB's glyburide?

   A. Lasix®
   B. Avapro®
   C. Atenolol
   D. Verapamil
   E. Allopurinol

7. TB is concerned that her current diabetes regimen may not be appropriate and asks for your opinion. Which of the following is the most appropriate recommendation?

   A. Keep her on the current regimen.
   B. Initiate Actos® 30 mg every day.
   C. Initiate nateglinide 60 mg once a day.
   D. Initiate miglitol 50 mg three times a day.
   E. Increase the glyburide to 15 mg twice a day.

8. Which patient characteristic does TB exhibit that would result in metformin not being an appropriate addition to her therapy?

   A. Age
   B. Obesity
   C. Hypertension
   D. Dyslipidemia
   E. Use of contrast dye

9. Which of the following medications can cause excess gas and is not an appropriate addition to TB's therapy?

    A. Starlix®
    B. Acarbose
    C. Repaglinide
    D. Tolbutamide
    E. Rosiglitazone

10. Which of the following has a similar mechanism of action to glyburide and is not an appropriate option to add to TB's therapy?

    A. Actos®
    B. Glyset®
    C. Prandin®
    D. Tolinase®
    E. Glucophage®

PATIENT PROFILE 42

DIABETES MELLITUS

PRESENTATION

LT is a 19-year-old man who visited his primary care physician because of polyuria and polydypsia. LT is allergic to peanuts (anaphylaxis). He takes acetaminophen 325 mg po prn for headache. His father has type II diabetes mellitus; his maternal grandmother is deceased and had type II diabetes mellitus. LT is a freshman in college, and his major is marketing. The physical findings are unremarkable. LT weighs 60 kg.

QUESTIONS

1. Appropriate tests are performed, and the results are consistent with diabetes mellitus. Insulin therapy is started. Which of the following is an appropriate starting dose of insulin for LT?

    A. 1–5 units/day
    B. 10–20 units/day
    C. 30–60 units/day
    D. 80–100 units/day
    E. 110–130 units/day

2. You recommend a dosing schedule that involves administration of regular insulin and NPH insulin twice daily (once in the morning and once in the evening). Which of the following statements is true?

    A. The morning dose should be given ½ hour after breakfast.
    B. This regimen is an appropriate dosing regimen and is designed to mimic the activity of a functioning pancreas.
    C. The evening dose should be given 1 hour after the evening meal.

    D. The morning regular insulin dose will lower the postprandial serum glucose level after lunch.
    E. The evening NPH insulin dose will lower the postprandial serum glucose level after supper.

3. Which of the following sequences is the correct way to mix regular insulin and NPH insulin?

    I. The NPH insulin should be drawn into the syringe.
    II. The amount of air equivalent to the NPH dose should be injected into the NPH vial.
    III. The amount of air equivalent to the regular insulin dose should be injected into the regular vial.
    IV. The plunger of the syringe should be drawn to the level of insulin to be injected (regular plus NPH).
    V. The regular insulin should be drawn into the syringe.

    A. IV → II → III → V → I
    B. IV → III → V → II → I
    C. IV → II → I → III → V
    D. III → V → II → I (IV is not part of the procedure to mix insulin)
    E. II → I → III → V (IV is not part of the procedure to mix insulin)

4. When administering insulin subcutaneously, which of the following is false?

    A. Anatomic injection sites include the buttocks, arms, thighs, and abdomen.
    B. The needle should be inserted into the skin at a 90° angle. If the patient has little subcutaneous fat, the needle may be inserted at a 45° angle.

C. The patient should be instructed to firmly pinch up the skin to be injected and to quickly insert the needle all the way.

D. The area in which the injection is given should be massaged for a moment once the needle is removed.

E. The skin should be released before the needle is withdrawn.

5. Which of the following describes how LT may feel if he becomes hyperglycemic because of lack of adherence to the prescribed insulin regimen?

A. More tired than usual
B. Hungrier than usual
C. Having problems seeing clearly
D. A and B
E. A, B, and C

PATIENT PROFILE 43

SOLUTIONS (PHARMACEUTICALS)

PRESENTATION

A patient presents a prescription to the pharmacist for 50 mEq of KCl per day, to be taken daily for 30 days. The pharmacy stocks 20 mEq/15 mL of KCl liquid.

1. How many mL of KCl are required to dispense the prescription?

A. 1500
B. 1125
C. 2000
D. 1000
E. 675

2. What will the daily dosage be?

A. 2 tablespoonfuls per day
B. 7½ teaspoonfuls per day
C. 37.5 mL per day
D. Both A and C are correct.
E. Both B and C are correct.

3. How many mg of KCl are there in one tablespoonful of the solution? (MW of KCl = 74.6)

A. 149.2
B. 268
C. 3.73
D. 1492
E. 373

4. What is the percentage strength of the KCl?

A. 9.95%
B. 14.92%
C. 24.87%
D. 19.89%
E. 55.95%

5. If a 15% KCl solution were available, how much would be required to achieve an equivalent daily dose to that required for this patient?

A. Approximately 18 mL
B. Approximately 99 mL
C. Approximately 45 mL
D. Approximately 10 mL
E. Approximately 25 mL

6. What is the osmolarity of the 15% KCl solution? (Assume 100% dissociation.)

A. 300 Osm/L
B. 2.01 Osm/L
C. 4.02 Osm/L
D. 150 Osm/L
E. 1.75 Osm/L

7. How much KCl would need to be added to 100 mL the KCl solution to make it isoosmotic? (The sodium chloride equivalent for KCl is 0.76.)

A. 0.9 g
B. 0.84 g
C. 1.68 g
D. 1.18 g
E. 2.36 g

8. How many mEq of Cl^- are there in each teaspoonful of the stock KCl? (MW K = 39.1, Cl = 35.5)

A. 13.3
B. 6.67
C. 1.33
D. 20.0
E. 3.99

9. How many mg of Cl⁻ are there in each teaspoonful of the stock KCl?

   A. 47.1
   B. 708.0
   C. 354.0
   D. 78.7
   E. 236.0

10. Approximately how many 10 mEq KCl capsules are required to prepare 100 mL of a stock 15% KCl solution?

   A. 10
   B. 15
   C. 35
   D. 20
   E. 40

PATIENT PROFILE 44

SEIZURE DISORDERS

PRESENTATION

UB is a 26-year-old woman with a long history of a complex partial seizure disorder with secondary generalization. When her husband brings her to the emergency department, she is in a semiconscious state. The husband states that UB has had three tonic-clonic seizures, each lasting approximately 4 minutes, over the past 45 minutes without fully recovering consciousness between "attacks." Her current antiepileptic drug (AED) regimen, which she has been using for almost 2 years, is a combination of carbamazepine (400 mg tid) and valproic acid (500 mg tid). The most recent serum drug concentrations are unavailable. UB's medication history includes phenytoin, which she stopped taking many years ago because of hirsutism. UB's husband thinks she may not be taking her medications regularly, because the seizures have been occurring more frequently (at least once a week) over the past several weeks.

QUESTIONS

1. What is this patient most likely experiencing?

   A. Carbamazepine toxicity
   B. Valproic acid toxicity
   C. Status epilepticus
   D. Absence seizures
   E. Complications of a drug-drug interaction

2. With which anticonvulsant would it be most appropriate to treat UB in the emergency department?

   A. Intravenous lorazepam
   B. Oral diazepam
   C. Oral carbamazepine

   D. Intravenous phenobarbital
   E. All of the above

3. After initial therapy, the emergency department resident wants to administer IV phenytoin. What is the maximum recommended rate of administration?

   A. 5 mg/min
   B. 10 mg/min
   C. 25 mg/min
   D. 50 mg/min
   E. 100 mg/min

4. The emergency department now stocks only Cerebyx® (fosphenytoin). Compared with parenteral phenytoin, fosphenytoin

   A. is more water soluble.
   B. is more rapidly absorbed after IM administration.
   C. may be administered more rapidly IV.
   D. A and B
   E. A, B, and C

5. When the seizure resolves, UB admits that she stopped taking her valproic acid because of an undesirable side effect of the drug. Which of the following side effects is associated with valproic acid therapy and can affect compliance?

   A. Gingival hyperplasia
   B. Weight gain
   C. Hirsutism
   D. Marked decrease in cognition
   E. Peripheral neuropathy

PATIENT PROFILE 45

ALCOHOL WITHDRAWAL AND DEPENDENCE

[handwritten notes: BAC = 0.13 ↑ gross motor impairment ↓ euphoria start dysphoria,]

PRESENTATION

LJ is a 50-year-old man who presents to the detoxification clinic complaining of feeling sick to his stomach and uncontrolled shaking.

LJ states that he was released from jail yesterday after spending 24 hours there for driving while intoxicated (BAC at time of arrest = .13%). He states that he has been drinking at least one 750-mL bottle of whiskey per day for the past 7 to 8 years. He has had short periods of sobriety during this time (none lasting more than 2 to 3 months) and has had numerous detoxifications from alcohol. He has become increasingly depressed over the past year because his wife left him. He states that he was drinking "more than usual" for the 7 days before being arrested; he has not had any alcohol since his arrest.

LJ has a history of depression and was given Zoloft years ago, but was noncompliant with doctor visits and medication. He has had hypertension for 10 years (currently untreated) and was diagnosed with BPH 5 years ago (also currently untreated). He has not seen his primary care physician in over 4 years. LJ is currently unemployed and lives alone. He has been divorced twice. He has two children from his first marriage whom he has not seen in 5 years. His father died of a myocardial infarction at age 60. His mother is alive but has had no contact with LJ in over 5 years.

He complains of sweating, shaking, and vomiting since his release from jail. He denies headache, seizures, constipation, or urinary incontinence.

LJ is currently taking no medications and has been noncompliant with medications in the past.

Patient name: Lee Jones
Address: 1145 Park Avenue
Age: 50
Height: 5'10"
Gender: M
Race: White
Weight: 84 kg
Allergies: NKDA
Social History:
Tobacco use: 2 packs per day × 20 years
Alcohol use: 750 ml whiskey/day × 7 to 8 years
Denies illicit drug use
Caffeine use: One to two cups of coffee per day; (–) tea, soda
Physical Examination:
Gen: LJ is a well-developed, well-nourished man lying on a gurney. He is sweating, looks anxious, has a tremor in both hands, and there is an odor of sweat and urine in the room.
VS: BP 151/115, P 115, R 22, T 100°F
HEENT: WNL
Chest: CTA; no crackles
Cardiac: Normal S_1 and S_2; no murmurs or gallops; occasional premature beats
Abd: Soft, obese, nontender; (+) BS; (+) hepatomegaly; (–) splenomegaly
Skin/Ext: Moist secondary to diaphoresis; tremor in both hands (R > L)
Neuro: A&O × 3 (but fluctuating from confusion to coherence during the examination); (+) tremor in both hands; CN II to XII intact; DTRs are exaggerated; patient states that he heard "female voices" talking to him last night.
Laboratory and Diagnostic Tests: Na 139 mEq/L, AST 254 IU/L, Ca 9.8 mg/dL, K 3.7 mEq/L, ALT 113 IU/L, Mg 1.2 g/dL, Cl 108 mEq/L, Alk Phos 41 IU/L, Phos 2.5 mg/dL, CO_2 25.5 mEq/L, GGT 265 IU/L, UA 10.8 mg/dL, BUN 9 mg/dL, LHD 321 IU/L, Alb 4.3 g/dL, SCr 1.4 mg/dL, T bili 1.1 mg/dL, PT 12.2 sec, Glu 136 mg/dL, D bili 0.4 mg/dL, INR 1.03
Tox Screen: (–) illicit drugs; (–) alcohol

QUESTIONS

1. What stage of alcohol withdrawal is LJ currently experiencing?

   A. Stage I
   B. Stage II
   C. Stage III
   D. Stage IV
   E. Stage V

2. Which of the following statements regarding the use of benzodiazepines in alcohol withdrawal is true?

   I. Benzodiazepines have proven efficacy in preventing agitation and seizures.
   II. All benzodiazepines appear to be equally effective in managing alcohol withdrawal symptoms when given in equivalent doses. ✓
   III. Benzodiazepines can be administered orally or parenterally for the management of alcohol withdrawal symptoms.

   A. I only
   B. III only

C. I and II only

B. II and III only

E. I, II, and III

3. Which one of the following is a reliable and validated scale used to evaluate patients with symptoms of alcohol withdrawal and initiate individualized therapy?

A. CAGE

B. CIWA-Ar

C. AIMS

D. PANSS

E. BPRS

4. The physician decides to start LJ on a benzodiazepine. Which one of the following statements best describes the most appropriate reason for the use of a specific benzodiazepine?

A. The physician should use diazepam because it has a short half-life and lacks oxidative metabolism to active metabolites.

B. The physician should use chlordiazepoxide because it has a rapid onset and has predictable absorption after intramuscular (IM) administration.

C. The physician should use lorazepam because it lacks oxidative metabolism to active metabolites and has predictable absorption after IM administration.

D. The physician should use diazepam because it has a long half-life and predictable absorption after IM administration

E. The physician should use lorazepam because it has a long half-life owing to oxidative metabolism to active metabolites.

5. Which of the following statements regarding β-blockers in the treatment of alcohol withdrawal are true?

A. β-Blockers have been shown to decrease the onset of delirium tremens.

B. β-Blockers cause an increase in diaphoresis and tremor.

C. β-Blockers have been shown to have anticonvulsant properties.

D. β-Blockers can help decrease the adrenergic manifestations of alcohol withdrawal.

E. β-Blockers work at the benzodiazepine receptor subunit.

6. LJ is successfully withdrawn from alcohol and is referred to an alcohol treatment program where he is started on ReVia. Which of the following statements regarding ReVia are true?

I. ReVia is a μ-opioid antagonist.

II. ReVia has been found to reduce ethanol craving and blocks the reinforcing effects of ethanol in patients who drink.

III. A prescription for ReVia can be filled with naloxone.

A. I only

B. III only

C. I and II only

D. II and III only

E. I, II, and III

7. Acamprosate is a medication used to manage chronic alcohol use by decreasing craving as a result of withdrawal. Which of the following statements best describes acamprosate?

A. Acamprosate is an antidepressant that blocks the reuptake of serotonin.

B. Acamprosate is an antipsychotic that blocks the rewarding effects of dopamine in the brain.

C. Acamprosate is an amino acid derivative that affects GABA and glutamine transmission.

D. Acamprosate is a μ-opioid antagonist that blocks the rewarding effects of ethanol.

E. Acamprosate is a form of aversion therapy and blocks the enzyme aldehyde dehydrogenase.

8. Medical complications of chronic alcoholism include which of the following?

I. Hepatitis

II. Hematologic complications

III. Gastritis and ulcer disease

A. I only

B. III only

C. I and II only

D. II and III only

E. I, II, and III

9. Which of the following agents causes its clinical effect by causing an aversive reaction when ethanol is coingested?

A. Acamprosate

B. ReVia

C. Disulfiram

D. Naltrexone

E. Clonidine

10. Wernicke-Korsakoff syndrome can be described best as:

I. A neurologic disorder caused by thiamine deficiency

II. A medical emergency that involves psychosis

III. A cardiomyopathy that develops after years of excessive alcohol use

A. I only

B. III only

C. I and II only

D. II and III only

E. I, II, and III

BACTEREMIA AND SEPSIS

PRESENTATION

JB is a 74-year-old white woman who received a flu shot 2 weeks before admission who reports progressive weakness. JB is diagnosed with Guillain-Barré syndrome. Despite hospitalization and supportive care, the weakness progresses. Plasmapheresis is considered. Before the first course of plasmapheresis, the muscle weakness is so severe that JB loses control of her glottis and proceeds to aspirate. Now in respiratory distress, JB is taken to the intensive care unit, and an endotracheal tube is inserted.

QUESTIONS

1. Antibiotic therapy was not started immediately. She had been in the hospital for 5 days before the ICU admission. There are no immediate radiographic changes, and the problem is believed to be chemical pneumonitis. The day after JB is admitted to the ICU, the chest radiograph blossoms with infiltrate in the right middle lobe, suggesting aspiration. A fever spikes to 39°C. Sputum cultures are suctioned deep from the endotracheal tube, blood and urine culture specimens are obtained, a nasogastric tube is placed, and administration is begun of ceftriaxone Ig IV q24h and metronidazole 500 mg NG q8h for presumed aspiration pneumonia. The preliminary blood cultures are 2/2 bottles positive for lactose-fermenting gram-negative bacilli. Empiric antibiotic therapy should be directed against which of the following organisms?

   A. *Staphylococcus aureus*
   B. *Klebsiella pneumoniae*
   C. *Enterobacter* species
   D. A and B
   E. B and C

2. Which of the following is the best choice to cover lactose-fermenting gram-negative bacilli?

   A. Ceftizoxime
   B. Cefazolin
   C. Ampicillin
   D. Vancomycin
   E. Penicillin

3. Defervescence occurs over the next 3 days, but JB is producing large amounts of chunky, green, foul-smelling sputum. A temperature spikes again, and the blood pressure begins to drop, necessitating fluid resuscitation and vasopressor support. Cultures of blood, sputum, and urine are obtained and show 3+ non–lactose-fermenting gram-negative bacilli growing from the sputum and blood. The antibiotic coverage should be changed to which of the following?

   A. Piperacillin 3 g IV q4h and gentamicin per dosing protocol
   B. Vancomycin 1 g IV q12h and gentamicin per dosing protocol
   C. Ceftriaxone 1g IV q24h and tobramycin per dosing protocol
   D. Unasyn® (ampicillin-sulbactam) 3 g IV q6h and amikacin per dosing protocol
   E. Levofloxacin 500 mg IV q24h

4. Culture and sensitivity testing of the organism on sputum and blood showed *Stenotrophomonas maltophilia*. After discontinuing the previously chosen therapy, which antibiotic would be the drug of choice for *S. maltophilia* infection?

   A. Clindamycin
   B. Vancomycin
   C. Trimethoprim-sulfamethoxazole
   D. Cefotaxime
   E. Penicillin

5. This particular strain of *S. maltophilia* has become resistant very rapidly to the previous choice. The treatment of choice once the primary therapy has failed should be

   A. amikacin.
   B. trovafloxacin.
   C. sparfloxacin.
   D. piperacillin-tazobactam and ciprofloxacin.
   E. ceftazidime and tobramycin.

PATIENT   PROFILE   4 7
CONSTITUTION AND FLOW RATES

PRESENTATION

The manufacturer's instructions for a 1-g vial of antibiotic state that the addition of 4.6 mL of sterile water for injection makes a solution with a resultant concentration of 200 mg/mL. The medication order calls for the addition of 600 mg antibiotic to 150 mL 5% dextrose injection to be administered over 30 minutes at a rate of 60 drops per minute.

QUESTIONS

1. How many milliliters (cubic centimeters) of powder volume does 1 g of the antibiotic occupy in the constituted solution?

    A. 0.0
    B. 0.4
    C. 1.0
    D. 1.4
    E. 4.6

2. How many milliliters of constituted solution have to be removed to obtain 600 mg of the antibiotic?

    A. 0.6
    B. 2.8
    C. 3.0

D. 4.6
E. 5.0

3. What is the approximate concentration of drug in the finished IV container?

    A. 0.4% w/v
    B. 1:400 w/v
    C. 0.4 mg/mL
    D. 0.4 mg %
    E. A and D

4. Which of the following calibrated (drops per milliliter) IV administration sets should be used for this patient?

    A. 8
    B. 12
    C. 16
    D. 20
    E. 24

5. Approximately how many milligrams of antibiotic will be delivered in one drop of the IV solution?

    A. 0.02
    B. 0.2
    C. 0.33
    D. 3
    E. 4

PATIENT   PROFILE   4 8
HYPERCHOLESTEROLEMIA

PRESENTATION

JW is a 54-year-old white woman with no history of hypercholesterolemia, who reports to her primary care physician to follow-up on her health fair number.

CC: "I was told my total cholesterol was 248 at a health fair last week"

PMH: Mild asthma (4 years), HTN (12 years), post-menopausal

FH: Noncontributory

SH: Smokes 1/2 ppd; married with two children; occasional EtOH use

MH: Metoprolol 50 mg BID, Albuterol inhaler two puffs PRN (three times per week), occasional ibuprofen use, NKDA

ROS: Noncontributory

PE: BP 132/88, P 63, RR 16, T 37.0 C, Wt 57.6 kg, Ht 168 cm

Labs: Total cholesterol (TC) 245 mg/dL, triglycerides (TG) 175 mg/dL, HDL cholesterol (HDL) 40 mg/dL, low-density lipoprotein (LDL) cholesterol 170 mg/dL, glucose 98 mg/dL

QUESTIONS

1. What formula was used to calculate JW's LDL?

    A. $LDL = TC + HDL + TG/5$
    B. $LDL = TC - HDL + TG/5$
    C. $LDL = TC - TG/5 + HDL$
    D. $LDL = TC - HDL - TG/5$
    E. $LDL = TC - HDL - TG/10$

2. How many coronary heart disease (CHD) risk factors, excluding LDL levels, does JW have?

    A. 1
    B. 2
    C. 3
    D. 4
    E. 5

3. What is the target goal for JW's LDL assuming his 10-year risk factor is less than 20%?

    A. <130 mg/dL
    B. <100 mg/dL
    C. <160 mg/dL
    D. <70 mg/dL
    E. <120 mg/dL

4. The doctor has initiated therapeutic lifestyle changes (TLC) and wants to start drug therapy. What is the best class of drugs with which to start therapy?

    A. Fibrates
    B. HMG CoA-reductase inhibitors (statins)
    C. Niacin
    D. Bile acid-binding resins
    E. Ezetimibe

5. Which of the following statins has the potential to lower LDL by the greatest percentage?

    A. Fluvastatin
    B. Pravastatin
    C. Lovastatin
    D. Simvastatin
    E. Rosuvastatin

6. Which of the following laboratory tests is required at baseline to monitor for the safe use of statins?

    A. Liver function tests (LFTs)
    B. Serum creatinine
    C. Complete blood count
    D. Red blood count
    E. Electrolytes

7. You recommend that the patient use atorvastatin to treat her hypercholesterolemia. What is the lowest starting dose for this drug?

    A. 20 mg QD
    B. 40 mg QD
    C. 10 mg QD
    D. 40 mg BID
    E. 20 mg QOD

8. Which of the following is considered a major adverse effect of statins for which the patient needs to be monitored?

    A. Headache
    B. Loss of vision
    C. Renal dysfunction
    D. Myopathy
    E. Asthma

9. Which of the following is an absolute contraindication of statins?

    A. Concomitant use of macrolide antibiotics
    B. Active and chronic liver disease
    C. Concomitant use of cylclosporine
    D. Chronic renal disease
    E. Chronic obstructive pulmonary disease

10. Which of the following maximum FDA-approved doses for statins is incorrect?

    A. Lovastatin 60 mg QD
    B. Atorvastatin 80 mg QD
    C. Simvastatin 80 mg QD
    D. Pravastatin 80 mg QD
    E. Fluvastatin 80 mg QD

PATIENT PROFILE 49

SEXUALLY TRANSMITTED DISEASES

PRESENTATION

CD, a 28-year-old woman, arrives in the emergency department with vaginal discharge, mild abdominal pain, and dysuria. Her medical history reveals recurrent gonococcal and nongonococcal urethritis and cervicitis. Gram stain of the vaginal discharge shows gram-negative diplococci and many neutrophils. The culture and susceptibility results are pending. CD has no known drug allergies. When questioned about her medication history, CD admits that she has been given prescriptions of an antibiotic in the past, does not remember the name of it, and has never completed the 7-day course of therapy. The intern consults with you about an appropriate treatment regimen for CD. The pregnancy test result is negative.

QUESTIONS

1. Which of the following regimens is most appropriate for CD?

   A. Ceftriaxone 125 mg IM once and azithromycin 1 g orally once
   B. Cefixime 400 mg orally once and ofloxacin 400 mg orally once
   C. Spectinomycin 2 g IM once and ofloxacin 400 mg orally once
   D. Ceftriaxone 125 mg IM and erythromycin base 500 mg orally qid
   E. Ofloxacin 400 mg once and cefotetan 1 g IM once.

2. If CD had been pregnant, which of the following regimens would have been most appropriate?

   A. Ceftriaxone 125 mg IM once and doxycycline 100 mg bid for 7 days
   B. Ceftriaxone 125 mg IM once and erythromycin base 500 mg orally qid for 7 days
   C. Azithromycin 1 g orally once and erythromycin base 500 mg orally qid for 7 days
   D. Azithromycin 1 g oral once and ofloxacin 300 mg orally bid for 7 days
   E. Ceftriaxone 125 mg IM once and ofloxacin 300 mg oral bid for 7 days

3. Which statement concerning doxycycline is true?

   A. Doxycycline is adequate coverage for chlamydia and trichomoniasis.
   B. Doxycycline is adequate coverage for chlamydia.
   C. Doxycycline is adequate coverage for chlamydia and gonorrhea.
   D. Doxycycline is adequate coverage for gonorrhea.
   E. Doxycycline is adequate coverage for chlamydia, gonorrhea, and trichomoniasis.

4. Which statement concerning ceftriaxone is true?

   A. Ceftriaxone should not be administered intramuscularly.
   B. Ceftriaxone is adequate coverage for chlamydia.
   C. Ceftriaxone is adequate coverage for chlamydia and gonorrhea.
   D. Ceftriaxone is adequate coverage for gonorrhea.
   E. Ceftriaxone is adequate coverage for chlamydia, gonorrhea, and trichomoniasis.

5. Which of the following statement(s) is/are true concerning appropriate treatment of CD?

   A. CD should be encouraged to refer her sex partner or partners for diagnosis, treatment, and counseling.
   B. CD should be offered HIV counseling and HIV testing.
   C. CD should be informed of the results of testing at this admission, and prevention strategies should be reinforced.
   D. CD should receive education on how to reduce the risk of transmission.
   E. All of the above

PATIENT PROFILE 50

SOFT TISSUE INFECTIONS

PRESENTATION

AD is a 15-year-old girl who was walking down the street to retrieve the mail when a dog came running out of the woods and bit her hand. The bite punctured the skin. Thinking nothing of the bite, the girl had gone home, cleaned the wound thoroughly, and put antiseptic ointment and a bandage on her hand. The next day AD sought medical attention for pain, purulent discharge, and swelling.

QUESTIONS

1. Which of the listed organisms is *most concern* in dog bite wounds?

   A. *Pseudomonas aeruginosa*
   B. *Pasteurella multocida*
   C. *Streptococcus pneumoniae*
   D. *Acinetobater baumannii*
   E. Enterococci

2. It is standard practice to thoroughly irrigate a wound with a sterile saline solution or chlorhexidine scrub solution. In addition to the irrigation, which of the following therapies should be considered routinely for a bite from an animal that has not been captured?

   A. Rabies vaccination
   B. Tetanus vaccination
   C. Hepatitis vaccination
   D. A and B
   E. B and C

3. AD has no known drug allergies. With this in mind, choose the *best* empirical antibiotic therapy for a mild wound infection from a dog bite?

   A. Metronidazole 500 mg PO bid
   B. Vancomycin 125 mg PO qid
   C. Amoxicillin-clavulanate 875/125 mg PO bid
   D. Cephalexin 500 mg PO qid
   E. Piperacillin-tazobactam 3.375 g IV q6h

4. Alternative oral therapy in patients who cannot tolerate β-lactam antibiotics for a mild wound infection from a dog bite might be which of the following?

   A. Clindamycin 300 mg PO qid and levofloxacin 500 mg PO qd
   B. Gentamicin 80 mg IV q8h and ceftazidime 1 g IV q8h
   C. Vancomycin 1 g IV q12h and ciprofloxacin 400 mg IV q12h
   D. Cefuroxime azetil 500 mg PO bid
   E. Loracarbef 40 mg PO bid and metronidazole 500 mg PO tid

5. Prophylactic antibiotic therapy in bite wounds should be administered for how long?

   A. 21 days
   B. 10 days
   C. 7 days
   D. 14 days
   E. 3 days

PATIENT PROFILE 51

ONCOLOGY: COLON CANCER

PRESENTATION

RR is a 63-year-old man admitted to the hospital with considerable rectal bleeding. He has been having intermittent abdominal pain for the past month. He has lost about 15 lb in the past 2 months. The rectal bleeding started 3 days ago. His medical history is significant for hypertension managed with metoprolol and lisinopril, hyperlipidemia managed with simvastatin, and new-onset angina controlled with diltiazem CD. He has no known drug allergies.

The family history is positive for colon and lung cancer. RR has never smoked and drinks one or two glasses of wine with dinner almost every night.

PHYSICAL EXAMINATION

BP: 110/65, RR: 24, HR: 88, T: 100°F
Ht: 5'10", Wt: 155 lb
HEENT: Dry mucous membranes

COR: S_1, S_2, and $+S_3$
ABD: Tender to palpation
RECT: Stool grossly positive for blood, no hemorrhoids

LABS

Hgb: 10.5
Hct: 32
RBC: 3.2
CEA: 24
Sigmoidoscopy: 3-cm lesion in the sigmoid colon

QUESTIONS

1. Surgical resection of the tumor is completed. The tumor is classified as Dukes B. RR and his physician discuss treatment and decide that RR will undergo adjuvant antineoplastic therapy with continuous infusion 5-FU and leucovorin. What is the dose-limiting toxicity of this regimen?

   A. Neurotoxicity (tingling and numbness of hands and feet)
   B. Bone marrow suppression
   C. GI toxicity (mucositis, diarrhea)
   D. Folic acid toxicity
   E. Thrombotic stroke

2. RR is not tolerating the 5-FU and leucovorin regimen because of the side effects, but the carcinoembryonic antigen (CEA) level is stable at 8. Which alternative therapy would be most appropriate?

   A. 5-FU with levamisole
   B. Paclitaxel with leucovorin
   C. Cisplatin, etoposide, and vinblastine

   D. Leucovorin as a single agent
   E. High-dose methotrexate with leucovorin rescue

3. What is the primary purpose of CEA monitoring in RR's care?

   A. Monitoring for treatment toxicity
   B. Monitoring for disease progression or treatment efficacy
   C. Prognostic indicator of survival
   D. Indicator of hepatic metastases
   E. Monitoring for need for changes in the dosages of antineoplastic agents

4. RR is tolerating the new treatment regimen but he is not eating enough food to maintain his weight. He states that he does not feel like eating. Which agent would be the most appropriate appetite stimulant for RR?

   A. Sertraline
   B. High-dose megestrol acetate
   C. Diphenhydramine
   D. High-dose meclizine
   E. Sugar-free gum

5. The colon cancer spreads to the liver and has not been responsive to IV antineoplastic therapy. RR and his physician decide to pursue aggressive therapy. Which treatment would be the most appropriate for hepatic metastases?

   A. Radiation to the liver
   B. Hepatic arterial infusion of 5-FU
   C. Insertion of radioactive implants in the liver
   D. Systemic intravenous infusion of doxorubicin
   E. There is no effective therapy for hepatic metastases.

PATIENT   PROFILE   52

CHLAMYDIA AND EMERGENCY CONTRACEPTION

PRESENTATION

BH is a 28-year-old Hispanic woman who complains of vaginal discharge at an outpatient clinic appointment.

BH started to experience "significant amounts of yellow discharge" over the past week or two. She relates this to when a condom slipped off of her partner during intercourse. At that time she went to the emergency department for emergency contraception.

PMH: Vaginal candidiasis; TB exposure, documented by a
    positive PPD test
Allergies: none
Current Meds: isoniazid 300 mg po qd
PE:
BP: 92/60, HR 72, RR 12, T afebrile
GEN: Young woman in no apparent distress
HEENT: TMs intact, oral mucosa clear

CHEST: Clear to auscultation
COR: RRR
GU: Normal external genitalia, cervix is normal and mobile with mucopurulent discharge, no uterine or ovarian masses
EXT: normal range of motion

LABS

Wet prep: (+) Polys >25
            (−) Whiff test
            (−) Clue cells
            (−) Hyphae
            (−) *Trichomonas*
            (−) Yeast
Pap smear: (+) *Chlamydia trachomatis*
BH is diagnosed with chlamydia.

QUESTIONS

1. Which of the following best describes *Chlamydia trachomatis*?

   A. Gram-negative bacteria
   B. Gram-positive bacteria
   C. Parasite
   D. Spirochete
   E. Virus

2. Which of the following is the only single-dose therapy that is effective in treating *C. trachomatis*?

   A. Amoxicillin
   B. Azithromycin
   C. Doxycycline
   D. Erythromycin
   E. Ofloxacin

3. Which of the following is accurate patient counseling information for azithromycin?

   A. Do not take with magnesium or aluminum containing antacids.
   B. The 1-g dose packet for oral suspension can be given without regard to meals.
   C. The tablet formation should be taken 1 hour before or 2 hours after meals.
   D. A and C only
   E. A, B, and C

4. Which of the following is a possible adverse effect of doxycycline?

   A. Arthropathy
   B. Disulfiram reaction with alcohol ingestion
   C. Kernicterus
   D. Permanent discoloration of the teeth during tooth development
   E. Red man syndrome

5. Which of the following is accurate patient counseling information for doxycycline?

   A. You may take it with food if it upsets your stomach.
   B. Use a sunscreen when exposed to sunlight.
   C. Contact your prescriber if you develop a rash.
   D. A and C only
   E. A, B, and C

6. BH asks if her partner needs to be treated. Which of the following is the best response?

   A. No, it is never necessary for your partner to be treated.
   B. It is necessary to treat your partner only if he has symptoms.
   C. Treatment is for the partner and is not routinely recommended.
   D. Yes, your partner should be treated with oral therapy.
   E. Yes, your partner should be treated with topical therapy.

7. BH had emergency contraception in the recent past. Which of the following is an FDA-approved product packaged for this indication?

   A. Ovral®
   B. Plan B®
   C. Preven®
   D. A and C only
   E. B and C only

8. Which of the following best defines when the first dose of emergency contraception should be administered?

   A. Within 72 hours of unprotected intercourse
   B. Within 7 days of unprotected intercourse
   C. Within 2 weeks of unprotected intercourse
   D. Within 72 hours of missing the first day of menses
   E. Once pregnancy is confirmed

9. Which of the following best defines when the second dose of emergency contraception should be administered?

   A. One hour after the first dose
   B. Twelve hours after the first dose
   C. Twenty-four hours after the first dose
   D. Two days after the first dose
   E. One week after the first dose

10. Which of the following are potential adverse effects of emergency contraception?

    A. Breast tenderness
    B. Nausea
    C. Vomiting
    D. A and B only
    E. A, B, and C

PATIENT PROFILE 53

MEDICINAL CHEMISTRY

PRESENTATION AND QUESTION

You have just started a new job in the university medical center hospital. Part of your responsibility is supervising the IV unit. Your first IV prescription includes Valium® (diazepam, structure 53.1) and dextrose (structure 53.2). Diazepam is used to stabilize the patient's condition against clonic seizures, and dextrose is used as a nutrient. The nurse asks, "Why give the patient two separate injections? I will infuse Valium into the dextrose bag."

1. You give the following answer:

   A. Yes, why not? That will be more convenient for the patient.

   B. No, do not do that. Dextrose can pharmacologically antagonize the actions of Valium.
   C. No, do not do that. The chemistry of diazepam indicates the presence of a ketone functional group that may interact chemically with the aldehyde function of the sugar.
   D. No, do not do that. If you do, Valium will precipitate out of the solution.
   E. Yes, you can do that if the Valium ampule is cooled in ice before use.

53.1

53.2

PATIENT PROFILE 54

SEIZURE DISORDERS

PRESENTATION

DG is a 9-year-old boy with a history of epilepsy. DG's mother comes to the pharmacy monthly for refills on his antiepileptic medication. DG has had a history of tonic-clonic seizures that began with an episode of status epilepticus at age 9. At the time of his initial diagnosis he was treated with valproic acid. His mother states that DG has had four breakthrough seizures in the last 9 months; two of these seizures were prolonged and were determined to be status epilepticus. Each time a seizure occurred, the dose of DG's valproic acid was increased. Once the dose of Depakote® was maximized, lamotrigine was added. He is currently treated with Depakote® (divalproex sodium delayed release) 500 mg tid and lamotrigine 50 mg bid. DG's mother reports that DG has been seizure free since the last dose adjustment. DG also has a prescription for diazepam rectal gel (Diastat®) 10 mg to be used for status epilepticus as needed.

PMH: Epilepsy. Tonic-clonic seizure and three incidents of status epilepticus.

MH: Divalproex sodium delayed release (Depakote®) 500 mg tid

Refill history: Depakote® 125 mg sprinkles bid: filled 1/15/04

Depakote® 250 mg bid: 2/15/04 filled monthly, until increased on 6/20/04 to 250 mg tid filled monthly, until increased 500 mg tid on 8/20/04

Lamotrigine 50 mg bid filled on 10/10/04

Diazepam 10 mg rectal gel UUD, PRN: dispensed 1/15/04 and 8/23/04

Allergies: NKDA

FH: Mother age 35 and father age 35 alive with no medical problems. Brother age 8 has seasonal allergies.

SH: DG attends public school and is currently in the fourth grade. DG is a bright, active 9 year old who likes to play baseball and roller blade. He has trouble keeping his grades up because of his seizure history and the side effects of the medication, which cause him to miss school sometimes. His seizures often frighten his friends and they sometimes do things without him.

Labs: Unavailable

PE: Est wt 60 lbs (27 kg), est ht 4'10"

PROBLEM LIST

1. Tonic-clonic seizure disorder
2. History of status epilepticus

QUESTIONS

1. Which of the following conditions can lead to seizure disorders?

   A. Head trauma
   B. Fever
   C. Lack of sleep
   D. All of the above

2. Which of the following is a first-choice drug therapy for tonic-clonic seizures?

   A. Ethosuximide
   B. Lamotrigine
   C. Valproic acid
   D. Phenobarbital

3. Which of the following is an adverse effect of valproic acid?

   A. Gastrointestinal (GI) upset
   B. Gingival hyperplasia
   C. Ataxia
   D. Nystagmus

4. Which of the following can increase the concentration of free valproic acid?

   A. Warfarin
   B. Aspirin
   C. Disulfiram
   D. Isoniazid

5. The mechanism of action of valproic acid is best described by its effects on which of the following?

   A. Potassium channels
   B. GABA
   C. Sodium channels
   D. Calcium channels

6. What is a benefit of Depakote® as compared with Depakene®?

   A. Dosing interval
   B. Available in an intravenous formulation
   C. Less GI distress
   D. Available as a sprinkle

7. The mechanism of action of lamotrigine is best described by its effect on which of the following?

   A. Sodium channels
   B. Calcium channels
   C. Glutamate
   D. All of the above

8. Which of the following is an adverse effect of lamotrigine?

   A. Insomnia
   B. Nausea
   C. Diarrhea
   D. Diplopia

9. What is the rationale for using a lower dose of lamotrigine in combination therapy with valproic acid?

   A. Lamotrigine inhibits the clearance of valproic acid through enzyme inhibition.
   B. Valproic acid inhibits the clearance of lamotrigine through enzyme inhibition.
   C. Valproic acid and lamotrigine have similar adverse effects.
   D. There is no need to lower the dose of lamotrigine.

10. What is the preferred benzodiazepine for status epilepticus?
    A. Diazepam
    B. Midazolam
    C. Lorazepam
    D. Clonazepam

PATIENT PROFILE 55

MAJOR DEPRESSION

PRESENTATION

BC is a 23-year-old woman who feels "sad all the time." Over the last few months she has felt a decrease in energy and a decrease in appetite. She had been rather social but has recently preferred to stay at home by herself. She says that nothing tragic has happened in her life, but there have been times over the last 5 years when she has felt withdrawn and sad but recovered after a few weeks, and it was never serious enough to prevent her from going to school. She has been going to work most of the time but has been leaving early most days because of lack of energy.

The medical history includes GERD. BC has no known drug allergies. Her medication history includes Tri-Levlen® (levonorgestrel and ethinyl estradiol) 1 tablet qd and famotidine 20 mg qd.

BC is single and lives alone. She is a recent college graduate who works as an administrative assistant. She says she uses alcohol occasionally ("a couple glasses of wine on weekends"). She denies tobacco use.

PHYSICAL EXAMINATION

BP sitting R arm: 118/78, HR: 68, T: 98.2°F, RR: 20

LABS

Na: 140 mEq/L	Cl: 98 mEq/L
K: 4.3 mEq/L	BUN: 18 mg/dL
CO_2: 26 mEq/L	SCr: 0.7 mg/dL
Gluc: 106 mg/dL	AST: 45 U/L
TSH: 5.4 μg/mL	ALT: 40 U/L
T_4: 4.0 μg/dL	Alk Phos: 40 U/L
T_3: 70.0 ng/dL	

A/P: A 23-year-old woman reports decreased appetite, anhedonia, and a decrease in energy. She is seeking help for these conditions.

QUESTIONS

1. Which of the following are symptoms of depression?

   A. Decrease in sleep
   B. Decrease in appetite
   C. Anhedonia
   D. A and B
   E. A, B, and C

2. Which of the following may be causing the depression?

   A. Oral contraceptives
   B. Hypothyroidism
   C. GERD
   D. A and B
   E. A, B, and C

3. After the addition of levothyroxine 0.05 mg qd the thyroid function test results are reported to be within normal limits. However, BC's mood has not improved appreciably. Which antidepressant is most appropriate for BC?

   A. Fluoxetine
   B. Amitriptyline
   C. Amoxapine
   D. Paroxetine
   E. Desipramine

4. How long after initiation of an antidepressant is a full response usually seen?

   A. Within hours
   B. 2 to 3 days later
   C. 1 to 2 weeks later
   D. 2 to 3 weeks later
   E. 4 to 6 weeks later

5. How long should BC be treated with an antidepressant?

   A. For 6 months after resolution of depressive symptoms
   B. For 10–12 months after resolution of depressive symptoms
   C. For 20–24 months after resolution of depressive symptoms
   D. Forever
   E. Until depressive symptoms disappear

PATIENT PROFILE 5 6

PEDIATRIC IMMUNIZATIONS

PRESENTATION

JB is an 8-month-old girl who is being seen in the pediatric clinic for the first time for follow-up of a recent visit to the hospital for community-acquired pneumonia. Three weeks ago the child had a fever, extreme lethargy, loss of appetite, dehydration, and a productive cough. She was seen in the ED with a temperature of 103.6°F. On physical examination, crackles were heard in the lungs bilaterally. The infant was discharged from the hospital after 2 days with a diagnosis of pneumonia, for which she was prescribed a 5-day course of azithromycin.

PMH: The patient received minimal prenatal care; was delivered at 38 weeks' gestation by routine vaginal delivery weighing 6 pounds 13 ounces. According to the mother, the child has been otherwise healthy, with no other illnesses, and has not required any medical care. She had no contact with the medical system until the emergency department visit and hospitalization 3 weeks ago. No previous immunizations have been given, except hepatitis B vaccine, which was given immediately after birth.

CC: "My daughter is here for a check-up."

FH: Noncontributory

SH: Mother, age 20, and father, age 21, work full time. They live in a government subsidized two-bedroom apartment. There were no recent illnesses among household members. There are no pets at home. The father smokes cigarettes in the home.

Meds: None

All: NKDA

ROS: Negative at this time, pneumonia is resolved

PE: Gen: Alert, happy, relatively small, appropriately developed 8-month-old infant in NAD; Wt 6.8 kg; Length 65 cm

VS: BP 100/62, P 140, RR 28, T 36.6°C (axillary)

HEENT: PERRLA, ears, nose, and throat clear

COR: RRR, no murmurs

Lungs: CTA B/L

Abd: Soft, NT, no masses or organomegaly

Genit: Normal

Ext: skin cool and dry

Neuro: Alert, normal DTRs b/l

QUESTIONS

1. Which of the following statements regarding DTaP is false?

   A. The acellular form of pertussis is given to reduce the risk of fever.

   B. DTaP is contraindicated in children with a family history of seizure.

   C. Common adverse effects include mild to moderate tenderness and redness at the injection site.

   D. The pertussis component protects against the development of "whooping cough."

   E. DTaP can be given by either intramuscular injection.

2. MMR vaccine administration is associated with all except which of the following?

   A. Autism

   B. Rash

   C. Fever

   D. Arthralgias

   E. Malaise

3. Which of the following immunizations contains a live-attenuated organism?

   A. Influenza vaccine

   B. Pneumococcal polysaccharide vaccine

   C. Meningococcal polysaccharide vaccine

   D. Varicella vaccine

   E. Diphtheria toxoid/tetanus toxoid/acellular pertussis vaccine

4. Live attenuated vaccines are contraindicated in which of the following patient populations?

   I. Pregnant women

   II. Patients with chronic renal failure

   III. Patients receiving inhaled corticosteroids

   A. I only

   B. III only

   C. I and II only

   D. II and III only

   E. I, II, and III

5. All of the following immunizations should be recommended to immunize JB at this time except which of the following?

   I. OPV

   II. MMR

   III. HiB

   A. I only

   B. III only

   C. I and II only

D. II and III only
E. I, II, and III

6. Patients with allergies to which of the following medications should not receive the inactivated polio vaccine (IPV)?

A. Clindamycin
B. Tetracycline
C. Streptomycin
D. Amoxicillin
E. Erythromycin

7. The MMR vaccine should not be given to which of the following patients?

I. Pregnant women
II. Cancer patients receiving chemotherapy
III. Patients with a history of egg allergy

A. I only
B. III only
C. I and II
D. II and III only
E. I, II, and III

8. Which of the brand name represents the *Haemophilus influenzae* type B vaccine?

A. Engerix-B
B. Recombivax-HB
C. Varivax
D. ProHIBiT
E. Havrix

9. Which of the following immunizations interferes with the Mantoux tuberculin skin test?

A. Inactivated polio vaccine
B. Influenza vaccine
C. Measles vaccine
D. Hepatitis B vaccine
E. Tetanus toxoid

10. Which of the following best describes the rationale for the addition of aluminum salts to inactivated bacterial toxin and vaccines?

A. Preserve against bacterial growth
B. Enhance their immunogenicity
C. Reduce local irritation associated with the injection
D. To stabilize the vaccine solution
E. All of the above

PATIENT PROFILE 57
RENAL TRANSPLANTATION

PRESENTATION

Residence	Community
Patient	CN
Age	61
Sex	Male
Allergies	Radiocontrast dye (anaphylactoid reaction)
Race	African American
Height	5'8"
Wt	162 lb
Diagnosis	Primary

Diagnosis Primary
1. s/p living related donor kidney transplant 1997
2. HTN
3. Hyperuricemia
4. Hypercholesterolemia

Secondary 1. Rheumatoid arthritis

	Date	Rx No.	Physician	Drug and Strength	Quantity	Sig	Refills
Medication record (prescription and OTC)	08/11	55629	AL	Cyclosporine (Neoral®) 100 mg	100	1 po bid	2

08/11	55630	AL	Mycophenolate mofetil (CellCept®) 250 mg	180	1 po bid	2
08/11	55631	AL	Prednisone 10 mg	30	1 po qd	3
08/11	55632	AL	Diltiazem (Cardiazem CD®) 240 mg	30	1 po qd	3
09/30	62100	AL	Allopurinol 100 mg	60	1 po bid	6
10/13	71213	AL	Atorvastatin 10 mg	30	1 po qd	2
11/01	OTC		Acetaminophen 325 mg	100	2 po every 4–6 h for pain	

| Dietary considerations | 10/13 | Patient received cholesterol dietary restriction counseling by dietician at clinic; patient will record food intake in diary |
| Pharmacist notes and other patient information | 10/13 | Asked patient whether baseline liver function tests and CBC count were done Patient counseling was offered and accepted (oral and written). |

QUESTIONS

1. What is the side effect that may occur with HMG-CoA reductase inhibitors and is closely monitored in the care of patients who are also receiving cyclosporine?

   A. Gingival hyperplasia
   B. Hallucinations
   C. Intermittent claudication
   D. Myopathy
   E. Seizures

2. Which of the following HMG-CoA reductase enzyme inhibitors has the least propensity for side effects when given with Neoral® (cyclosporine)?

   I. Simvastatin
   II. Lovastatin
   III. Atorvastatin

   A. I only
   B. II only
   C. I and II only
   D. II and III only
   E. I, II, and III

3. How would you advise a patient who reports gastrointestinal discomfort associated with use of CellCept® (mycophenolate mofetil)?

   A. Stop taking the drug.
   B. Take one-half the daily dose.
   C. Combine the drug with an antacid.
   D. Contact the physician.
   E. Take the drug at bedtime only.

4. The patient reports severe hip pain. Use of which of the following is associated with necrosis of the hip?

   A. Prednisone
   B. CellCept® (mycophenolate mofetil)
   C. Neoral® (cyclosporine)
   D. Atorvastatin
   E. Allopurinol

PATIENT PROFILE 58

ACNE

PRESENTATION

DW is a 17-year-old woman who presents to the pharmacy to ask you for advice on her acne. DW has several visible comedones, open and closed on her forehead, nose, and chin. She is distressed because her mother had "bad" acne when she was DW's age, and as an adult her mother has visible scarring and pitting on her cheeks. DW "broke out" approximately 2 weeks ago, and states that her current cleansing regimen is only making it worse. She has also tried tanning at a salon; she believes that a tan complexion helps camouflage the pimples; she admits to using tanning oil to help speed up the process. DW recently became sexually active and worries that this may have something to do with her acne.

CC: "What can you recommend for these pimples on my face?"

MedHx: Phenytoin 100 mg po bid

Albuterol MDI 2p QID prn

Acetaminophen 1000 mg po q6 prn HA

PMH: Seizure disorder

Mild asthma

Tension headaches (approximately 1 each month)

PSH: Tonsillectomy at age 7

FH: DW's mother had severe acne in high school

SH: DW is a junior in high school, and still lives at home with her parents and her two younger sisters. DW plays field hockey and is a member of the symphony (she plays both the piano and violin). She is always on the honor roll. She denies tobacco, alcohol, and illicit drug use.

Allergies: NKDA

PE:

BP 116/72, HR 60, T 38.5°C

Weight = 122; Height = 5'2"

GEN: WDWN young woman

SKIN: Approximately 4 closed and open comedones on her forehead, two closed comedones on the bridge of her nose, and three open comedones on her chin.

Labs: Not obtained

Medication record (prescription and OTC):

Date	Drug and Strength	Quantity	Sig	Refills
11/3	Phenytoin 100 mg	60	1 bid	11
11/3	Albuterol MDI	17	2p QID	5
12/1	Phenytoin 100 mg	60	1 bid	10
12/1	APAP 500 mg	120	2 q6 PRN	3
1/4	Phenytoin 100 mg	60	1 bid	9

QUESTIONS

1. Which factors may be exacerbating DW's acne?

   I.   Phenytoin ✓
   II. Oil from the tanning salon ✓ ✓
   III. Helmet from field hockey ✓

   A. I only
   B. III only
   C. I and II
   D. II and III
   E. I, II, and III

2. What nonpharmacologic methods would you recommend to help minimize DW's acne?

   A. Avoid chocolate.
   B. Exfoliate the skin by washing more vigorously at least three to four times a day.

C. Refrain from sexual activity.
D. Squeeze the pimples to express the excess sebum to help prevent further development of the lesion.
E. Play the piano instead of the violin.

3. DW would like to start taking oral contraceptives; which of the following would you recommend?

   A. Micronor®
   B. Loestrin Fe® 1.5/30
   C. Norlestrin® 1/50
   D. Ortho Tri-Cyclen®
   E. Ovral®

4. What is the medical/clinical term for a "white head?"

   A. Closed comedone
   B. Macrocomedone
   C. Open comedone
   D. Papule
   E. Pustule

5. DW would like you to recommend an over-the-counter product. Which of the following is available without a prescription?

   A. Accutane®   isotretinoin
   B. Azelaic acid – Azelex / Finacea
   C. Benzoyl peroxide
   D. Cleocin® – clindamycin
   E. Tretinoin – Retin A   soln > gel > cream

6. Two weeks have past since DW began using the product you recommended, she complains that her acne is not improving to her satisfaction. What should you recommend?

   A. Try a more potent agent or a higher strength.
   B. Wait at least 1 month before modifying the regimen.
   C. Switch to another dosage form.
   D. Review proper administration, DW must not be using the product correctly.
   E. Increase the frequency of use.

7. DW's friend is taking isotretinoin; she would like clarification regarding all the publicity about this drug. Which of the following are possible adverse effects of isotretinoin?

   I.   Teratogenicity ✓
   II. Cheilitis
   III. Infertility

A. I only
B. III only
C. I and II
D. II and III
E. I, II, and III

8. What is the brand name of isotretinoin?

A. Accutane® ✓
B. Benzamycin®
C. Differin® _ Adapalene
D. Minocin® _ minomycin .
E. Retin-A® _ tretinoin.

9. Which of the following statements is/are true regarding prescription orders for isotretinoin?

I.   No refills are allowed. ✓
II.   Telephone orders cannot be accepted. ✓
III. The prescription is only valid for 7 days. ✓

A. I only
B. III only
C. I and II
D. II and III
E. I, II, and III

10. Which of the following statements regarding topical
preparations to treat acne are true?

I.   Resorcinol is not effective unless it is combined
with sulfur preparations. ✓
II.   Products containing sulfur may cause skin discoloration. ✓
III. Salicylic acid is equally as effective as benzoyl
peroxide.

A. I only
B. III only
C. I and II
D. II and III
E. I, II, and III

PATIENT PROFILE 59

CORONARY ARTERY DISEASE

PRESENTATION

SB is a 65-year-old man who arrives at the general medicine clinic with a 1-week history of nausea, agitation,
tremors, and increased number of angina attacks associated with palpitations. The history of the present illness
is that SB has been treated in a smoking cessation clinic
and had his last cigarette 1 month ago. SB recently was
treated with colchicine 1 week ago for an acute attack of
gout.

The past medical history includes angina for 5 years. The
condition has been stable with isosorbide dinitrate, but SB
lately reports chest pain with exertion. He has had hypertension for 10 years that is controlled with hydrochlorothiazide and has had COPD for 3 years that is stable with
theophylline and albuterol prn through an inhaler.

SB has smoked one pack of cigarettes per day for 30
years and uses alcohol occasionally. His mother has
COPD, and his father has CAD and gout.

MEDS

Hydrochlorothiazide 50 mg po qd
KCl 20 mEq po qd
Isosorbide dinitrate 30 mg po tid
Theophylline SR 300 mg po bid
Albuterol inhaler 2 puffs q4h prn
Nitroglycerin .4 mg SL prn for chest pain
EC aspirin 325 mg po qd
NKDA

PHYSICAL EXAMINATION

GEN: Well-developed man in mild distress
BP: 155/95, HR: 100, RR: 16, T: 37.5°C
Ht: 177.8 cm, Wt: 70 kg
HEENT: Mild AV nicking
COR: S_1, S_2, no S_3, sinus tachycardia
CHEST: Barrel chest, increased accessory muscle use
ABD: Soft, nontender
GU: WNL
RECT: Heme negative
EXT: MTP of left toe erythematous, tender, warm to
touch 1 week ago, now WNL
NEURO: A/O × 3

LABS

Na: 139   Ca: 8.1
K: 4.6   PO$_4$: 3.2

Cl: 96
BUN: 19
WBC: 9.5
Hgb: 13.5
SCr: 1.2
Total chol: 245

HCO₃: 27
Mg: 1.8
Plts: 253,000
Hct: 40
Gluc: 110

HCO_3: 27
Mg: 1.8
Plts: 253,000
Hct: 40
Gluc: 110

WBC differential: WNL
Theophylline: 21
Urinalysis: WNL
Chest x-ray: Clear
EKG: Sinus tachycardia, occasional PVCs

QUESTIONS

1. Which of the following is the most likely reason for the recent increase in angina episodes?

    A. Subtherapeutic theophylline level leading to exacerbation of COPD
    B. Inadequate blood pressure control
    C. High cholesterol
    D. Theophylline toxicity
    E. Recent gout attack

2. Which of the following interventions would be most appropriate to manage the angina?

    A. Decrease isosorbide dinitrate to 20 mg po tid
    B. Add metoprolol 50 mg po bid
    C. Add diltiazem 120 mg po qd
    D. Add atenolol 50 mg po qd
    E. Increase hydrochlorothiazide to 100 mg po qd

3. Which of the following medications could have contributed to the acute attack of gout 1 week ago?

    A. Hydrochlorothiazide
    B. Albuterol
    C. Theophylline
    D. Isosorbide dinitrate
    E. KCl

4. Which of the following interventions would not be appropriate for SB to initiate to modify risk factors for coronary artery disease?

    A. Starting simvastatin 10 mg po qd
    B. Smoking cessation
    C. Starting niacin SR 500 mg po bid
    D. Limiting alcohol intake to not more than one drink per day
    E. Adherence to a step 1 diet

5. In 6 months, SB is found to have a peptic ulcer likely caused by aspirin. Which of the following is the most appropriate choice to replace aspirin in SB's antiischemia drug regimen?

    A. Enoxaparin 30 mg sq bid
    B. Dipyridamole 50 mg po qid
    C. Clopidogrel 75 mg po qid
    D. Warfarin 5 mg po qd
    E. Amlodipine 5 mg po qd

PATIENT PROFILE 60

INHALATION ANTHRAX

PRESENTATION

LM is a 36-year-old man presenting to the emergency department with nonspecific flulike symptoms for the past 24 to 48 hours. LM's wife states he has had a fever of 102°F, a nonproductive cough, sore throat, headache and fatigue, and general feelings of malaise. The wife denies any nasal congestion or runny nose. He presented to the emergency department today in respiratory distress with pleuretic pain.

CC: LM is complaining of shortness of breath and flulike symptoms.

PMH: LM has had no past medical problems and no medication allergies.

SH: The patient denies tobacco and illicit drug use. His wife states LM may drink one or two beers a week and drinks one cup of caffeinated coffee per day. LM lives at home with his wife and two children (ages 7 and 5). LM is a postal worker at the central distribution center (4 years).

FH: Both of LM's parents are still alive. His mother has osteoarthritis and his father has no medical conditions.

Gen: Well-nourished man in mid-thirties in apparent respiratory distress

VS: BP 110/65, RR 19, Pulse 116 bpm, Temp 102°F, Wt: 180 lbs

HEENT: With in normal limits (wnl)

Chest: Rhonchi present

CV: No murmurs, gallops or rubs

Abd: NT/ND

Skin: wnl

Laboratory:

WBC: 10,000 mm^3 (5 to 10,000 mm^3)

Chest x-ray: Shows mediastinal widening with pleural effusion

Blood smear: Positive for gram-positive rods after 12 hours

Diagnosis: Inhalation anthrax

MN: Patient in severe respiratory distress and with abrupt spike in temperature. Patient expired in 2 days.

QUESTIONS

1. The Centers for Disease Control and Prevention (CDC) categorizes pathogens into categories according to their accessibility, potential for morbidity and mortality, and level of contagiousness. Anthrax is what category according to the CDC guidelines?

   A. Category A
   B. Category B
   C. Category C
   D. Not on the CDC list

2. A positive diagnosis of inhalation anthrax includes a clinical presentation and a positive history of exposure to anthrax. A diagnosis must be made quickly; therefore, other diagnostic tools also are used in confirming the diagnosis. What other physical signs can be used for a positive diagnosis of inhalation anthrax?

   A. Mediastinum widening shown on a chest x-ray
   B. Mediastinal adenopathy or pleural effusions
   C. Blood smear of gram-positive rods
   D. A and C only
   E. All of the above

3. The gram-positive rods found on the blood smear were most likely which of the following?

   A. *Yersinia pestis*
   B. *Coxiella burnetii*
   C. *Bacillus anthracis*
   D. *Francisella tularensis*

4. Treatment protocols per the CDC guidelines for inhalation anthrax include which of the following?

   A. Amoxicillin 500 mg PO QID
   B. Doxycycline 100 mg IV q12 hours
   C. Rifampin 600 mg PO QD
   D. A and B
   E. B and C

5. According to the CDC guidelines, what is the recommend length of treatment for inhalation anthrax?

   A. 10 days
   B. 20 days
   C. 60 days
   D. 120 days

6. What is the typical incubation period for inhalation anthrax?

   A. 1 to 14 days
   B. 3 to 5 days
   C. 6 to 10 hours
   D. 1 to 14 hours

7. Prophylactic treatment of all postal employees and first responders is necessary. According to the CDC guidelines, exposure prophylaxis treatment in a possible biological attack includes which of the following?

   A. Ciprofloxacin 500 mg PO q12 hours
   B. Doxycycline 100 mg PO q12 hours
   C. Tetracycline 500 mg PO QID
   D. A or B treatment options are acceptable.
   E. All of the above are suitable treatment options.

8. An anthrax vaccine is available for prophylaxis of military personnel (pre-exposure). What is the correct dosing regimen?

   A. 0, 2, 4 weeks, then yearly booster
   B. 0, 2, 4, 6 weeks only
   C. 0, 2, 4, 6 weeks, then 6 months, then yearly boosters
   D. 0, 2, and 4 weeks, then 6, 12, and 18 months, then yearly boosters

9. What are the most important counseling points to tell the postal employees about their prophylactic medication?

   I. The agent is an antibiotic and must be taken for the full course of therapy.
   II. The medication should be taken with a full (8-oz) glass of water.
   III. Avoid antacids or iron products within 2 hours *after* taking the medication.
   IV. The patient should completely avoid products containing caffeine.

   A. I only
   B. I and II only
   C. I, II, and III
   D. IV only
   E. All of the above

10. All of the following are true about anthrax except which of the following?

   A. There are multiple forms of anthrax: inhalation, oropharyngeal, cutaneous, and gastrointestinal.

B. An acellular vaccine is available and the CDC controls distribution.
C. Cutaneous anthrax is the most deadly form of anthrax

D. Inhalation anthrax has two phases: the initial presentation followed by an improvement in symptoms followed by a second phase of a rapid progression to respiratory failure and death.

PATIENT PROFILE 61

DIABETES MELLITUS

PRESENTATION

AB is a 48-year-old woman with a history of psoriasis and hypercholesterolemia who visits her primary care physician because of polyuria and polydypsia. She has no allergies. Her medications include hydrocortisone 2.5% cream applied to the affected skin bid prn and simvastatin 10 mg po qd. Her father has hypertension and CAD and has had one MI. Her mother has diabetes mellitus type II. AB does not use ethanol, tobacco, or illicit drugs. The physical examination findings are unremarkable.

LABS

Na: 138 mEq/L
K: 3.9 mEq/L
Fasting plasma glucose: 162 mg/dL

The physician suspects that AB may have diabetes mellitus and repeats the fasting plasma glucose measurement the next day. The measurement is 132 mg/dL.

QUESTIONS

1. AB is found to have diabetes mellitus. A fasting plasma glucose greater than or equal to which of the following amounts confirms the diagnosis of diabetes mellitus?

    A. 115 mg/dL
    B. 126 mg/dL
    C. 135 mg/dL
    D. 140 mg/dL
    E. 156 mg/dL

2. In addition to exercise and diet modification, drug therapy is warranted. Which of the following would be reasonable for initial monotherapy? Select the best answer.

    A. Glipizide
    B. Glyburide
    C. Glucagon
    D. A and B only
    E. A, B, and C

3. Migraine headaches develop, and AB is given propranolol 20 mg po qid for prophylaxis. You know that β-adrenergic blockers may alter the severity of or block the warning signs of hypoglycemia. What sign of hypoglycemia may remain as the only warning signal? Select the best answer.

    A. Palpitations
    B. Tachycardia
    C. Tremor
    D. Confusion
    E. Sweating

4. AB is picking up a prescription in the pharmacy where you work. She states, "I feel like my sugar is very low. What should I do?" Which of the following responses is/are appropriate?

    A. Take three glucose tablets.
    B. Drink ½ cup of juice, such as apple or orange, or ½ cup of regular soda, not sugar-free.
    C. Drink 1 cup of milk.
    D. A and B only
    E. A, B, and C

PATIENT PROFILE 62

DEPRESSION

PRESENTATION

JK is a 54-year-old single white man. He was admitted to the psychopharmacology clinic after an inpatient alcohol detox and 3-week residential program.

HPI: 20+ year ETOH use/abuse and chronic depressive symptoms. He finds that his alcohol use is secondary to his depressive mood. He has had periods of abstinence in the past but as stressors increased so did alcohol use. Symptoms of depression include insomnia, psychomotor retardation, depressed mood, and decreased appetite. He denies suicidal ideation, auditory hallucinations, visual hallucinations, and mania. A previous trial of nefazodone may have been helpful; a trial of gabapentin produced some relief from anxiety. His current use of mirtazapine is not helping.

PMH: DM2

s/p MI × 4 years

GERD

Hypertension

Hypercholesterolemia

Anemia

Alcohol dependence

Dysthymia

Meds: Mirtazapine 45 mg HS

Trazodone 100 mg HS

Metformin 850 mg BID

Lisinopril 10 mg QD (not taking)

Simvastatin 20 mg QH

Rabeprazole 20 mg QD

Nitro 0.4 mg sl PRN

Thiamine 100 mg q.a.m.

Folic acid 1 mg q.a.m.

Vitamin C 500 mg q.a.m.

Ferrous sulfate 324 mg q.a.m.

PE: v/s 128/81, 20, 37.1, 93; Ht 170.2 cm, Wt 80.8 kg

Labs: tchol 193, trig 248 H, albumin 3L, other lfts wnl, tsh wnl, hbA1C 8.9 H, Fe 38 L, TIBC 161 L, chem7 wnl, hgb 11.8 L, hct 34.9 L, rbc 3.7 L

QUESTIONS

1. Which of the following antidepressants could result in a drug–disease interaction if used to treat JK's dysthymia?

   A. Fluoxetine
   B. Sertraline
   C. Venlafaxine
   D. Citalopram

2. Which of the following would worsen JK's GERD if used to treat his dysthymia?

   A. Escitalopram
   B. Duloxetine
   C. Venlafaxine
   D. Amitriptyline

3. What pharmacodynamic drug interaction could occur if mirtazapine and clonidine are coadministered?

   A. Opposing effects on the α_2 receptor
   B. Synergistic effects on the histamine 1 receptor
   C. Additive antagonistic effects on the muscarinic receptor
   D. Opposing effects on the dopamine 2 receptor

4. What is the mechanism of action for sleep with trazodone?

   A. α_1 Receptor antagonism
   B. Histamine 1 receptor antagonism
   C. Serotonin 2 receptor antagonism
   D. α_2 Receptor antagonism

5. Which of the following antidepressants has the potential for worsening the patient's hypercholesterolemia?

   A. Mirtazapine
   B. Escitalopram
   C. Duloxetine
   D. Venlafaxine

SEIZURE DISORDERS

PRESENTATION

BC is a 2-year-old boy brought to the emergency department by his parents after having a tonic-clonic seizure that lasted approximately 10 minutes. The child has no history of a seizure disorder. During the examination the child is alert but has a temperature of 39.5°C and has evidence of an upper respiratory tract infection.

QUESTIONS

1. What type of seizure disorder does BC most likely have?

   A. Generalized tonic-clonic seizure disorder
   B. Absence seizures
   C. Complex partial seizure disorder
   D. Febrile seizure
   E. Simple partial seizure disorder

2. An appropriate treatment strategy at this point would include which of the following?

   A. Reduction of fever
   B. Administration of IV phenytoin
   C. Administration of IV diazepam
   D. A and B
   E. A, B, and C

3. In the care of young children, seizure prophylaxis with phenobarbital may be associated with a reduction in

   A. height.
   B. weight.
   C. intelligence quotient.
   D. A and B
   E. B and C

4. Which of the following agents may be administered rectally to manage subsequent seizures?

   A. Phenobarbital
   B. Phenytoin
   C. Fosphenytoin
   D. Lamotrigine
   E. Diazepam

5. Because of reports of serious hepatotoxicity and aplastic anemia, which of the following agents should be reserved for seizures refractory to other agents?

   A. Lamotrigine
   B. Topiramate
   C. Tiagabine
   D. Gabapentin
   E. Felbamate

BACTEREMIA AND SEPSIS

PRESENTATION

DL is a 40-year-old man with a history of rheumatic heart disease. DL visited his dental hygienist for a routine cleaning approximately 1 week before his hospital admission. DL's usual practice had been to take erythromycin before having his teeth cleaned; however, he lost his prescription and didn't think much of it. DL was healthy until 2 days ago, when he spiked a fever to 39.5°C, which was unrelieved with acetaminophen. On the morning of admission, the fever persists, and DL reports abnormalities of his hands (Janeway lesions). At admission, two specimens for blood cultures are drawn from peripheral sites, and a transthoracic echocardiogram reveals valvular vegetation consistent with endocarditis.

QUESTIONS

1. Choose an empiric antibiotic regimen for DL.

   A. Nafcillin 2 g IV q4h and gentamicin 1 mg/kg IV q8h
   B. Ceftazidime 2 g IV q8 hours and ciprofloxacin 400 mg IV q8h
   C. Trovafloxacin 300 mg po q24h
   D. Aztreonam 1 g IV q8h and gentamicin 1 mg/kg IV q8h
   E. Cefoxitin 1 g IV q6h

2. If cultures results show methicillin-resistant *Staphylococcus aureus*, the drug of choice becomes IV vancomycin.

What additional drug from the following list can be added for synergy?

A. Isoniazid
B. Ciprofloxacin
C. Azithromycin
D. Clindamycin
E. Rifampin

3. Nafcillin is the mainstay of therapy for *Staphylococcus aureus* infections, which of the following can be attributed to nafcillin?

A. Pain and irritation with IV infusion
B. Hypokalemia with doses of 200-300 mg/kg/d
C. Reversible neutropenia with more than 3 weeks of treatment
D. Interstitial nephritis
E. All of the above

4. DL had been taking erythromycin for endocarditis prophylaxis for years. Knowing that DL is not allergic to β-lactam antibiotics and is capable of taking oral therapy, which would be the best regimen for DL?

A. Amoxicillin 2 g po 1 h before dental procedure
B. Ampicillin 2 g IM or IV 30 minutes before dental procedure
C. Cephalexin 2 g po 1 h before dental procedure
D. Azithromycin 500 mg po 1 h before dental procedure
E. Clindamycin 600 mg IV within 30 minutes before procedure

5. All of the following statements are true regarding penicillin-resistant strains of *Streptococcus* in endocarditis except:

A. Penicillin can be used to manage infection with penicillin-resistant strains of *Streptococcus*.
B. There are no differences in dosing of penicillin for patients who have penicillin-susceptible strains of *Streptococcus* and those with penicillin-resistant strains.
C. Ampicillin in combination with gentamicin can be used to control streptococci with a high level of penicillin resistance.
D. Cefazolin may be used to treat patients who are allergic to penicillin.
E. Vancomycin may be used to treat patients with high-level penicillin resistance.

PATIENT PROFILE 65

DIABETES

PRESENTATION

JP is a morbidly obese 29-year-old woman with established type II diabetes. She is visiting her family doctor because of new tingling in her hands and feet. JP has missed the last four scheduled appointments. She was diagnosed with type II diabetes while being evaluated for hypothyroidism 8 years ago. She was diagnosed with schizoaffective disorder at 19 years old and has been well controlled with risperidone. Later, she was diagnosed with depression at 25 years old. JP initially began diet modifications and exercise to control her weight, but then quickly found that she was experiencing generalized diffuse pain in the areas of her upper back, lower back, shoulders, quadriceps, and calves. Further evaluations could find no specific locus for her pain and subsequent evaluations could find no other causes. JP was then diagnosed with fibromyalgia, which limits her to low impact aerobics, walking, or swimming. Recently, JP had a routine EKG with QT prolongation of 500 msec.

FH: Parents are divorced: Mother, age 55, has long history of multiple hospitalizations in state psychiatric hospitals with schizophrenia over the last 40 years. Father, age 65, lives alone and has hypertension and diabetes.

SH: Recently employed as stock room manager at local warehouse, just received her GED 6 months ago. Involved in long-term relationship with coworker × 2 years. She drinks 6 cups of coffee per day, has a 10-pack year tobacco history, denies EtOH and illicit drug use.

Allergies: Penicillin
Risperidone 2 mg po HS
Sertraline 100 mg po HS
Glimepiride 4 mg po HS (started 4 years ago)
Levothyroxine sodium 125 μg QD
Gen: Morbidly obese white female appearing anxious but alert, smelling of cigarette smoke.
Vitals: BP 100/66 mm Hg, HR 72 bpm, RR 14 breaths/min, T 98.1°F, Wt 297 lbs, Ht 5'7", BMI 46.5 kg/m^2
HEENT: PERRLA, funduscopic findings reveal normal retina, EOMI, mucous membranes moist
Chest: Clear to auscultation and percussion
Cor: Normal S$_1$ and S$_2$ sounds, RRR

Abd: Grossly obese, nontender, +BS, no hepatosplenomegaly

Ext: 2+ Pitting edema BL, cool diaphoretic skin

Neuro: Cranial nerves II to XII intact

Labs: Na 138 mEq/L, K 4.4 mEq/L, Cl 99 mEq/L, HCO_3 24 mEq/L, BUN 18 mg/dL, SCr 0.9 mg/dL, fasting glucose, 162 mg/dL, WBC 7.8 cells/mm^3, platelets 275 cells/mm^3, Hgb 13 g/dL, HCT 39%, HbA1c 8.3%

QUESTIONS

1. JP is complaining of new tingling sensations in her hands and feet consistent with neuropathy resulting from uncontrolled diabetes. Which is the safest option for peripheral neuropathy that minimizes potential drug interactions or drug toxicity?

   A. Desipramine 25 mg po QD
   B. Topiramate 25 mg po QD
   C. Amitriptyline 10 mg po QD
   D. Fluphenazine 1 mg po tid
   E. Capsaicin 0.025% applied to fingers and toes tid

2. Which of the following statements is true of glimepiride?

   A. Glimepiride is an effective hypoglycemic agent approved for type I and II diabetes.
   B. Glimepiride should be used alone without changes in diet and lifestyle to manage hyperglycemia.
   C. Glimepiride is a major substrate of CYP 2C8/2C9 and concentrations can increase in the presence of CYP 2C8/2C9 inhibitors.
   D. Glimepiride is a major substrate of CYP 3A4 and concentrations can increase in the presence of CYP 3A4 inhibitors.
   E. Glimepiride stimulates the release of glucagon from pancreatic β islet cells and induces hepatic gluconeogenesis.

3. Three months later JP returns for a follow-up visit. JP's fasting plasma glucose is 157 mg/dL with dietary modification and limited exercise because of fibromyalgia. She has gained 6 lbs since her last visit. What is the most appropriate strategy for improving her glucose control?

   A. Increase her glimepiride dose to 6 mg daily.
   B. Increase her glimepiride dose to 8 mg daily.
   C. Discontinue glimepiride and add metformin 500 mg daily for 2 weeks, then increase to 500 mg twice daily.
   D. Continue glimepiride and add metformin 500 mg daily for 2 weeks, then increase to 500 mg twice daily.

   E. Continue glimepiride and nateglinide 120 mg taken 10 to 15 minutes before each meal.

4. A fasting lipid panel returns with the following data: HDL-C 50 mg/dL, TC 250 mg/dL, TG 300 mg/dL. What is JP's LDL-C based on these values?

   A. 135 mg/dL
   B. 140 mg/dL
   C. 145 mg/dL
   D. 150 mg/dL
   E. 155 mg/dL

5. Considering that JP has diabetes and risk factors for coronary disease, what is the optimal LDL-C goal according to the 2004 ATP III updates?

   A. 70 mg/dL
   B. 80 mg/dL
   C. 100 mg/dL
   D. 120 mg/dL
   E. 130 mg/dL

6. JP has received a trial of lifestyle modification and has limited ability for exercise. The likelihood of JP achieving her goal LDL-C without drug therapy is remote. Which is the most effective pharmacotherapeutic intervention for cholesterol reduction?

   A. Gemfibrozil 600 mg po BID
   B. Ezetimibe 10 mg po QD
   C. Niacin XR 500 mg po QD to start, then titrate by 500 mg every 4 weeks as tolerated to a maximum of 2000 mg
   D. Colestipol 5 g dissolved in 90 mL po BID
   E. Simvastatin 40 mg po QD

7. JP is back for a follow-up of her HbA1c, fasting glucose, and fasting lipid panel. She has lost 12.5 lbs, BMI 44.5 kg/m^2, HbA1c 7%, fasting glucose 132 mg/dL, TC 185 mg/dL, HDL-C 55 mg/dL, TG 200 mg/dL, LDL-C 90 mg/dL. AST and ALT are wnl and JP reports that she is tolerating her medication without any side effects. JP smells of cigarette smoke at this visit. What is the most cost-effective intervention to modify JP's risk of heart disease with diabetes?

   A. Counsel JP on smoking cessation at every visit, discuss risks of CHD, and refer for cognitive behavioral therapy.
   B. Counsel JP about resuming her lifestyle and diet modifications, including a membership at a local fitness facility.
   C. Recommend increasing the dose of her simvastatin to 80 mg to achieve an additional 5% to 7% LDL-C reduction.

D. Add ezetimibe to achieve an additional 30% reduction of LDL-C.
E. Add gemfibrozil to reduce TG by 35%.

8. How often does JP need to have LFTs and muscle enzymes checked as part of routine monitoring?

A. At baseline, then yearly
B. At baseline, 3 months, 6 months, and 12 months after start of therapy
C. At baseline, then every 3 months routinely
D. At baseline, then every 6 months routinely
E. At baseline, 3 months, then every 6 months routinely

9. JP returns in 4 months and is diagnosed with an upper respiratory tract infection (URI). She receives a 10-day course of clarithromycin. How will this short course of clarithromycin affect JP?

A. Clarithromycin and simvastatin have no clinically significant drug interaction. This combination is safe and does not increase the risk of drug-induced adverse affects.
B. Clarithromycin inhibits CYP 2C9, resulting in higher intracellular concentrations of unmetabolized simvastatin and greater risk for statin-induced myopathy.
C. Clarithromycin induces CYP 2C19, resulting in higher intracellular concentrations of unmetabolized simvastatin and greater risk for statin-induced myopathy.

D. Clarithromycin inhibits CYP 3A4, resulting in higher intracellular concentrations of unmetabolized simvastatin and greater risk for statin-induced myopathy.
E. Clarithromycin induces CYP 3A4, resulting in higher intracellular concentrations of unmetabolized simvastatin and greater risk for statin-induced myopathy.

10. What is the most appropriate strategy to manage this interaction between clarithromycin and simvastatin?

A. Advise JP to avoid clarithromycin and allow the sinus infection to remit spontaneously. Tell her that 9 out of 10 URIs are viral; therefore, antibiotics do not ultimately shorten the course or severity of an infection.
B. Advise JP to discontinue simvastatin permanently. She has received the drug for at least 4 months and her lipid panel is likely to show dramatic improvements in her LDL.
C. Advise JP to temporarily stop taking simvastatin while she is taking clarithromycin. The day after finishing her course of clarithromycin she can resume taking simvastatin.
D. Advise JP to stop clarithromycin. Call the doctor to recommend dirithromycin for 14 days instead for the URI and continue to take simvastatin.
E. Advise JP to stop clarithromycin. Call the doctor to recommend azithromycin for 10 days instead for the URI and continue to take simvastatin.

PATIENT PROFILE 66
RADIOPHARMACEUTICALS

PRESENTATION

A technetium generator is used to produce a solution of radioactive sodium pertechnetate. The activity after generation is 15 mCi/mL (555 MBq/mL). The half-life of technetium Tc 99m is 6.0 hours. The patient is to be given a dose of 9 mCi/mL (333 MBq/mL) 10 hours after generation of the sodium pertechnetate.

QUESTIONS

1. How many megabequerels (MBq) are there in 100 mCi of a radioactive substance?

A. 2.7×10^{-4}
B. 2.7

C. 3.7×10^3
D. 3.7×10^6
E. 3.7×10^9

2. What is the disintegration rate constant for the decomposition of technetium Tc 99m?

A. $3.208 \times 10^{-5} \sec^{-1}$
B. $0.1155 h^{-1}$
C. $8.658 h^{-1}$
D. A and B
E. A and C

3. Ten hours after generation of the sodium pertechnetate, what would be the activity of the solution?

A. 175 MBq/mL
B. 7.50 mCi/mL
C. 4.73 mCi/mL
D. A and B
E. A and C

4. How many milliliters of the sodium pertechnetate solution should be used to administer the dose 10 hours after generation?

A. 0.5
B. 0.6

C. 1.2
D. 1.0
E. 1.9

5. What radioactive substance is used as the substrate in the technetium generator to produce sodium pertechnetate?

A. ^{98}Tc
B. ^{99m}Tc
C. ^{99}Mo
D. ^{100}Ru
E. ^{111}In

PATIENT PROFILE 67

DOG BITE WOUND

PRESENTATION

AA is a 6-year-old boy brought to the emergency department by his mother. This morning (approximately 3 hours ago), AA experienced a dog bite to the "fleshy" portion of his right forearm while wrestling with his friend. The patient's mother witnessed the attack; it appeared to her that the dog was agitated by the wrestling of the children. The bite episode was brief; the dog removed its grip immediately after the bite. The dog does not have a history of previous biting episodes; it is a 3-year-old healthy female Rotweiler with a documented up-to-date vaccination schedule.

CC: Dog bite wound on right forearm
PMH: Premature birth at 30 weeks without residual sequelae; he spent 3 weeks in neonatal intensive care unit. Immunizations are up to date. His last DTaP vaccine (fifth dose in the series) was administered just prior to his fifth birthday.
MH: MVI with fluoride
ALL:NKDA
FH: His mother has asthma. His father is healthy.
SH: He lives at home with both parents and attends first grade. There are no pets in the home.
ROS: AA complains of pain and stiffness in his forearm. He has a slight headache and is fatigued.
VS: BP 128/78 mm Hg, HR 120, RR 18, Temp 36°C, Wt 25 kg, Ht 115 cm
Gen: NAD, appears fatigued and anxious
HEENT: PERRLA, no lymphadenopathy, neck supple
Skin: Dry, occasional bruises and healing abrasions
Chest: Clear, normal breath sounds
CV: Tachycardia
Abd: Soft, nontender, +BS

Ext: Three puncture wounds on the dorsal and medial aspects of the right forearm. The wounds appear clean without any evidence of infection. He has full ROM at the wrist and elbow.
Neuro: Alert but fatigued
Labs and diagnostics tests: Labs are not available. A right forearm x-ray suggests that the bite did not penetrate bone.

QUESTIONS

1. Assess AA's need for rabies and tetanus immunization:

   I. A tetanus vaccine booster (DTaP or DT) should be administered.
   II. Tetanus immune globulin should be administered.
   III. The rabies vaccine schedule should be initiated.
   IV. Rabies immune globulin should be administered.

   A. I is needed; II, III, and IV are not needed.
   B. I and II are needed; III and IV are not needed.
   C. I and III are needed; II and IV are not needed.
   D. There is no apparent indication for rabies or tetanus immunization at this time.

2. After appropriate wound cleansing and dressing, AA is discharged from the emergency department. Should he receive a course of antibiotic treatment now to prevent infection of the wound?

   A. No. The wound does not appear infected.
   B. No. Although it is too early to see signs of infection, the wound should be watched and antibiotic therapy started if it becomes infected.

C. Yes. The wound is likely contaminated with potential pathogens. The patient should receive oral antibiotic therapy for 3 to 5 days.

D. Yes. The wound is likely contaminated with potential pathogens. The patient should receive oral antibiotic therapy for 14 days.

3. If AA develops an infection associated with this bite wound, initial empirical antibiotic therapy should be directed toward which of the following organisms?

I. *Staphylococcus aureus*
II. *Pasteurella multocida*
III. *E. coli*
IV. Anaerobic flora of the dog

A. I; no need to cover for II, III, and IV
B. II; no need to cover for I, III, and IV
C. I and II; no need to cover for III and IV
D. I, II, and IV; no need to cover for III

4. Which of the following antibiotics would be most appropriate for use in AA if he needed antibiotic prophylaxis for this bite wound?

A. Ciprofloxacin
B. Erythromycin
C. Tetracycline
D. Amoxicillin/clavulanate (Augmentin)

5. What does the inclusion of clavulanic acid (in Augmentin) do to enhance the activity of amoxicillin?

A. It increases the serum concentrations of amoxicillin.
B. It irreversible binds to β-lactamase.
C. It enhances the interaction of amoxicillin with its binding site.
D. Its own intrinsic antibacterial activity results in synergy with amoxicillin.

6. AA's mother also was bitten in an attempt to protect her child. Her medical history includes asthma, for which she takes Advair 500/50 bid, Uniphyl 400 mg QD, and pra albuterol. She also requires chronic anticoagulation with warfarin because of a history of idiopathic recurrent deep vein thromboses. She has had an anaphylactic reaction to penicillins in the past.

If the mother's physician was considering a short course of ciprofloxacin and clindamycin for prophylaxis of her bite wound, a pharmacokinetic interaction could occur with her theophylline therapy. What is the nature of this interaction?

A. Ciprofloxacin inhibits the hepatic metabolism of theophylline.
B. Ciprofloxacin inhibits the absorption of theophylline.

C. Theophylline inhibits the absorption of ciprofloxacin.
D. Theophylline inhibits the renal elimination of ciprofloxacin.

7. An interaction also may be observed between ciprofloxacin and the mother's chronic warfarin therapy. What is the nature of this interaction?

A. Ciprofloxacin possesses anticoagulant properties and may place her at a higher risk of bleeding.
B. Ciprofloxacin inhibits the metabolism of warfarin and may place her at a higher risk of bleeding.
C. Ciprofloxacin reduces the absorption of warfarin and may reduce the efficacy of her anticoagulation.
D. Ciprofloxacin induces the metabolism of warfarin and may reduce the efficacy of her anticoagulation.

8. If Ciprofloxacin was prescribed for the mother, why should she not take it with milk?

A. Administration with milk may cause her to become nauseous.
B. The absorption of the Ciprofloxacin may be reduced.
C. The absorption of the Ciprofloxacin may be increased.
D. Administration with milk may cause her to develop diarrhea.

9. Before prescribing Ciprofloxacin for the mother, it would be prudent to know about any history of serious cardiac conduction defects. Why is this important?

A. Fluoroquinolone use may cause QTc prolongation and torsades de pointes in patients at risk for this adverse effect.
B. Ciprofloxacin inhibits the absorption of many antiarrhythmic medications.
C. Ciprofloxacin inhibits the metabolism of many antiarrhythmic medications.
D. Ciprofloxacin induces the metabolism of many antiarrhythmic medications.

10. If tetracycline was prescribed for the mother, why should she not take it with milk?

A. Administration with milk may cause her to become nauseous.
B. The absorption of the tetracycline may be reduced.
C. The absorption of the tetracycline may be increased.
D. Administration with milk may cause her to develop diarrhea.

PATIENT PROFILE 68
SEXUALLY TRANSMITTED DISEASE, HIV

PRESENTATION

SC is a 28-year-old woman who comes to the clinic with a recent history of rather profuse, loose, yellow vaginal discharge with vaginal irritation. When asked about her medical history, SC states that she has a history of syphilis and that she received treatment 2 years ago. At that time, HIV testing was recommended, but SC refused. SC has had multiple sex partners for the past 5 years; she denies intravenous drug use. The intern sends specimens for culture and sensitivity testing. The Gram stain of the vaginal discharge does not reveal gram-negative diplococci, and the chlamydia test result is negative. A wet mount examination of the vaginal discharge reveals numerous trichomonads and large numbers of white blood cells. The diagnosis is trichomoniasis. SC currently takes ibuprofen as needed and Triphasil® (levonorgestrel and ethinyl estradiol).

QUESTIONS

1. Which of the following is an appropriate treatment regimen for SC and her partners?

   A. Doxycycline 100 mg bid for 7 days
   B. Amoxicillin 500 mg tid for 7 days
   C. Metronidazole 2 g orally once
   D. Azithromycin 1 g orally once
   E. Ceftriaxone 125 mg IM once

2. The intern reviewing SC's medical history finds the history of syphilis. He asks you what is the drug of choice for syphilis. You correctly reply

   A. parenteral penicillin G.
   B. ciprofloxacin.
   C. ceftriaxone.
   D. erythromycin.
   E. tetracycline.

3. The intern offers SC HIV testing, and she accepts this time. HIV testing is scheduled during a follow-up visit after completion of therapy for trichomoniasis. HIV antibody testing results are positive, and SC is found to have HIV infection. Why is it important to establish the diagnosis of HIV infection early in the course of disease?

   A. Treatment regimens are available to slow the decline of immune function.
   B. Persons with HIV infection are at increased risk of infections for which preventive measures are available.
   C. HIV infection affects the diagnosis, evaluation, management, and follow-up of many other diseases, including in some cases sexually transmitted diseases.
   D. Obtaining an early diagnosis of HIV enables health care providers to counsel such patients and to assist in preventing HIV transmission.
   E. All of the above

4. The intern asks you to recommend the initial antiretroviral regimen for SC. Her viral load is high, and initiation of antiretroviral therapy would be beneficial. After careful discussion with the patient, you recommend initiation of the following regimen: stavudine (Zerit®, d4T), lamivudine (Epivir®, 3TC), and nelfinavir (Viracept®). Which of the following statement(s) is/are true concerning nelfinavir (Viracept®)?

   A. SC should be counseled that nelfinavir may cause loose stools and mild to moderate diarrhea, which can be managed with antidiarrheal agents such as loperamide.
   B. Nelfinavir and other currently approved protease inhibitors are substrates of and metabolized by the cytochrome P450 3A4 isoenzyme, and drug interactions with other agents metabolized by this pathway should be carefully assessed.
   C. The main toxicity of nelfinavir is agranulocytosis. A baseline white blood cell count and differential should be obtained before initiation of therapy, and monthly monitoring should be performed.
   D. A and B
   E. All of the above

5. What is the main dose-limiting toxicity of stavudine (Zerit®, d4T)?

   A. Granulocytopenia
   B. Anemia
   C. Nephrotoxicity
   D. Peripheral neuropathy
   E. Hepatotoxicity

SOFT TISSUE INFECTIONS

PRESENTATION

CM is a 43-year-old man who visits the clinic in which your pharmacy is located. His chief complaint is pain on his right shin. The story is as follows: During the most recent snowstorm, CM was shoveling snow. When he came to the concrete stairs leading into his house, he slipped on some ice and fell into the stairs, banging his shin on the corner of the concrete stairs. When he looked at the wound, CM found that the skin was broken, and he proceeded to treat the wound superficially. One week has passed, and CM now has a fever and has swelling at the wound site with red lines streaking toward the groin area that suggest infection. CM has no known drug allergies.

QUESTIONS

1. Which type of organism is *most likely* growing in the leg?

    A. Lactose-fermenting gram-negative enteric bacilli
    B. Ayptical pathogens
    C. Gram-positive clusters of cocci
    D. Anaerobes
    D. Non-lactose-fermenting gram-negative rods

2. Which organism would you *most commonly* find growing in this patient's leg?

    A. *Staphylococcus aureus*
    B. *Escherichia coli*
    C. *Bacteroides fragilis*
    D. *Legionella pneumophilia*
    E. *Enterobacter cloacae*

3. Which of the following antibiotics would *best* control this patient's infection?

    A. Erythromycin
    B. Clindamycin
    C. Cefotaxime
    D. Nafcillin
    E. Metronidazole

4. Which of the following is the *most appropriate* drug for CM if a rash develops in reaction to penicillins?

    A. Aztreonam
    B. Cefazolin
    C. Gentamicin
    D. Ceftazadime
    E. Imipenem

5. If CM has an anaphylactic reaction to a β-lactam antibiotic, which of the following drugs would be the *most appropriate* for managing cellulits?

    A. Vancomycin
    B. Penicillin
    C. Gentamicin
    D. Rifampin
    E. Ciprofloxacin

ONCOLOGY: LUNG CANCER

PRESENTATION

HP is a 48-year-old man who visits his physician because of a sore right shoulder. He cannot recall any specific injury in the past few weeks. The shoulder is not red or swollen, and the pain is not reproduced with application of pressure. HP has been managing the pain with acetaminophen 650 mg q4h ATC. On this regimen the pain stays at about 3 on a 10-point scale. The medical history includes elevated cholesterol managed with gemfibrozil. HP has no known drug allergies but does have seasonal allergies. He has a 60 pack-year smoking history and drinks two beers a couple nights a week.

PHYSICAL EXAMINATION

BP: 140/85, HR: 84, RR: 20
Ht: 6'2", Wt: 220 lb
ROS: No headache, vision changes, cough, chills, or abdominal pain

LABS

Na: 138   K: 4.1
Ca: 9.2   Alb: 3.8

BUN: 20

SCr 1.1

WBC: 5.3

Hgb 13.8

Hct: 42

Plts: 260,000

Shoulder x-ray: Not definitive

Chest x-ray: Peripheral lesion in the right upper lobe confirmed with chest

CT

Head CT: Evidence of lesions on the brain

HP is found to have stage IV non-small cell lung cancer. He will receive chemotherapy.

QUESTIONS

1. HP's primary risk factor for lung cancer is

   A. increased use of acetaminophen.
   B. increased cholesterol.
   C. social alcohol use.
   D. smoking.
   E. actual body weight greater than ideal body weight.

2. HP will receive an antineoplastic drug regimen that includes cisplatin 100 mg/m^2 on day 1 and etoposide 100 mg/m^2 on days 1–3. This cycle will be repeated every 28 days. The primary dose-limiting toxicity of cisplatin is

   A. neurotoxicity.
   B. nephrotoxicity.
   C. bone marrow suppression.
   D. headache.
   E. glove and stocking paresthesia.

3. Appropriate information to convey to the nurse administering the etoposide would include the following:

   A. Determine predose heart rate and monitor for bradycardia during the infusion.
   B. Monitor ECG during the infusion for possible ventricular arrhythmia.
   C. Determine predose blood pressure and monitor for hypotension during the infusion.
   D. Infuse as rapidly as possible to minimize blood pressure changes.
   E. Infuse over 24 hours to avoid nephrotoxicity.

4. Because of the presence of brain metastasis, prophylaxis against seizures is recommended. Which therapy would be most appropriate?

   A. Phenytoin and dexamethasone
   B. Phenobarbital and gabapentin
   C. Brain irradiation
   D. Divalproex and prednisone
   E. Carbamazepine

5. HP returns for his third course of therapy (cisplatin and etoposide). Routine laboratory monitoring reveals a calcium level of 12.4. Which of the following is the most likely explanation for the elevated calcium?

   A. Previously undiagnosed bone metastasis
   B. Increased intake of dairy products
   C. Decreased intake of nutritional supplements
   D. Paraneoplastic syndrome
   E. Rapid decrease in total protein

PATIENT PROFILE 71

INSOMNIA

PRESENTATION

CC: "I can't seem to fall asleep at night. I stay up for hours."

HPI: AT is a 23-year-old woman who reports trouble falling asleep when she goes to bed every evening, usually around 11 PM. She often stays awake until 3 or 4 AM. She is exhausted on rising at 7 AM. AT complains of exhaustion for the past week leading to trouble during her daily routine of classes and work. She also asks about using St. John's wort to help her sleep because she would prefer "something more natural" rather than another prescription medication, and she has concerns about becoming addicted to a sleep aid.

PMH: Depression × 6 years, started selective serotonin reuptake inhibitors (SSRIs) 6 weeks ago; gastroesophageal reflux disease (GERD) × 2 years

SH: Student at local college; caffeine: 2 cups coffee and 2 colas daily; alcohol: 8 to 10 drinks per weekend; illicit drugs: denies

FH: Mother with mild depression; father with hypertension; sister with GERD × 6 months; brother alive and well

MH: Paxil CR 12.5 mg qam, Protonix 40 mg qd, Lo Ogesterel 1 tablet qd, ibuprofen 200 mg (2 tablets) PO q6h PRN

Allergies: NKDA

PHYSICAL EXAMINATION

Gen: Young Asian female in NAD
VS: Blood pressure: 120/80 mm Hg; heart rate: 68 beats per minute; height: 5 ft, 4 in; weight: 135 lb; temperature: 98.4°F
ROS: Noncontributory
Laboratory data: Noncontributory

QUESTIONS

1. Which of the medications on AT's profile should *not* be use concurrently with St. John's wort?

   A. Paxil; may cause serotonin syndrome.
   B. Lo Ogesterel; may result in contraceptive failure.
   C. Ibuprofen; may result in nonsteroidal anti-inflammatory drug (NSAID) toxicity.
   D. Protonix; may cause gastric upset.
   E. Both A and B are correct.

2. Which of the following is *true* regarding the use of St. John's wort?

   I. Its use has been associated with insomnia and restlessness.
   II. It is used most often to treat depression and anxiety.
   III. It is believed to modulate the neurotransmitters serotonin, norepinephrine, and dopamine.

   A. I only
   B. II only
   C. I and II
   D. II and III
   E. I, II, and III

3. No longer wanting to take St. John's wort, AT says that she has a friend who takes kava and asks if this is an option for her. What should AT be told about kava?

   A. Kava is safe and effective as an antianxiety agent.
   B. Kava is safe to use but proven to be ineffective as an antianxiety agent.
   C. Kava may be an effective antianxiety agent but possibly damages the liver.
   D. Kava is ineffective as an antianxiety agent and has many adverse effects.
   E. Kava is only used to treat attention-deficit/hyperreactivity disorder (ADHD).

4. Use of the amino acid L-tryptophan as a sleep aid

   I. is no longer recommended.
   II. is associated with eosinophila-myalgia syndrome.
   III. is associated with depression.

   A. I only
   B. II only

   C. III only
   D. I and II
   E. I, II, and III

5. All the following statements are *true* about the use of valerian as a sleep aid *except:*

   A. It reduces time to sleep onset.
   B. It improves quality of sleep.
   C. It can be taken up to 2 hours before bedtime.
   D. It should not be used with alcohol.
   E. Its long-term use is well established.

6. Which of the following statements about melatonin is *true*?

   I. It is commonly taken in supplements and used for jet lag and insomnia.
   II. It is a hormone endogenously synthesized in the pituitary gland.
   III. It is available as a parenteral product.

   A. I only
   B. II only
   C. I and II
   D. I and III
   E. I, II, and III

7. Pharmacologically induced insomnia is seen commonly with all the following *except*

   A. Diuretics
   B. Steroids
   C. SSRIs
   D. Anticonvulsants
   E. HMG Co-A reductase inhibitors

8. What is the mechanism of action by which diphenhydramine exerts its effect?

   A. Blockade of histamine receptors
   B. Blockade of muscarinic receptors
   C. Stimulation of muscarinic receptors
   D. Both A and B are correct.
   E. Both A and C are correct.

9. Which of the following is the *proper* way to initiate diphenhydramine as a sleep aid?

   A. Take 50 mg before bedtime for 3 nights and then reevaluate sleep.
   B. Take 50 mg before bedtime for 7 nights and then reevaluate sleep.
   C. Take 50 mg 1 to 2 h before bedtime for 3 nights and then reevaluate sleep.
   D. Take 50 mg 1 to 2 h before bedtime for 7 nights and then reevaluate sleep.

E. Take as needed; diphenhydramine is safe, and there is no need to reevaluate.

10. All the following products contain diphenhydramine *except*

A. Unisom Nighttime Sleep Aid
B. Sominex
C. Nytol
D. Tylenol P.M.
E. Alka-Seltzer P.M. Effervescent Tablets

PATIENT PROFILE 72

MEDICINAL CHEMISTRY

PRESENTATION AND QUESTION

TG, a 50-year-old man, has an uncomplicated urinary tract infection. His doctor prescribes co-trimoxazole (sulfamethoxazole, structure 72.1 and trimethoprim, structure 72.2). TG tolerates the medication, which seems to be working in fighting the infection and reducing the severity of symptoms. During therapy, TG is scheduled for outpatient surgery on his knee, which necessitates use of a local anesthetic. The physician asks for your help.

1. Which local anesthetic would you recommend for this patient?

A. Procaine (structure 72.3)
B. Bupivacaine (structure 72.4)
C. Tetracaine (structure 72.5)
D. Lidocaine (structure 72.6)
E. Any of the above

72.1

72.2

72.3

72.4

72.5

72.6

CHRONIC NONMALIGNANT PAIN

PRESENTATION

CR is a 40-year-old man who presents to his primary care physician with complaints of constant pain in his lower back. He works in a factory and spends most of his day lifting large, heavy materials. About 6 weeks ago, he was loading materials into a delivery truck when he felt "excruciating" pain in his back that radiated to his left leg. He immediately had to lay flat on his stomach for 1 hour before the pain lessened. A coworker took him to the emergency room (ER), where he was given a prescription for Vicodin. Imaging studies of his back and leg revealed no abnormalities. He was told to schedule a visit with his primary care physician and was sent home. He states that the pain in his left leg has subsided but that his lower back is still "killing" him. CR has not been able to return to work since the incident and has been collecting Worker's Compensation. He is able to do light yard work but cannot lift objects such as garbage pails or grocery bags. He states that he has been feeling very "down" because he has not been helpful "around the house" and "can't even take his two sons fishing." He has taken all the Vicodin that was prescribed in the ER and presents today seeking more pain medicine.

CR has no chronic diseases. He had been taking four Vicodin tablets per day with relief. He has not taken any medications today. He uses ibuprofen for occasional headaches. He has no allergies to medications. He does not drink and has a 20 pack-year history of tobacco use. CR is 6 ft, 4 in tall and weighs 220 lb. His vital signs are blood pressure = 130/76 mm Hg; heart rate = 65 beats per minute; and a pain score of 8. He appears to be in mild distress. His physical examination reveals tenderness and pain to touch at the L4 to L5 vertebrae. CR completed a sit-to-stand test in 32 seconds (normal = 7 to 10 s).

The physician refers CR for further imaging studies and physical therapy. A prescription is written for Vicodin 1 to 2 tablets PO q4–6h PRN. CR will return in 3 months for a follow-up visit.

QUESTIONS

1. Which of the following statements regarding CR's pain management regimen is *correct*?

   A. CR was previously taking more than the recommended daily dose of Vicodin, and liver function tests should be performed to assess for liver damage.

   B. Because hydrocodone can cause constipation, CR should be given a prescription for a stool softener and stimulant laxative.

   C. Vicodin can be used for the long-term management of CR's pain because it lacks a ceiling effect.

   D. CR is receiving an appropriate regimen to manage his pain, and there is nothing more that can be done for him at this time.

2. Which of the following parameters must be assessed continuously during the management of CR's pain?

   A. Level of analgesia
   B. Adverse effects to medications
   C. Activities of daily living
   D. Signs of aberrant drug-taking or drug-seeking behavior
   E. All the above

3. Which of the following medications may be beneficial as adjunctive therapy in the management of CR's pain?

   A. Ibuprofen
   B. Acetaminophen
   C. Percocet
   D. Meperidine

4. CR returns for his 3-month follow-up. He has completed a series of MRIs that confirmed the absence of abnormalities. He also attempted to work with a physical therapist, but the exercises were too painful to complete. He states that his Vicodin requirement has increased since his last visit. His pain score today is 8, and he has already taken two Vicodin tablets. Which of the following is the *most likely* explanation for CR's current response to Vicodin therapy?

   A. Opioid tolerance
   B. Opioid intolerance
   C. Opioid addiction
   D. Opioid diversion

5. The physician is now considering long-term treatment options for CR. He would like to initiate extended-release morphine. If CR is currently taking six Vicodin tablets per day, which of the following is the appropriate equivalent morphine dosing regimen?

   A. Extended-release morphine 5 mg PO bid
   B. Extended-release morphine 15 mg PO bid
   C. Extended-release morphine 20 mg PO bid
   D. Extended-release morphine 30 mg PO bid

6. CR returns to his primary care physician 1 month later and is complaining that the morphine doses do not last long enough. He takes his morning dose at 8 AM, and it begins to "wear off" by 1 PM. Which of the following statements regarding CR's response to his pain management regimen is *correct*?

  A. CR may be addicted to morphine and should be referred to an addiction specialist for further management.
  B. CR may require the addition of a short-acting opioid to manage breakthrough pain.
  C. CR may be tolerant to morphine and should be switched to a fentanyl patch.
  D. CR should continue with the same dosing regimen because he is already on the maximum dose of morphine per day and the dose cannot be increased.

7. Since his last visit, CR reports that his new regimen is working well except for a few bothersome side effects. Which of the following side effects do patients generally build tolerance to during opioid therapy?

  A. Constipation
  B. Nausea
  C. Sedation
  D. B and C only
  E. All the above

8. Which of the following are considered to be signs of addiction in a patient being managed on chronic opioid therapy?

  A. Multiple episodes of "lost" prescriptions
  B. Doctor shopping
  C. Frequent calls and visits to the physician's office
  D. All the above

9. Since the origin of CR's pain is still unknown, the physician would like to send CR for a nerve conduction study. If it is determined that CR has pain that is neuropathic in nature, which of the following medications would be beneficial in treating this?

  A. Cyclobenzaprine
  B. Clonazepam
  C. Gabapentin
  D. Acyclovir

10. Which of the following organizations has created standardized guidelines for the use of opioids in the management of patients with chronic nonmalignant pain?

  A. JCAHO
  B. WHO
  C. American Pain Society
  D. DEA
  E. None of the above

PATIENT PROFILE 74

MAJOR DEPRESSION

PRESENTATION

CB is a 68-year-old white man recently found to have major depression. The pharmacy has been consulted regarding new antidepressant medications and any drug or disease interactions that may exist in the patient's profile.

The patient has had an increase in depressive symptoms such as irritability, an increase in sleep, anhedonia, and pessimism over the last few months. He is now spending much of his time in bed or watching television. The medical history includes atrial fibrillation for 8 years, hypertension for 10 years, and hypercholesterolemia. CB has not undergone any surgical procedures. He is allergic to penicillin (rash) and cephalexin (rash).

Pravastatin 20 mg qd
Multivitamin 1 tab qd
Tums EX 2 tabs qd

CB's father died at 57 years of age of MI. His mother died at 69 of lung cancer. CB quit smoking tobacco 15 years ago. He uses alcohol occasionally. He is a retired electrical engineer and lives at home with his wife.

PHYSICAL EXAMINATION

GEN: Quiet, disheveled elderly man who looks his stated age BP sitting R arm: 110/68, HR: 60, T: 97°F, RR: 18

MEDS

Warfarin sodium 2.5 mg qd
Clonidine 0.1 mg qd

LABS

Na: 141 mEq/L   Cl: 98 mEq/L
K: 4.0 mEq/L CO_2: 16 mEq/L

BUN 24 mg/dL   SCr: 1.1 mg/dL
Gluc: 130   INR: 2.4
AST: 37 U/L L   ALT: 35 U/L
Alk Phos: 80 U/L

A/P: CB is a 68-year-old white man with a history of fibrillation, hypertension, and hypercholesterolemia. He has recently been found to have major depression and is about to
start antidepressant medication.

QUESTIONS

1. Which antidepressant should be avoided by a patient
   with cardiac arrhythmias?

   A. Sertraline
   B. Bupropion
   C. Venlafaxine
   D. Amitriptyline
   E. Fluoxetine

2. Which of CB's medications should be changed because of its potential to cause depression?

   A. Warfarin
   B. Clonidine
   C. Pravastatin
   D. Multivitamin
   E. Tums EX

3. Which selective serotonin reuptake inhibitor has the
   least effect on pharmacokinetic drug interactions
   through the CYP450 enzyme system?

   A. Fluoxetine
   B. Paroxetine
   C. Sertraline
   D. Fluvoxamine
   E. They all effect CYP450 equally.

4. Which selective serotonin reuptake inhibitor has the
   least effect on INR for a patient whose condition is
   stabilized with warfarin?

   A. Fluoxetine
   B. Sertraline
   C. Paroxetine
   D. Fluvoxamine
   E. They all affect INR to an equal degree.

5. What are the most common symptoms associated
   with abrupt cessation of a selective serotonin reuptake
   inhibitor?

   A. Fatigue, nausea, dizziness, tremor, chills, and di-
      aphoresis
   B. Tonic-clonic seizure, coma, death
   C. Hypertensive emergency, stroke
   D. A and B
   E. A, B, and C

PATIENT PROFILE 75

DIABETES AND PERIPHERAL NEUROPATHY

PRESENTATION

CC: DR is a 78-year-old man who presents to your pharmacy complaining of worsening pain in his legs, especially at night.

HPI: DR was diagnosed with type 2 diabetes 15 years ago
and suffers from peripheral neuropathy. He is currently
being treated with gabapentin 400 mg PO tid. The pain
has gotten so severe that he has difficulty sleeping at
night and often takes temazepam to help him fall
asleep. He has suffered from back pain for years and
had surgery 6 months ago for a slipped disk. His back
pain has been controlled by oxycodone/APAP as
needed for the past 3 months. His leg pain, however,
remains uncontrolled and has worsened over the past
month.

PMH: Hypertension, dyslipidemia, herniated disk (L4–5),
type 2 diabetes, peripheral neuropathy, insomnia,
PVD

ALL: NKDA

MH: Lisinopril 20 mg PO qd, oxycodone/APAP 5/325
mg PO q6h PRN, gabapentin 400 mg PO tid,
temazepam 15 mg PO qhs PRN, atorvastatin 10 mg
PO qd, hydrochlorothiazide 25 mg PO qam, metformin 850 mg PO tid, glyburide 10 mg PO qam (increased recently from 5 mg PO qd)

FH: Father deceased, stroke, at age 70. Mother deceased,
breast cancer, at age 66.

SH: Married with no children. Lives at home and cares for
wife suffering from Alzheimer's disease. Smokes occasionally (<1 pack per day)

PSH: Status post L4–5 diskectomy 01/04
VS: Blood pressure: 132/88 mm Hg; height: 5 ft, 11 in; weight: 206 lb
Labs: 143 99 19 total cholesterol: 178 mg/dL; low-density lipoprotein (LDL) cholesterol: 108 mg/dL; 143; high-density lipoprotein (HDL) cholesterol: 44 mg/dL; triglycerides: 148 mg/dL; 4.7 25 1.3; HgA1C: 7%

VISIT NOTES

DR tests his blood sugar one to two times daily when he wakes in the morning and 2 hours after lunch. He brings his log book in for you to review about once a month. His fasting readings have been averaging 130 mg/dL, and his postprandial readings are averaging 170 mg/dL. He appears to be in good control of his blood sugar and picks up his refills on time. He states that his legs feel fine during the day but worsen considerably at night. He states that his oxycodone/APAP controls his back pain but makes it difficult for him to focus during the day. He feels unsteady on his feet after he takes the medication.

QUESTIONS

1. According to the JNC VII, what is DR's goal blood pressure?

   A. <125/75 mm Hg
   B. <120/80 mm Hg
   C. <130/80 mm Hg
   D. <140/90 mm Hg

2. Which of the following is *not* a risk factor for a foot ulcer in DR?

   A. Smoking
   B. Hypertension
   C. Length of diabetes
   D. Peripheral neuropathy

3. Which of the following are *contraindications* to metformin therapy?

   I. Age > 65
   II. Serum creatinine >1.5 mg/dL in males
   II. Circulatory dysfunction

   A. I only
   B. I and II only
   C. II and III only
   D. I, II, and III

4. What is DR's goal LDL?

   A. <200 mg/dL
   B. <160 mg/dL
   C. <130 mg/dL
   D. <100 mg/dL

5. DR has been feeling "funny" lately, ever since his glyburide was increased. This happens prior to dinner, after a short walk. When you question him, he tells you that he eats an early lunch and does not snack in the afternoon. You suspect hypoglycemia. Which of the following is(are) symptom(s) of hypoglycemia?

   I. Sweating
   II. Tremor
   III. Dizziness

   A. I only
   B. I and II only
   C. III only
   D. I, II, and III

6. According to the United Kingdom Prospective Diabetes Study (UKPDS), which of the following observations is *true*?

   A. Intensive control of blood glucose has little affect on the development of diabetes complications.
   B. Intensive control of blood glucose was associated with a significant reduction in the microvascular complications of diabetes.
   C. Intensive control of blood glucose was associated with a significant reduction in both the macro- and microvascular complications of diabetes.
   D. Intensive control of blood glucose was associated with a significant reduction in the macrovascualr complications of diabetes.

7. Hypoglycemia is defined as a blood glucose concentration less than what?

   A. 100 mg/dL
   B. 70 mg/dL
   C. 60 mg/dL
   D. 50 mg/dL

8. Which medications in DR's profile are *most likely* being used to treat pain associated with peripheral neuropathy?

   A. Metformin
   B. Atorvastatin
   C. Gababpentin
   D. Temazepam

9. Which of the following strategies is *appropriate* to help alleviate the pain associated with DR's peripheral neuropathy?

   A. Increase his oxycodone/APAP dose to 2 tablets every 6 hours as needed.

B. Increase his evening gabapentin dose to 800 mg.

C. Begin tramadol at a dose of 50 mg PO q4h PRN.

D. Begin fluoxetine at a dose of 20 mg PO qd.

10. What is the *most appropriate* counseling point for DR concerning his gabapentin?

A. This medication is likely to cause tremor.

B. This medication may cause drowsiness, especially at higher doses.

C. This medications is likely to cause insomnia, especially at higher doses.

D. This medication may cause serotonin syndrome when taken at high doses.

PATIENT PROFILE 76

URINARY TRACT INFECTION

PRESENTATION

Residence	Community	
Patient	FL	
Age	25	
Sex	Female	
Allergies	ASA, penicillin	
Race	White	
Ht	5'2"	
Wt	125 lb	
Diagnosis	Primary	1. Uncomplicated UTI 2. NIDDM
	Secondary	1. Migraine headaches

	Date	Rx No.	Physician	Drug and Strength	Quantity	Sig	Refills
Medication record (prescription and OTC)	11/15	24298	AJ	Ortho-Novum® (norethin-drone-mestranol) 1/35-28	1	As directed	6
	11/29	25467	BM	Imitrex® (sumatriptan succinate) 25 mg tabs	12	2 as directed	1
	12/02	25999	CB	Bactrim DS® (trimethoprim-sulfamethoxazole)	3	3 × 1 as SD	0

QUESTIONS

1. What is the most likely pathogen causing UTI in this patient?

A. *Serratia*

B. *Staphylococcus*

C. *Klebsiella*

D. *Escherichia coli*

E. *Proteus*

2. Which of the following is/are true regarding the use of Bactrim DS® (trimethoprim-sulfamethoxazole) in the management of uncomplicated UTI?

I. Bactrim DS® (trimethoprim-sulfamethoxazole) is never prescribed empirically.

II. Bactrim DS® (trimethoprim-sulfamethoxazole) may be effective when given as a single daily dose (3 tabs × 1).

III. Bactrim DS® (trimethoprim-sulfamethoxazole) can safely be administered to patients who are allergic to penicillin.

A. I only

B. III only

C. I and II only

D. II and III only

E. I, II, and III

3. Bactrim DS® (trimethoprim-sulfamethoxazole) single dose should not have been administered to FL because

    A. she is allergic to ASA.
    B. she has a history of migraine headaches.
    C. she takes oral contraceptives.
    D. she has diabetes mellitus.
    E. she is allergic to penicillin.

4. Auxiliary labels and patient information when dispensing Bactrim® (trimethoprim-sulfamethoxazole) should include all of the following except:

    A. Store in refrigerator
    B. To be taken on an empty stomach

    C. Take with full glass of water
    D. Photosensitivity may occur
    E. Use sun block and wear sunglasses while outdoors

5. When a rash develops after administration of Bactrim DS® (trimethoprim-sulfamethoxazole) and the patient has a severe allergy to penicillin, which of the following drugs may be recommended to manage uncomplicated UTI?

    A. Amoxicillin and clavulanate potassium
    B. Sulfisoxazole
    C. Doxycycline
    D. Clindamycin
    E. Ciprofloxacin

PATIENT PROFILE 77

KIDNEY TRANSPLANTATION

PRESENTATION

HPI: KT is a 43-year-old man who was admitted yesterday for a living unrelated renal transplant. He tolerated the procedure very well and today complains of pain and nausea.

PMH: Diabetes mellitus type II with nephropathy, retinopathy, and neuropathy; hemodialysis three times per week since October 2003; hyperlipidemia; hypertension

SH: Single man who works as a mechanic. Reports occasional alcohol use. Smoked one pack per day for 15 years but quit when he started on hemodialysis.

FH: Father is healthy. Mother has diabetes and hypertension. Has four healthy siblings.

VS: Temperature: 36.3°C; blood pressure: 143/88 mm Hg; heart rate: 58 beate per minute; respiratory rate: 17 breaths per minute; weight: 86 kg

LABORATORY AND DIAGNOSTIC TESTS

Sodium: 138 mEq/L	Potassium: 4.9 mEq/L
Chloride: 98 mEq/L	CO_2: 30 mEq/L
Blood urea nitrogen (BUN): 24 mg/dL	Serum creatinine: 2.8 mg/dL
Glucose: 197 mg/dL	Calcium: 8.5 mg/dL
Magnesium: 1.6 mEq/L	Phosphorus: 2.1 mg/dL
White blood cell Count: 10,800/mm^3	Hematocrit: 31.7%
Platelets 359,000/mm^3	Tacrolimus trough: < 3 ng/mL

PRETRANSPLANTATION LABORATORY VALUES

Donor: Cytomegalovirus (CMV) IgG: positive; herpes simplex virus (HSV) 1 IgG: positive; Epstein-Barr virus (EBV) IgG: positive

Recipient: CMV IgG: negative; HSV 1 IgG: positive; EBV IgG: negative

Urine culture from day of transplant positive for *Candida*

CURRENT MEDICATIONS

Basiliximab 20 mg IV given in the OR prior to reperfusion
Cyclosporine (Neoral) 200 mg PO bid
Famotidine 20 mg PO bid
Methylprednisolone 40 mg IV q6h (tapering dose)
Metoprolol 100 mg PO bid
Mycophenolate mofetil 1000 mg PO bid
Nystatin 500,000 units swish and swallow qid
Valgancyclovir 900 mg PO qd
Hydromorphone PCA as needed for pain
Regular insulin sliding scale AC and HS

QUESTIONS

1. KT's physician wants to restart the atorvastatin 10 mg daily that KT was taking prior to transplant. Which of the following describes the *most significant*

risk associated with restarting atorvastatin at this time?

A. Increased risk of rhabdomyolysis
B. Increased risk of elevated liver function tests
C. Decreased atorvastatin efficacy
D. Elevated cyclosporine levels
E. Decreased cyclosporine levels

2. Which of the following is the *best choice* to manage KT's hypertension?

A. Increase metoprolol to 150 mg PO bid
B. Initiate verapamil SR 240 mg PO qd
C. Initiate lisinopril 10 mg PO qd
D. Initiate labetalol 100 mg PO tid
E. Initiate amlodipine 5 mg PO qd

3. Which of the following would be the *best choice* to manage this patient's hypophosphatemia?

A. Initiate K-Phos Neutral
B. Initiate Neutra-Phos
C. Initiate Neutra-Phos-K
D. Initiate any of the preceding medications. They are equivalent.
E. Hypophosphatemia is rare in a renal transplant recipient, and it does not require treatment.

4. Which of the following are risk factors for developing CMV disease in this patient?

A. He received induction immunosuppression with a polyclonal antibody.
B. His donor was positive for CMV IgG.
C. Virus carried by the recipient prior to transplantation may reactivate.
D. A and B
E. All the above

5. Which of the following *best describes* cyclosporine's mechanism of action?

A. Inhibits T-cell activation by inhibiting interleukin-2 production
B. Inhibits T-cell activation by inducing calcineurin
C. Blocks costimulation by attaching to the CD3 receptor of T cells
D. Prevents proliferation of T cells by intercalating into the DNA
E. Causes apoptosis of activated, mature cytotoxic T cells

6. Which of the following adverse effects could be attributed to cyclosporine?

A. Gingival hyperplasia, hypoglycemia, and tremor
B. Hirsutism, hypercalcemia, and rhabdomyolysis
C. Renal dysfunction, leukocytosis, and hyperphosphatemia

D. Gingival hyperplasia, renal dysfunction, and hypertension
E. Hair loss, tremor, and hyperkalemia

7. Basiliximab is treatment- and cost-effective when used for which of the following?

A. Treatment of acute rejection
B. Induction immunosuppression
C. Long-term maintenance immunosuppression
D. A and B
E. B and C

8. All *except for* which of the following would be effective for prophylaxis of *Pneumocystis carinii* pneumonia?

A. Atovaquone 1500 mg PO daily
B. Dapsone 100 mg PO daily
C. Doxycycline 100 mg PO daily
D. Pentamadine 300 mg inhaled once by month
E. Sulfamethoxazole-trimethoprim 800/160 mg PO daily

9. Fluconazole 200 mg PO daily is ordered to treat the yeast in the urine. Which of the following is true regarding drug interactions?

A. No interaction is present.
B. Fluconazole inhibits the metabolism of cyclosporine, resulting in elevated blood cyclosporine levels.
C. Fluconazole induces the metabolism of cyclosporine, resulting in decreased blood cyclosporine levels.
D. Cyclosporine and fluconazole, when used in combination, are associated with increased rates of hepatic toxicity.
E. Fluconazole prevents elimination of mycophenolate mofetil, resulting in elevated levels of mycophenolic acid in the blood.

10. Prior to discharge, the outpatient pharmacy fills a 30-day supply of all of KT's medications. Included is a medication labeled "cyclosporine, modified release" that was substituted for Neoral. Which of the following is *true* regarding this medication?

A. This is an error. Generic cyclosporine may never be substituted for a Neoral prescription.
B. This is an error. Cyclosporine, modified release, is the generic equivalent of Sandimmune, which is not bioequivalent to Neoral.
C. This is an error. Cyclosporine, modified release, has an absorption that is approximately 20% less than that of Neoral.
D. No error was made. Cyclosporine, modified release, is a generic formulation of Neoral and may be dispensed in the absence of a "NDPS."
E. No error was made. All cyclosporine formulations are interchangeable.

PATIENT PROFILE 78

CORONARY ARTERY DISEASE

PRESENTATION

JS is a 64-year-old woman who visits her primary care physician because of chest pain and shortness of breath while walking. JS states that recently she has been experiencing mild chest pain and "breathlessness" while she takes her daily walk. She states her symptoms do not start until she is three-fourths of the way through her 1-mile walk. JS states that rest usually alleviates the discomfort and that this is the first time she has experienced these problems. The medical history includes diabetes mellitus for 5 years, asthma, degenerative joint disease, and ulcerative colitis.

MEDS

Glyburide 5 mg po qd
Azmacort® (triamcinolone acetonide) 4 puffs bid
Albuterol 2 puffs prn
Atrovent® (ipratropium bromide) 2 puffs qid
Naproxen 375 mg po bid

JS does not smoke, use alcohol, or abuse drugs. Her family history has no relevant findings.

PHYSICAL EXAMINATION

BP: 152/95, P: 78, RR: 16, T: afebrile
Ht: 66", Wt: 185 lb
GEN: Pleasant elderly female, mildly obese
HEENT: Normal
COR: Normal S_1 and S_2; no murmurs, gallops, or rubs
Chest: Clear to ascultation
ABD: Soft, nontender
EXT: No edema

LABS

Na: 137   K: 3.9
Cl: 100 CO_2: 26
BUN: 27   SCr: 1.3
Glucose: 210   WBC: 4.8
Total chol: 250 Hct: 38.4

HDL chol: 44   Plts: 234,000
LDL chol: 170   Hgb: 12.5
Trig: 243

QUESTIONS

1. Which of the following would be inappropriate to initiate for JS at this time?

    A. Increase glyburide to 10 mg po qd
    B. Start atenolol 50 mg po qd
    C. Start amlodipine 5 mg po qd
    D. Start Imdur® (isosorbide mononitrate) 30 mg po qd
    E. Start aspirin 81 mg po qd

2. Which of the following may interfere with blood pressure control?

    A. Naproxen
    B. Albuterol inhaler
    C. Azmacort® (triamcinolone acetonide) inhaler
    D. Glyburide
    E. Atrovent® (ipratropium bromide) inhaler

3. Which of the following would be the best choice for JS to prevent angina pain before her daily walk?

    A. Take one aspirin, 325 mg
    B. Administer 2 puffs of albuterol
    C. Take an extra dose of nifedipine, 30 mg
    D. Administer 0.4 mg SL nitroglycerin
    E. Administer 2 puffs of Atrovent® (ipratropium bromide)

4. Which of the following would be an appropriate intervention for JS in managing CAD?

    A. Vitamin E 400 IU po qd
    B. Premarin® (conjugated estrogen) 0.625 mg po qd and Provera® (medroxyprogesterone) 2.5 mg po qd
    C. Aspirin 325 mg po qd
    D. Nifedipine 30 mg po tid
    E. Sotalol 80 mg po bid

SOFT TISSUE INFECTIONS

PRESENTATION

DW is a 58-year-old white man who comes to the clinic with fever and chills that have lasted for several days and are unrelieved with acetaminophen. The course over the past couple of days is as follows: Three days ago DW's wife trimmed his toenails, as she has been doing for years. DW put on a new pair of boots and ventured onto his property to prepare it for the coming winter. That night after removing his boots, DW noticed that both feet were a bit discolored from the rubbing of his new boots. The following morning DW noticed that his wife had trimmed the toenail on his right great toe too close. Clear fluid had begun to drain from that toe. Later that day DW felt feverish and had chills, which eventually led him to the clinic. The medical history includes diabetes mellitus, hypertension, renal insufficiency, and diabetic neuropathy. DW is admitted to the hospital with a diabetic foot infection.

QUESTIONS

1. Choose the *best* answer regarding the type of organisms found in diabetic foot infections.

   A. Because diabetic food infections are considered "skin" infections, *Staphylococcus* and *Streptococcus* species are the most common organisms isolated.

   B. On average, only one organism is isolated in a diabetic foot infection.

   C. *Proteus mirabilis,* group D streptococci, *Escherichia coli, Staphylococcus aureus, Bacteroides fragilis, Peptococcus,* and *Peptostreptococcus* are all pathogens that can be isolated from a diabetic foot ulcer.

   D. Patients with diabetes typically have a normal immunologic response to infection. This explains why most patients who come to medical attention as DW did receive oral antibiotics for the duration of infection.

   E. The correlation between results of superficial cultures taken from the wound site and deep aspiration of the wound is strong, which rules out the need for deep wound cultures.

2. All the following about DW's diabetic foot infection are *true* except

   A. Today's broad-spectrum antibiotics easily allow us to use antibiotic therapy for osteomyelitis infec-

tions, which are infrequent among patients with diabetes.

   B. DW may have had this infection sooner than he reported. Diabetic neuropathy often masks the clinical signs and symptoms of infection.

   C. Foot infections common among persons with diabetes are infection of the soft tissue adjacent to the nail, infection of the middle foot secondary to painless trauma, infection of the toe web space, and infection of the sole over the head of the metatarsals.

   D. Necrotizing skin infections and osteomyelitis are common complications of diabetic foot ulcers.

   E. Specimens for culture and sensitivity testing should be obtained initially for a diabetic patient with a lesion on the foot.

3. Because DW will be admitted to the hospital, antibiotic therapy should be started immediately after cultures are obtained from DW's foot. Which of the following therapies would be the *best* choice for empirical management of this infection?

   A. Monotherpay with nafcillin 1 g IV q6h
   B. Monotherapy with aztreonam 1 g IV q8h
   C. Combination therapy with nafcillin 2 g IV q6h and penicillin 3 million units IV q4h for increased streptococcal coverage
   D. Monotherapy with piperacillin-tazobactam 3.375 g IV q6h
   E. Monotherapy with metronidazole 500 mg PO q8h

4. Osteomyelitis is ruled out. Which statement involving DW's therapeutic decisions is *most truthful*?

   A. Culture and sensitivity results indicate standard diabetic foot flora sensitive to the antibiotic panel against which it was tested. Therapy should continue for 10 to 12 weeks.

   B. In an attempt at pharmacoeconomic consciousness, 72 hours of IV antibiotic therapy is completed, and you recommend switching to an oral agent in an effort to facilitate this patient's discharge.

   C. Seventy-two hours have passed, and not much improvement has occurred. You consider modifying antibiotic therapy to include coverage for *Pseudomonas aeruginosa.*

D. Right foot amputation is the only alternative available for DW.

E. You suspect that DW has been colonized with vancomycin-resistant enterococci, and therapy for this infection will resolve the symptoms.

5. Osteomyelitis is ruled out. Which statement involving DW's therapeutic decisions is *most truthful*?

A. Inspect the feet daily for the presence of cuts, blisters, or scratches. Look between all toes, and examine the bottom of the foot.

B. Use tepid water to wash the feet daily and dry them thoroughly.

C. Apply lotion to the feet to prevent calluses and cracking.

D. Wear properly fitting shoes.

E. All the above

PATIENT PROFILE 80
DIABETES MELLITUS

PRESENTATION

PB is an obese 42-year-old man with a history of hypothyroidism, depression, and hypercholesterolemia. He sees his physician for a follow-up visit after starting atorvastatin (he was noncompliant with dietary modifications and exercise) and to get the results of an Hb A_{1c} test. A finger stick at his last visit was 150 mg/dL. PB has an allergy to penicillin that manifests as a rash. He is currently taking paroxetine 30 mg po qd, atorvastatin 10 mg po qd, and levothyroxine 112 μg po qd. PB's mother died at age 67. His father is alive, has hypertension, CAD, and carcinoma of the prostate, and has had an MI. There is no family history of diabetes mellitus. PB does not smoke, use illicit drugs, or drink alcohol. Vitals signs are BP: 130/80, HR: 72, and RR: 18. Physical examination findings are within normal limits. The Hb A_{1c} result is 13.5%.

QUESTIONS

1. The pharmacist recommends starting metformin. When making this decision, the pharmacist needed to consider the contraindications to metformin. Which of the following are contraindications to metformin therapy?

A. Renal disease or dysfunction suggested by a serum creatinine level greater than 1.5 mg/dL for men and greater than 1.4 mg/dL for women

B. Congestive heart failure necessitating pharmacologic management

C. Elevation of liver enzymes two times the upper limit of normal

D. A and B only

E. A, B, and C

2. Which of the following is the most common side effect of metformin?

A. Drowsiness

B. Diarrhea

C. Paresthesia

D. Lactic acidosis

E. Tinnitus

3. To minimize this adverse effect (answer selected in question 2), how should therapy be initiated?

A. Start with 500 mg po bid, with the morning and evening meals. Make dosage increases in increments of 500 mg every week, given in divided doses, up to 2500 mg/day.

B. Start with 850 mg po qd, with morning meal. Make dosage increases in increments of 850 mg every other week in divided doses up to 2550 mg/day.

C. Start with 1000 mg po bid, with morning and evening meals. Make dosage increases in increments of 250 mg every week in divided doses up to 2500 mg/day.

D. A and B

E. B and C

4. Several months later, PB is involved in a car accident and is brought to the emergency department. He is admitted to the hospital for the management of severe abdominal pain. The physician orders abdominal CT with intravenous administration of a contrast agent to be performed at 10 A.M. the next day. One hour before CT scan and intravenous administration of the contrast agent, PB takes his 9 A.M. metformin dose.

(PB's condition is stabilized on a dose of 1000 mg po bid.) What do you recommend?

A. Cancel the 10 A.M. CT scan with the intravenous contrast agent. Metformin should be held for 48 hours before a radiographic procedure with an intravenous contrast agent. Metformin can be restarted 48 hours after the CT scan is obtained.

B. Reschedule CT with intravenous administration of the contrast agent for 3 P.M. (6 hours after the morning metformin dose). Metformin should be held for 24 hours after the CT scan and then restarted.

C. PB should go to the scheduled 10 A.M. CT scan with intravenous administration of a contrast agent. Metformin should be held for 48 hours after CT and restarted after renal function is assessed and determined to be normal.

D. PB should go to the scheduled 10 A.M. CT scan with the intravenous contrast agent. Metformin therapy should not be interrupted and should continue at 1000 mg po bid.

E. PB should go to the scheduled 10 A.M. CT scan with the intravenous contrast agent. Metformin therapy should not be interrupted, but the dose should be reduced by 50% (500 mg po bid) for 48 hours. After 48 hours, therapy can resume at 1000 mg po bid.

PATIENT PROFILE 81

DIABETES MELLITUS

PRESENTATION

RL is a 42-year-old woman seen in the primary care clinic for routine follow-up. Her past medical history includes type 1 diabetes mellitus for 30 years, white coat hypertension, and diabetic neuropathy. She denies side effects from any of her medications. She had a rash after taking Bactrim (trimethoprim-sulfamethoxazole) as a child. Bactrim is the only medication to which she has had an allergic reaction.

RL states that her diabetic neuropathy has worsened since her last visit 3 months ago. She describes intermittent burning pain that radiates throughout the soles of her feet. She states that at times it is unbearable and that she finds herself calling in sick to work so that she does not have to walk. She is a receptionist at a local marketing firm and generally does not have to walk extensively for her job. However, she states that when the burning pain begins, even walking short distances is extremely painful. She states that the pain when it is at its worst is 8 on a scale of 10 (0–10 pain scale). In the past, she had experienced similar pain, but it occurred with less frequency and intensity. She generally does not like to take medication unless it is necessary, but given the increasing intensity of her pain, she would like to try something that might help. She has never taken any prescribed pain medication except for two doses of Tylenol with codeine 30 mg after she had her wisdom teeth removed several years ago, which she was able to tolerate without any problems.

She has been checking her blood pressures at home. Her systolic blood pressures have been running in the 120s and her diastolic blood pressures have been running in the 80s according to her log book. She has brought her home blood pressure machine with her today, and her primary care provider has confirmed its accuracy.

RL's average blood sugar readings from her glucose meter are as follows: 7 AM fasting blood sugars: 120 mg/dL; and 6 PM predinner blood sugars: 240 mg/dL. She states that she is compliant with her medications and has not been skipping any meals. She has been less active lately because of the increased pain in her feet.

None of RL's relatives have type 1 diabetes mellitus. However, both her parents have heart disease and hypertension. She is an only child. She denies tobacco use, illicit drug use, or alcohol use. She has been married for 20 years and has one son who is a senior in high school. She has been working at the marketing firm for over 10 years and enjoys her job. She belongs to a knitting club and has noticed that the sensitivity in several of her fingers has diminished. She is concerned that her peripheral neuropathy is progressing to beyond her feet. She checks her feet every day.

RL confirmed that she fasted 12 hours before her blood was drawn at the laboratory today. RL's height is 5 ft, 1 in. RL's weight is 130 lb. MB's vital signs are as follows: blood pressure: 168/88 mm Hg; heart rate: 80 beats per minute; respiratory rate: 20 breaths per minute; and temperature: 98.6°F. MB's laboratory values today are as follows: A1c: 8.1%; Na: 134 mEq/L; K: 4.2 mEq/L; blood urea nitrogen (BUN): 18 mg/dL; serum Cr: 0.6 mg/dL; glucose: 105 mg/dL; total cholesterol: 198 mg/dL; low-density lipoprotein (LDL) cholesterol: 98 mg/dL; high-density lipoprotein (HDL) cholesterol: 80 mg/dL; and triglycerides: 100 mg/dL.

All liver function tests and components of her complete blood count are within normal limits. On review of her medical chart, you note that both of her previous spot urine microalbumin: creatinine ratios were around 8 µg/mg creatinine, which is consistent with normoalbuminuria.

On visual inspection of RL's feet, no areas of cracking, redness, or inflammation are noted. Her dorsalis pedis and posterior tibial pulses are palpable. Except for areas of diminished sensation on her fingers and feet, all other physical examination findings are within normal limits.

QUESTIONS

1. Which of the following medications would be *most appropriate* to recommend for treatment of RL's burning foot pain?

   A. Ibuprofen 400 mg qid as needed
   B. Acetaminophen 325 mg, 1 to 2 tablets qid as needed
   C. Amitriptyline 25 mg at bedtime
   D. Percocet (oxycodone 5 mg/acetaminophen 325 mg), 1 to 2 tablets qid as needed
   E. MS Contin (morphine, sustained release) 15 mg, 1 tablet twice daily

2. RL's primary care provider decides to initiate Neurontin (gabapentin) for the treatment of RL's burning foot pain. Which of the following is the *most appropriate* treatment plan when initiating gabapentin therapy?

   A. 100 mg at bedtime for 2 weeks; then evaluate for efficacy
   B. 100 mg at bedtime for 8 weeks; then evaluate for efficacy
   C. 300 mg at bedtime for 1 day, then 300 mg twice daily for 1 day, then 300 mg three times daily for a total of 8 weeks; then evaluate for efficacy
   D. 300 mg three times daily for 2 weeks; then evaluate for efficacy
   E. 600 mg three times daily for 8 weeks; then evaluate for efficacy

3. Which of the following is a common side effect of gabapentin that RL should be counseled on?

   A. Drowsiness
   B. Dry mouth
   C. Constipation
   D. Vision changes
   E. Hair loss

4. RL is unable to tolerate gabapentin. Her primary care provider decides to try a trial of Ultram (tramadol) for her pain. Which of the following doses is an *appropriate* dose to initiate tramadol treatment?

   A. 25 mg once daily

   B. 25 mg once daily for 1 day, then 25 mg twice daily for 1 day, then 25 mg three times daily for 1 day, then 25 mg four times daily
   C. 100 mg once daily
   D. 100 mg twice daily for 1 week, then 100 mg four times daily
   E. 100 mg four times daily as needed

5. Which of the following disease states may using tramadol exacerbate?

   A. Heart failure
   B. Diabetes mellitus
   C. Gout
   D. Hypertension
   E. Epilepsy

6. RL's blood pressure when checked by her primary care provider is 168/88 mm Hg. Given her past medical history and her home blood pressure readings, which of the following recommendations is most appropriate for the treatment of her blood pressure?

   A. Add furosemide 20 mg once daily
   B. Add lisinopril 40 mg once daily
   C. Add atenolol 12.5 mg once daily
   D. Add verapamil sustained release 120 mg once daily
   E. No treatment is needed at this time because her blood pressures at home are at goal.

7. Which of the following medication regimens would be the *most appropriate* to treat RL's diabetes mellitus?

   A. Repaglinide 0.5 mg tid with each meal
   B. Glyburide 40 mg bid
   C. Metformin 500 mg once daily
   D. Rosiglitazone 4 mg twice daily
   E. Insulin 70/30, 20 units in the morning and 10 units in the evening

8. If insulin treatment is initiated in RL, which of the following is an *appropriate* daily dose?

   A. 5 units
   B. 10 units
   C. 30 units
   D. 50 units
   E. 100 units

9. Several years later RL is seen in the pharmacy clinic. She is currently on Humalog (insulin lispro) 5 units three times daily before meals and Lantus (insulin glargine) 24 units at bedtime. Her average home glucose meter blood sugars are as follows: fasting before breakfast and morning insulin: 320 mg/dL; before noontime insulin: 150 mg/dL; before evening insulin: 120 mg/dL; and before bedtime: 68 mg/dL. Which of the following interventions is most appropriate?

A. Recommend that she checks a 2 AM blood sugar to make sure that she is not becoming hypoglycemic overnight

B. Recommend that she increase her bedtime insulin glargine dose to 30 units

C. Recommend that she take her insulin glargine in the morning instead of at bedtime

D. Recommend that she increase her breakfast insulin lispro dose to 8 units

E. Recommend that she increase her noontime insulin lispro dose to 8 units

10. RL is at a community pharmacy picking up her prescriptions. She states that she has a painful wart on the bottom of her foot and asks you, the pharmacist, if you would recommend that she use an over-the-counter product containing salicylic acid. Which of the following responses is the *most appropriate*?

A. Any topical medication containing salicylic acid is appropriate to use. Apply twice daily to wart for up to 12 weeks.

B. Topical solutions generally are less effective than topical plasters containing salicylic acid. Apply plaster to wart over night, and then change the plaster as needed every 24 hours until the wart is removed

C. These topical solutions are not recommended for patients with diabetes mellitus. Consult with your primary care provider or podiatrist for other options.

D. These topical solutions are not recommended for patients with diabetes mellitus. Using a pumice stone to scrap off the wart is a good alternative.

E. Topical salicylic acid solutions are seldom effective. A prescription for an oral antiviral may be necessary. Contact your primary care provider.

PATIENT PROFILE 8 2

ASTHMA CASE

PRESENTATION

BH is a 17-year-old girl with asthma who arrives at the ambulatory clinic with increasing wheezing and shortness of breath. She has been using her prn albuterol inhaler at least 3 times daily over the past week. She takes no other asthma medication. During the visit, the FEV_1 is 60% of the predicted value.

QUESTIONS

1. According to current NHLBI guidelines for management of asthma, what would be the most appropriate strategy at this time?

   A. Increase the dose of albuterol inhaled
   B. Add a long-acting oral β_2 selective agonist to the regimen
   C. Add an inhaled corticosteroid to the regimen
   D. Replace albuterol with an inhaled corticosteroid
   E. Replace albuterol with an oral corticosteroid

2. BH's physician advises her to monitor her disease using an ambulatory peak flow meter. Peak expiratory flow rates (PEFR) correlate most closely with which of the following pulmonary function tests?

   A. FVC
   B. FEV_1

   C. FEF_{25-75}
   D. FEV_1/FVC
   E. All of the above

3. An optimal PEFR for BH should be

   A. >40% of personal best.
   B. >50% of personal best.
   C. >60% of personal best.
   D. >70% of personal best.
   E. >80% of personal best.

4. BH is advised to keep a diary to record her PEFR readings. If therapy has the asthma under good control, BH should be in which color zone?

   A. Red
   B. Blue
   C. Yellow
   D. White
   E. Green

5. How often should BH be advised to monitor her PEFR?

   A. At least once a day
   B. At least once a week
   C. At least once a month
   D. Whenever she has symptoms
   E. Whenever she uses her albuterol inhaler

PATIENT PROFILE 83

HYPERLIPIDEMIA

PRESENTATION

JF is a 72-year-old woman referred to the lipid clinic for optimization of her therapy for hyperlipidemia. JF states that she takes her medications and has tolerated gemfibrozil well. She was unable to tolerate several statins in the past. Cost is an issue for this patient because she currently has no prescription medication coverage. JF is active and walks 30 minutes per day. Past medical history includes hyperlipidemia, diabetes mellitus type 2, and angina. Her diabetes is controlled with a strict diet. Current medications are gemfibrozil 600 mg PO bid, ecasa 325 mg PO qd, atenolol 50 mg PO qd, and multivitamin 1 PO qd. JF's father died from a myocardial infarction (MI) at age 68. She is a smoker and a social drinker.

PHYSICAL EXAMINATION

Blood pressure: 130/68 mm Hg; heart rate: 60 beats per minute; respiratory rate: 17 breaths per minute; temperature: afebrile
General: Alert, oriented, and pleasant patient.
HEENT: Unremarkable
Chest: Heart reveals regular rhythm.
Neuro: Unremarkable
ABD: Soft and nontender
EXT: No edema

LABORATORY VALUES

Na: 138 mEq/L	K: 3.7 mEq/L
Cl: 111 mEq/L	CO_2 content: 26 mEq/L
Blood urea nitrogen (BUN): 14 mg/dL	Glucose: 90 mg/dL
Serum Cr: 0.8 mg/dL	Total cholesterol: 321 mg/dL
High-density lipoprotein (HDL) cholesterol: 34 mg/dL	Triglycerides: 93 mg/dL
Low-density lipoprotein (LDL) cholesterol: 175 mg/dL	AST: 23 mg/dL
ALT: 24 mg/dL	HbA1c: 7.8%
Uric acid: 6 mg/dL	

QUESTIONS

1. Which of the following conditions confers high risk for coronary heart disease (CHD) events (CHD risk equivalent)?

    A. Diabetes
    B. Hypertension
    C. Asthma
    D. Gout
    E. All the above

2. What is the current LDL cholesterol goal for patients with existing cardiovascular disease or a CHD risk equivalent such as with JF?

    A. <200 mg/dL
    B. <180 mg/dL
    C. <160 mg/dL
    D. <130 mg/dL
    E. <100 mg/dL

3. In addition to a complete lipid profile, which of the following laboratory values should be monitored before and after initiating HMG-CoA reductase inhibitor therapy?

    A. Serum glucose
    B. Liver function tests
    C. White blood cell count
    D. Complete blood cell count
    E. Serum uric acid level

4. Based on the National Cholesterol Education Program's Adult Treatment Panel III, which of the following are JF's positive risk factors for heart disease?

    A. Hypertension, low HDL cholesterol, age
    B. Hypertension, high HDL cholesterol, age
    C. Hypertension, high HDL cholesterol, family history of premature CHD
    D. Hypertension, high HDL cholesterol, family history of premature CHD
    E. Hypertension, low HDL cholesterol, family history of premature CHD

5. A pharmacy student with you on rotation concludes that JF's current LDL cholesterol goal is less than 130 mg/dL. Do you agree or disagree with this assessment?

    A. Agree; her LDL cholesterol goal is correct, and follow-up should be in 12 months.
    B. Agree; her LDL cholesterol goal is correct, and follow-up should be in 6 months.
    C. Agree; her LDL cholesterol goal is correct, and follow-up should be in 6 weeks.

D. Disagree; her LDL cholesterol goal is less than 100 mg/dL, and follow-up should be in 6 weeks.

E. Disagree; her LDL cholesterol goal is less than 100 mg/dL, and follow-up should be in 12 months.

6. Given JF's HMG-CoA reductase history, the medical staff is concerned about the patient's risk of myositis. What is an appropriate definition of myositis, and what type of monitoring should we follow with regard to myositis patients?

A. Myositis is myalgia and an increase in serum creatine phosphokinase (CPK) of greater than 10 times the upper limit of normal. We should monitor CPK levels routinely.

B. Myositis is myalgia and an increase in serum creatine phosphokinase (CPK) of greater than 5 times the upper limit of normal. We should monitor CPK levels when there are unexplained symptoms of muscle aches.

C. Myositis is myalgia and an increase in serum creatine phosphokinase (CPK) of greater than 10 times the upper limit of normal. We should monitor CPK levels when there are unexplained symptoms of muscle aches.

D. Myositis is myalgia and an increase in serum creatine phosphokinase (CPK) of greater than 5 times the upper limit of normal. We should monitor CPK levels routinely.

E. Myositis is muscle pain and an increase in liver function tests of greater than 5 times the upper limit of normal.

7. The physician wants to increase JF's LDL lowering but does not want to use gemfibrozil and discontinues it. He looks to you for your opinion. Which would be considered the *best recommendation* at this time?

A. Given her age and risk of adverse events, you would not want to add other medications. The patient should be limited to lifestyle modifications.

B. Because she is a smoker, the only recommendation would be to focus on her smoking cessation.

C. Revisit and emphasize lifestyle modifications and smoking cessation but also add atorvastatin 10 mg PO qd.

D. Revisit and emphasize lifestyle modifications and smoking cessation but also add ezetimibe 10 mg PO qd.

E. Refer the patient to another physician who will prescribe gemfibrozil.

8. In general, what effect does hydrochlorothiazide have on a lipoprotein profile?

A. Increases total cholesterol
B. Decreases total cholesterol
C. Decreases HDL cholesterol
D. Decreases triglycerides
E. Has no effect

9. Given JF's medication experience, she is apprehensive regarding drug therapy and wants to know the side effects of ezetimibe. You counsel her that ezetimibe has which of the following side effects?

A. Flatulence
B. Fatigue
C. Flushing
D. All the above
E. None of the above

10. A therapeutic lifestyle change (TLC) diet is comprised of which of the following?
A. A limit of saturated fat of less than 7% of calories
B. Increased viscous (soluble) fiber (10–25 g/day)
C. Increased plant stanols/sterols (2 g/day)
D. All the above
E. None of the above

PATIENT PROFILE 84

ANTACID SUSPENSIONS

PRESENTATION

An antacid suspension contains a 540 mg/5 mL formulation of magaldrate with a formula of $Al_2H_{14} Mg_4O_{14} \cdot 2 H_2O$. Particles of magaldrate (0.5 μm diameter, 5 g/mL density) in water (1.00 g/mL density, 0.8904 cps viscosity) have a rate of settling of 5.29 cm/day. The particles are insoluble in water, alcohol, and mineral oil.

QUESTIONS

1. Find the molecular weight of magaldrate.

A. 68
B. 71
C. 352
D. 388
E. 424

2. In extemporaneous compounding suspensions, which of the following methods can be used to slow the rate of settling?

   A. Add methyl cellulose to the vehicle
   B. Make a paste of magaldrate particles with mineral oil
   C. Reduce particle size by grinding the particles in a mortar and pestle
   D. Use syrup instead of water as a vehicle
   E. All of the above

3. To what viscosity (in centipoises) should the suspension be adjusted to achieve a rate of settling of 0.01 μm/s?

   A. 0.00168
   B. 0.00612
   C. 0.0145
   D. 61.2
   E. 471

4. How many mEq of magnesium can be found in 1 g of magaldrate?

   A. 2.0
   B. 2.4
   C. 4
   D. 8
   E. 18.9

5. Why are magaldrate suspensions packaged in opaque or translucent containers?

   A. To protect against light sensitivity of the drug
   B. To provide drug chemical stability
   C. To provide for the maintenance of color and flavor
   D. Because of the pharmaceutical inelegance of a settled suspension
   E. A and C

PATIENT PROFILE 85

ASTHMA

PRESENTATION

TK is a 4-year-old girl brought to the emergency room by her parents. She is experiencing severe dyspnea and coughing. On physical examination, she is noted to be very anxious and in some respiratory distress with periodic coughing. She also exhibits a hyperinflated chest with accessory muscle breathing. Examination of lung sounds reveals bilateral expiratory wheezes. She is on no medications, and her medical history is remarkable for having several episodes of acute bronchitis since she was 2 years old. A preliminary diagnosis of asthma is made.

VITAL SIGNS

Respiratory rate: 32 breaths per minute
Blood pressure: 112/78 mm Hg
Heart rate: 120 beats per minute
Temperature: 98°F

QUESTIONS

1. Asthma is best characterized how?

   A. As an obstructive disease
   B. As a restrictive disease
   C. As an inflammatory disease
   D. A and C
   E. B and C

2. Which of the following agents would be *most appropriate* to treat TK's acute symptoms?

   A. Hydrocortisone
   B. Salmeterol
   C. Albuterol
   D. Theophylline
   E. Ipratropium

3. What is the *preferred method* to administer β-agonists for patients who are acutely ill in TK's age group?

   A. Orally
   B. Intravenously
   C. Subcutaneously
   D. Via nebulizer
   E. Via meter-dose inhaler

4. All the following would be considered a β_2-selective agonist except

   A. Terbutaline
   B. Isoproterenol
   C. Salmeterol
   D. Bitolterol
   E. Albuterol

5. What is the relative advantage of administering a β_2-selective agent as compared with a nonselective agent for TK?

A. More rapid improvement in symptoms
B. Less potential for cardiotoxicity
C. Less potential for developing tolerance
D. These agents treat the underlying cause of asthma.
E. There is no relative advantage.

6. In 3 weeks, TK exhibits symptoms consistent with mild persistent disease. In addition to as-needed inhaled β-agonist therapy, National Institutes of Health (NIH) guidelines for children in her age group recommend which daily medication for control of her disease?

A. Oral low-dose corticosteroid
B. Inhaled low-dose corticosteroid
C. Oral β-agonist
D. Oral theophylline
E. Inhaled ipratropium

7. Spacer devices may be used to assist children with the use of meter-dose inhalers. Which of the following is an example of a spacer device?

A. Aerolizer
B. Aerochamber
C. Diskus
D. A and B
E. A, B, and C

8. The type of device that uses sound waves to administer aerosolized medications is called what?

A. A metered-dose inhaler
B. An air-jet nebulizer
C. A peak-flow meter
D. An ultrasonic nebulizer
E. A spacer device

9. Which of the following statements concerning the role of cromolyn and nedocromil in managing childhood asthma is *most correct*?

A. They are considered alternative agents to inhaled corticosteroids for daily control of mild persistent asthma.
B. They are both administered orally.
C. They are considered leukotriene modifiers.
D. They are associated with generally serious side effects.
E. They are effective for treating acute brochospasm.

10. What is one concern with the use of chronic oral corticosteroids specifically in children?

A. Downregulation of β_2 receptors
B. Cognitive impairment
C. Hyperactivity
D. Growth suppression
E. Cardiac arrhythmias

PATIENT PROFILE 86

METASTATIC BREAST CANCER

PRESENTATION

CC: "I'm having pain in my hips and back, and I am very tired."

HPI: TD is a 65-year-old white woman presenting with 6 out of 10 pain in her hips and lower back. She began noticing the pain about 3 weeks ago and treated it herself with Aleve. She initially had good results with Aleve but no longer sees any effect. She also notes mild increasing dyspnea on exertion and has experienced increasing fatigue.

PMH: Breast cancer: stage IIIB breast cancer diagnosed 7 years ago; menopause (15 years ago); hypothyroidism; type 2 diabetes mellitus

FH: No significant cancer history; mother alive and well at 89 years of age; father died from myocardial infarction (MI) at age 50.

SH: Married; mother of two grown children; currently retired living with husband; no tobacco history or alcohol use.

ALL: NKDA

MH: Levothyroxine 188 μg PO qd, metformin 500 mg PO bid, Lantus 30 units qpm, Humalog pen 10 units ac, Aleve 1 tab PO q12h

ROS: Significant pain in hips and lower back; mild SOB.

VS: Temperature: 99°F; blood pressure: 140/90 mm Hg; heart rate: 68 beats per minute; respiratory rate: 20 breaths per minute; O_2 saturation: 95% RA

Height: 63 in; weight: 160 lb

General: Pleasant, slightly confused, overweight woman, in mild distress

HEENT: PERRLA, EOMI

Neck: Supple; no LAD or thyromegaly

Lungs: ↓ BS at right base

Heart: Mild tachycardia, RR, no MRG
ABD: Soft, nontender/nondistended, positive bowel
  sounds
EXT: No C/C/E
Neuro: A&O $\times$ 3

LABORATORY DATA

Na: 142 mEq/L	K: 4.0 mEq/L
Cl: 107 mEq/L	CO_2: 26 mEq/L
Blood urea nitrogen (BUN): 10 mEq/L	Serum Cr: 0.8 mg/dL
Glucose: 137 mg/dL	Ca: 12.5 mg/dL
Mg: 2.4 mg/dL	PO_4: 3.0 mg/dL
Total bilirubin: 0.8 mg/dL	ALP 120 IU/mL
Low-density lipoprotein (LDH) cholesterol: 570 IU/mL	Albumin: 3.0 mg/dL
Hgb: 13 g/dL	Hct: 37%
Platelets: 150,000/mm³	White blood cell (WBC) count: 6000/mm³ 70% P, 23% L, 6% M, 1% E

DIAGNOSTIC TESTS

CT scan: Solitary nodule in right lung
Lung biopsy: Metastatic adenocarcinoma consistent with
  breast primary
Bone scan: Abnormal localization in right pelvis and lower
  lumbar spine
Bone biopsy: Metastatic adenocarcinoma consistent with
  breast primary
Echocardiogram: LVEF ~ 50% with mild hypokinesis

ASSESSMENT/PLAN

TD is a 65-year-old woman with stage IV breast cancer
with metastatic disease to the lung, lower lumbar spine,
and right pelvis. TD will be treated with IV fluid and zoledronic acid. She also will receive vinorelbine plus
trastuzumab. TD also will begin treatment with OxyContin
10 mg PO bid with OxyIR 5 mg PO q3–4h PRN for breakthrough pain.

QUESTIONS

1. TD is given zoledronic acid for which of the following
   indications?

   A. Hypercalcemia
   B. Bone metastases
   C. Bone pain
   D. All the above

2. What is TD's corrected calcium level?

   A. 12.7 mg/dL
   B. 12.9 mg/dL
   C. 13.3 mg/dL
   D. 14 mg/dL

3. What is the most appropriate dose of zoledronic acid
   in this patient?

   A. 4 mg IV over 2 hours every week
   B. 4 mg IV over 15 minutes every week
   C. 4 mg IV over 2 hours every 4 weeks
   D. 4 mg IV over 15 minutes every 4 weeks

4. Which of the following adverse events is associated
   with trastuzumab?

   A. Infusion reactions
   B. Nephrotoxicity
   C. Endometrial cancer
   D. Mood changes

5. TD has been requiring increasing amounts of Oxy-
   Contin and complains of persistent constipation.
   What is the most appropriate recommendation for
   you to make to TD?

   A. Drink plenty of water and exercise regularly.
   B. Take Colace twice a day every day.
   C. Take Colace and Senokot twice a day every day.
   D. Ignore the constipation; it will go away in a few
      days.

6. TD has been requiring OxyContin 100 mg PO bid
   with no breakthrough medication to control her pain.
   Her prescription insurance no longer covers OxyContin, and the physician asks you to recommend a dose
   of MS Contin. What do you recommend?

   A. MS Contin 15 mg PO q12h
   B. MS Contin 60 mg PO q12h
   C. MS Contin 100 mg PO q12h
   D. MS Contin 180 mg PO q12h

7. TD is eventually stabilized on MS Contin 100 mg PO
   q12h and requires hospitalization. She will not be able
   to receive anything by mouth for the next several days.
   You are asked to convert her outpatient pain medication to an equivalent dose of intravenous morphine to
   be given over the day. What do you recommend?

   A. 1 mg IV q4h
   B. 5 mg IV q4h
   C. 10 mg IV q4h
   D. 15 mg IV q4h

8. Vinorelbine belongs to which class of antineoplastics?

   A. Alkylating agent
   B. Vinca alkaloid

C. Anthracycline

D. Taxane

9. Which of the following is a dose-limiting toxicity of vinorelbine?

A. Ototoxicity

B. Hepatotoxicity

C. Myelosuppression

D. Nausea and vomiting

10. Vinorelbine arrests cell division by which of the following methods?

A. Intercalation between DNA base pairs

B. Cross-linking DNA strands

C. Promoting the assembly of microtubules

D. Inhibiting microtubule formation

PATIENT PROFILE 87

RESPIRATORY TRACT INFECTION

PRESENTATION

PJ is a 51-year-old white man who is homeless. He has a fever, cough, and chills that have lasted for 2 days. PJ reports bronchitis for 2 weeks before admission and had a dry cough that resolved without drug treatment. Two days before admission PJ had an onset of fever, chills, and sweats and was treated at a clinic for the homeless with Tylenol® (acetaminophen), which provided some relief.

PJ had pneumonia in May of 1994 and had rheumatic fever at the age of 4 or 5. He has a resultant heart murmur. PJ has no known drug allergies. PJ is homeless, unemployed, and lives on the street. He is single and has no children. He became homeless 2 years ago after his mother died of a long illness for which he cared for her. He has smoked 1 pack of cigarettes per day for 25 years, uses alcohol occasionally (likes to drink beer), and has gone without a drink for 1 week. PJ is a disheveled looking 51-year-old man who appears far older than his stated age. He complains of a cough and states that if he can't get a cigarette he will hold someone hostage until he does.

PHYSICAL EXAMINATION

BP: 130/90, HR: 108; RR: 12, T: 39°C, Sao_2: 95%
Chest: note E to A egophony and fremitus

LABS

Na: 131	K: 3.5
Cl: 97	CO_2: 20
WBC: 16.1	Hgb: 12.9
Plts: 157	Hct: 38
BUN: 18	Neut: 84
SCr: 0.99	Lymph: 4
Gluc: 123	Bands: 5

A/P: PJ is a 51-year-old homeless, unemployed man who has a history of drinking and smoking who presents with a community-acquired pneumonia.

QUESTIONS

1. Which of the following pathogens is most likely the organism that caused the pneumonia?

A. *Streptococcus pneumoniae*

B. *Legionella pneumophila*

C. *Pseudomonas aeruginosa*

D. *Bacteroides fragilis*

E. *Peptostreptococcus* species

2. According to criteria, PJ can be treated for pneumonia as an outpatient. PJ has enrolled in an indigent care program and is eligible for pharmaceutical samples free of charge. He has shown in the past that he is largely non-compliant. Which of the following antibiotics would be the most appropriate for PJ to take orally as an outpatient?

A. Ceftazidime

B. Amoxicillin and clavulanate

C. Azithromycin

D. Erythromycin

E. Cefaclor

3. The culture and sensitivity results from a sputum sample indicate that pneumococci have grown and are sensitive to penicillin, doxycycline, cefuroxime, and erythromycin. The result of a urine *Legionella* antibody

test is positive. Which choice would you consider the best therapeutic decision?

A. Discontinue the azithromycin because there is a pharmacoeconomic advantage to using penicillin 500 mg po qid in its place.

B. Continue azithromycin therapy because this macrolide antibiotic will cover both pneumococci and *Legionella* species.

C. Consider the addition of gentamicin 300 mg IV q24h to cover the gram-negative organism *Legionella*.

D. Switch the current therapy to cefuroxime 500 mg po bid for better pneumococcal coverage.

E. Add metronidazole to the current therapy for additional gram-positive coverage.

4. PJ returns to the emergency department 10 days later with similar symptoms. He admits to not finishing his prescribed course of azithromycin. The *Streptococcus pneumoniae* infection is now thought to be penicillin resistant at an intermediate level. Knowing his financial and compliance concerns remain largely the same, select an antibiotic from the following list that would be the most useful to PJ.

A. Trovafloxacin 300 mg po qd is necessary to treat this patient. Its broad spectrum will cover both *Pseudomonas aeruginosa* and *Bacteroides fragilis*, which may be causing the pneumonia.

B. Ampicillin 500 mg po qid would be useful to PJ because of its extended gram-negative spectrum.

C. A switch from azithromycin to clarithromycin 500 mg po bid should be enough to eradicate the resistant pneumococcal infection.

D. Intravenous vancomycin 1g q12h is deemed necessary for intermediate-resistance *Streptococcus pneumoniae*.

E. Levofloxacin 500 mg po qd should be sufficient to control the penicillin-resistant strain of *Streptococcus pneumoniae*.

5. PJ becomes noncompliant with the regimen. He returns to the emergency department with pleuritic chest pain. A chest x-ray shows dense, bilateral infiltrates, which are worse than those on previous radiographs. PJ is hypoxic and is intubated because of respiratory failure. He is admitted to an intensive care unit with the diagnosis of severe community-acquired pneumonia. PJ has no drug allergies. Which of the following antibiotic regimens would be the best choice to treat PJ?

A. Doxycycline 500 mg IV q12h and metronidazole 500 mg IV q12h

B. Ceftriaxone 1 g IV q24h and azithromycin 500 mg IV q24h

C. Gentamicin 50 mg IV q24h and imipenem 500 mg IV q12h

D. Ampicillin 2 g IV q6h, metronidazole 500 mg IV q8h, and gentamicin 70 mg IV q24h

E. Bactrim® (trimethoprim-sulfamethoxazole) 10 mg/kg/d IV in 3 divided doses as the only antibiotic

PATIENT PROFILE 88

DIABETES MELLITUS: COMPLICATIONS

PRESENTATION

CC: "I seem to be thirsty all the time, which makes me feel the need to visit the restroom multiple times during the work day."

HPI: WV is a 50-year-old man who was diagnosed recently with diabetes mellitus type 2. WV was diagnosed with elevated blood glucose levels during a routine visit to his primary care physician (PCP). WV has recent complaints of wanting to drink liquids all the time. WV also complains of intermittent headaches and leg cramps. Based on the results of a full physical examination, WV's PCP reports signs and symptoms of autonomic neuropathy. Owing to WV's poor blood glucose control, WV was initiated on combination therapy for his diabetes. WV was sent to a pharmacist-run outpatient clinic for counseling on general diabetes education and self-monitoring strategies.

Medications: Metformin 500 mg PO bid, glyburide 10 mg PO qd, regular insulin 10 units SC 30 minutes before meals, lisinopril 40 mg PO qd, atenolol 25 mg PO qd, aspirin 81 mg PO qd

PMH: Hypertension diagnosed 1 year ago

PSH: None

FH: Father (98 years old) diagnosed with type 2 diabetes; mother deceased at age 72 from fall complication owing to osteoporosis; brother (44 years old) diagnosed with diabetes type 2 and hypertension.

SH: Single; denies alcohol or illicit drug use.
Allergies: NKDA

PHYSICAL EXAMINATION

General: Overweight white man; appearance reflects apparent age.

VS: Blood pressure: 132/90 mmHg; heart rate: beats per minute; respiratory rate: 22 breaths per minute; temperature: 37°C

Height: 5 ft, 5 in; weight: 113 kg

Skin: Normal skin turgor

HEENT: PERRLA; EOM intact; mucous membranes dry.

COR: RRR; no murmur, rubs, or gallops; posterior tibial and dorsalis pedis pulses normal

Chest: Lungs CTA

ABD: Soft, nontender, normal bowel sounds

GU: Increased urinary output

RECT: Normal anus

EXT: No edema; no calluses or ulcers on foot

NEURO: Normal

ECG: Normal

LABORATORY VALUES

Na: 122 mEq/L

Cl: 98 mEq/L

Blood urea nitrogen (BUN): 23 mg/dL

Glucose: Pending

Hct: 46.8%

PT: N/A

Triglycerides: 120 mg/dL

High-density lipoprotein (HDL) cholesterol: 40 mg/dL

K: 5.9 mEq/L

HCO_3: 6.0 mEq/L

Serum Cr: 1.2 mg/dL

Hgb: 14.8 g/dL

Platelets: $300 \times 10^3/mm^3$

aPTT: N/A

Total cholesterol: 210 mg/dL

Low-density lipoprotein (LDL) cholesterol: 110 mg/dL

QUESTIONS

1. Which of the following *most likely* represents the blood glucose level that WV may have had for the diagnosis of diabetes during his visit to the physician?

   A. Fasting plasma glucose level of 110 mg/dL
   B. Fasting plasma glucose level of 128 mg/dL
   C. 2-hour postload glucose level of 126 mg/dL
   D. 2-hour postload glucose level of 140 mg/dL
   E. 2-hour postload glucose level of 185 mg/dL

2. Which of the following is a symptom that WV reported that may indicate hyperglycemia?

   A. Leg cramps
   B. Polydipsia
   C. Polyphagia

   D. Diaphoresis
   E. Tachycardia

3. Which medication(s) from WV's medication history may precipitate a hypoglycemic event?

   A. Metformin only
   B. Atenolol only
   C. Regular insulin only
   D. Glyburide and regular insulin
   E. Metformin and regular insulin

4. Which of the following is an *appropriate* recommendation for treating a hypoglycemic event?

   A. Two Life Savers
   B. One glucose tablet
   C. Four to six ounces of fruit juice
   D. Eight to ten chocolate candies
   E. One-half tube of glucose gel

5. What is the first symptom that WV would most likely experience if he is having a hypoglycemic reaction?

   A. Seizure
   B. Confusion
   C. Sweating
   D. Palpitations
   E. Tachycardia

6. When should WV be screened for diabetic complications?

   A. WV should be screened immediately.
   B. WV should be screened in 5 years.
   C. WV should be screened in 10 years.
   D. WV should be screened in 20 years.
   E. WV does not need to be screened.

7. Which of the following complications is WV *less likely* to experience?

   A. Retinopathy
   B. Nephropathy
   C. Cardiovascular complications
   D. Diabetic ketoacidosis (DKA)
   E. Hyperglycemic, hyperosmolar, nonketotic syndrome (HHNS)

8. Which of the following describes a complication that WV may be currently experiencing based on WV's diagnosis of autonomic neuropathy?

   A. Foot ulcer
   B. Hyperactive bladder
   C. Erectile dysfunction
   D. Loss of protective sensation of the feet
   E. Increased intestinal and gastric peristalsis

9. In order to prevent cardiovascular-related complications, WV should try to maintain which of the following goals?

 A. Blood pressure of 120/80 mm Hg
 B. Blood pressure of 130/80 mm Hg
 C. Fasting plasma glucose level of 140 mg/dL
 D. LDL level of 110 mg/dL
 E. 2-hour postprandial plasma glucose level of 200 mg/dL

10. Which of the following is a risk factor that WV currently has that places him at risk for metabolic syndrome according to the Adult Treatment Panel (ATP) III guidelines?

 A. Triglycerides
 B. Blood pressure
 C. Total cholesterol
 D. Low-density lipoprotein
 E. High-density lipoprotein

PATIENT PROFILE 89

MEDICINAL CHEMISTRY

PRESENTATION AND QUESTION

MJ, a 28-year-old woman, decides to use birth control pills because she already has two girls and a boy, ages 3, 4, and 5. The physician prescribes pills that contain ethinyl estradiol (structure 89.1) as the main active ingredient. A recent plasma lipid profile indicates that MJ has a high cholesterol level that is not controlled with diet alone. MJ presents a prescription to you in the pharmacy for cholestyramine (structure 89.2), which is a relatively safe cholesterol-lowering agent.

What would be your advice to MJ?

 A. Take the resin with the birth control pills together in the evening.
 B. Cholestyramine is not a good choice for you. Consult your physician to change your prescription to lovastatin (structure 89.3).
 C. If you must use cholestyramine, ask your physician about alternatives to oral contraceptives.
 D. B and C
 E. There is no reason to be alarmed, both agents can be taken concurrently.

89.1

89.2

89.3

PATIENT PROFILE 90
TUBERCULOSIS

PRESENTATION

AJ, a 25-year-old woman, arrives in the emergency department with fever, chills, night sweats, fatigue, weight loss, and a productive cough. These symptoms have persisted for a few weeks. She is a full-time pharmacy student and works on weekends in a hospital. Her medical history includes a seizure disorder. She was HIV-negative when tested 1 year ago. Medications on admission are phenytoin 300 mg/day, ibuprofen prn, multivitamins daily, and Os-Cal® (calcium carbonate) 1000 mg/day. The purified protein derivative (PPD) skin test result is positive, and three sputum specimens contain acid-fast bacilli. Culture and susceptibility results are pending. A chest x-ray reveals extensive pulmonary consolidation. Lab data on admission include AST 22 IU/L, serum creatinine 0.8 mg/dL, BUN 7 mg/dL, and albumin 3.8 mg/dL. The phenytoin serum level at admission is 15 mg/L.

QUESTIONS

1. Which of the following statement(s) is/are true regarding the proper administration and interpretation of the purified protein derivative (PPD) skin test for this patient?

    A. Administer an intradermal injection of 5 tuberculin units (5 TU) of PPD of killed tubercle bacilli on the inner forearm.
    B. The delayed-type hypersensitivity response to the PPD skin test should be examined and interpreted by a trained health care provider 48 to 72 hours after the injection.
    C. The delayed-type hypersensitivity response to the PPD skin test should be examined and interpreted by a trained health care provider 6 to 12 hours after the injection.
    D. A and B
    E. A and C

2. Which of the following statement(s) concerning isoniazid therapy is/are true?

    A. AJ should receive pyridoxine (vitamin B_6) with isoniazid.
    B. AJ should be counseled that isoniazid may impart an orange discoloration to urine, stool, sputum, saliva, tears, and sweat and that soft contact lenses may be permanently discolored.
    C. AJ should receive baseline examination of visual acuity before initiation of isoniazid therapy, followed by monthly eye examinations.
    D. A and B
    E. All of the above

3. The most toxic effect of ethambutol is

    A. hepatotoxicity.
    B. nephrotoxicity.
    C. ototoxicity.
    D. optic neuritis.
    E. tinnitus.

4. The addition of rifampin therapy to a patient taking phenytoin may _____ phenytoin serum concentrations because of the _____ effect of rifampin.

    A. increase, inhibitory
    B. decrease, induction
    C. decrease, inhibitory
    D. increase, induction
    E. None of the above

5. The most toxic effect of pyrazinamide is

    A. hepatotoxicity.
    B. optic neuritis.
    C. nephrolithiasis.
    D. peripheral neuropathy.
    E. ototoxicity.

OSTEOPOROSIS

PRESENTATION

A 70-year-old postmenopausal white women presents with left hip fracture. She fell out of bed at the nursing home and also sustained a femoral neck fracture.

PMH: Hypertension, diabetes, osteoporosis, rheumatoid arthritis, hypothyroid
SH: Lives in a nursing home. Husband died 3 years ago. She has one son who is active in her health care
FH: Noncontributory
ALL: NKDA

PHYSICAL EXAMINATION

VS: Blood pressure: 130/80 mm Hg; heart rate: 60 beats per minute; respiratory rate: 10 breaths per minute; temperature: 99.2°F
Weight: 60 kg
General: Frail-looking women; looks appropriate for her age; in acute distress status post fracture
HEENT: PERRLA, EOMI
Heart: NSR, murmur
Lungs: Crackles at the bases
GU: Urinary incontinence
GI: Normal bowel sounds
EXT: Some bruises on arms and legs

LABORATORY VALUES

$$\frac{130 \mid 112 \mid 1.2}{3.7 \mid 38 \mid 20} \diagdown 80$$

Phos: 2.5
White blood cell (WBC) count: 5
Hgb: 12
Total cholesterol: 180 mg/dL
Low-density lipoprotein (LDL) cholesterol: 120 mg/dL
High-density lipoprotein (HDL) cholesterol: 40 mg/dL

Ca: 10.8
Albumin: 3
Hct: 36%
Platelets: 150

Triglycerides: 150 mg/dL

T score from last year: > −2.5
Radiology: Left femoral neck fracture

MEDICATIONS

Aspirin 81 mg PO qd
Lopressor 50 mg PO bid
Hydrochlorthiazide 25 mg PO qd
Pravachol 20 mg PO qd
Metformin 500 mg PO bid
Lantus 10 Uints qhs
Prednisone 20 mg PO qd
Levoxyl 75 µg PO qd
Levofloxicin 500 mg PO bid

QUESTIONS

1. According to the National Institute of Health (NIH), which of the following defines osteoporosis?

   A. T score > −2.5 SD
   B. T score < −2.5 SD
   C. T score < −1.5 SD
   D. Developing a fracture

2. Postmenopausal women should receive

   A. 500 mg elemental iron per day.
   B. 500 mg elemental calcium per day.
   C. 1000 mg elemental calcium per day.
   D. 1500 mg elemental calcium per day.

3. The patient in this profile has which of the following risk factors for osteoporosis?

   A. Low calcium
   B. Premenopausal
   C. Overweight
   D. Not on calcium supplementation

4. Which of the following medications is the patient currently taking that could have contributed to her osteoporosis risk?

   A. Metformin
   B. Aspirin
   C. Levoxyl
   D. Lopressor

5. What is the major difference between alendronate 70 mg every week and 35 mg every week?

   A. The 35-mg dose is associated with fewer adverse effects.
   B. The 70-mg dose is used for treatment of osteoporosis.
   C. The 70-mg dose should not be used in elderly patients.
   D. The 35-mg dose costs substantially less than the 70-mg dose.

6. What is the major difference between the Z score and the T score?

   A. The Z score is the bone mineral density (BMD) result compared with a person of the same age and sex; the T score is the BMD result compared with a "young normal" person of the same sex.
   B. The Z score is a BMD result compared with a "young normal" person of the same sex; the T score is a BMD result compared with a person of the same age and sex.
   C. The Z score can detect only osteopenia.
   D. The T score can detect only osteoporosis.

7. Which of the following would be counseling points for a patient taking Fosamax?

   I. Drink at least 8 ounces of water with each dose.
   II. Do not eat for 30 minutes after ingesting a dose.
   III. Take at bedtime

   A. I
   B. III
   C. I and II
   D. II and III

8. Which of the following is(are) contraindication(s) to starting a a bisphosphonate?

   I. CrCl < 60
   II. History of esophageal erosion
   III. Patients who are NPO

   A. I
   B. III
   C. I and II
   D. II and III

9. Forteo (teriparatide) has been associated with which of the following?

   A. Osteosarcoma
   B. Liver chrosis
   C. Corneal deposits
   D. Pulmonary fibrosis

10. The patient's physician has decided to start her on a calcium/vitamin D regimen. Which medication should be spaced at least 3 hours around the calcium?

   A. Lopressor
   B. Aspirin
   C. Levaquin
   D. Metformin

PATIENT PROFILE 92

URINARY TRACT INFECTION

PRESENTATION

Institution	Nursing Home	
Patient	KY	
Age	77	
Sex	Female	
Allergies	NKA	
Race	Asian	
Height	5'4"	
Wgt	138 lb	
Diagnosis	Primary	1. Nosocomial UTI
		2. Stable angina
		3. HTN
	Secondary	1. s/p breast Ca

	Date	Test
Lab and diagnostic tests	11/24	Stress test
	11/24	CK 400 IU/mL
	11/24	Cardiac isoenzymes pending
	11/24	SCr 1.4 mg/dL and BUN 23 mg/dL
	11/24	Blood glucose 157 mg/dL

	11/24	Potassium 5.1 mEq/mL		
	11/24	Echocardiogram pending		
	11/24	Urine C & S pending		

	Date	Drug and Strength	Route	Sig
Med orders	11/24	Lisinopril 10 mg	PO	qd
	11/24	Diltiazem CD 240 mg	PO	qd
	11/24	Isosorbide dinitrate 10 mg	PO	tid
	11/24	Ranitidine 150 mg	PO	bid
	11/26	Gentamicin 100 mg	IV	1 dose
	11/27	Gentamicin 60 mg	IV	q12h
	11/27	Ampicillin Ig	IV	q6h
Additional orders	11/26	WBC 15,300 mm^3		
	11/27	Gentamicin trough conc. 2.5 mg/L		
	11/26	Gentamicin peak conc. 14 mg/L		
Pharmacist notes	11/26	Monitor SCr and BUN and gentamicin blood conc.		
	11/26	Adjust gentamicin dose according to renal function		
	11/27	Urinary pathogens identified and sensitive to prescribed antibiotics		

QUESTIONS

1. Which of the following is/are true about hospital-acquired acute UTI?

   I. The sensitivity to antibiotics of community-acquired bacteria differs from that of hospital-acquired bacteria.
   II. *Escherichia coli*, *Proteus* species, and *Pseudomonas* species are the predominant pathogens in hospital acquired UTI.
   III. Antibiotic-resistant organisms occur more frequently with hospital-acquired UTI.

   A. I only
   B. III only
   C. I and II only
   D. II and III only
   E. I, II, and III

2. The pharmacist who receives the November 26 drug order for gentamicin should recognize that the dose is

   A. a test dose.
   B. a loading dose.
   C. the therapeutic dose.
   D. the recommended dose for patients with renal impairment.
   E. not a recommended dose.

3. The potential toxic effects associated with elevated gentamicin trough levels include

   A. nephrotoxicity and ototoxicity.
   B. hyperlipidemia and kidney stones.
   C. rash and tinnitus.
   D. arrhythmia and cardiac arrest.
   E. Stevens-Johnson syndrome and hyperuricemia.

4. The elevated gentamicin blood concentrations may have been caused by

   A. declining renal function.
   B. hepatic failure.
   C. septicemia.
   D. anemia.
   E. drug interaction with lisinopril.

5. The physician asks you to recommend an antibiotic that is on formulary and is as effective as ampicillin and gentamicin in control of nosocomial UTI caused by susceptible organisms. Which of the following antibiotics would you recommend?

   A. Tetracycline
   B. Amoxicillin
   C. Bactrim® (trimethoprim-sulfamethoxazole)
   D. Metronidazole
   E. Cefotaxime

6. Which of the following is not a criterion for converting from IV to oral antibiotic therapy?

   A. Signs and symptoms of UTI should be improving.
   B. WBC and vital signs should be normal.
   C. The patient should be afebrile 12 to 24 hours before the switch.
   D. The patient should be younger than 60 years.
   E. The patient should have a functioning GI tract.

ONCOLOGY: OVARIAN CANCER

PRESENTATION

JP is a 60-year-old woman who visits her physician because of abdominal fullness, bloating, nausea, and general malaise. Eight months ago, her routine physical examination had been without abnormal findings. JP's medical history includes hypertension and congestive heart failure managed with lisinopril and furosemide, fibrillation managed with digoxin and quinidine, and NIDDM managed with metformin. JP is allergic to sulfa drugs (full body rash). She is married and had one child (age 30). She does not smoke and never drinks alcohol.

PHYSICAL EXAMINATION

BP: 135/80, RR: 18, HR: 60
Ht: 5'3", Wt: 130 lb

LABS

Na: 142
K: 5.1
Dig: 1.6
FBS: 130
CA-125: 80 (normal <35)

Abdominal ultrasonography reveals a 3 cm × 5 cm mass on the right ovary. Exploratory laparotomy confirms the diagnosis of ovarian cancer, and the patient undergoes total abdominal hysterectomy with bilateral oophorectomy.

QUESTIONS

1. Which of the following is the best description of CA-125?

   A. Nonspecific tumor marker used primarily to detect hematologic malignant tumors
   B. Tumor marker specific for cervical cancer
   C. Tumor marker specific for metastatic disease
   D. Tumor marker specific for ovarian cancer
   E. Nonspecific tumor marker used primarily in the diagnosis of malignant disease

2. JP is scheduled to begin a chemotherapy regimen 3 weeks after her operation. The initial plan is to use a regimen containing carboplatin, cyclophos-phamide, and doxorubicin. Which of the following statements is the most appropriate critique of the regimen suggested?

   A. The regimen is appropriate as described
   B. Recommend changing the carboplatin to cisplatin to reduce nephrotoxicity.
   C. Recommend adding mesna to the regimen to reduce nephrotoxicity.
   D. Recommend changing doxorubicin to mitoxantrone to reduce cardiotoxicity.
   E. Recommend changing doxorubicin to daunorubicin to prevent discoloration of urine.

3. The CA-125 level begins to rise after three courses of the first regimen. Therapy is adjusted to include paclitaxel. To minimize adverse effects during the infusion, pretreatment is recommended. Which of the following regimens will be most effective in preventing an adverse reaction during the infusion?

   A. Dexamethasone alone
   B. Dexamethasone and ondansetron
   C. Diphenhydramine, ranitidine, and dexamethasone
   D. Ranitidine alone
   E. No pretreatment if the appropriate tubing is used for infusion

4. The dose limiting toxicity of a paclitaxel is

   A. alopecia.
   B. bone marrow suppression.
   C. peripheral neuropathy.
   D. nausea and vomiting.
   E. anaphylaxis.

5. To maximize antineoplastic drug concentrations at the tumor site, which route of administration would be most appropriate?

   A. Intravenous
   B. Intraarterial
   C. Intrathecal
   D. Intraperitoneal
   E. Intramuscular

P A T I E N T   P R O F I L E   9 4

ASTHMA

PRESENTATION

LT is a 50-year-old asthmatic man who regularly uses inhalation medications to control acute asthma attacks. In addition to asthma, LT suffers from glaucoma, for which he is using eye drops of carbachol (Structure 94.1).

94.1

QUESTIONS

1. Which of the following agents is *likely* to be among LT asthma medications?

   A. Ipratropium bromide (Structure 94.2)
   B. Colterol (Structure 94.3)
   C. Cromolyn (Structure 94.4)
   D. A or B
   E. A, B, or C

94.2

94.3

94.4

2. Assuming that cromolyn is useful in treating asthma, what is its role?

   A. Directly dilates the bronchial smooth muscles
   B. Treats the inflammatory component of asthma
   C. Inhibits mast cells degradation

3. Assuming that ipratropium bromide is useful in treating asthma, what is its role?

   A. Directly dilates the bronchial smooth muscles by an adrenergic mechanism
   B. Inhibits histamine binding
   C. Treats the inflammatory predisposing factors of asthma
   D. Inhibits mast cell degradation
   E. Directly dilates the bronchial smooth muscles by an antimuscarinic mechanism

4. What is the exact pharmacologic classification of colterol?
   A. Nonselective β agonist
   B. Selective β_1 antagonist
   C. Selective β_2 agonist
   D. Selective β_1 agonist

5. Which of the following drugs has(have) the same mechanism of action of colterol?

   I. Albuterol
   II. Terbutaline
   III. Metoprolol
   IV. Metapreteronol

   A. I and IV
   B. I and III
   C. II and III
   D. I, II, and IV
   E. All the above

94.5

6. Bitolterol (Structure 95.5) is a prodrug for colterol as the diester with *p*-methylbenzoic acid (toluic acid). What is the rationale of manufacturing colterol as bitolterol?

   A. To improve colterol absorption through lung tissues
   B. To improve colterol stability toward metabolism
   C. To produce more volatile material for aerosol applications
   D. A and B
   E. A, B, and C

7. Considering that LT suffers from glaucoma in addition to his asthma problem, which of the preceding antiasthmata agents is(are) expected to exacerbate the glaucoma problem?

   A. Bitolterol
   B. Cromolyn
   C. Ipratropium bromide
   D. A and B
   E. B and C

8. If LT becomes hypertensive, which of the following antihypertensive drugs should be contraindicated considering his asthma problem?

   A. Atenolol
   B. Propranolol
   C. Clonidine
   D. Prazosin
   E. Lisinopril

9. The bronchodilator isoproteronol (Structure 94.6) should be contraindicated as antiasthmata agent if LT is suffering from hypertension.

   A. Yes
   B. No

94.6

10. Why are corticosteroids useful in asthma management?

    A. Corticosteroids have β_2-agonist bronchodilating effects.
    B. Corticosteroids act as central respiratory stimulants.
    C. Corticosteroids are anti-inflammatory agents.
    D. None of the above

PATIENT PROFILE 9 5

BIPOLAR DISORDER

PRESENTATION

LM is a 57-year-old woman with a diagnosis of bipolar type I disorder. Her husband has brought her to the crisis intervention unit. She is dressed in a miniskirt and T-shirt that seem inappropriate for her age. LM's husband claims that within the last couple of weeks LM slept only a few hours a night, was constantly talking, and went on a couple of shopping sprees during which she spent thousands of dollars. Before the onset of these symptoms, LM increased her coffee intake from 2 cups to 8 cups a day because of her need to prepare for a party she was hosting.

LM had been found to have bipolar type I disorder after a manic episode at age 33. Since then she has been hospitalized more than 20 times while being treated with lithium carbonate. The medical history includes hypertension for 10 years and hypothyroidism. She is allergic to erythromycin (rash). The family history includes a sister with diagnosed bipolar disorder treated with valproic acid. LM is unemployed and has two adult children.

MEDS

Lithium carbonate 450 mg bid × 20 years
Hydrochlorothiazide 50 mg qd × 10 years
Levothyroxine 0.05 mg qd × 5 years

PHYSICAL EXAMINATION

GEN: 57-year-old woman who is uncooperative, very talkative, and inappropriately dressed
BP sitting R arm: 190/98, HR: 80, RR: 24, T: 99.0°F

LABS

Na: 140 mEq/L	Cl: 100 mEq/L
K: 3.6 mEq/L	CO_2 20 mEq/L
SCr: 0.6 mg/dL	Gluc: 145 mg/dL
WBC: 8.7 × 10^3/mm^3	Hct: 36%
Hgb 11 g/dL	Plts 195 × 10^9/L
Li: 0.4 mEq/L	

A/P: LM is a 57-year-old woman with a history of bipolar type I disorder, hypertension, and hypothyroidism. She was brought to the crisis intervention unit by her husband because of symptoms of decreased sleep, increased talkativeness, increased spending, and increased activity.

QUESTIONS

1. Which of the patient's sign(s) is/are characteristic of a manic episode?

   A. Decreased need for sleep
   B. Spending sprees
   C. Coffee intake
   D. A and B
   E. A, B, and C

2. What is the most likely cause of the patient's most recent manic episode?

   A. Use of hydrochlorothiazide 50 mg qd
   B. Increased use of caffeinated coffee
   C. Missed doses of levothyroxine
   D. Extra doses of lithium
   E. Hypertension

3. What is the best option for managing this patient's manic episode?

   A. Continue lithium at 450 mg bid
   B. Discontinue lithium and start valproic acid 500 mg bid
   C. Add nortriptyline 50 mg HS
   D. Add carbamazepine 400 mg bid
   E. Add fluoxetine 20 mg qam

4. Which of the following antihypertensive medications can cause lithium toxicity?

   A. Captopril
   B. Hydrochlorothiazide
   C. Propranolol
   D. A and B
   E. A, B, C

5. What is considered the therapeutic serum drug level of lithium in the treatment of patients with bipolar disorder?

   A. 10–20 mEq/L
   B. 4–12 mEq/L
   C. 1–2 mEq/L
   D. 0.6–1.0 mEq/L
   E. 0.1–0.5 mEq/L

PATIENT PROFILE 96
ACUTE ON CHRONIC RENAL FAILURE

PRESENTATION

CC: Primary care physician referral

HPI: An 83-year-old woman is referred to the hospital for a renal workup. The patient had complaints of decreased urine output (UO) and a 10-lb weight gain 1 week PTA according to her daughter. On examination by the medical housestaff, the patient denies chest pain, palpitations, dyspnea, or abdominal pain.

PMH: Congestive heart failure (CHF), hypertension (HTN), urinary incontinence, gout (no active medications), mild dementia, moderate renal insufficiency (baseline serum creatinine 1.3)

Medications on admission: Nitroglycerin (10 mg) transdermal 0.4 μg/h qam, ramipril (Altace) 2.5 mg qd, hydrochlorothiazide (Hydrodiuril) 25 mg qd, multivitamin 1 tab qd, oxybutynin (Ditropan) 5 mg qd

ALL: Penicillin

FH: Not available

SH: Patient lives with daughter; no alcohol use; 30 pack-year history of tobacco use

PE: Patient looks younger than stated age, lying in bed, comfortable and in NAD.

ROS: Significant findings: MMM, cardiac murmur, 2(+) pedal edema BL, A&O × 2

VS: Temperature: 98.2°F; heart rate: 90 beats per minute; blood pressure: 140/90 mm Hg; respiratory rate: 18 breaths per minute; O_2 saturation: 97% RA

Weight: 129 lb (baseline 119 lb); height: 5 ft, 2 in

LABORATORY VALUES

Na: 130
Cl: 107
Blood urea nitrogen (BUN): 82
BG: 88

Hct: 30.4%
Platelets: 212

K: 6.4
Total CO_2: 18
Serum Cr: 4.0

White blood cell (WBC) count: 10.1
Hgb: 10.0

U/A: C&S pending; SG. 1.015; pH 7.5, Na: 20, Cr: 52, /hpf RBC: 0–2; WBC: 6–10,

Bacteria (occ); yeast (–)

UO: < 10 mL/h

ECG: No QRS widening or T-wave elevations

Chest x-ray: Bilateral pleural effusions; no evidence of pneumonia

Medications administered in emergency room: Regular insulin 10 units and 50% dextrose 50 mL IV × 1, ciprofloxacin (Cipro) 400 mg IV q12h

QUESTIONS

1. Choose the *first* or *highest-priority problem* on the list from the following assessments for this case.

   A. Hyperkalemia most likely owing to acute renal failure (ARF) with no significant ECG changes
   B. Oliguric ARF probably owing to cardiac decompensation, thiazide diuretic or ACE inhibitor use, or medication noncompliance
   C. Decreased total CO_2 may indicate non–life-threatening metabolic acidosis.
   D. Elevated blood pressure most likely owing to volume overload
   E. Hyponatremia most likely owing to fluid overload: 2(+) pedal edema BL; 10-lb weight gain 1 week PTA

2. Identify the *most important* missing patient-specific information needed to properly evaluate, treat, and monitor renal insufficiency.

   A. Specific allergy history
   B. Medication compliance, including over-the-counter (OTC) and herbals medications, Na, and dietary and fluid intake
   C. At home blood pressure measurements, baseline mental status
   D. Baseline serum creatinine, BUN, EF, arterial blood gases (ABGs), blood pH
   E. Urine C&S results

3. Choose the factor that is associated with improved patient outcomes in ARF.

   A. Nonoliguria
   B. Advanced age
   C. Hospitalization
   D. Comorbidity
   E. All the above

4. What are the most clinically significant distinguishing features associated with ARF reported in this case?

   A. Elevated serum creatinine, BUN, and K^+
   B. Accumulation of H^+
   C. Hyperphosphatemia/hypocalcemia
   D. Low Hct and Hgb
   E. Urinary sediment

5. The patient's calculated FeNa is 1.8%. All the following statements are true *except*

   A. FeNa helps to establish the diagnosis of ARF.
   B. Prerenal azotemia may be differentiated from intrinsic renal failure when the FeNa value is < 1%.
   C. Prerenal azotemia may be differentiated from intrinsic renal failure when the FeNa value is ≥ 1%.
   D. Confounding variables such as diuretic use may influence the calculated FeNa, leading to a false-positive value.
   E. Both urinary and serum sodium and creatinine values are needed to calculate FeNa.

6. Regular insulin has a quick onset of action in the management of hyperkalemia, whereby it reduces serum K^+ by promoting K^+ movement from the extracellular to the intracellular space. What other agent would you recommend if the patient experiences persistent hyperkalemia?

   A. Sodium polysterene sulfonate (Kayexalate)
   B. Calcium gluconate IV
   C. Calcium chloride IV
   D. Sodium bicarbonate IV
   E. Albuterol IH

7. Recommend the *most appropriate* agent in this case to convert the patient from oliguria to nonoliguria.

   A. Nesiritide IV
   B. Furosemide IV
   C. Metolazone PO
   D. Chorothiazide IV
   E. Hydrochlorothiazide PO

8. All the following statements are *true* regarding medication use in renal failure pertaining to this patient *except*

   A. Thiazide diuretics such as hydrochlorothiazide worsen renal failure in the presence of ClCr < 30 mL/min.
   B. The dose of fluoroquinolones such as ciprofloxacin should be reduced in the presence of renal failure to avoid nephrotoxicity.
   C. Angiotensin-converting enzyme (ACE) inhibitors such as ramipril should be discontinued temporarily in the presence of renal failure and hyperkalemia.
   D. Combination therapy with two different diuretics may be successful in patients resistant to a single agent.
   E. The calcium channel blocker nifedipine should be added to the antihypertensive regimen.

9. The patient remains oliguric on hospital day 2 despite aggressive diuretic therapy with adequate IV hydration to avoid volume depletion. Serum creatinine and BUN are still elevated at 3.0 and 61, respectively. Serum K^+ is 5.0. Provide a plausible explanation for worsening renal perfusion in this patient.

   A. Higher than usual doses of diuretics are necessary in the presence of ARF.
   B. Worsening CHF
   C. Volume overload
   D. Hypoalbuminemia
   E. All the above

10. What is the *most likely* indication for combination use of a loop and thiazide diuretic regimen in this patient?

   A. Hyperuricemia
   B. Diuretic resistance
   C. Hyponatremia
   D. Nephrotic syndrome
   E. Hyperkalemia

PATIENT PROFILE 97

CORONARY ARTERY DISEASE

PRESENTATION

SK is a 45-year-old man brought to the emergency room by two friends. Although confused and severely short of breath, SK is able to complain loudly of crushing chest pain radiating to the neck, jaw, and left arm. The friends state that SK was in his usual state of health when they arrived to watch a football game. They ate pizza and shared a six-pack of beer during the game. At halftime, SK said he felt sick, took a couple swigs of antacid, stuck a tablet under his tongue, and seemed better. At the end of the fourth quarter, when his team failed to make a game winning field goal, SK, red-faced and sweating, jumped out of his chair yelling, grabbed his chest, and fell back. His friends stuck two of his nitroglycerin tablets under his tongue and brought him the emergency department. SK's medical history includes CAD, NIDDM, hypertension, and hyperlipidemia.

MEDS

Regular insulin 10 units sq qam and qpm
NPH insulin, 10 units sq qam and qpm

Verapamil SR 120 mg po qd
Nitroglycerin 0.4 mg SL prn
ISDN 10 mg po tid
Lovastatin 20 mg po qd
Cholestyramine 4 g po tid

PHYSICAL EXAMINATION

GEN: Confused, anxious, well-developed, well-nourished in moderate distress; tachypneic and diaphoretic; 9/10 chest pain
BP: 180/100, HR: 120, RR: 45, T: 38.3°C
Ht: 5'5", Wt: 78 kg
HEENT: AV nicking and narrowing
COR: Positive S_3 gallop
CHEST: Bilateral clear to ascultation
ABD: Central obesity
GU: WNL
RECT: Guaic negative
EXT: Edema to midcalf
NEURO: Mildly confused, A/O × 3
ECG: Sinus tachycardia, ST segment elevation to 4 mm in leads I, II, and V_2 through V_6

LABS

Na: 135	K: 3.0
Cl: 105	HCO$_3$: 20
BUN: 24	SCr: 1.3
Gluc: 220	Hgb: 13
Hct: 40	Plts: 170
PT: 11.5	aPTT: 28.2

QUESTIONS

1. SK is having an acute MI, and the physician determines that reperfusion of the occluded coronary artery is needed. Which of the following is not indicated at this time?

   A. Streptokinase
   B. Tissue-plasminogen activator (tPA)
   C. Aspirin
   D. Clopidogrel
   E. Unfractionated heparin

2. SK has signs of left ventricular failure. Which of his long-term medications should be discontinued?

   A. Isosorbide dinitrate
   B. Verapamil
   C. Lovastatin
   D. Cholestyramine
   E. Regular insulin

3. Which of the following agents is not indicated for use in acute MI

   A. Unfractionated heparin
   B. Metoprolol
   C. Nitroglycerin
   D. Diltiazem
   E. Morphine sulfate

4. SK recovers without complications. The ejection fraction is found to be 35% on echo. Which of the following medications will help prevent LV remodeling and progression to CHF?

   A. Lisinopril
   B. Atenolol
   C. Isosorbide dinitrate
   D. Aspirin
   E. Amiodarone

5. Which of the following has not been shown to decrease mortality during or after acute MI?

   A. Aspirin
   B. Metoprolol
   C. Enalapril
   D. Isosorbide dinitrate
   E. Streptokinase

PATIENT PROFILE 98

BACTEREMIA AND SEPSIS

PRESENTATION

TN is a 77-year-old, 80-kg white male who was admitted to the intensive care unit after resection of colon cancer. Other problems TN is experiencing include atrial fibrillation, *Staphylococcus aureus* pneumonia, gastrointestinal (GI) bleeding, and a question of bowel ischemia. His past medical history includes a myocardial infarction (MI) with an ejection fraction of 25%, ischemic heart disease, an international normalization ratio (INR) of greater than 8, atrial fibrillation, benign prostatic hypertrophy, right lower lobectomy, and colon cancer. Laboratory values are consistent with infection. Culture results are as follows:

10/2	Sputum: 1 + *Aspergillus fumigatus*
10/12	Blood: Enterococci sensitive to ampicillin, gentamicin (in combination with ampicillin), and vancomycin
10/12	Sputum: 4 + *Staphylococcus aureus* sensitive to tetracycline, Bactrim (trimethoprim-sulfamethoxazole), levofloxacin, cefazolin, clindamycin, erythromycin, and oxacillin
10/15	Gallbladder: 3 + enterococci sensitive to ampicillin, gentamicin (in combination with ampicillin), and vancomycin

Active infections include the enterococcal bacteremia, *S. aureus* pneumonia, and enterococcal gallbladder infection.

QUESTIONS

1. Which of the following antibiotic regimens would you consider the *best choice* to manage TN's gallbladder infection?

   A. Because vancomycin covers all gram-positive infections including enterococci, it should be considered the standard of therapy in all enterococcal infections. Dose at 1g IV q12h.
   B. Metronidazole traditionally is considered to cover infections below the diaphragm. By anatomic design, the gallbladder lies below the diaphragm and should be covered by 500 mg IV q8h.
   C. The culture and sensitivity results can be used to guide your antibiotic therapy. Ampicillin 2 g IV q6h + gentamicin 80 mg IV q12h for synergy against the enterococci should be the therapy of choice.
   D. A second-generation cephalosporin such as cefotetan 1 g IV q12h can be used to manage this enterococcal infection below the diaphragm.
   E. A third-generation cephalosporin such as ceftriaxone, which is eliminated partially through the hepatobiliary tree, can be used to manage this gallbladder infection.

2. Further laboratory reporting of the culture results shows the strain of *S. aureus* in TN's sputum to be methicillin resistant. TN has normal renal function. After discontinuing the selected antibioitcs, which antibiotic should be used to treat TN for methicillin-resistant *S. aureus* (MRSA)?

   A. Imipenem 500 mg IV q6h
   B. Vancomycin 1 g IV q12h
   C. Imipenem 500 mg IV q12h
   D. Vancomycin 1g IV q6h
   E. Nafcillin 2 g IV q6h

3. TN has severe diarrhea with green, foul-smelling stool. A stool sample for *Clostridium difficile* toxin and fecal leukocytes has been sent to the microbiology laboratory for identification. Which therapy and dose would you select, if any, for empirical management of *C. difficile* colitis?

   A. Two *Lactobacillus* packets mixed in apple sauce before each meal
   B. Vancomycin 1 g IV q12h
   C. Yogurt with activated cultures tid
   D. Metronidazole 500 mg PO tid
   E. Wait for culture results before beginning treatment.

4. Which of the following statements is the *most correct* regarding vancomycin monitoring for TN?

   A. In general, a peak level between 20 and 50 mg/dL and a trough level of less than 10 mg/dL are considered therapeutic.
   B. The sample for the peak vancomycin level should be drawn immediately after the infusion has been completed.
   C. Vancomycin should be infused over 15 to 30 minutes.
   D. Vancomycin dosing is based on ideal body weight.
   E. All these statements regarding vancomycin are true.

5. All the following can be considered toxicities of vancomycin except

   A. "Red-man syndrome" can occur with rapid infusion < 60 minutes.
   B. Trough accumulation over time may necessitate dose adjustment.
   C. Nephrotoxicity may occur when vancomycin is used in the absence of other nephrotoxic drugs.
   D. Nephrotoxicity may occur when vancomycin is used in combination with aminoglycosides.
   E. Ototoxicity may occur.

ASTHMA

124   PATIENT PROFILE 100, SKI...

PE: Slightly obese w...
BP 150/90 mm ...
Labs: Electr...
WBC 9.5 c...

QUE...

PRESENTATION

SS is a 16-year-old hockey player with exercise-induced asthma. He has no other symptoms.

QUESTIONS

1. Which of the following agents would be appropriate for SS to use for prophylaxis before exercise?

    A. Albuterol inhaler
    B. Cromolyn inhaler
    C. Fluticasone inhaler
    D. A or B
    E. A, B, or C

2. Should SS have an acute asthmatic attack while playing hockey, which of the following would be appropriate to control bronchospasm?

    A. Albuterol inhaler
    B. Cromolyn inhaler
    C. Fluticasone inhaler
    D. A or B
    E. A, B, or C

3. SS's physician now prescribes salmeterol for prevention of exercise-induced asthma. How should SS be counseled on the use of this agent?

    A. Salmetero...
        exercising...
    B. Salmeter...
        exercising...
    C. Salmeter...
        before exe......
    D. Salmeterol should be inhaled 2 hours ....
        exercise.
    E. Salmeterol should be inhaled 4 hours before exercise.

4. SS is concerned about potential side effects of use of the inhaler. Which of the following is a common side effect of inhalation of selective β_2 agonists?

    A. Weight gain
    B. Growth suppression
    C. Oral thrush
    D. Muscle tremors
    E. Gastric ulceration

5. Cardiovascular effects are more commonly associated with less selective β-agonists. Of the following β_2 agonists, which is the least selective agent?

    A. Albuterol
    B. Isoproterenol
    C. Bitolterol
    D. Pirbuterol
    E. Salmeterol

SKIN AND SOFT TISSUE INFECTIONS AND OSTEOMYELITIS

PRESENTATION

HG is a 65-year-old woman who consults her primary care provider (PCP) because of pain, redness, and swelling in her left ankle that has gotten progressively worse over the last 24 hours. She tells the PCP that the day before the onset of these symptoms she had done major "spring cleaning" in her garden and had sustained several sometimes bleeding deep scratches when trimming her thorny hedges. She had cleaned the wounds with water and soap but soon the pain started, and now she can barely lift her leg. The PCP diagnoses cellulitis and asks for your advice in managing this patient.

PMH: Peripheral vascular disease
Hypertension (currently not treated)
Medications: Multivitamins
ASA 325 mg PO QD
SH: Regular alcohol use (2 glasses of wine/day)
Allergies: Sulfa drugs (rash)

oman in no acute distress
Hg, HR 80 beats/min, Temp 37.4°C
olytes WNL
lls/mm³, no differential done

TIONS

1. Which of the following are the most common microorganisms associated with cellulitis?

A. Staphylococci
B. Streptococci
C. Staphylococci and streptococci
D. Gram-negative bacteria
E. Gram-negative and -positive bacteria

2. Which of the following should be used to treat HG?

A. PO Bactrim for 7 to 14 days and analgesics as needed, and she should elevate and immobilize her leg.
B. PO cefixime for 7 to 14 days, analgesics as needed, and she should apply ice packs to the leg.
C. PO ciprofloxacin for 7 to 14 days, and analgesics as needed, and she should elevate and immobilize her leg and apply cool saline dressings.
D. PO dicloxacillin for 7 to 14 days, and analgesics as needed, and she should elevate and immobilize her leg and apply cool saline dressings.
E. PO ampicillin for 7 to 14 days, and analgesics as needed, and she should elevate and immobilize her leg and apply cool saline dressings.

3. A few weeks later, HG returns to her PCP and claims that after initial improvement with the prescribed antibiotic (and subsequently discontinuation of the drug), her symptoms returned. She has now a very swollen and inflamed ankle and lower leg that is extremely painful to touch with several superficial lesions. She is also complaining of chills and a fever of 38.5°C. It is decided to hospitalize HG, and a wound culture is ordered. A suitable treatment could include any of the following agents *except*:

A. Nafcillin 1 to 1.5 g IV q 6H
B. Ceftriaxone 1 g IV q 24H
C. Cefazolin 1 to 2 g IV q 8H
D. Clindamycin 600 mg IV q 8H
E. Aztreonam 1 g IV q 8H

4. The wound culture shows MRSA sensitive to all antibiotics that were tested on the panel in the microbiology laboratory. Appropriate treatment options for MRSA infections may include any of the following agents *except*:

A. Vancomycin
B. Daptomycin

C. Linezolid
D. Quinupristin/dalfopristin
E. Imipenem

The medical intern taking care of the patient HG wants to know characteristic potential adverse drug reactions (ADR) associated with some of the drugs mentioned in Question 4. Match the following drugs with the correct ADR.

5. Vancomycin   A. Neutropenia, thrombocytopenia, MAO inhibition
6. Linezolid   B. Red man syndrome, ototoxicity, phlebitis
7. Imipenem   C. Seizures, allergies

8. HG's therapy is subsequently changed to an appropriate drug for MRSA. Two days after starting her intravenous (IV) therapy the swelling on her leg has somewhat decreased but her pain continues, and localized tenderness, erythema, as well as drainage from an open wound on her lower leg adjacent to the ankle are noticed. An x-ray of her lower leg shows a skin abscess. The physician intends to open and drain the abscess and also wants to initiate therapy for anaerobes. A suitable treatment at this point would be to add which of the following?

A. Metronidazole
B. Ceftazidime
C. Clindamycin
D. A or C
E. A or B

9. After appropriate management of the abscess it turns out that the longstanding infectious process has affected HG's ankle bone, and plain bone films and bone scan results are consistent with the diagnosis of secondary osteomyelitis (contiguous spread). With respect to managing this disease, which of the following statements is/are correct?

I. Antibiotics need to be given intravenously and in high doses to achieve adequate concentrations in the bone.
II. New treatment approaches consider oral therapy for 4 to 6 weeks as follow-up to an initial 2-week IV treatment.
III. Empiric therapy for contiguous-spread osteomyelitis should include coverage against gram-positive and -negative organisms as well as anaerobes.

A. I only
B. II only
C. III only
D. I and II
E. All of the above statements are correct.

10. A bone biopsy shows *Pseudomonas aeruginosa* as the causative agent in HG's osteomyelitis. Assuming the organism is sensitive to all antipseudomonal drugs on the hospital formulary, and the renal function of the patient is normal, the physician wants to know if the combination of gentamicin 2 mg/kg IV q 8 to 12 hours plus ceftazidime 2 g IV q 8h (both given for at least 4 weeks) is a suitable synergistic treatment regimen for HG. You tell him which of the following?

A. This regimen is synergistic and appropriate.
B. This regimen is not synergistic and inappropriate.

PATIENT PROFILE 101
OINTMENTS

PRESENTATION

A commercially available 1-lb ointment product contains drug in a concentration of 0.5% w/w.

QUESTIONS

1. How many grams of drug are present in 1 lb of the commercial product?

    A. 0.0005
    B. 2.27
    C. 200
    D. 227
    E. 908

2. How many grams of ointment base should be added to 1 lb of the commercial product to produce a drug concentration of 1:1000 w/w?

    A. 114
    B. 454
    C. 568
    D. 1816
    E. 2270

3. How many grams of pure drug powder should be added to 1 lb of the commercial product to produce a drug concentration of 3% w/w?

    A. 11.4
    B. 11.7
    C. 13.6
    D. 73.4
    E. 75.7

4. Express the concentration of drug in 1 lb of the commercial product in terms of milligrams drug per gram of ointment.

    A. 0.0005
    B. 0.5
    C. 2
    D. 5
    E. 200

5. Which of the following is true regarding the compounding of an ointment dosage form by the addition of drug powder to ointment?

    A. The compounded product is a dosage form that is softer in texture than the original ointment itself.
    B. The compounded product is a dosage form that is stiffer in texture than the original ointment itself.
    C. The addition of mineral oil (a nonsolvent) to the drug powder facilitates incorporation of the powder into the ointment.
    D. A and C
    E. B and C

PATIENT PROFILE 102
OPPORTUNISTIC INFECTIONS

PRESENTATION

TC is a 32-year-old, 64-kg, white, homosexual man admitted to the hospital with shortness of breath, fever, and a dry cough of 2 weeks duration. A chest radiograph reveals bilateral interstitial markings, and arterial blood gas analysis reveals hypoxemia with a PaO_2 of 55 mm Hg, $PaCO_2$ of 44 mm Hg, and a pH of 7.3. Hypertonic saline nebulization of sputum induction and subsequent bronchoalveolar lavage were performed. Examination of the specimens revealed intracystic bodies and extracystic trophozoites. TC is given the diagnosis of moderate *Pneumocystis carinii* pneumonia (PCP). He had never been tested for HIV infection, and this episode of PCP is his AIDS-defining illness. He has NKDA. Ibuprofen, acetaminophen on an as-needed (PRN) basis, and antibiotics for bacteria pneumonia are the only medications that he has taken in the past.

QUESTIONS

1. Which the following is the most appropriate treatment regimen for TC?

   A. Initiate trimethoprim-sulfamethoxazole (TMP-SMZ) therapy and corticosteroid therapy for approximately 21 days.
   B. Initiate dapsone therapy with corticosteroid therapy for approximately 21 days.
   C. Initiate trimetrexate therapy and folinic acid along with corticosteroid therapy for approximately 21 days.
   D. Initiate TMP-SMZ therapy for approximately 21 days; corticosteroid therapy is not warranted in the treatment of this patient.
   E. Initiate dapsone therapy for approximately 21 days; corticosteroid therapy is not warranted in the treatment of this patient.

2. TC responds well to 21 days of therapy for PCP. This patient needs secondary prophylaxis. Which is the preferred prophylactic regimen for TC?

   A. Trimethoprim-sulfamethoxazole (TMP-SMZ)
   B. Dapsone
   C. Aerosolized pentamidine
   D. Atovaquone
   E. Dapsone, pyrimethamine, and leucovorin

3. Once the acute PCP infection resolved, TC's physician ordered viral load studies and a CD4+ cell count. The results were as follows: viral load 300,000 copies/mL (Quantiplex™ HIV RNA assay and CD4+

cell count 45 mm^3). The physician wants to initiate antiretroviral therapy with two nucleoside reverse transcriptase inhibitors and one protease inhibitor. He wants to avoid choosing agents that have similar toxicity profiles. Which of the following regimens has at least two agents with similar toxicity profiles and would not be a good initial regimen?

   A. Zidovudine (Retrovir®, AZT), lamivudine (Epivir®, 3TC), and indinavir (Crixivan®)
   B. Didanosine (Videx®, ddI), zalcitabine (Hivid®, ddC), and nelfinavir (Viracept®)
   C. Zidovudine (Retrovir®, AZT), didanosine (Videx®, ddI), and saquinavir (Fortovase®)
   D. Lamivudine (Epivir®, 3TC), abacavir (Ziagen™), and nelfinavir (Viracept®)
   E. Stavudine (Zerit®, d4T), lamivudine (Epivir®, 3TC), and nelfinavir (Viracept®)

4. Which of the following agents is matched appropriately with its class and potential adverse effect?

   A. Stavudine (Zerit®); nucleoside reverse transcriptase inhibitor; peripheral neuropathy
   B. Atazanavir (Reyataz); non-nucleoside reverse transcriptase inhibitor; anemia
   C. Abacavir (Ziagen®); protease inhibitor; nephrolithiasis
   D. Nelfinavir (Viracept®); nucleoside reverse transcriptase inhibitor; hyperthyroidism
   E. Zalcitabine (Hivid®); protease inhibitor, anemia

5. The physician also wants to initiate *Mycobacterium avium-intracellulare* complex (MAC) prophylaxis because TC's CD4+ count is low. Which of the following is/are appropriate prophylactic therapy for MAC?

   A. Clarithromycin (Biaxin®)
   B. Azithromycin (Zithromax®)
   C. Ciprofloxacin (Cipro®)
   D. A and B
   E. All of the above

6. Cryptococcal meningitis is an opportunistic infection that can occur in patients with AIDS. Which of the following is the appropriate therapy of choice for treatment of acute cryptococcal meningitis in patients with AIDS?

   A. Clarithromycin (Biaxin®)
   B. Amphotericin B, plus flucytosine

C. Ketoconazole (Nizoral®)
D. Azithromycin (Zithromax®)
E. Ciprofloxacin (Cipro®)

7. Cytomegalovirus (CMV) retinitis is an opportunistic infection that can occur in patients with AIDS. One of the antiviral agents, ganciclovir, has been used to treat CMV retinitis. Which of the following statements is the dose-limiting toxicity of this agent?

A. Hepatitis
B. Neutropenia
C. Retinopathy
D. Hyperkalemia
E. Cardiac arrhythmias

8. Which of the statements is true about the antiviral agents listed in the following?

A. Cidofovir is a nucleotide analogue that is well absorbed (bioavailability approximately 80%).
B. Cidofovir has a long intracellular half-life resulting in less frequent administration (e.g., once weekly therapy).
C. Ganciclovir is a prodrug of valganciclovir.
D. Hepatotoxicity is the dose-limiting toxicity of cidofovir.
E. Hepatotoxicity is the dose-limiting toxicity of foscarnet.

9. Toxoplasma encephalitis is an opportunistic infection that can occur in patients with AIDS. One of the options of treatment is sulfadiazine and pyrimethamine plus leucovorin. Which of the following statements is true about management with sulfadiazine, pyrimethamine plus leucovorin?

A. Sulfadiazine is a para-aminobenzoic acid (PABA) analogue that competitively inhibits dihydropteroate synthase and prevents synthesis of folic acid in bacteria.
B. Pyrimethamine is a PABA analogue that competitively inhibits dihydropteroate synthase and prevents synthesis of folic acid in bacteria.
C. Leucovorin is an inhibitor of dihydrofolate reductase.
D. Sulfadiazine is an inhibitor of dihydrofolate reductase.
E. Pyrimethamine inhibits DNA synthesis, primarily by interfering with the biosynthesis of thymidylate.

10. A patient with AIDS is receiving intravenous amphotericin B therapy for an opportunistic antifungal infection. Which of the following is the correct dose-limiting toxicity of this agent?

A. Hepatitis
B. Hemorrhagic cystitis
C. Nephrotoxicity
D. Congestive heart failure
E. Cardiac arrhythmias

PATIENT PROFILE 103
RESPIRATORY TRACT INFECTION

PRESENTATION

MK is a 34-year-old white man who comes to the emergency department because of shortness of breath, pleuritic chest pain, and a 2-day history of diarrhea. He is not bringing up much sputum, but a chest x-ray shows bilateral patchy infiltrates that suggest pneumonia.

QUESTIONS

1. Which would be the most likely choice of antibiotic for this hospitalized patient with community-acquired pneumonia?

A. Ceftazidime and tobramycin
B. Ceftriaxone and azithromycin
C. Penicillin and erythromycin
D. Clindamycin and metronidazole
E. Trimethoprim-sulfamethoxazole

2. After 1 day of therapy, a rash develops. An alternative single agent that can be used intravenously or orally to manage pathogens that cause community-acquired pneumonia (Streptococcus pneumoniae and atypical pathogens) would be which of the following?

A. Levofloxacin
B. Clindamycin
C. Imipenem
D. Cefixime
E. Loracarbef

3. A *Legionella* urine antigen assay comes back negative. This can be translated into which of the following clinical manifestations?

   A. Macrolide therapy should be discontinued because this patient does not have *Legionella* infection.
   B. Discontinue the β-lactam therapy and continue the macrolide because the patient most likely does not have pneumococcal pneumonia.
   C. Switch antibiotic therapy primarily to cover anaerobes.
   D. A negative urine antigen test result does not confirm that a patient does not have *Legionella* infection, and macrolide therapy should be continued.
   E. Discontinue all antibiotic therapy and follow chest x-rays and the fever curve.

4. Erythromycin is likely to be used to manage community-acquired pneumonia, and administration of this antibiotic does not necessitate hospitalization. Which is the most common adverse reaction associated with both IV and oral administration of erythromycin?

   A. Prolonged QT interval leading to torsades de pointes when used with nonsedating antihistamines such as astemizole
   B. Motilin activation in the GI tract that initiates uncoordinated peristalsis resulting in anorexia, nausea, or vomiting
   C. Transient reversible deafness or tinnitus with doses higher than 4 g/d among patients with hepatic or renal dysfunction
   D. Cholestatic hepatitis among adults but not children
   E. Rash

5. Culture shows a highly resistant strain of *Streptococcus pneumoniae* with an MIC >2. Which of the following IV antibiotics will provide coverage against this highly resistant strain?

   A. Vancomycin and rifampin
   B. Vancomycin as a single agent
   C. Cefotaxime
   D. Ceftriaxone
   E. All of the above

PATIENT PROFILE 104

ASTHMA

PRESENTATION

MM is a 44-year-old woman who presents to your outpatient clinic complaining of chest pain, shortness of breath, wheezing, and cough. This is the first time you have seen MM as she was referred to you. She states that this problem started about a year ago and forced her to see her primary care physician. At that time she was given an inhaler that she uses if she needs it. MM states that she has not been using the inhaler for the past 4 months because the prescription has run out and she has not been able to contact her physician for a new one. MM states that even after the appointment she suffered from shortness of breath occasionally, but the inhaler did help while she had it. She states that difficulty breathing has become more recurrent over the past month or so. MM has never smoked; she drinks about 4 glasses of wine per week, and enjoys running when she has time and is physically able to do so. She has one dog that she has had for about 15 years. MM states that the only over the counter or herbal medications she is taking are a daily multivitamin, Lamisil® for athlete's foot,

and ibuprofen for occasional aches and pains. She states that her only other medical condition besides asthma is insomnia. She currently is a single mother of one and works in a textile factory in Fall River. She is an only child and her mother and father are both alive and healthy with no known medical conditions. During your work-up it is determined that she is experiencing the mentioned symptoms approximately 3 times per week with no nighttime symptoms. Her FEV1 is 80% of personal best, with normal white blood cells and sputum. An FEV1/FVC has yet to be calculated.

Medication History:
Daily multivitamin
Lamisil® apply twice a day for 14 days
Ibuprofen 200 mg as needed for occasional aches and pains
Albuterol inhaler one or two puffs by mouth every 4 to 6 hours as needed
Ambien® 5 mg by mouth every night at bedtime

Medical History:
Athlete's foot
Asthma
Insomnia

QUESTIONS

1. Based on MM's information what classification of asthma is most appropriate?

   A. Step 0, at risk for asthma
   B. Step 1, mild intermittent asthma
   C. Step 2, mild persistent asthma
   D. Step 3, moderate persistent asthma
   E. Step 4, severe persistent asthma

2. What nonpharmacologic therapy is the best recommendation for MM?

   A. Give away the dog.
   B. Increase her exercise.
   C. Receive the influenza vaccine.
   D. Remove any rugs in the house.
   E. Decrease alcohol consumption.

3. Which of MM's medications has the potential to exacerbate an asthma attack?

   A. Daily multivitamin
   B. Lamisil® apply twice a day for 14 days
   C. Ambien® 5 mg by mouth every night at bedtime
   D. Ibuprofen 200 mg as needed for occasional aches and pains
   E. None of the above

4. What is the best option for first-line chronic therapy for MM?

   A. Albuterol MDI as needed and one prednisone 5-mg tablet every day for 10 days
   B. Albuterol MDI as needed and salmeterol discus one puff by mouth two times a day
   C. Albuterol MDI as needed and Qvar® 40-µg inhaler four puffs by mouth four times a day
   D. Albuterol MDI as needed and ipratropium inhaler two puffs by mouth every 4 to 6 hours
   E. Albuterol MDI as needed and fluticasone 88-µg inhaler one puff by mouth two times a day

5. Which of the following is the most appropriate counseling point for MM concerning her albuterol MDI?

   A. It should never be primed.
   B. You must wash your mouth out after use.
   C. Approximately 90% of the dose will reach your lungs.

   D. Actuation should occur 1 to 2 seconds prior to inhalation.
   E. The dose of the medication can "tail off" toward the end of the canister.

6. Which of the following is a common side effect of the albuterol MM is taking?

   A. Cough
   B. Tremor
   C. Glaucoma
   D. Oral thrush
   E. Hypokalemia

7. Which of the following is an advantage of a dry powder inhaler over the albuterol MDI that MM has been using?

   A. Smaller size
   B. More portable
   C. Increased sturdiness
   D. Concomitant use with a spacer
   E. Less patient technique dependent

8. MM inquires if an asthmatic medication is available in tablet form. She has had a difficult time using the inhalers and is looking for an alterative. Which of the following medications is most appropriate to recommend for MM?

   A. Pirbuterol
   B. Formoterol
   C. Montelukast
   D. Theophylline
   E. Nedocromil sodium

9. MM returns to your clinic 6 months later and complains of shortness of breath while she is sleeping. She states that this occurs two to three times weekly. What is the next appropriate step taken to better manage MM's asthma?

   A. Initiate Singulair® 10 mg every night at bedtime.
   B. Initiate theophylline 400 mg by mouth four times a day.
   C. Initiate cromolyn sodium inhale one puff by mouth every day.
   D. Initiate Serevent Diskus® inhale one puff by mouth twice a day.
   E. Increase the albuterol dose to four inhalations by mouth every 6 hours.

10. When should MM be evaluated to determine if the most recent addition to her therapy can be discontinued?

    A. 1 to 3 months
    B. 3 to 6 months
    C. 6 to 9 months
    D. 9 to 12 months
    E. Over a year

PATIENT PROFILE 105

TUBERCULOSIS

PRESENTATION

CS is a 31-year-old woman who comes to the clinic and states, "I feel tired and weak, and I've lost weight over the past few weeks." She also has had a cough and fever over the past few weeks. She thought she had the flu but did not improve and feels worse. Her medical history includes diabetes, which is well controlled with insulin. She also takes oral contraceptives and a multivitamin daily. She does not drink or smoke. When questioned about her occupation, CS answers that she works in a nursing home as a nursing assistant. A PPD skin test is administered, and sputum specimens are obtained. The PPD skin test result is positive, and chest radiography and clinical evaluation support the diagnosis of tuberculosis. Baseline laboratory values are within normal limits. The patient is placed in isolation, and treatment with isoniazid, rifampin, pyrazinamide, and streptomycin is initiated.

QUESTIONS

1. Tuberculosis is spread mainly by

   A. contact with items touched by an infected patient.
   B. inhaling infectious airborne particles coughed by an infected patient.
   C. contact with animals with tuberculosis.
   D. skin contact with an infected patient.
   E. none of the above.

2. A potentially life-threatening adverse effect of isoniazid is

   A. congestive heart failure.
   B. hepatotoxicity.
   C. renal failure.
   D. stroke.
   E. pulmonary embolism.

3. Which of the following statement(s) concerning isoniazid is/are true?

   A. This patient should receive pyridoxine with isoniazid.
   B. Isoniazid is a potent inducer of hepatic microsomal enzymes.
   C. Hyperuricemia occurs frequently with this drug, and a baseline uric acid concentration should be measured before initiation of therapy.
   D. A and B
   E. All of the above

4. The intern wants to know which toxicities are possible with streptomycin. You reply that the main toxicity/toxicities associated with this agent is/are:

   A. nephrotoxicity.
   B. ototoxicity.
   C. hepatitis.
   D. A and B.
   E. all of the above.

5. Which of the following statement(s) concerning rifampin therapy is/are true?

   A. CS should be counseled to use alternative forms of birth control while taking rifampin.
   B. CS should be counseled that rifampin may impart an orange discoloration to urine, stool, sputum, saliva, tears, and sweat and that soft contact lenses may be permanently discolored.
   C. Rifampin is primarily eliminated through the kidneys. The dose must be adjusted if renal impairment occurs to prevent accumulation of the drug.
   D. A and B
   E. All of the above

PATIENT PROFILE 106
^{32}P CONSIDERATIONS

PRESENTATION

A pharmacist has three 10-mL ^{32}P-chromic phosphate vials, each containing four mCi/mL. They are dropped in the hood, and break open, spilling the contents. Presuming the contents can be left to decay, and decay for 10 half-lives is considered to "background," answer the following:

$$(t_{1/2} \; ^{32}P = 14.3 \; days)$$

QUESTIONS

1. How long will it take until 80% of the ^{32}P is decayed?

   A. 4.6 days
   B. 11.4 days
   C. 22.7 days
   D. 33.2 days
   E. 73.4 days

2. How long will it take to reach background levels?

   A. 14.3 days
   B. 71.5 days
   C. 143 days
   D. 286 days
   E. It will never entirely reach background.

3. What type of emission does ^{32}P have?

   A. Alpha
   B. Beta
   C. Gamma
   D. Positron
   E. X-ray

4. Which type of material should be used to shield the spill area?

   A. Lucite
   B. Lead
   C. Steel
   D. Uranium
   E. Gold

5. How many atoms of ^{32}P are represented by 12 mCi?

   A. 3.75×10^{22}
   B. 4.44×10^{8}
   C. 5.61×10^{7}
   D. 6.23×10^{12}
   E. 7.91×10^{14}

6. How many MB of ^{32}P are present at the time of the spill?

   A. 4.44×10^{3}
   B. 3.24×10^{3}
   C. 1.11×10^{3}
   D. 4.44×10^{6}
   E. 3.24×10^{6}

7. In reference to Question 4 (which type of material should be used), *why* is that material best?

   A. To decrease gamma emission
   B. To decrease Auger electron emission
   C. To increase x-ray emission
   D. To decrease Bremsstrahlung emission
   E. To decrease positron emission

8. One week after the spill and original assay, it is discovered one vial still contains 1.2 mL of volume. What activity remains in this volume at this time?

   A. 2.4 mCi
   B. 3.4 mCi
   C. 12.0 mCi
   D. 24 mCi
   E. 1.2 mCi

9. Which of the following is considered a normal dose of ^{32}P-chromic phosphate for treatment of pleural effusion?

   A. 10 μCi
   B. 100 μCi
   C. 1 mCi
   D. 10 mCi
   E. 100 mCi

10. The above dose is given

   A. By mouth
   B. By instillation
   C. By inhalation
   D. By intravenous injection
   E. By intramuscular injection

PATIENT PROFILE 107

ONCOLOGY: HODGKIN'S LYMPHOMA

PRESENTATION

ED is a 38-year-old man who visits his physician with vague symptoms of malaise, night sweats, intermittent fever, and swollen cervical lymph nodes. ED had been otherwise healthy his entire life. The only significant finding in the medical history is surgery for a torn ACL in his left knee. ED takes no scheduled medications. He uses acetaminophen for minor aches and pains. He has no known allergies.

PHYSICAL EXAMINATION

BP: 118/74, HR: 68, T: 100.6°F
Ht: 5'11", Wt: 170 lb
HEENT: Enlarged, nontender cervical lymph nodes
ABD: No palpable masses, nondistended, nontender

LABS

Electrolytes: WNL
Radiologic evaluation: Chest and abdominal CT findings suggest nodal involvement on both sides of the diaphragm

ED is found to have stage III Hodgkin's disease and will undergo chemotherapy and radiation therapy.

QUESTIONS

1. Chemotherapy will consist of alternating courses of MOPP (mechlorethamine, vincristine, prednisone, and procarbazine) and ABVD (doxorubicin, bleomycin, vinblastine, and dacarbazine). After six cycles of therapy, ED reports shortness of breath. Which agent is most likely responsible for this effect?

   A. Vincristine
   B. Bleomycin
   C. Vinblastine
   D. Procarbazine
   E. Doxorubicin

2. With this combination of antineoplastic agents, ED will experience bone marrow suppression. An attempt is made to use agents with different toxicities, because some of the agents do not cause severe bone marrow suppression. Which agents in the regimen are least likely to affect the bone marrow?

   A. Prednisone and vinblastine
   B. Procarbazine and doxorubicin
   C. Vincristine and bleomycin
   D. Prednisone and doxorubicin
   E. Vinblastine and dacarbazine

3. Which component of the treatment regimen will most likely increase ED's risk of doxorubicin-induced cardiotoxicity?

   A. Concurrent use of bleomycin
   B. Concurrent chest irradiation
   C. Sequential treatment with procarbazine
   D. Sequential treatment with prednisone
   E. Concurrent inguinal node irradiation

4. Treatment to control nausea and vomiting will be an important component of therapy. In the antineoplastic regimen described, which antiemetic regimen would be most appropriate for control of acute nausea and vomiting?

   A. Prochlorperazine 10 mg IM q4h
   B. Metoclopramide 10 mg IV q8h
   C. Perphenazine 5 mg IM q4h prn with diphenhydramine 50 mg IV q4h prn
   D. Ondansetron 24 mg po and dexamethasone 10 mg IV before treatment
   E. Granisetron 1 mg IV q6h prn

5. ED completes treatment. Long-term effects of this treatment regimen will most likely include

   A. increased risk of a secondary malignant tumor
   B. increased risk of coronary artery disease.
   C. decreased risk of hyperlipidemia.
   D. decreased risk of COPD.
   E. increased risk of male pattern baldness.

OBSESSIVE COMPULSIVE DISORDER

PRESENTATION

TP is a 19-year-old man who has been referred to a psychiatric clinic by a dermatologist. TP states that his skin is red, dry, and flaking. Upon further questioning, he states that he washes his hands approximately 150 times per day and that it takes him, on average, 4 hours to complete his morning shower. He states that he knows this does not make sense, but he has intrusive thoughts about dirt and germs and cannot get through the rest of his day unless he takes a 4-hour shower. He is in danger of failing his first semester of college because his cleaning behaviors take 8 to 9 hours per day, leaving him very little time to attend classes and study.

PE: Height 6'2", Weight 220 lb
Allergies: NKDA
PMH: Noncontributory
SH: Denies tobacco, alcohol, and illicit drug use
Caffeine: Three to four cups of coffee per day; two to
   three caffeinated sodas per day. (He states that he
   needs the caffeine to stay awake in class.)
FH: No known family history of medical or psychiatric
   disorders
ROS/PE: TP is a freshman at a local college. He denies
   headache, seizures, chest pain, nausea, vomiting, diarrhea, constipation, shortness of breath, or urinary incontinence. His physical examination is noncontributory except his skin is dry, with some desquamation
   and redness, primarily involving the hands.
Laboratory and Diagnostic Tests: No laboratory information is available at this time.
Diagnosis: Obsessive compulsive disorder (OCD)
CM: TP is currently taking no medications.

QUESTIONS

1. TP asks for an explanation of OCD. Which of the following statements regarding OCD is/are true?

    I.   OCD is classified as an anxiety disorder.
    II. OCD requires the presence of obsessions or compulsions that cause marked distress or significantly interfere with daily functioning.
    III. Adults with OCD usually realize that their obsessions and compulsions are excessive or unreasonable.

    A. I only
    B. II only
    C. I and II only
    D. II and III only
    E. I, II, and III

2. The compulsion that TP is experiencing can best be described by which one of the following statements?

    A. Intrusive or recurrent thoughts of dirt and germs
    B. Intrusive or recurrent thoughts of failing his first semester of college
    C. Washing his hands 150 times per day and showering for 4 hours per day
    D. Seeing a dermatologist to treat his dry, red, flaking skin
    E. Finding other activities to do instead of studying

3. Which of the following is the leading hypothesis for the etiology of OCD?

    A. Dopaminergic dysfunction
    B. Serotonergic dysfunction
    C. Noradrenergic dysfunction
    D. Anticholinergic dysfunction
    E. GABAergic dysfunction

4. Which one of the following tricyclic antidepressants (TCA) is Food and Drug Administration (FDA) approved for the treatment of OCD?

    A. Amitriptyline
    B. Nortriptyline
    C. Doxepin
    D. Imipramine
    E. Clomipramine

5. First-line medication treatments for OCD include which of the following medications?

    I.   Fluvoxamine, fluoxetine, paroxetine, sertraline
    II. Clomipramine, fluvoxamine, fluoxetine, paroxetine
    III. Venlafaxine, clomipramine, fluvoxamine, fluoxetine

    A. I only
    B. III only
    C. I and II only
    D. II and III only
    E. I, II, and III

6. Which of the following statements regarding the use of benzodiazepines in the treatment of OCD is/are true?

    I.   In general, benzodiazepines are not helpful in treating OCD.
    II. Drug interactions can occur between benzodiazepines and medications used to treat OCD.

III. Benzodiazepines can interfere with the effectiveness of cognitive behavioral therapy (CBT) and should not be used concurrently.

A. I only
B. III only
C. I and II only
D. II and III only
E. I, II, and III

7. The use of a selective serotonin reuptake inhibitor (SSRI) to treat TP's OCD is proposed. TP asks whether the medication will completely eliminate his obsessions and compulsions. Which one of the following is the most appropriate response to TP's questions?

A. Complete elimination of obsessions and compulsions can be expected within the first month of therapy.
B. Complete elimination of obsessions and compulsions can be expected within 8 to 12 weeks of the start of therapy.
C. Response to medication treatment in OCD is gradual; complete elimination of obsessions and compulsions may take as long as 5 to 6 months.
D. Complete elimination of obsessions and compulsions in OCD is rare with available treatments.
E. Medication for the treatment of OCD completely eliminates only the compulsions, not the obsessions.

8. The physician wants to start fluvoxamine for the treatment of OCD in TP. Which one of the following is the most appropriate initial recommended dosage for TP?

A. 25 mg per day
B. 50 mg per day
C. 100 mg per day
D. 150 mg per day
E. 200 mg per day

9. Fluvoxamine belongs to which one of the following medication classes?

A. Monoamine oxidase inhibitor
B. Tricyclic antidepressant
C. Selective serotonin reuptake inhibitor
D. Serotonin/norepinephrine reuptake inhibitor
E. Norepinephrine reuptake inhibitor

10. Which one of the following scales is used to monitor the response of OCD symptoms to pharmacologic and nonpharmacologic treatment?

A. BPRS (Brief Psychiatric Rating Scale)
B. PANSS (Positive and Negative Symptom Scale for Schizophrenia)
C. Y-BOCS (Yale-Brown Obsessive-Compulsive Symptom Checklist)
D. AIMS (Abnormal Involuntary Movement Scale)
E. CIWA-Ar (Clinical Institute Withdrawal Assessment-Alcohol, Revised)

PATIENT PROFILE 109

MEDICINAL CHEMISTRY

PRESENTATION AND QUESTION

While working in the pharmacy, you received a telephone call from TJ, a 50-year-old man who says he is unable to wake up in the morning to go to work. If he does awaken, he says he feels sleepy most of the day. The discussion reveals that TJ is taking Valium® (diazepam) (structure 109.1) at bedtime to help him fall asleep quickly.

1. Which of the following would you recommend to TJ?

A. Stop taking Valium® (diazepam), and ask your physician to consider changing the prescription to butabarbital (structure 109.2).

B. Continue taking Valium® (diazepam) but drink a full glass of orange juice with it as a urine acidifier to increase urinary elimination of the drug.
C. Continue taking Valium® (diazepam) but take it with soda as a urine alkalinizer to increase urinary elimination of the drug.
D. Stop taking Valium® (diazepam), and ask your physician to consider prescribing oxazepam instead (structure 109.3)
E. Continue taking Valium® (diazepam), but immediately before you go to sleep, drink a cup of coffee so that the caffeine will pharmacologically antagonize the effects of the drug during the night.

109.1   **109.2**   **109.3**

PATIENT PROFILE 110
MIXED DYSLIPIDEMIA

PRESENTATION

SS is a 68-year-old black man who was noted to have an elevated total cholesterol level (280 mg/dL) during a community screening program 2 months ago. Follow-up lipid levels performed at his physician's office upon routine examination revealed the following.

PMH: Hypertension for 9 years
SH: Smokes one pack per day; active (on local tennis club); retired school teacher; EtOH (12 oz/mo)
FH: Father died of a heart attack at 52 years of age; mother died at 78 years of age from unknown causes; 59-year-old sister is alive and well
MH: HZTC 25 mg po QD for 5 years; no pertinent OTC use; NKDA
ROS: Noncontributory
PE: BP 156/86 right arm, seated (average of three readings), Wt 63.5 kg, Ht 158 cm, rest of examination unremarkable

LABORATORY VALUES

Fasting glucose 145 mg/dL, Na+ 137 mEq/L, Cl⁻ 95 mEq/L, BUN 16 mg/dL, serum creatinine 1.4 mg/dL, TC 320 mg/dL, TG 390 mg/dL, HDL cholesterol 58 mg/dL, LDL cholesterol 184 mg/dL

QUESTIONS

1. How many independent coronary heart disease (CHD) risk factors (other than LDL) does SS have?

   A. 1
   B. 3
   C. 2
   D. 4
   E. 5

2. The physician wants to treat SS for hypercholesterolemia and hypertriglyceridemia. What drug combination is best for SS?

   A. HMG CoA: reductase inhibitor (statin) and fibrate
   B. Statin and niacin
   C. Statin and bile acid sequestrants
   D. Statin and ezetimibe
   E. Statin and fish oil

3. Which of the following fibrates is/are not available in the United States?

   A. Gemfibrozil
   B. Fenofibrate
   C. Ciprofibrate
   D. Clofibrate
   E. All of the above are available in the United States.

4. The physician has decided to use the fibrate fenofibrate in combination with a statin to treat SS. What is the usual daily dose of fenofibrate?

   A. 600 mg/day
   B. 600 mg bid
   C. 200 mg bid
   D. 200 mg/day
   E. 2000 mg/day

5. Which of the following adverse effects is not a potential major adverse effect of fenofibrate?

   A. Myopathy
   B. Cholesterol gallstones

C. Upper gastrointestinal complaints
D. Dyspepsia
E. Acute renal insufficiency

6. In which of the following diseases is fibrates contraindicated?

   A. Elevated complete blood count
   B. Asthma
   C. Severe hepatic insufficiency
   D. Congestive heart failure
   E. Seizures

7. When using fibrates in combination with statins there is an increased risk of developing which of the following?

   A. Glucose intolerance
   B. Myopathy
   C. Gallstones
   D. Heart failure
   E. Arrhythmias

8. If niacin is combined with the statin to treat SS a number of potential problems could arise. Which of the following laboratory values may be elevated because of niacin?

A. Sodium
B. LDL
C. Serum creatinine
D. Potassium
E. Glucose

9. What is the usual daily dose of crystalline (regular release) niacin?

   A. 0.5 to 1.0 g/day
   B. 1.5 to 3.0 g/day
   C. 0.5 to 1.0 mg/day
   D. 1.5 to 3.0 mg/day
   E. 3.0 to 4.5 g/day

10. Which of the following side effects of niacin can be alleviated by giving two 325-mg aspirins about 30 to 45 minutes before giving the niacin?

    A. Flushing
    B. Hyperuricemia
    C. Hepatotoxicity
    D. Dyspepsia
    E. Hyperglycemia

PATIENT PROFILE 111

BIPOLAR DISORDER

PRESENTATION

DW is a 20-year-old man who has been admitted to the psychiatric unit for what appears to be a manic episode. During the week before admission, the patient had been increasingly agitated, and his sleep had decreased to about 2 hours a night. During the interview DW states that he will be asked by the president to be a cabinet advisor for all diplomatic matters and that he needs to get ready to move to Washington, DC. DW also has been landscaping his yard and has been outside working on it through the night. Unfortunately, the yard is a mess with many unfinished projects. The patient is pacing the unit and asking all the staff to release him because he has to get to Washington to work for the president.

The patient has had as many as four of these episodes in the last year, yet the family has never had him admitted to the hospital because he seemed to return to normal within a week or two. This time, however, the neighbors called the police because of the late night yard work and because when the police arrived DW became very loud and belligerent, screaming that they were KGB officials trying to kidnap him to Russia.

The medical history is normal, and there are no known drug allergies. DW was taking no medications before ad-

mission. Since admission the previous night, DW has been given 4 mg lorazepam in 1-mg doses with fair effect. The family history provides no relevant findings. DW states that he drinks about 4 beers a day just to calm himself. He lives with his parents, attends community college, and is not working.

PHYSICAL EXAMINATION

BP sitting R arm: 130/80, HR: 80, T: 99°F

LABS

AST: 40 U/L
ALT: 44 U/L
Alk Phos: 60 U/L
Tox screen negative for cocaine, marijuana, opiates, barbiturates
Blood alcohol level 160 mg/dL

A/P: Since admission last night the patient has slept very little. He has received a total of 4 mg lorazepam over a 16-hour period with little effect. The patient continues to be very talkative and demanding at times. Thoughts are tangential and grandiose.

QUESTIONS

1. Which of the patient's symptom(s) is/are characteristic of a manic episode?

   A. Decreased sleep
   B. Grandiosity
   C. Tangential thinking
   D. A and B
   E. A, B, and C

2. Because it is possible that the patient has had up to four of these manic episodes, labeling him a rapid cycler, which medication is the drug of choice?

   A. Valproic acid
   B. Lithium
   C. Clonazepam
   D. Chlorpromazine
   E. Gabapentin

3. Which monitoring parameters are recommended when valproic acid is used?

   A. Liver function tests
   B. Serum valproic acid level
   C. Complete blood cell count
   D. A and B
   E. A, B, and C

4. What monitoring parameters are recommended when lithium is used?

   A. Thyroid function tests
   B. Serum lithium level
   C. Liver function tests
   D. A and B
   E. A, B, and C

5. Valproic acid toxicity has occurred with therapeutic dosage of which of the following drug(s)?

   A. ASA
   B. Phenobarbital
   C. Furosemide
   D. A and B
   E. A, B, and C

PATIENT PROFILE 112

CONTRACEPTION

PRESENTATION

TH is a 37-year-old woman who presents to her family physician complaining of increased weight gain since the initiation of Depo-Provera® (medroxyprogesterone) 8 months ago (Table 112-1). TH reports an increase of 11 pounds since starting Depo-Provera®.

There was no complaint of adverse effects at the 1-month follow-up visit. She now requests oral contraception and wishes to discontinue Depo-Provera®. She denies spotting, abdominal pain, or other adverse effects. TH states that she will consider an intrauterine device if an oral contraceptive is not tolerated.

PMH: Seasonal allergic rhinitis
Allergies: None
Current Meds: Depo-Provera® (dose and frequency not documented)
loratadine 10 mg po qd
ibuprofen 400 mg po qid prn for back pain

Table 112-1. Depo-Provera ® Use History

Time	First Dose	One-Month Follow-up	Second Dose	Third Dose	Fourth Dose	Wishes to Discontinue Therapy Before Fifth Dose
Weight (pounds)	115	115	118	118	123	126
BP (mm Hg)	100/70	100/60	112/64	110/80	100/72	110/70

FH: Noncontributory
SH: Denies alcohol, tobacco, and recreational drug use; lives with daughter
PE: BP: 110/70, HR 72, RR 16, Wt 126 lbs, Height 5'1"
Gen: Well appearing, comfortable, in no apparent distress
HEENT: Postnasal drip, uvula midline, no maxillary or frontal tenderness, neck supple, no lymphadenopathy
Chest: Clear to auscultation, no wheezing
COR: RRR, no murmurs
Musculoskeletal: Mild palpable left side tenderness at C5-C6, full range of movement, strength 5/5, DTR 2/2
Skin: No lesions

LABORATORY RESULTS

Lipid profile: TC 165 mg/dL, HDL 59 mg/dL; pap smear: (−) chlamydia, (−) gonorrhea; pregnancy test (−)

QUESTIONS

1. Which of the following best describes when the first dose of Depo-Provera® must be given for contraception?

   A. The first 5 days of a normal menstrual cycle
   B. The day that menses stops during a normal menstrual cycle
   C. The first 2 weeks of a normal menstrual cycle
   D. The day of ovulation during a normal menstrual cycle
   E. Anytime during a normal menstrual cycle

2. Which of the following best describes the frequency in which Depo-Provera® should be administered?

   A. Every week
   B. Every month
   C. Every 3 months
   D. Every 6 months
   E. Every 12 months

3. By which of the following routes should Depo-Provera® be administered?

   A. Intramuscular
   B. Intravaginal
   C. Intravenous
   D. Oral
   E. Subcutaneous

4. Which of the following is/are an adverse effect(s) of Depo-Provera®?

   reast tenderness
   pression
   ight gain
   nd C only
   , and C

5. Which of the following is a contraindication to combined oral contraceptives?

   A. Deep vein thrombosis
   B. Epilepsy
   C. Family history of breast cancer
   D. Infection with HIV
   E. Mild headache

6. Which of the following best describe(s) when to initiate oral contraceptive therapy when the patient is without current contraceptive methods?

   A. The first day of the next menses
   B. The first Sunday after the onset of menses
   C. At any time during the cycle
   D. A and B only
   E. A, B, and C

7. Which of the following reduce(s) the contraception effect of oral contraceptives and consequently require(s) the concomitant use of a back-up contraceptive method?

   A. Ethanol
   B. Tetracycline
   C. Warfarin
   D. A and B only
   E. A, B, and C

8. Which of the following is accurate patient counseling information about when menses will occur during a cycle with a monophasic oral contraceptive product?

   A. During week one of the active pills
   B. During week two of the active pills
   C. During week three of the active pills
   D. Every other week
   E. Within 1 to 3 days after the last active pill

9. Which of the following symptoms, which may indicate a serious illness, should TH report to her prescriber if it/they occur(s)?

   A. Blurred vision
   B. Calf pain
   C. Severe headache
   D. A and B only
   E. A, B, and C only

10. Which of the following oral contraceptives is administered to provide expected menstrual bleeding once every 3 months rather than the traditional every month, as with the 28-day regimens?

    A. Mircette® (desogestrel/ethinyl estradiol)
    B. Ortho-TriCyclen® (norgestimate/ethinyl estradiol)
    C. Ovcon 50® (norethindrone/ethinyl estradiol)
    D. Seasonale® (levonorgestrel/ethinyl estradiol)
    E. Tri-Norinyl® (norethindrone/ethinyl estradiol)

URINARY TRACT INFECTIONS

PRESENTATION

Patient	MK
Age	27
Sex	Female
Allergies	NKA
Race	White
Height	5'7"
Wt	128 lb
Diagnosis	Primary

1. Asymptomatic bacteriuria
2. First trimester pregnancy

	Date	Rx No.	Physician	Drug and Strength	Quantity	Sig	Refills
Medication record	1/15	30965	EL	Ferro-Folic™ 500 mg	100	1 qd	6
(prescription	2/23	31790	EL	Ampicillin 500 mg	40	1 q6h	0
and OTC)							

QUESTIONS

1. Which of the following is/are false regarding asymptomatic bacteriuria in pregnancy?

   I.   Asymptomatic bacteriuria does not necessitate antibiotic treatment of pregnant women who have no evidence of mechanical obstruction or renal insufficiency.
   II. Asymptomatic bacteriuria in pregnancy may lead to pyelonephritis if the patient is not treated.
   III. Asymptomatic bacteriuria may cause low birth weight.

   A. I only
   B. III only
   C. I and II only
   D. II and III only
   E. I, II, and III

2. Which of the following drugs is a folic acid antagonist and is considered teratogenic during the first trimester of pregnancy?

   A. Nitrofurantoin
   B. Tetracycline
   C. TMP-SMX
   D. Gentamicin
   E. Ciprofloxacin

3. Which of the following is/are true regarding ampicillin and pregnancy?

   I.   The drug may be safely administered during each trimester of pregnancy.
   II. The drug may be excreted in breast milk and cause hemolytic anemia in the newborn.
   III. The drug may cross the placental barrier during the third trimester and cause kernicterus in the newborn.

   A. I only
   B. III only
   C. I and II only
   D. II and III only
   E. I, II, and III

4. Which of the following is/are true regarding duration of antibiotic therapy for a pregnant patient?

   I.   Cure rates with single-dose administration are superior to those with a 7-day course of treatment.
   II. Eradication of bacteriuria occurs only with intravenously administered antibiotics.
   III. Seven and 10-day regimens are equally effective in the management of UTI in pregnancy.

   A. I only
   B. III only
   C. I and II only
   D. II and III only
   E. I, II, and III

PATIENT PROFILE 114
PARKINSON'S DISEASE

PRESENTATION

JB is a 48-year-old man presenting to the pharmacy to refill his amantadine prescription. JB has refilled his prescription for amantadine 100 mg bid every month for the past 6 months. While filling the original prescription the dispensing pharmacist questioned the use of this agent in such a young patient (without a history of psychosis). This prompted the pharmacist to ask JB about his condition. JB stated that he had complained to his physician about a slight tremor in his left hand when he was watching TV or reading a book. JB was diagnosed with early to mild Parkinson's disease. JB was quite surprised because he felt that he was too young to have developed this disease. He did not report the symptom initially because he thought that he was just imagining things and could not understand why it was happening. He states that his tremor does not interfere with his functioning at work yet but is afraid that he will not be able to continue in his job as the symptoms progress.

PMH:
Parkinson's disease
Hyperlipidemia
Seasonal allergies
MH:
Amantadine 100 mg bid; refilled monthly since 1/15/04
Atorvastatin 10 mg qd: refilled monthly since 7/10/02
Benadryl 25 mg q6h during the autumn
Allergies: NKDA, seasonal allergies in the autumn
FH: JB's mother is alive and well and takes no medication at age 69. His father is alive with hypertension and hypercholesterolemia at age 75. His sister is alive and takes no medication at age 42.
SH: JB is married with two children (ages 17 and 19) and is employed as a lawyer. His wife is also a lawyer. His younger child is in high school and his older child is currently enrolled in college. JB denies cigarette smoking but does drink wine with his dinner at night. He also attends many functions during work and drinks a couple of beers at these functions.
PE: BP 125/75 mm Hg, pulse 65

PROBLEM LIST

1. Parkinson's disease
2. Hyperlipidemia
3. Seasonal allergies

QUESTIONS

1. The lack of which of the following neurotransmitters is thought to be primarily responsible for Parkinson's disease?

   A. Dopamine
   B. Serotonin
   C. Norepinephrine
   D. MAO-B

2. The clinical presentation of Parkinson's disease is characterized by which of the following?

   A. Bradykinesia
   B. Tremor at rest
   C. Postural instability
   D. All of the above

3. JB's physician prescribed amantadine. What is the reasoning behind this choice of therapy?

   A. It is useful against the depression associated with Parkinson's disease.
   B. It has a limited side-effect profile.
   C. It is effective against tremor.
   D. It is effective for long-term therapy.

4. Which of the following side effects is associated with amantadine therapy?

   A. Sleep apnea
   B. Diarrhea
   C. Livedo reticularis
   D. Wearing off

5. JB's physician would like to switch JB's drug therapy. Which of the following is the best choice?

   A. Carbidopa/levodopa
   B. Benztropine
   C. Selegiline
   D. Pergolide

6. JB's physician decides to switch JB to Benztropine. What side effects might JB experience?

   A. Dry mouth
   B. Constipation
   C. Blurred vision
   D. All of the above

7. JB takes Benadryl® for his seasonal allergies. What is the role of Benadryl® in Parkinson's therapy?

   A. As a sleep agent
   B. To prevent falls
   C. As an anticholinergic agent
   D. As a dopamine agonist

8. Why should JB discontinue his use of Benadryl®?

   A. It results in increased anticholinergic effects when combined with Benztropine.
   B. It results in increased drowsiness when combined with Benztropine.
   C. It results in decreased anticholinergic effects when combined with Benztropine.
   D. JB should not discontinue Benadryl®.

9. What should you tell JB about his fear of not being able to function as a lawyer?

   A. Parkinson's disease is curable so he should not worry.
   B. Parkinson's disease is not curable so he should retire.
   C. Because his job does not require fine motor coordination he should be able to continue working.
   D. None of the above.

10. Which of the following is a good monitoring tool for JB?

    A. DSM-IV
    B. Hoehn and Yahr Staging
    C. Frequent blood tests
    D. PET scanning

PATIENT PROFILE 115

CORONARY ARTERY DISEASE

PRESENTATION

SB is a 76-year-old woman who arrives in the emergency department with shortness of breath, fatigue, dizziness, increased sputum production, and chest pain. She characterizes the chest pain as sternal, radiating to the left jaw, and 7/10 in severity. The pain had developed several hours ago while SB was watching television. SB states the pain is consistent with her typical anginal pain but that the severity is increased.

MEDICAL HISTORY

CAD × 10 years
s/p AMI in 1988 and 1993
s/p CABG in 1993
Hypertension × 15 years
Gastritis
Crohn's disease
CHF × 5 years, EF: 30% 1 year ago
UTI

MEDS

Amlodipine 10 mg po qd
Aspirin EC 325 mg po qd
Lisinopril 10 mg po qd
Sulfasalizine 500 mg po qid
Prednisone 5 mg po qd
Lasix® (furosemide) 40 mg po qd
Digoxin 0.125 mg po qd

PHYSICAL EXAMINATION

GEN: Elderly woman in moderate respiratory distress and somewhat confused
BP: 90/50, HR: 110, RR: 32, T: afebrile
HEENT: Unremarkable
COR: S_1, S_2, and S_3 heard; tachycardia
CHEST: Rales one-third of the way up bilaterally
ABD: Unremarkable
EXT: Mild edema at the ankles
NEURO: Mildly confused, A/O × 3
ECG: ST-segment depression and T-wave inversion in leads V_2 through V_4

The patient continues to become confused in the emergency department, and blood pressure drops to 80/40. A Swan–Ganz catheter is placed, and the following readings are obtained:

CI: 1.9 L/min
PCWP: 24 mm Hg
SVR (calculated): 1020 (800–1200)

QUESTIONS

1. Which of the following is the most likely cause of the low blood pressure?

   A. Vasodilatation secondary to infection
   B. Low intravascular volume
   C. Decreased cardiac output

D. Increased intravascular volume
E. Adverse drug effect from digoxin

2. Which of the following is the most appropriate choice to help stabilize hemodynamic status?

A. Milrinone drip
B. 1 L normal saline solution
C. Norepinephrine drip
D. Dobutamine drip
E. Nitroglycerin drip

3. One hour after arriving in the CCU, SB goes into ventricular tachycardia (VT) at a rate of 170 beats/min. Which of the following is the drug of choice to treat VT in the acute MI setting?

A. Procainamide
B. Bretylium
C. Amiodarone
D. Metoprolol
E. Lidocaine

4. The physician decides to provide continuing amiodarone therapy to prevent any recurrences of VT. With which of the following medications will amiodarone interact?

A. Lasix® (furosemide)
B. Amlodipine
C. Aspirin
D. Digoxin
E. Lisinopril

5. SB recovers with no further complications. Which of the following interventions is the most appropriate in her long-term therapy for CAD?

A. Discontinue amlodipine, start metoprolol, and slowly titrate to 50 mg po bid
B. Increase digoxin to 0.250 mg po qd
C. Discontinue aspirin, start Ticlopidine 250 mg po bid
D. Discontinue amlodipine, start hydralazine 10 mg po qid
E. Increase amlodipine to 20 mg po qd

PATIENT PROFILE 116

ADULT IMMUNIZATIONS

PRESENTATION

AJ is a Korean War veteran who presents to the Veterans' Administration ambulatory clinic for routine follow-up. He is a 69-year-old man who suffered a myocardial infarction (MI) 2 years ago. This is his first visit to this clinic. His medical records dating back to 1980 indicate no immunizations.

CC: "I'm here today to get a refill for my heart medicine."
PMH: COPD × 5 years, hospitalized once this year for an exacerbation
HTN × 10 years
Type 2 diabetes mellitus (DM) × 8 years
MI 2 years ago
FH: Father died of cardiac arrest at age 65, brother died at age 60 of MI, sister age 71 alive with DM and Afib.
SH: Retired engineer, married, lives with wife. Smokes tobacco 1.5 ppd × 50 years, denies alcohol or recreational drug use.
Meds: Metoprolol XL 100 mg qd
Lisinopril 20 mg qd
Glipizide 10 mg bid

ASA 81 mg qd
NTG 0.4 mg prn CP
Atrovent MDI 2 puff qid
Flovent MDI 2 puff bid
Albuterol 2 puff qid prn
All: PCN
ROS: No palpitations, dizziness, cough, chest pain, or blood in urine or stool. He uses albuterol two to three times per week. There are no signs or symptoms of hypoglycemia.
PE:
Gen: Well-developed and well nourished man in NAD
VS: BP 154/90, pulse 80, RR 12, Temp 37°C, Ht 6'1," Wt 94 kg
HEENT: PERRLA, EOMI, TMs intact
Neck: No lymphadenopathy, masses, or JVD
Cor: RRR, no murmurs
Lungs: Barrel chest, expiratory wheeze b/l, no rales or rhonchi
Abd: NT/ND, no HSM, normal BS
Ext: No CCE
Neuro: Alert, CN II-XII intact, normal DTRs b/l

LABORATORY VALUES

Na 142 mEq/L, Hbg 14.0 mg/dL, K 4.2 mEq/L, Hct 39.5%, Cl 106 mEq/L, WBC $6.4 \times 10^3/mm^3$, CO_2 26 mEq/L, Plat $210 \times 10^3/mm^3$, BUN 22 mg/dL, HbA_1C 9.8%, SCr 1.2 mg/dL, glucose (fasting) 180 mg/dL

QUESTIONS

1. Which of the following statements about the dosing and frequency of the influenza vaccine is true?

   A. A booster dose should be given every 10 years.
   B. A second dose should be given if it has been more than 5 years since the first dose.
   C. A dose should be given annually because of the short immunity and changing virus.
   D. Only a one-time dose should be given.
   E. None of the above

2. What is the optimal time period for influenza vaccine administration?

   A. May–September
   B. April–June
   C. October–December
   D. January–July
   E. The vaccine can be given any time of year.

3. The influenza vaccine is contraindicated in which of the following?

   I.   Patients with an allergy to eggs
   II. Patients with an allergy to neomycin
   III. Pregnant patients

   A. I only
   B. III only
   C. I and II only
   D. II and III only
   E. I, II, and III

4. Which of the following medications is approved for the prevention on outbreak of influenza A infection in a nursing home?

   A. Amantadine
   B. Acyclovir
   C. Ciprofloxacin
   D. Penicillin G
   E. Ketoconazole

5. Which of the following is/are indications for the Hepatitis B vaccine?

   I.   Hemodialysis patients
   II. Healthcare workers

   III. Homosexual men

   A. I only
   B. III only
   C. I and II only
   D. II and III only
   E. I, II, and III

6. Which of the following vaccines should be specifically considered in college students living in dormitories because of the fast spreading nature of the illness?

   A. Inactivated polio vaccine
   B. Varicella vaccine
   C. Pneumococcal polysaccharide vaccine
   D. Meningococcal polysaccharide vaccine
   E. Tetanus toxoid

7. The pneumococcal polysaccharide vaccine is indicated in which of the following patient populations?

   I.   Patients with DM
   II. Patients with CVD
   III. Infants under 2 years of age

   A. I only
   B. III only
   C. I and II only
   D. II and III only
   E. I, II, and III

8. The bacille Calmette-Guérin (BCG) vaccine protects against which of the following infections?

   A. Tetanus
   B. Tuberculosis
   C. HIV
   D. Hepatitis C
   E. Measles

9. Which of the following neurologic conditions has been associated with the influenza vaccine?

   A. Neuroleptic malignant syndrome
   B. Guillain-Barré syndrome
   C. Pseudoparkinsonism
   D. Normal pressure hydrocephalus
   E. Senile dementia

10. AJ should receive a booster dose of which of the following immunizations every 10 years?

    A. Influenza vaccine
    B. Hepatitis B vaccine
    C. Pneumococcal polysaccharide vaccine
    D. Tetanus toxoid
    E. Hepatitis A vaccine

PATIENT PROFILE 117

HYPERCHOLESTEROLEMIA

PRESENTATION

XX is a 27-year-old man who visits his primary care physician for a physical examination before starting a new job. He reports that he has had a dry cough on and off for approximately 1 month but otherwise has been in his usual state of health. His medical history includes GERD diagnosed 5 weeks earlier and a fracture of the right arm in 1993. XX is allergic to penicillin (rash) and takes omeprazole 20 mg po qd. XX's father has hypertension and diabetes mellitus. His mother died at the age of 62 years of acute myocardial infarction. XX has smoked 1½ packs of cigarettes a day for 7 years.

PHYSICAL EXAMINATION

BP: 136/82, HR: 70, RR: 14, T: 99.8°F
HEENT: Normal
COR: RRR, S_1 and S_2 are present
CHEST: Clear to ascultation
ABD: Soft, abnormal bowel sounds
NEURO: Intact

LABS

Na: 136 mEq/L
Cl: 101 mEq/L
BUN: 12 mg/dL
SCr: 0.6 mg/dL
Total cholesterol: 194 mg/dL
K: 4.5 mEq/L
CO_2: 26 mEq/dL
Gluc: 98 mg/dL
WBC: 8.7 K/μL with normal differential
HDL chol: 58 mg/dL

QUESTIONS

1. What are XX's risk factors for coronary heart disease?

   A. He smokes.
   B. His mother died at the age of 62 years from an acute MI.
   C. His father has hypertension.
   D. A and B only
   E. A, B, and C

2. How would you recommend managing XX's cholesterol level?

   A. The total cholesterol is at the desired level. Teach XX about diet and exercise to keep his cholesterol at a desirable level and repeat total cholesterol and HDL measurements in 5 years.
   B. The total cholesterol level is borderline high. XX should be referred to a nutritionist to start a step 1 diet. He should return in 6 months for repeat total cholesterol and HDL measurements.
   C. The total cholesterol level is borderline high. Before treatment is chosen, lipoprotein analysis should be performed.
   D. The total cholesterol level is high. Niacin should be started. XX should return in 6 months for repeat total cholesterol and HDL measurements.
   E. The total cholesterol level is high. Cholestyramine resin should be started. XX should return in 6 months for total cholesterol and HDL measurements.

3. The next time XX undergoes cholesterol screening, a lipoprotein analysis is performed and provides the following information: total cholesterol 238 mg/dL, triglycerides 140 mg/dL, HDL 54 mg/dL, LDL 176 mg/dL. Repeated results reveal similar values. Dietary therapy is initiated. What is the goal LDL level with dietary therapy?

   A. <160 mg/dL
   B. <130 mg/dL
   C. <100 mg/dL
   D. <70 mg/dL
   E. <40 mg/dL

4. If XX were a 50-year-old man with coronary heart disease, what modality of treatment would you recommend?

   A. Diet
   B. Exercise
   C. Drug therapy
   D. A and B only
   E. A, B, and C

5. If XX were a 50-year-old man with a history of coronary heart disease, what would be the goal LDL level with therapy?

   A. <160 mg/dL
   B. <130 mg/dL
   C. <100 mg/dL
   D. <70 mg/dL
   E. <40 mg/dL

PATIENT PROFILE 118

ACNE

PRESENTATION

AA is a 15-year-old boy who presents to his dermatologist with complaints about acne. AA is concerned about his recent eruption of acne; he has approximately seven visible closed comedones on his forehead only. The acne began appearing about 15 days ago. This is AA's first visit with a dermatologist; his mother scheduled this appointment when she noticed that AA was feigning illness to avoid going to school. Apparently, AA's classmates have been teasing AA about his oily skin and acne. AA has already missed several days of school because of several episodes of asthma exacerbations and his mother is worried that he will fall behind his classmates. His mother also wants to be sure to treat AA's acne before he develops pitting scars like his older brother.

MH:
Albuterol MDI 2p qid prn
Salmeterol Diskus 1p bid   *Steroid use*
Fluticasone 44 µg 2p bid
Methylphenidate 10 mg bid
PMH: Severe asthma
Attention deficit hyperactivity disorder (ADHD) (predominantly inattentive)
FH: DW's older brother has severe, nodular acne. DW's father had ADHD as a child but "outgrew it" as an adult.
SH: AA is a freshman in high school and lives at home with his parents and one older brother (age 17). AA is a member of the chess club and the ski club in the winter. He denies alcohol and illicit drug use. He admits to sneaking cigarettes from his mother (approximately eight per week).
Allergies: Sulfa (AA developed Steven-Johnson's syndrome after taking SMZ-TMP)
PE: BP 102/66, HR 68, T 38.5°C, Wt 130, Ht 5'1"
Gen: WDWN young man
Skin: Approximately seven visible open comedones on his forehead   *mild*
Labs: Not obtained (Table 118-1)

QUESTIONS

1. Which of AA's medication may be exacerbating his acne?

   I. Prednisone ✓
   II. Methylphenidate
   III. Salmeterol

   A. I only
   B. III only
   C. I and II
   D. II and III
   E. I, II, and III

2. The dermatologist classifies AA's acne as mild. Which of the following regimens should you recommend?

   A. Azelaic acid 2% cream: apply bid
   B. Clindamycin 1% solution: apply qid
   C. Erythromycin 2% gel: apply qod
   D. Tazarotene 1% gel: apply bid
   E. Tretinoin 0.01% gel: apply qod

3. Given his allergy history, which agent is contraindicated for AA?

   A. Azelex®
   B. A/T/S® *erythromycin topical*
   C. Benzamycin®
   D. Klaron® *sulfacetamide*
   E. Vibramycin®

4. AA's dermatologist decided to try benzoyl peroxide gel and would like you to counsel AA. Which of the following statements would you tell AA about his medication?

   I. Apply immediately after washing your face, while your skin is still moist.
   II. This may bleach fabric. ✓
   III. The most common side effects are burning and stinging. ✓

Table 118-1. Medication Record (Prescription and Over the Counter)

Date	Drug and Strength	Quantity	Sig	Refills
8/2	Prednisone 10 mg	30	tud	2
8/2	Albuterol MDI	17	2p qid prn	5
8/2	Salmeterol diskus	30	1p bid	5
8/2	Fluticasone 44 µg	13	2p bid	5
8/10	Methylphenidate 10	60	1 bid	0

A. I only
B. III only
C. I and II
D. II and III
E. I, II, and III

5. Which of the following is not an example of a topical retinoid?

A. Azelaic acid
B. Differin®
C. Tazorac®
D. Retin-A®
E. Tretinoin

6. What is an advantage of using adapalene instead of tretinoin?

A. It is more effective in treating severe acne.
B. It possesses more antimicrobial activity.
C. Its onset of action is much faster.
D. It is associated with less irritation.
E. There is no advantage to using adapalene instead of tretinoin.

7. After 6 months of therapy, AA's acne is getting worse. His acne is now classified as moderate; his dermatologist would like to prescribe an antibiotic. Which of the following is the most appropriate antibiotic regimen for AA?

A. Ciprofloxacin 500 mg bid
B. Doxycycline 50 mg bid
C. Erythromycin stearate 500 mg qid — too much.
D. Tetracycline 500 mg qd   BID - QID
E. Minocycline 50 mg qid

8. Which of the following has the most anti-inflammatory activity?

A. BenzaClin®   combination   BPO + clindamycin
B. Benzoyl peroxide
C. Cleocin 1%®
D. Minocin®
E. Tazarotene

9. For which of the following conditions is isotretinoin indicated?

A. Closed comedones
B. Macrocomedones
C. Nodules
D. Open comedones
E. Papules

10. Which of the following are potential side effects of isotretinoin?

I. Psychosis
II. Photosensitivity
III. Elevated triglycerides

A. I only
B. III only
C. I and II
D. II and III
E. I, II, and III

PATIENT PROFILE 119

ASTHMA

PRESENTATION

NJ is a 20-year-old woman with asthma. She takes both albuterol and beclomethasone to control moderately persistent asthma. She says she receives no benefit from the use of the beclomethasone inhaler and does not want to have the prescription refilled. She would prefer to use only the albuterol inhaler.

QUESTIONS

1. What would be the most appropriate response to NJ's concerns?

   A. Explain that beclomethasone is a bronchodilator that will help open her airways.
   B. Explain that beclomethasone is an anti-inflammatory agent that will help control the underlying disease.
   C. Explain that she should increase the use of albuterol if her symptoms continue to worsen.
   D. Explain that she should experience immediate relief of symptoms if she uses her beclomethasone inhaler correctly.
   E. Explain that she may need an oral corticosteroid to reduce the risk of steroid-induced side effects.

2. Which of the following is the most appropriate advice to give patients using both an albuterol and a steroid inhaler?

   A. When administering, the two are used together and the albuterol inhaler should be used first.
   B. Patient should rinse their mouths after using the steroid inhaler.
   C. The steroid inhaler should be used only as needed for relief of symptoms.

D. A and B
E. A, B, and C

3. To help control nocturnal symptoms, which of the following inhalers would be the most appropriate to use in the evening?

   A. Albuterol
   B. Ipratropium
   C. Salmeterol
   D. Pirbuterol
   E. Metaproterenol

4. NJ's physician is considering adding a medication that selectively targets a major mediator of inflammation in the pathogenesis of asthma. Which of the following agents most closely meets this criterion?

A. Ipratropium
B. Budesonide
C. Theophylline
D. Zafirlukast
E. Nedocromil

5. In counseling NJ on the proper use of the albuterol metered-dose inhaler, all of the following steps are correct except:

   A. Shake canister well.
   B. Exhale slowly before pressing down on canister.
   C. Open mouth wide and hold inhaler 2–3 finger breadths away from mouth.
   D. After inhaling, hold breath for approximately 10 seconds.
   E. Inhale second puff as soon as possible after first.

PATIENT PROFILE 120
CUTANEOUS ANTHRAX

PRESENTATION

DM is a 16-year-old boy presenting to the emergency department complaining of a sore on his right hand. He states that he had a fever, mild headache, and has not been feeling very well for 4 days. He noticed a spot on his right hand that was itchy approximately 4 days ago. He states that the spot formed ring of small "bubbles" on his hand 2 days ago, the "bubbles" are filled with fluid.

CC: DM has a sore on his right hand that was itchy and bubbly he thinks it's a spider bite.
PMH: DM's past medical history is insignificant other than seasonal allergic rhinitis. DM is allergic to Minocycline.
SH: Patient denies alcohol, tobacco, and illicit drug use. He states that he may drink one or two caffeinated soda per day, denies any coffee intake. He lives at home with his parents and has a sister age 10. DM works part-time at the postal distribution center after school 2 days a week.
FH: Both parents are alive and have no medical problems. Sister has no medical problems.
PE:
Gen: Young male in no apparent distress with an ulcerative lesion on his right hand.
VS: BP 116/78 mm Hg, pulse 52 bpm, Wt 160 lbs, Temp 101°F
HEENT: Within normal limits
Chest: Clear to auscultation
CV: RRR, no murmurs, gallops, or rubs
ABD: NT/ND

Skin: Ulcerative lesion on right hand with fluid-filled vesicles
Labs: Vesicle fluid sent to the laboratory for culture (gram-positive rods observed)
Electrolytes: Within normal limits
Diagnosis: R/O brown recluse bite
Meds: Loratadine 10 mg PO QD for seasonal allergies
MN: Vesicles ruptured and formed a depressed black eschar-positive diagnosis of cutaneous anthrax

QUESTIONS

1. Which of the following statements is false about cutaneous anthrax?

   A. Humans can be infected with bacillus anthracis spores through an abrasion on the skin or through a scratch.
   B. It is common for farmers who work with infected cattle outside of the United States to get cutaneous anthrax.
   C. If untreated, it has almost 100% fatality rate.
   D. It is not transmitted person to person by aerosol delivery.
   E. None of the above is a false statement.

2. Which of the following is the causative organism for cutaneous anthrax?

   A. Flavivirus
   B. Castor bean extract
   C. *Coxiella burnetii*
   D. Anthracis

3. What is the average incubation period for cutaneous anthrax once exposed?

    A. 1 to 3 days
    B. 1 to 12 days
    C. 3 to 5 days
    D. 5 to 10 days

4. Which of the following is the recommended drug of choice for the treatment of cutaneous anthrax (small lesions) for this patient?

    A. Ciprofloxacin 500 mg po q12 hours
    B. Doxycycline 100 mg po q12 hours
    C. Amoxicillin 1g po qd
    D. Levofloxacin 500 mg po q12 hours

5. In reference to Question 4, the chosen antibiotic is considered to be of which type?

    A. Tetracycline
    B. Penicillin
    C. Sulfonamide
    D. Quinolone

6. DM needs to be treated for how many days per the CDC guidelines?

    A. 10 days
    B. 20 days
    C. 60 days
    D. 120 days

7. The use of quinolone for DM's sister is often not recommended because of concerns with which of the following?

    A. Severe gastrointestinal upset
    B. Arthropathy
    C. Intense fatigue
    D. Will turn teeth blue

8. Prophylaxis therapy must be administered to all postal workers in the distribution center. What is the recommended length of treatment?

    A. 7 to 10 days
    B. 20 days
    C. 60 days
    D. 120 days

9. It is important to drink a full glass of water with Doxycyline and to remain upright to prevent which of the following?

    A. Esophagitis
    B. Photosensitivity
    C. Tooth discoloration
    D. Nausea

10. Planning a mass prophylaxis of those exposed requires public health officials and healthcare providers (including pharmacists) to do which of the following?

    A. Have well-communicated policies in place before an attack occurs.
    B. Have communication between public health officials and healthcare workers about who should receive prophylaxis and with what drugs.
    C. Have distribution centers identified with layouts that include security, traffic flow, and personnel needs.
    D. Have plans in place for follow-up, including assessment of adherence, adverse drug reactions, and illness.

PATIENT PROFILE 121

ELIXIRS

PRESENTATION

An elixir dosage form is to be manufactured such that ¼ oz of drug will be contained in each pint of solution. Formulation studies demonstrate a need for an ethyl alcohol concentration of 20% v/v. A 20% v/v ethyl alcohol solution has a density of 0.95 g/mL.

QUESTIONS

1. Which of the following is the concentration of drug in the solution dosage form?

    A. 0.015% w/v
    B. 1:150 w/v
    C. 15 mg/mL
    D. 15 mg%
    E. C and D

2. The purpose of alcohol in elixir dosage forms includes all of the following except:

    A. To buffer the solution to the pH of maximum stability

B.   Cosolvent to produce or maintain drug solubility
C.   To preserve the solution
D.   To provide a pharmacologic sedative effect
E.   A and D

3.   How much alcohol and how much water should be used to produce 1 pint of a 20% v/v ethyl alcohol solution?

A.   94.6 mL alcohol and 378.5 mL water
B.   94.6 mL alcohol and sufficient water to make 1 pint of solution
C.   99.6 mL alcohol and 373.5 mL water
D.   99.6 mL alcohol and sufficient water to make 1 pint of solution
E.   C and D

4.   The specific gravity of a 20% v/v ethyl alcohol solution at room temperature is 0.95. Express the ethyl alcohol concentration in terms of percentage strength weight-volume (% w/v).

A.   0.0475
B.   19.00
C.   20.00
D.   20.95
E.   21.05

5.   How many kilograms of drug are needed to produce 20 gallons of elixir?

A.   0.040
B.   1.13
C.   1.20
D.   40
E.   1134

PATIENT PROFILE 122

DEPRESSION

PRESENTATION

WM is a 59-year-old white man who is severely depressed and was admitted 3 days ago after trying to commit suicide via an overdose with acetaminophen. He states that he has felt depressed since he was a teenager but has never taken medications or sought treatment. He works as a manager of a 7/11 and claims that he puts in about 75 hours per week. He denies illicit drug use and states he only drinks socially (a couple of drinks if at a party or out to dinner).

PMH: Hypertension
BPH
Meds: Amlodipine 10 mg qd
Terazosin 4 mg hs
MVI qd
PE: v/s BP 132/88, pulse 84, R 18, Temp 37°C
Labs: WNL except for AST 88, ALT 94

QUESTIONS

1.   Which of the following choices is true about the use of desipramine in this patient?

A.   Desipramine can be fatal in small overdoses and this patient has proved that he may use overdose as a method of suicide.
B.   Desipramine is ineffective as an antidepressant in patients with hypertension.

C.   Desipramine is better tolerated than most other choices of antidepressants.
D.   Desipramine has a faster onset of action than other antidepressants.

2.   What is the drug interaction between nortriptyline and terazosin?

A.   Nortriptyline has opposite effects on the muscarinic receptors.
B.   Terazosin reverses the antidepressant effects of nortriptyline.
C.   Nortriptyline and terazosin have additive effects on the α_1 receptor.
D.   Nortriptyline and terazosin have opposite effects on the α_1 receptor.

3.   Why is lorazepam a poor choice for treating this patient's depression?

A.   It is deadly in small overdoses.
B.   Lorazepam is depressogenic and not an antidepressant.
C.   Lorazepam and amlodipine have a fatal drug–drug interaction.
D.   Patients with BPH should not use benzodiazepines.

4.   Which of the following could result in a fatal drug interaction with amlodipine?

A.   Nefazodone
B.   Paroxetine

C. Citalopram
D. Bupropion

5. Which of the following is the most likely explanation for this patient's increased AST and ALT?

A. He has recently binged on alcohol.
B. Amlodipine is hepatotoxic.
C. He has cirrhosis.
D. It is a residual effect of acetaminophen overdose.

P A T I E N T   P R O F I L E   1 2 3

RESPIRATORY TRACT INFECTION

PRESENTATION

When CM goes to pick up his child at the day-care center, a rambunctious child expectorates onto him. Not thinking too much of this, CM wipes off the goo and proceeds to eat some Cheerios®. The following morning, CM finds himself short of breath with a fever of 103°C. He takes some acetaminophen and goes to work. Six hours later the fever returns, and CM coughs up purulent, rust-colored sputum. He also notices that his heart is racing and thinks it might be a good idea to seek medical attention.

QUESTIONS

1. When CM gets to his primary care physician's office, he is asked to expectorate an induced sputum sample. CBC results yield a WBC count of 15.3 (high), lymphocytes 6 (low), and bands of 12 (high). A Gram stain on the sputum sample shows gram-positive cocci in chains. What is the most likely organism? Assuming CM had no underlying disease.

    A. *Legionella pneumophila*
    B. *Haemophilus influenzae*
    C. *Streptococcus pneumoniae*
    D. *Acinetobacter calcoaceticus*
    E. *Bacteroides fragilis*

2. While waiting for the culture and sensitivity results, you are asked to recommend an antibiotic for empiric treatment. Which of the following antimicrobial agents would be the best empiric choice for CM if he is admitted to the hospital?

    A. Ceftriaxone
    B. Gentamicin
    C. Metronidazole
    D. Tetracycline
    E. Aztreonam

3. While eating his eighth piece of apple pie, CM is found in his room choking. A slice of apple is halfway into the trachea before a nurse places her fingers in CM's mouth and removes the food. Because CM has aspirated the pie, it would be most prudent to add which of the following antibiotics to the regimen to improve anaerobic and gram-positive coverage?

    A. Vancomycin
    B. Ceftazidime
    C. Imipenem
    D. Clindamycin
    E. Metronidazole

4. It is well known that underlying diseases can predispose patients to lower respiratory tract infection. It is also known that among patients with aspiration pneumonia, anaerobic organisms (which commonly cannot be cultured) are responsible in part for the pneumonia. The presence of underlying disease among patients with pneumonia shifts the bacterial flora toward yielding which of the following types of bacteria in addition to the typical bacterial pathogens that occur among this patient population?

    A. Gram-positive cocci in clusters
    B. Gram-positive cocci in chains
    C. Lactose-fermenting gram-negative rods
    D. Non–lactose-fermenting gram-negative rods
    E. Atypical organisms

5. Of the nondrug therapies to augment management of pneumonia, which is designed to loosen mucous and secretions trapped in the lower airways?

    A. Pulse oximetry
    B. Measuring intake and output
    C. Nasotracheal suctioning
    D. Postural percussion and drainage
    E. Nasally applied saline mist

DIABETES

PRESENTATION

SP is a 61-year-old white woman with type I diabetes presenting for her monthly follow-up with disease state management and routine diabetes check-up. SP has been followed closely by the disease state management team (including a pharmacist) for 3 years. SP has maintained good control of her type I diabetes for the better part of 3 years with periodic diet and lifestyle indiscretion. Her last HbA1c from 3 months ago was 8.4%. SP typically maintains an HbA1c of 7% and fasting capillary glucose range of 120 to 160 mg/dL.

PMH: In 1974 SP was hospitalized with fever of unknown origin, epigastric pain, and watery stools. Gastroenterology and infectious disease specialists determined that SP was experiencing acute pancreatitis. She was treated acutely with antibiotics and since being hospitalized 30 years ago, SP had acute pancreatic flares again in 1979, 1987, and 1998. In 1998 a C-peptide test suggested very little endogenous pancreatic ß-islet cell activity, and effectively type I diabetes. In 1999 SP finally agreed to begin insulin. SP has managed insulin therapy with few problems over the last 5 years. Occasionally SP experiences nausea, abdominal pain, fever, and watery stools, which remind her of pancreatitis. During these times she stops all solid food and monitors her glucose four times per day.

FH: Mother deceased, diabetes-related complications with ESRD, father deceased, hemorrhagic stoke; sister, age 57, no medical problems

SH: SP is a recently retired postal supervisor who worked for 33 years. She's been married for 34 years. Her husband is a retired army veteran with multiple medical problems. Her daughter is 30 years old; she's morbidly obese with type II diabetes and depression. SP denies EtOH and illicit substances. She drinks one to two cups of coffee daily. She's a former smoker with a 15 pack-year history (she quit 20 years ago).

Allergies: Sulfonamides

Meds: Lisinopril 40 mg po qd
Atenolol 100 mg po qd
Amlodipine 10 mg po qd
Doxazosin 1 mg po qd
ASA 325 mg po qd
Lansoprazole 15 mg po qd
Amitriptyline 25 mg po qd
Atorvastatin 80 mg po qd
Fish oil capsules 1000 mg po bid
Insulin regular 15 to 25 units before each meal

Isophane insulin NPH 66 units each morning, 34 units with dinner

Gen: Pleasant middle-aged woman, relaxed and friendly

Vitals: 116/88 mmHg, RR 16 breaths/min, pulse 72 beats/min, Temp 98.0°F, Ht 62", Wt 187 lbs, BMI 34.5 kg/m^2

HEENT: Funduscopic findings reveal normal retina, EOMI, mucous membranes moist

Chest: Clear to auscultation and percussion

COR: normal S_1 and S_2 sounds

ABD: Nontender, + BS, no hepatosplenomegaly

GU: Deferred

RECT: Deferred

EXT: Good pulses 2 + BL

Neuro: Cranial nerves II-XII intact

LABORATORY VALUES

Na 144 mEq/L, K 4.9 mEq/L, Cl 107 mEq/L, HCO$_3$ 22 mEq/L, BUN 10 mg/dL, SCr 1.0 mg/dL, fasting glucose 153 mg/dL, WBC 9.1 K cells/mm^3, platelets 325 K cells/mm^3, Hgb = 12 g/dL, HCT 37%, HbA1c 7.7%, LDL 108 mg/dL (direct), HDL 40 mg/dL, TC 180 mg/dL, TG 275 mg/dL

QUESTIONS

1. SP mentions that she has been waking up in the middle of the night in a cold sweat over the last few days. She typically eats around 7:30 PM, goes to bed at 10:30 PM and wakes up hungry between 1 and 2 AM. When hunger strikes in the night, SP makes a peanut butter and jelly sandwich or snacks on leftovers. Over the last 3 days you notice the following waking morning blood glucose values: 189 mg/dL, 207 mg/dL, 170 mg/dL. How is her current insulin regimen contributing to nighttime hypoglycemia?

   A. The mealtime dose of regular insulin is peaking overnight, resulting in hypoglycemic symptoms of hunger and diaphoresis.

   B. The second NPH dose peaks overnight resulting in hypoglycemic symptoms of hunger and diaphoresis.

   C. The mealtime doses of regular insulin and NPH insulin are creating a "stacking" effect where excessive insulinization leads to nighttime hypoglycemic symptoms of hunger and diaphoresis.

   D. SP may have a lipodystrophic injection site that delays absorption of the NPH insulin causing it to peak overnight

E. SP's NPH insulin may have become denatured in extremes of heat or cold resulting in delayed absorption with an overnight peak

2. SP tells you she likes this regimen because she can combine insulin types and administer one injection twice daily. What is the most appropriate strategy to manage JP's nocturnal hypoglycemic symptoms?

   A. Counsel SP to administer her NPH at bedtime and continue to monitor morning fasting glucose.
   B. Reduce her evening dose of NPH by 10% and continue to monitor morning fasting glucose.
   C. Reduce her evening dose of regular insulin by 30% and continue to monitor morning fasting glucose.
   D. Eat a snack before bedtime consisting of at least 20 to 30 g of complex carbohydrates.
   E. Counsel SP to stop taking her evening dose of NPH to prevent future nocturnal hypoglycemia.

3. SP follows this recommendation and comes back in 2 weeks for a follow-up visit. She reports that she sleeps through the night more often but still experiences nocturnal hypoglycemic symptoms two to three times per week. SP still wants to try this regimen because she is familiar with insulin regular and NPH. SP comes back for another follow up 2 months later and has gained 7 lbs. She reports that she snacks occasionally before bed to prevent hypoglycemic symptoms and seldom wakes up in the night. At this time her HbA1c = 8%, BMI = 35.5 kg/m². When learning that her HbA1c is up to 8% SP wants to try other options to gain control. How would you adjust SP's insulin regimen to improve her glucose control?

   A. Discontinue NPH. Use Ultralente insulin as the basal insulin and continue regular insulin as the prandial insulin.
   B. Discontinue regular insulin. Continue NPH as the basal insulin and begin using insulin lispro as the prandial insulin
   C. Discontinue NPH. Use insulin glargine as the basal insulin and continue regular insulin as the prandial insulin.
   D. Discontinue regular and NPH insulin. Begin using insulin glargine as the basal insulin and use insulin lispro as the prandial insulin.
   E. Discontinue regular and NPH insulin. Begin using Ultralente insulin as the basal insulin and insulin aspart as the prandial insulin.

4. Which of the following statements about insulin lispro is false?

   A. Insulin lispro is used in combination with insulin glargine in a physiologic strategy for insulin replacement.

B. Insulin lispro may replace regular insulin used in insulin pumps or administered subcutaneously with a syringe.
C. Insulin lispro has an immediate onset and peaks within 15 minutes of administration.
D. Insulin lispro is approved for use in pen injectors.
E. Insulin lispro can be mixed with insulin glargine.

5. Which of the following statements about insulin glargine is true?

   A. Insulin glargine has not received an approval for use in pediatric patients with type I diabetes.
   B. Insulin glargine is release slowly over 20 to 24 hours and does not peak, making it an ideal basal insulin.
   C. Insulin glargine can be mixed with regular insulin and administered in one injection.
   D. Insulin glargine is associated with more hypoglycemia than insulin NPH or Ultralente insulin.
   E. Insulin glargine doses are converted from insulin NPH using a 1 : 1 ratio.

6. How would you convert SP's current regimen with insulin NPH and regular insulin to insulin glargine and insulin lispro?

   A. 50% insulin glargine (88 U) once daily at bedtime and 50% insulin lispro (87 U) allocated as 29 units with each meal
   B. 33% insulin glargine (59 U) once daily at bedtime and 66% insulin lispro (116 U) allocated as 38 units with each meal
   C. 66% insulin glargine (116 U) once daily at bedtime and 33% insulin lispro (60 U) allocated as 20 units with each meal
   D. 40% insulin glargine (70 U) once daily at bedtime and 60% insulin lispro (105 U) allocated as 35 units with each meal
   E. 60% insulin glargine (105 U) once daily at bedtime and 40% insulin lispro (69 U) allocated as 23 units with each meal.

7. How many vials of insulin glargine must be dispensed to provide a complete 28 days' supply?

   A. One vial
   B. Two vials
   C. Three vials
   D. Four vials
   E. Five vials

8. How many vials of insulin lispro must be dispensed to provide a complete 28-days' supply?

   A. One vial
   B. Two vials
   C. Three vials

D. Four vials

E. Five vials

9. SP tells you that she occasionally likes to snack between meals when she is out at a social event with friends or her husband. SP realizes it is important to maintain a tight glucose control but wants to partake socially. SP asks you how to use this new form of insulin to cover for additional carbohydrate intake. How would you recommend SP use insulin lispro to cover extra carbohydrate from snacks?

A. 1 U of insulin lispro per 100 g of carbohydrate

B. 1 U of insulin lispro per 75 g of carbohydrate

C. 1 U of insulin lispro per 50 g of carbohydrate

D. 1 U of insulin lispro per 25 g of carbohydrate

E. 1 U of insulin lispro per 10 g of carbohydrate

10. SP thanks you for your advice. She shows you her glucometer and you notice that her fasting capillary glu-

cose prior to meals can range from 150 to 300 mg/dL. SP asks how much insulin she needs to correct for high premeal glucose readings. How would you advise SP to begin adjusting for high premeal glucose?

A. For premeal glucose readings over 150 mg/dL, use 1 U of insulin lispro to reduce glucose 100 mg/dL.

B. For premeal glucose readings over 150 mg/dL, use 1 U of insulin lispro to reduce glucose 50 mg/dL.

C. For premeal glucose readings over 200 mg/dL, use 1 U of insulin lispro to reduce glucose 100 mg/dL.

D. For premeal glucose readings over 200 mg/dL, use 1 U of insulin lispro to reduce glucose 50 mg/dL.

E. For premeal glucose readings over 200 mg/dL, use 1 U of insulin lispro to reduce glucose 75 mg/dL.

PATIENT PROFILE 125

DERMATOLOGY

PRESENTATION

DR is a 20 year-old-woman who comes to your pharmacy with a prescription for benzoyl peroxide gel (Benzac® AC 2.5%). You notice several whiteheads on her forehead, and she has a few blackheads on her nose. No inflamed papules, pustules, or nodular lesions are apparent. DR states that she went to see a dermatologist and he prescribed a form of benzoyl peroxide for 2 weeks and had little success. The medical history includes recurrent sinusitis. DR was treated for the last episode with amoxicillin-clavulanate (Augmentin®). She also takes ibuprofen for menstrual cramps, norgestrel with ethinyl estradiol (Lo/Ovral®), and astemizole (Hismanal®).

QUESTIONS

1. The following should be emphasized to the patient concerning the initiation of benzoyl peroxide therapy:

A. Initial treatments should be applied once daily to decrease irritation.

B. The gel should be applied sparingly, and the periorbital, perinasal, and perioral skin should be avoided.

C. Mild erythema, burning, or stinging may occur with the initial application. If the medication is ap-

plied at bedtime, the erythema should be minimal by the next morning.

D. A and B

E. All of the above

2. What other information should be included in your counseling session with DR?

A. Tolerance to adverse effects should occur as therapy continues.

B. Because benzoyl peroxide can bleach hair and clothes, the preparation should be allowed to dry before coming into contact with fabrics.

C. The full therapeutic effect may not be apparent for 4 to 8 weeks, so compliance is important.

D. A and B

E. All of the above

3. DR responds fairly well to the benzoyl peroxide therapy and continues the therapy for approximately 7 months. At that time, however, DR notices worsening of her acne and inflamed lesions. The dermatologist decides to add systemic therapy with minocycline while continuing the benzoyl peroxide therapy. DR comes to your pharmacy with a prescription for minocycline. Which of the following statement(s) concerning minocycline is/are true?

A. This agent can cause esophagitis due to reflux; it should not be taken just before going to bed.
B. Minocycline should be avoided in pregnancy.
C. Vestibular side effects, such as dizziness, vertigo, and light-headedness, can occur with minocycline use, particularly at higher doses.
D. A and B
E. All of the above

4. DR was not aware of the cost of minocycline therapy and tells you that she cannot afford this therapy. She asks you to ask her dermatologist for an alternative agent that is less expensive. You notice on her medication profile that DR also takes astemizole (Hismanal®). Which combination should be avoided because of an interaction that could result in cardiac effects such as prolongation of the QRS or the QT interval?

A. Trimethoprim-sulfamethoxazole and astemizole
B. Erythromycin and astemizole
C. Tetracycline and astemizole
D. A and B
E. All of the above

5. If tetracycline had been the agent originally prescribed, which of the following statement(s) is/are true concerning this agent?

A. Photosensitivity can occur, and patients should be counseled to wear sunscreen with an SPF of at least 15 if planning to spend time in the sun.
B. Vaginal yeast infection is a common side effect of tetracycline.
C. Coadministration with dairy products, antacids, bismuth salts, sucralfate, and iron can decrease absorption of tetracycline, and administration should be separated.
D. A and B
E. All of the above

PATIENT PROFILE 126

HUMAN IMMUNODEFICIENCY VIRUS

PRESENTATION

LB is a 28-year-old woman presenting to her primary care physician with vaginal discharge and burning with urination.
PMH: Multiple episodes of gonococcal urethritis
Primary syphilis (treated with benzathine penicillin) 12 months ago
Chronic hepatitis C
HIV-positive, diagnosed 12 months ago
No history of AIDS-related opportunistic infections
MH: Methadone 40 mg qd
ALL: NKDA
SH: Smokes (1 ppd × 10 years)
Intravenous drug user (IVDU) for many years, but currently receiving chronic methadone maintenance
ROS: Burning with urination. She does not have any other complaints. She has not noted any recent weight gain, edema, abdominal pain, or abdominal girth enlargement.
PE: VS: BP 115/75 mm Hg, HR 100, RR 18, Temp 37.5°C, Ht 170 cm, Wt 55 kg
Gen: Pale, cachectic, ill-appearing woman, with some pelvic discomfort
HEENT: Drooping eyelids, otherwise normal
CV: Normal, no murmurs
Chest: Clear

ABD: Normal, no pitting edema
GU: Slight vaginal discharge; examination does not reveal any adnexal or cervical motion tenderness
Ext: Thin, but otherwise normal
Neuro: Lethargic but oriented ×3

LABORATORY VALUES

Hct 27%, CD4 150 cells/mm³ (500 6 months ago), Hgb 12 g/dL, HIV RNA 25,000 copies/mL (4000 6 months ago), WBC 3500 cells/mm³, PLTS 150,000 cells/mm³, BUN 20 mg/dL, AST 110 U/L, SCr 1.0 mg/dL, ALT 125 U/L, serum HCG positive

QUESTIONS

1. In light of her urethral signs and symptoms and her past history of sexually transmitted diseases, LB's physician would like to initiate treatment for infectious urethritis. To treat this condition, antibiotic coverage should include which of the following?
   I. *Chlamydia trachomatis*
   II. *Neisseria gonorrhoeae*
   III. *Streptococcus pneumoniae*
   IV. *Bacteroides fragilis*

A. I; no need to cover for II, III, and IV
B. II; no need to cover for I, III, and IV
C. I and II; no need to cover for III and IV
D. I, II, and IV; no need to cover for III

2. Listed below are four drug regimens. Which is the most appropriate regimen for treatment of LB's infectious urethritis?

A. One dose of ceftriaxone 125 mg intramuscularly (IM) plus erythromycin po 500 mg qid for 7 days
B. One dose of ciprofloxacin po 500 mg plus doxycycline po 100 mg bid for 7 days
C. One dose of ceftriaxone 125 mg IM
D. Azithromycin 1 g as a single oral dose

3. Which of the following is sufficient to establish an AIDS diagnosis in this HIV-positive patient?

A. Her HIV RNA is 25,000 copies/mL.
B. She has acquired several sexually transmitted diseases.
C. Her CD4 cell count is 150 cells/mm^3.
D. Her WBC count is 3500 cells/mm^3.

4. Which of the following antiretrovirals (ARTs) should be avoided in LB because of her pregnancy?

I. Combinations of d4T and ddI
II. Amprenavir oral solution
III. Saquinavir capsules
IV. Abacavir oral solution
V. Abacavir tablets
VI. Efavirenz capsules

A. I, II, and VI only
B. I, II, III, and IV only
C. I and II only
D. III and V only

5. If LB's physician were to prescribe ART therapy, which of the following regimens is least likely to produce a significant and sustained virologic, immunologic, and clinical response?

A. Nevirapine + lamivudine + d4T
B. Abacavir + lamivudine + zidovudine
C. Kaletra + lamivudine + stavudine
D. Efavirenz + 3TC + AZT

6. If LB's physician were to consider starting AZT therapy to prevent mother-to-child transmission of HIV, which of the following is included as components of this protocol?

I. Oral AZT is administered to the mother starting at 14 weeks of gestation.

II. IV AZT is administered to the mother at the start of labor and continued until delivery.
III. Oral AZT is administered to the infant for 6 weeks after delivery.
IV. Oral AZT is administered to the mother for 9 months after delivery.

A. The protocol includes I, II, III, and IV.
B. The protocol includes I and III only.
C. The protocol includes I, II, and IV only.
D. The protocol includes I, II, and III only.

7. If LB's physician wishes to initiate ART therapy, LB's maintenance methadone requirements may change. Which of the following ARTs is most likely to cause this change and what effect is likely to be observed?

A. Lopinavir/ritonavir (Kaletra®); increased methadone requirements
B. Zidovudine; decreased methadone requirements
C. Nelfinavir; decreased methadone requirements
D. Stavudine; increased methadone requirements

8. In light of LB's history of chronic hepatitis C and elevated liver enzymes, her physician should be cautious with dosing of some of her ARTs. Which of the following ART classes require a dose change or should be used with particular caution in patients with significant hepatic dysfunction?

I. Protease inhibitors
II. Fusion inhibitors
III. Nucleoside reverse transcriptase inhibitors
IV. Nonnucleoside reverse transcriptase inhibitors

A. I, II, III, and IV
B. I, II, and IV only
C. I and IV only
D. III and IV only

9. Which of the following ART classes is most likely to cause a lipodystrophy syndrome?

A. Protease inhibitors
B. Nucleoside reverse transcriptase inhibitors
C. Nonnucleoside reverse transcriptase inhibitors
D. Fusion inhibitors

10. Which of the following ART classes is most likely to cause lactic acidosis?
A. Protease inhibitors
B. Nucleoside reverse transcriptase inhibitors
C. Nonnucleoside reverse transcriptase inhibitors
D. Fusion inhibitors

PATIENT PROFILE 127

ONCOLOGY: PEDIATRIC ACUTE LYMPHOCYTIC LEUKEMIA

PRESENTATION

RB is a 3-year-old girl brought to the pediatrician by her mother because of fever, pallor, and leg pain. This is the second visit in 2 weeks for similar symptoms. There are no defined bumps or bruises on RB's legs, and the fever has been continually low grade. Blood is drawn for a CBC count, and the results are as follows:

WBC: 50,000

Differential: Neutrophils 15%, lymphocytes 75%, lymphoblasts 10%

Plts: 125,000

Hgb: 6%

Bone marrow biopsy shows more than 60% blast cells. Acute lymphocytic leukemia is diagnosed. Initial treatment is chemotherapy.

QUESTIONS

1. Before antineoplastic therapy is initiated, RB is treated with allopurinol. What is the most likely indication for treatment with allopurinol?

   A. Prevention of acute gout
   B. Maximization of effect of planned antineoplastic agents
   C. Prevention of elevation of uric acid level caused by cell destruction
   D. Minimization of antineoplastic drug toxicity
   E. Prevention of drug-drug interactions between vincristine and prednisone

2. RB begins induction therapy with prednisone, vincristine, and asparaginase. She tolerates the therapy fairly well but has not had a bowel movement in 5 days. What is the most likely cause of the constipation?

   A. Decreased fluid intake
   B. Exposure to vincristine
   C. Exposure to asparaginase
   D. Decrease in physical activity
   E. Use of ibuprofen used to control leg pain

3. RB achieves remission after induction therapy. Her therapy will continue with consolidation and maintenance phases of therapy. What is the most likely reason to extend maintenance therapy?

   A. To prevent disease recurrence
   B. To prevent spread of disease to the CNS
   C. To allow bone marrow to be harvesting for possible transplantation
   D. To prevent spread of disease to the liver
   E. To extend the close follow-up period

4. Which of the following treatments is most likely to be used to minimize the risk of spread of disease to the CNS?

   A. Cranial irradiation alone
   B. Low-dose, intravenous administration of methotrexate and cranial irradiation
   C. Intrathecal administration of methotrexate alone
   D. Intrathecal administration of methotrexate, hydrocortisone, and cytarabine
   E. Intravenous administration of hydrocortisone alone

5. What is the primary adverse effect of cranial irradiation?

   A. Headache
   B. Intractable nausea and vomiting
   C. Vision changes
   D. Cognitive impairment
   E. Ototoxicity

PATIENT PROFILE 128

OVER-THE-COUNTER PRODUCTS

PRESENTATION

CC: "I'm here for my yearly physical."

HPI: JA is a 72-year-old Caucasian woman who has come to her primary care physician for her annual physical examination.

PMH: Hypertension, hypothyroidism, osteoporosis, urinary incontinence, iron-deficiency anemia

Surgical history: Hysterectomy 20 years ago

ALL: NKDA

FH: Father died at age 89 of leukemia. Mother died at age 82 of natural causes. JA has one brother, two sisters, and four children with no health problems.

SH: JA is a retired Spanish teacher. She has lived alone since her husband's death 4 years ago. She is a non-smoker, does not drink alcohol, rarely has caffeine, and has never used illicit drugs.

MH: Lisinopril 10 mg PO qd, hydrochlorothiazide 25 mg PO qd, alendronate sodium 70 mg PO once weekly, conjugated estrogen 0.625 mg PO qd, tolteridine 2 mg PO bid; levothyroxine 0.1 mg PO qd, vitamin C 500 mg PO qd, calcium 600 mg plus vitamin D 200-IU tablets PO bid, Maalox suspension PO PRN for heartburn, ferrous sulfate 325 mg PO bid

PHYSICAL EXAMINATION

Gen: Well-nourished elderly woman in NAD who walks with a slight shuffle compared with previous years

VS: Blood pressure: 110/70 mm Hg; pulse: 64 beats per minute; respiration rate: 16 respirations per minute; temperature: 98.7°F; height: 60.5 in; weight: 120 lb

HEENT: PERRLA, fundi clear, ears clear

Neck: Supple without adenopathy or thyromegaly

Pulm: Clear to A&P

CV: RRR; normal S_1, S_2 sounds

Abd: Soft, nontender, positive bowel sounds

GU: Gynecologic examination deferred

Ext: Normal skin turgor; slight tenderness and swelling bilaterally in knees

Neuro: Reflexes are symmetric and active.

LABORATORY VALUES

Sodium: 138 mEq/L
Potassium: 4.1 mEq/L
Chloride: 95 mEq/L
Bicarbonate: 23 mEq/L
Blood urea nitrogen (BUN): 12 mg/dL
Serum creatinine: 1.5 mg/dL
Glucose (fasting): 85 mg/dL
Albumin: 4.0 mg/dL
Hemoglobin: 11 g/dL
Hematocrit: 36%
Platelets: 150 K/mm^3
White blood cell (WBC) count: 5000/mm^3
Thyroid-stimulating hormone (TSH): 2 μIU/mL (0.4–4 μIU/mL)
Total cholesterol: 211 mg/dL
Triglycerides: 172 mg/dL
High-density lipoprotein (HDL) cholesterol: 33 mg/dL
Low-density lipoprotein (LDL) cholesterol: 144 mg/dL

QUESTIONS

1. JA's doctor is concerned about her triglyceride level and would like to initiate atorvastatin 10 mg PO qd. However, JA is tired of taking prescription medications and would like to know if there is an over-the-counter (OTC) product that she could take instead. Which of the following OTC products could be used to reduce JA's triglyceride level?

   A. Vitamin E
   B. Selenium
   C. Vitamin A
   D. Nicotinic acid
   E. Aspirin

2. JA returns to her doctor 2 months later with symptoms consistent with those of community-acquired pneumonia. Her doctor prescribes levofloxacin 500 mg PO qd for 7 days. Which of JA's current medications is most likely to interact with the levofloxacin therapy?

   A. Tolteridine
   B. Maalox
   C. Lisinopril
   D. Alendronate
   E. Vitamin C

3. Which of the following OTC products should be used with caution in JA?

   A. Diphenydramine
   B. Senna
   C. Dextromethorphan
   D. Docusate
   E. Famotidine

4. JA is diagnosed with osteoarthritis. What would be an appropriate first-line therapy for her?

   A. Celecoxib
   B. Aspirin

    C. Ibuprofen
    D. Acetaminophen
    E. Naproxen

5. What vitamin is used to promote the absorption of iron?

    A. A
    B. B_6
    C. C
    D. D
    E. E

6. JA has been constipated for 3 days. She asks about using mineral oil because her mother used to give that to her as a child. Which of the following is(are) correct regarding the use of mineral oil in the management of JA's constipation?

    I. Mineral oil should not be administered at bedtime because it may result in lipid pneumonia.
    II. Absorption of fat-soluble vitamins is not altered by the administration of mineral oil.
    III. Mineral oil is a lubricant laxative that softens fecal contents by coating them and therefore preventing the colonic absorption of fecal water.

    A. I only
    B. III only
    C. I and III only
    D. II and III only
    E. I, II, and III

7. Which of the following statements is *not true* regarding JA's intake of calcium?

    A. Adequate vitamin D intake and taking the calcium source with a meal help to increase calcium absorption.

    B. Iron absorption is enhanced by high doses of calcium supplementation.
    C. Excessive ingestion of aluminum-containing antacids can result in a negative calcium balance.
    D. JA's osteoporosis is the result of an imbalance in the process of resorption and formation of the calcium content in one.
    E. The recommended daily amount of calcium for women over 50 years of age is 1200 mg.

8. Which of JA's medications may impair the absorption of the levothyroxine dose?

    A. Ferrous sulfate
    B. Conjugated estrogen
    C. Lisinopril
    D. Tolteridine
    E. Vitamin C

9. What is a frequent side effect of iron therapy?

    A. Cough
    B. Dizziness
    C. Headache
    D. Constipation
    E. Weight gain

10. Which of the following OTC products could lead to a possible increase in JA's serum level of estrogen?

    A. Ferrous sulfate
    B. Maalox
    C. Vitamin C
    D. Calcium
    E. Vitamin D

PATIENT PROFILE 129
MEDICINAL CHEMISTRY

PRESENTATION AND QUESTION

SK is a 45-year-old man with diabetes. His blood sugar has been adequately controlled with tolbutamide (struc-ture 129.1) administered tid. He says he sometimes forgets to take his medication and has asked his physician for help. The physician calls you and asks for your advice.

$CH_3-\bigcirc-SO_2NHCONHC_4H_9$

129.1

$Cl-\bigcirc-SO_2NHCONHC_3H_7$

129.2

You recommend that SK switch to chlorpropamide (structure 129.2), which can be taken once a day rather than two or three times a day. The physician immediately says, "You're right. Why didn't I think of that?" The physician continues, "Can you refresh my memory about why there is such a difference in duration of action between tolbutamide and chlorpropamide even though they are very similar in chemical structure?" Your explanation is as follows:

A. There is no scientific explanation for the difference. It is just the intrinsic properties of each sulfonylurea oral antidiabetic agent.

B. The butyl group in the tolbutamide molecule makes it less lipophilic, so it has a faster excretion rate than does chlorpropamide.
C. Chlorpropamide undergoes enterohepatic circulation and tolbutamide does not.
D. Chlorpropamide has more plasma protein binding than tolbutamide, which let it stay longer in the body.
E. Tolbutamide is easily metabolized through oxidation of the toluyl group into inactive carboxylic acid products, whereas chlorpropamide does not undergo oxidation at the chlorine atom site.

PATIENT PROFILE 130

IRRITABLE BOWEL SYNDROME

PRESENTATION

FP is a 65-year-old woman who presents to the clinic with new complaints about her diarrhea-predominant irritable bowel syndrome (IBS). She states that she was diagnosed with IBS "years" ago, for which she uses loperamide for relief. She has recently been having four loose, watery bowel movements per day (compared with her baseline of two per day) and has been taking more loperamide than usual. She complains that these symptoms have kept her awake at night. She denies weight loss or blood in her stool.

FP also has depression and osteoarthritis of the knee, and she is postmenopausal. Her current medication regimen includes Premarin 0.625 mg PO daily, fluoxetine 20 mg PO daily, calcium with vitamin D (dose unknown), multivitamin 1 tablet PO daily, loperamide 2 mg PO bid PRN, Aleve PRN, glucosamine and chondroitin (dose unknown), atenolol 50 mg PO daily, and hydrochlorothiazide 50 mg PO daily. She has had an anaphylactic reaction to penicillin in the past. Vital signs are blood pressure = 140/82 mm Hg; heart rate = 59 beats per minute; and temperature 37°C. She is currently not experiencing any pain from her IBS or osteoarthritis. Her physical examination is unremarkable. Blood chemistry and a complete blood count (CBC) have been ordered and are pending.

QUESTIONS

1. What additional information would be helpful in determining the cause of FP's IBS exacerbation?

A. Diet
B. Activity level
C. Stress level
D. A and C only
E. All the above

2. Which of the following are considered "alarm" symptoms in patients with IBS?

A. Weight gain
B. Loose stools
C. Gastrointestinal bleeding
D. Neutropenia

3. Which of the following medications in FP's regimen in combination with her IBS place her at risk for development dehydration and electrolyte abnormalities?

A. Fluoxetine
B. Premarin
C. Hydrochlorothiazide
D. Atenolol

4. Loperamide can decrease gastrointestinal motility and therefore could _____ of medications in FP's regimen.

A. Decrease the absorption
B. Increase the absorption
C. Increase the metabolism
D. Inhibit the metabolism

5. Which of the following statements regarding the use of loperamide is *correct*?

A. Loperamide should be used for no longer than 5 days.
B. Loperamide should be used for no longer than 1 week

C. The daily maximum dose of loperamide is 16 mg.

D. The daily maximum dose of loperamide is 8 mg.

E. There is no daily maximum dose or limitations to the duration of use for loperamide.

6. Diphenoxylate/atropine is considered a second-line agent in the treatment of diarrhea-predominant IBS. Which of the following statements regarding the use of diphenoxylate/atropine in FP is *correct*?

A. Diphenoxylate/atropine is not an appropriate treatment option for FP owing to its high incidence of anticholinergic side effects.

B. The combination of diphenoxylate/atropine and fluoxetine places FP at risk for developing serotonin syndrome.

C. Diphenoxylate/atropine is contraindicated in patients with hypertension.

D. Diphenoxylate/atropine is an appropriate treatment option for FP.

7. The physician would like to know about other treatment options for the management of diarrhea-predominant IBS. A literature search reveals that cholestyramine can be used in patients who are refractory to standard antidiarrheal therapy. Which of the following is(are) reason(s) not to use cholestyramine in FP?

A. Palatability

B. Risk of drug-drug interactions

C. Cost

D. A and B only

E. All the above

8. FP has seen television commercials recently promoting a new medication for IBS called Zelnorm. She would like to know if this medication could be helpful for her symptoms. Which of the following statements regarding the use of Zelnorm in FP is *correct*?

A. Zelnorm is approved for use in patients with constipation-predominant IBS and therefore is not an option for FP.

B. Zelnorm can cause severe diarrhea and should not be used in FP.

C. Zelnorm is currently not approved for use in women.

D. A and B only

E. All the above

9. The physician is still uncertain as to which medication would be most appropriate to use in FP. She had prescribed a drug named alosetron in the past for other patients, but it has been withdrawn from the market. A colleague told her that it was now available again. Which of the following statements regarding alosetron is *correct*?

A. Alosetron is a 5-HT_3-selective antagonist that is used to treat women with diarrhea-predominant IBS.

B. Alosetron was withdrawn from the market in 2000 because of several case reports of severe constipation and ischemic colitis.

C. Alosetron can be prescribed for women with diarrhea-predominant IBS, but the physician must register with the manufacturer, and the patient must sign an agreement for use.

D. All the above

10. Alosetron should be discontinued immediately in patients experiencing which of the following symptoms?

A. Severe constipation

B. Rectal bleeding

C. Headache

D. A and B only

E. All the above

PATIENT PROFILE 131

SCHIZOPHRENIA

PRESENTATION

JB is a 24-year-old man with paranoid-type schizophrenia diagnosed 6 months ago. He reports muscle rigidity and neck stiffness. JB has a history that began when he was 20 years of age of hearing voices that tell him that others are evil. Six months ago he started therapy with chlorpromazine 50 mg bid and titrated up to the present dose of 150 mg bid. The hearing of voices is well controlled, although JB now reports muscle rigidity and a stiff neck.

The medical history includes schizophrenia. JB underwent an appendectomy at age 14. He had no known drug allergies. JB takes chlorpromazine 150 mg bid. He lives with his parents. He denies use of alcohol or illicit drugs. He smokes two packs of cigarettes per day.

PHYSICAL EXAMINATION

BP sitting R arm: 132/88, HR: 76
BP standing R arm: 100/68, HR: 110
RR: 22
T: 99°F

LABS

Na: 139 mEq/L
Cl: 99 mEq/L
CO_2 20 mEq/L
Gluc: 120 mg/dL
K: 4.2 mEq/L
BUN 32 mg/dL
SCr 0.9 mg/dL

A/P: JB is a 24-year-old man with schizophrenia who appears well nourished and well kept. Since a recent increase in chlorpromazine dose to manage auditory hallucinations, the patient has experienced a stiff nick and muscle rigidity. The patient also reports feeling dizzy when he stands quickly.

QUESTIONS

1. Chlorpromazine controls auditory hallucinations through which supposed pharmacologic mechanism?

   A. Antagonism of muscarinic receptors
   B. Agonism of α_1 receptors
   C. Antagonism of dopamine-2 receptors
   D. Antagonism of serotonin reuptake
   E. Antagonism of histamine-1 receptors

2. The stiff neck and muscle rigidity can be labeled as what?

   A. A positive symptom of schizophrenia
   B. A negative symptom of schizophrenia
   C. An extrapyramidal symptom
   D. Tardive dyskinesia
   E. Serotonin syndrome

3. Which of the following is considered first-line therapy for the stiff neck and muscle rigidity?

   A. Benztropine 0.5 mg bid
   B. Increasing the chlorpromazine dose to 175 mg bid
   C. Clonidine 0.1 mg tid
   D. Fluoxetine 10 mg qd
   E. Multivitamin 1 tab qd

4. The orthostatic hypotension is most likely caused by antagonism of chlorpromazine at which receptor?

   A. Dopamine 2
   B. Histamine 1
   C. Serotonin 2
   D. α_1
   E. α_2

5. Which antipsychotic agent is associated with the greatest risk of seizures?

   A. Haloperidol
   B. Fluphenazine
   C. Clozapine
   D. Olanzapine
   E. Risperidone

PATIENT PROFILE 132

DIABETES AND NEPHROPATHY

PRESENTATION

CC: GP is a 59-year-old woman who presents to your pharmacy for a refill of her quinapril.

HPI: GP is a long-time patient at your pharmacy. She was diagnosed with type 2 diabetes 24 years ago and has been struggling to control her blood glucose for years. She is hypertensive, has been diagnosed recently with open-angle glaucoma, and has neuropathy in her hands and feet. The pain is minimal, although she often feels "pins and needles" if she sits for too long in one position. Recent blood work confirmed microalbuminuria (102 mg/24 hours), and her blood pressure is still uncontrolled.

PMH: Hypertension, type 2 diabetes, dylipidemia, peripheral neuropathy, glaucoma, depression

ALL: PCN, codeine

MH: Quinapril 10 mg PO qd, glyburide 10 mg PO qd, metformin 850 mg PO bid, rosiglitazone 4 mg PO qd, simvastatin 10 mg PO qhs, hydrochlorothiazide 25 mg PO qd, amitriptyline 25 mg PO qhs, fluoxetine 20 mg PO qd, conjugated estrogens 0.625 mg PO qd

FH: Mother deceased, history of type 2 diabetes, died of stroke at age 60. Father alive, age 86, Alzheimer's disease

SH: Married, homemaker, three children. Smokes (1 pack per day for 30 years)

PSH: Hysterectomy, 05/99; status post coronary artery bypass surgery (CABG), 11/02

VS: Blood pressure: 150/92 mm Hg; height: 5 ft, 5 in; weight: 145 lb

Labs: 143 108 29; 185; total cholesterol: 207 mg/dL; low-density lipoprotein (LDL) cholesterol: 144 mg/dL; 5.0 25 1.9; triglycerides: 145 mg/dL; high-density lipoprotein (HDL) cholesterol: 43 mg/dL; HgA1C: 11%; U/A: microalbuminuria

---

VISIT NOTES

According to her blood glucose log book, GP's blood glucose levels have not been controlled over the past 6 months, which is reflected in her HgA1C. She has difficulty taking her medications as directed, especially those which are dosed more than twice daily.

QUESTIONS

1. According to the JNC VII, what is GP's goal blood pressure?

   A. < 125/75 mm Hg
   B. < 130/70 mm Hg
   C. < 130/80 mm Hg
   D. < 140/90 mm Hg

2. Which of the following classes of medications has *not* been shown in clinical trials to delay the progression of nephropathy in diabetic patients?

   A. ARBs
   B. β-Blockers
   C. Dihydropyridine calcium channel blockers
   D. Nondihydropyridine calcium channel blockers

3. What is GP's creatinine clearance?

   A. 20 mL/min
   B. 27 mL/min
   C. 33 mL/min
   D. 43 mL/min

4. Which of the following medications should be adjusted because of GP's creatinine clearance?

   A. Quinapril
   B. Fluoxetine
   C. Rosiglitazone
   D. Conjugated estrogens

5. Which of the following medications is contraindicated in GP based on her laboratory values?

   A. Fluoxetine
   B. Metformin

   C. Simvastatin
   D. Rosiglitazone

6. What is GP's goal HDL?

   A. < 40 mg/dL
   B. < 50 mg/dL
   C. > 30 mg/dL
   D. > 50 mg/dL

7. What is GP's LDL goal?

   A. < 200 mg/dL
   B. < 160 mg/dL
   C. < 130 mg/dL
   D. < 100 mg/dL

8. Which of the following is considered a coronary heart disease (CHD) risk equivalent in GP?

   A. Smoking
   B. Dyslipidemia
   C. Hypertension
   D. Existing CHD

9. GP's ophthalmologist would like to start an eye drop to treat her glaucoma. Which of the following medications is the *most appropriate* to treat GP's glaucoma?

   A. Latanoprost
   B. Brimonidine
   C. Dorzolamide
   D. Pilocarpine solution

10. GP's physician would like to start insulin therapy with glargine insulin to replace the oral medication that was discontinued. Which of the following is *true regarding glargine*?

    A. Insulin glargine will act as a bolus to cover GP's meal-related hyperglycemia.
    B. Insulin glargine can be used in an insulin pump to provide long-term blood glucose control.
    C. Insulin glargine is a long-acting, peakless insulin that will mimic endogenous basal insulin.
    D. Insulin glargine can be mixed in the same syringe with a rapid-acting insulin if needed to cover meal-related hyperglycemia.

P A T I E N T   P R O F I L E   1 3 3

PARKINSON'S DISEASE

PRESENTATION

Patient	CS	
Age	67	
Allergies	NKA	
Race	White	
Height	5'6"	
Wt	125 lb	
Diagnosis	Primary	1. Parkinson's disease
		2. Depression
		3. BPH
	Secondary	1. Memory loss
		2. Insomnia

	Date	Rx No.	Physician	Drug and Strength	Quantity	Sig	Refills
Medication record	3/05	11256	NM	Benztropine 2 mg	60	1 bid	6
(prescription and OTC)	3/05	11257	NM	Sinemet® (carbidopa-levodopa) 10/100	90	1 tid	6
	3/05	11258	NM	Sertraline 50 mg	30	1 hs	2
Pharmacist notes and other patient info	3/05	Patient is forgetful and lives alone. Medications were placed in blister pack with day and time of administration.					
	3/05	Follow-up call to VNA about med compliance.					
	3/06	VNA notifies us patient has a Rx from another pharmacy for Hytrin® (terazosin)					
	3/06	Urinary retention may be a problem for this patient; waiting for return call from physician.					

QUESTIONS

1. Why are anticholinergics such as benztropine prescribed for a patient in the early stages of Parkinson's disease?

   A. To control insomnia
   B. To control tremor
   C. To control forgetfulness
   D. To control constipation
   E. All of the above

2. Why should benztropine be avoided by patients with benign prostatic hypertrophy (BPH)?

   A. It may cause urinary retention.
   B. It may interact with Hytrin® (terazosin).
   C. It may cause hyponatremia.
   D. It may cause insomnia.
   E. It may increase uric acid concentrations.

3. Dose-limiting side effects of levodopa are minimized when the drug is used in combination with the dopa decarboxylase inhibitor, carbidopa. Which of the following statement(s) is/are true?

   I. Carbidopa inhibits the peripheral conversion of levodopa to dopamine.
   II. Carbidopa does not penetrate the blood-brain barrier but increases the amount of dopamine to the brain.
   III. Carbidopa allows the dose of levodopa to be decreased by 80%.

   A. I only
   B. III only
   C. I and II only
   D. II and III only
   E. I, II, and III

4. Sinemet® (carbidopa-levodopa) contains a 1:10 fixed ratio of carbidopa and levodopa in which of the following formulations?

   I. Sinemet® 10/100
   II. Sinemet® 25/250
   III. Sinemet® 25/100

   A. I only
   B. III only
   C. I and II only

D. II and III only
E. I, II, and III

5. The initial response to levodopa is quite favorable and is termed the *honeymoon phase*. How long does this phase usually last?

A. 2 weeks
B. 12 months
C. 2 years
D. 10 years
E. 20 years

PATIENT PROFILE 134

KIDNEY TRANSPLANTATION

PRESENTATION

CC: EC is a 45-year-old man who presents to the transplant clinic complaining of headaches and new-onset tremor. He was asked to make this unscheduled appointment today because of an acute rise in his serum creatinine (baseline $S_{Cr} \approx 1.2$ mg/dL).

HPI: About 1 week ago, he went to his primary care physician (PCP) and was diagnosed with a gastric ulcer. He was given a prescription for Prevpak, filled it, and started taking it 2 days ago.

PMH: Cadaveric kidney transplant 4 years ago; polycystic kidney disease, hypertension, and coronary artery disease; had a myocardial infarction (MI) in 1999.

SH: Married with two children. Reports occasional alcohol use. Denies smoking. Works in an office as an investment accountant.

FH: Significant for polycystic kidney disease (mother and two of his three siblings)

VS: Temperature: 36.8°C; blood pressure: 110/64 mm Hg; heart rate: 88 beats per minute; respiratory rate: 16 breaths per minute

LABORATORY AND DIAGNOSTIC TESTS

Sodium: 141 mEq/L	Potassium: 4 mEq/L
Chloride: 112 mEq/L	CO_2: 26 mEq/L
Blood urea nitrogen (BUN): 16 mg/dL	Serum creatinine: 2.8 mg/dL
Glucose: 119 mg/dL	Calcium: 8.7 mg/dL
Magnesium: 1.3 mEq/L	Phosphorus: 3.2 mg/dL
White blood cell (WBC) count: 3800/mm^3	Hematocrit: 24.7%
Platelets 125,000/mm^3	Tacrolimus trough (7:30 AM): 21.4 ng/mL

CURRENT MEDICATIONS*

Aspirin 81 mg PO qd

*Takes all medications on an 8 AM/8 PM schedule

Lisinopril 10 mg PO qd
Magnesium oxide 400 mg PO bid
Metoprolol XL 100 mg PO qd
Oyster shell calcium with vitamin D 400 units PO bid
Prednisone 5 mg PO qd
Tacrolimus 2 mg PO bid
Lansoprazole 30 mg PO bid × 14 days (started 2 days ago)
Amoxicillin 500 mg PO bid × 14 days (started 2 days ago)
Clarithromycin 500 mg PO bid × 14 days (started 2 days ago)

QUESTIONS

1. Which of the following complications may cause an acute rise in the serum creatinine concentration?

   A. Acute rejection
   B. Dehydration
   C. Cyclosporine-induced nephrotoxicity
   D. A and B
   E. All the above

2. If this patient were diagnosed with acute cellular rejection, which of the following would be *appropriate* first-line therapy?

   A. Increase tacrolimus and mycophenolate mofetil doses
   B. Start high-dose intravenous methylprednisolone
   C. Start intravenous thymoglobulin
   D. Start intravenous Atgam
   E. Start intravenous OKT3

3. Which of the following changes in laboratory values might you expect as a result of administering high-dose methylprednisolone?

   A. Elevated potassium
   B. Elevated WBC count
   C. Decreased hematocrit and hemoglobin
   D. Elevated platelet count
   E. Decreased blood glucose

4. Which of the following complications are associated with long-term steroid use?

   A. Osteoporosis
   B. Hypertension
   C. Hypoglycemia
   D. A and B
   E. All the above

5. Which of the following is the *most likely* reason for EC's acute rise in the blood tacrolimus concentration?

   A. Acute rejection
   B. Dehydration
   C. Cyclosporine toxicity
   D. A and B
   E. All the above

6. Which of the following medications have been associated with renal dysfunction?

   A. Cyclosporine
   B. Sirolimus
   C. Tacrolimus
   D. A and B
   E. A and C

7. This patient's physician wishes to switch him from tacrolimus to sirolimus. Which of the following would you expect to be affected by sirolimus use?

   A. Pulmonary function tests
   B. Liver function tests
   C. Blood glucose levels
   D. Lipid panel
   E. Blood pressure and heart rate

8. What is the most likely reason for EC's elevated tacrolimus level?

   A. Drug interaction with lansoprazole
   B. Drug interaction with amoxicillin
   C. Drug interaction with clarithromycin
   D. The blood was drawn at the wrong time
   E. The patient took the wrong dose

9. Which of the following would be an *appropriate* treatment regimen for the gastric ulcer in this patient?

   A. Amoxicillin, clarithromycin, and lansoprazole as ordered
   B. Amoxicillin and lansoprazole
   C. Amoxicillin, metronidazole, and pantoprazole
   D. Clarithromycin, metronidazole, and omeprazole
   E. Clarithromycin, tetracycline, rabeprazole, and bismuth

10. During this clinic visit, EC requests a flu shot for the upcoming winter. Which of the following would be the *most appropriate* response?

   A. You are not a candidate for vaccines because immunosuppressed patients are unable to mount any response to them.
   B. You are not a candidate for live virus vaccines such as the flu shot.
   C. You are not a candidate for all types of vaccines, but an annual flu shot is safe and is strongly recommended.
   D. All vaccines are safe for use and strongly recommended in an immunosuppressed patient such as yourself.
   E. All vaccines are safe for use but not usually effective in an immunosuppressed patient such as yourself.

PATIENT PROFILE 135

CONGESTIVE HEART FAILURE

PRESENTATION

PN is a 55-year-old man who visits the clinic because of increasing shortness of breath when he walks up the stairs to his office. He states that over the past 3 weeks his shortness of breath has become progressively worse, to the point at which he cannot walk a full flight of stairs without pausing to catch his breath. PN states that this problem is new and that he did not have any limitations in physical activity until about 1½ to 2 months ago. On further questioning he states he also has problems sleeping flat on his back and that he needs two pillows to be comfortable. He also has noticed a 5-kg weight gain over the past month. He says that he eats a good diet and attempts to maintain a healthy lifestyle. The medical history includes hypertension, peptic ulcer disease (treated for *Helicobacter pylori* infection 2 years ago), and coronary artery disease (acute myocardial infarction 5 years ago). A review of systems shows nocturia (1 time per night) and chronic lower back pain.

MEDS

Diltiazem CD 300 mg po qd
Ibuprofen 800 mg prn for back pain
Pepcid® (famotidine) 20 mg po qhs
Clonidine 0.2 mg po bid
Nitroglycerin SL 0.4 mg prn for chest pain
Ticlid® (ticlopidine) 250 mg po bid

PHYSICAL EXAMINATION

BP: 145/90, HR: 85, RR: 20, T: afebrile
Ht: 5'11", Wt: 78 kg
HEENT: JVD 7 cm
COR: S_1, S_2, and positive S_3
PULM: Inspiratory rales
ABD: Slight hepatomegaly
EXT: 2+ pitting edema

LABS

Na: 132	K: 3.5
Cl: 95	CO_2: 28
BUN: 30	SCr: 1.0
Gluc: 120	WBC: 5.3
Hgb: 12.6	Hct: 39.3
Plts: 250,000	

QUESTIONS

1. Which of the following long-term medications may be exacerbating CHF by causing fluid overload?

   A. Ibuprofen
   B. Diltiazem
   C. Clonidine
   D. Ticlid® (ticlopidine)
   E. Pepcid® (famotidine)

2. Which of the following medications may be exacerbating PN's CHF by reducing the contractility of the myocardium?

   A. Ibuprofen
   B. Diltiazem
   C. Clonidine
   D. Ticlid® (ticlopidine)
   E. Pepcid® (famotidine)

3. Which of the following medications should be administered to PN at this time to manage the exacerbation of CHF?

   A. Enalapril
   B. Captopril
   C. Carvedilol
   D. Furosemide
   E. Isosorbide dinitrate with hydralazine

4. Which of the following interventions is going to provide the greatest benefit in terms of decreasing mortality from CHF?

   A. Digoxin 0.125 mg po qd
   B. Lasix® (furosemide) 20 mg po qd
   C. Enalapril 5 mg po bid
   D. Isosorbide dinitrate 30 mg po tid
   E. Amlodipine 5 mg po qd

5. Which of the following would you want to avoid if chronic renal insufficiency were to develop?

   A. Lasix® (furosemide)
   B. Metoprolol
   C. Hydralazine
   D. Lisinopril
   E. Carvedilol

PATIENT PROFILE 136

DIABETES MELLITUS

PRESENTATION

RG is a 72-year-old Asian woman who brings a new prescription for ibuprofen 600 mg qid for arthritis pain to the HMO outpatient pharmacy where you work. She states that she has tried Tylenol for the pain, but it was not effective. Her pain is primarily in her knees although occasionally the joints in her hands bother her as well. She states that when the pain is at its worst, it is 5 on a scale of 10 (0–10 pain

scale). The pain rarely wakes her up at night. This tends to happen on days when she has been more active than usual, such as when she goes shopping all day with her daughter-in-law. She experiences some pain in her knees every day.

She has a cold and is considering purchasing some Alka-Seltzer Cold Plus for her symptoms of runny nose, cough, and headache. She denies fevers or chills. She has had the symptoms for about a day. She states that owing to the congestion, she has not been able to sleep well at night.

Her past medical history includes heart failure (LVEF = 30% on echocardiogram), obesity, osteoarthritis, type 2 diabetes mellitus, status post myocardial infarction 4 years ago, and hyperlipidemia. Her current medications are aspirin 81 mg once daily, glipizide 10 mg once daily, fosinopril 80 mg once daily, metoprolol XL 25 mg once daily, and lovastatin 40 mg once daily. She uses a medication box to keep track of her pills and is compliant with her medication regimen.

RG lives with her husband of 50 years. She has two children, both of whom are married and live nearby. She has one grandchild who is 3 years old. She does not drink alcohol or use tobacco products. Her only exercise is the work she does around the house. In general, she is fairly sedentary.

She denies any signs or symptoms of hypoglycemia or hyperglycemia, although her fasting morning blood sugar from her home glucose meter today was 150 mg/dL, which is a little higher than usual. She states that her blood sugars usually run in the 100s. She only checks her blood sugar once a day in the morning before she takes her medication and before she eats breakfast.

She is concerned about her weight and is considering trying a product she heard about on the radio. She has met with a dietician several times but does not feel that she can follow the recommendations that were made. She did not discuss her concerns with the dietician but decided not to go to her follow-up appointment with the dietician. In particular, she remembers being told to decrease the amount of rice that she eats. However, RG states that rice is a central part of her diet and culture and that she finds eating rice comforting.

RG's height is 5 ft, 1 in. RG's weight is 180 lb. RG's vital signs per her primary care provider's progress note are as follows: blood pressure: 150/88 mm Hg; heart rate: 55 beats per minute; respiratory rate: 17 breaths per minute; and temperature: 98.6°F. RG's laboratory values today are as follows: A1c: 7.1%; Na: 134 mEq/L; K: 3.8 mEq/L; blood urea nitrogen (BUN): 17 mg/dL; serum Cr: 1.3 mg/dL; glucose: 148 mg/dL; total cholesterol: 175 mg/dL; low-density lipoprotein (LDL) cholesterol: 98 mg/dL; high-density lipoprotein (HDL) cholesterol: 52 mg/dL; and triglycerides: 125 md/dL. All liver function tests and components of her complete blood count are within normal limits. RG confirmed that she fasted 12 hours prior to her blood being drawn.

You review RG's medical chart and note that at his last visit 3 months ago her vital signs were as follows: blood pressure: 156/82 mm Hg; heart rate: 60 beats per minute; respiratory rate: 18 breath per minute; and temperature: 98.6°F. Her past urine microalbumin:albumin ratios were less than 10 μg/mg creatinine, which is consistent with normoalbuminuria.

QUESTIONS

1. Given RG's age, current medications, and past medical history, which of the following conditions is RG at risk of developing owing to the addition of ibuprofen to her medication regimen?

   A. Renal failure
   B. Constipation
   C. Orthostatic hypotension
   D. Insomnia
   E. Hair loss

2. Alka-Seltzer Cold Plus contains the following active ingredients per tablet: acetaminophen 250 mg, chlorpheniramine 2 mg, and phenylephrine 5 mg. This product does not contain sugar. The manufacturer recommends taking 2 tablets every 4 hours without exceeding 8 tablets in a 24-hour period. RG asks you if it would be okay to try this cold remedy. Based on the information provided in the case presentation, which of the following statements is the *most appropriate* response?

   A. This medication is an appropriate medication to use because your blood sugars are controlled.
   B. This medication is not an appropriate medication to use because your blood sugars are not controlled.
   C. This medication is an appropriate medication to use because your blood pressure is controlled.
   D. This medication is not an appropriate medication to use because your blood pressure is not controlled.
   E. This medication is an appropriate medication to use because your cholesterol is controlled.

3. RG's primary care provider is considering adding an agent for treatment of RG's blood pressure. Which of the following recommendations is the *most appropriate*?

   A. Add captopril 50 mg tid
   B. Add furosemide 20 mg once daily
   C. Add amlodipine 5 mg once daily
   D. Add Catapres-TTS (clonidine patch) 0.1 mg/24 hours; change patch every 7 days
   E. Add terazosin 1 mg once daily

4. RG's primary care provider is considering adding hydrochlorothiazide to her medication regimen. Which of the following is an adverse effect of hydrochlorothiazide?

   A. Hyperkalemia
   B. Elevated liver function tests
   C. Pulmonary fibrosis
   D. Weight gain
   E. Glucose intolerance

5. Twice a week RG takes care of her grandchild. On those days she sometimes misses her noon meal and

has been becoming hypoglycemic. RG's care provider decides to discontinue her glipizide and try Prandin (repaglinide). Which of the following is the *most appropriate* way to initiate Prandin drug therapy?

A. Repaglinide 0.5 mg once daily a half hour before morning meal
B. Repaglinide 0.5 mg twice daily a half hour before morning and evening meals
C. Repaglinide 0.5 mg once daily with evening meal
D. Repaglinide 0.5 mg twice daily with morning and evening meals
E. Repaglinide 0.5 mg three times daily with first bite of each meal. If meal is skipped, skip dose of medication as well.

6. Which of the following adverse effects should RG be counseled about on initiation of Prandin (repaglinide)?

A. Hypoglycemia
B. Gastritis
C. Cough
D. Urinary retention
E. All the above

7. Several years later, RG's glycemic control worsens. Her primary care provider is considering adding metformin to her medication regimen. Which of the following laboratory values are the *most appropriate* to review before initiation of metformin therapy?

A. Creatinine
B. Liver function tests
C. Albumin
D. A and B
E. A, B, and C

8. Metformin is added to RG's medication regimen. Which of the following is the *most appropriate* dose for initiation of metformin therapy?

A. Metformin 1000 mg tid
B. Metformin 1000 mg twice daily
C. Metformin 850 mg tid
D. Metformin 500 mg bid
E. Metformin 125 mg once daily

9. Several years later, RG is seen in the emergency department of a local hospital with severe abdominal pain. An abdominal CT scan with intravenous radiocontrast material is ordered for this afternoon. In addition to other medications, RG is taking metformin 1000 mg twice daily. She took her last dose this morning at 9 AM. It is currently 11 AM. Which of the following is the *most appropriate* recommendation?

A. Delay the CT scan with intravenous radiocontrast material until the evening so that the metformin will be out of her system prior to the procedure. Then resume metformin immediately after the CT scan has been completed.
B. Suggest that the physician order a CT scan without intravenous radiocontrast material because using radiocontrast material is an absolute contraindication with metformin use.
C. Hold the metformin until 48 hours after the CT scan with intravenous radiocontrast material. After 48 hours, check renal function and resume metformin only if renal function is normal.
D. Decrease RG's metformin dose by 50% to 500 mg twice daily until 48 hours after the CT scan with intravenous radiocontrast material has been completed. Resume her usual metformin dose only if renal function is normal.
E. Hold the metformin for 2 weeks after the CT scan with intravenous radiocontrast material. Check renal function and resume metformin only if renal function is normal.

10. Several months later, RG is considering purchasing an alternative medication for weight loss and asks you for advice. She lists the active ingredient as country mallow. You conduct a search on country mallow and find that it is an ephedra-like substance. Which of the following statements is the *most appropriate* response?

A. Although minimal data exist on the efficacy of these agents on weight loss, they have not been documented to cause harm and are worth a trial.
B. Substantial data exist on the efficacy of these agents on weight loss. However, they tend to increase blood sugar levels and should not be used in patients with diabetes mellitus.
C. These agents may be effective at reducing weight but have been associated with elevations in blood pressure and fatalities.
D. These agents are known to increase levels of your medications for diabetes mellitus. Consult with your physician before initiating therapy. You may need a reduction in your doses so that you do not experience hypoglycemia.
E. These agents tend to mask the signs and symptoms of a low blood sugar reaction. Because a low blood sugar reaction, if not treated promptly, potentially could be fatal, these agents should not be used in patients with diabetes mellitus on medications that can cause hypoglycemia.

PATIENT PROFILE 137

HYPERCHOLESTEROLEMIA

PRESENTATION

AL is a 46-year-old woman with a history of hyperthyroidism and migraine headaches. She is visiting her primary care physician for a yearly routine examination. AL has no known drug allergies and takes methimazole 30 mg po qd and naproxen 500 mg po bid prn. There is no family history of coronary artery disease or diabetes mellitus. AL's mother died of breast cancer, her father has hypertension, and her sister had cervical cancer. AL is married, has four children, and works in a school kitchen. She does not smoke cigarettes, drink alcohol, or use illicit drugs. She consumes no specific diet and does not exercise.

PHYSICAL EXAMINATION

BP: 120/70, HR: 68, RR: 20
Ht: 63.5", Wt: 160 lb

LABS

Electrolytes: WNL
SCr: 0.6 mg/dL
Total chol: 257 mg/dL
HDL chol: 42 mg/dL
LDL chol: 204 mg/dL
Trig: 56 mg/dL

BUN: 14 mg/dL
WBC: 5.63 K/μL
Hct: 40.6%
Hgb: 13.8g/dL
Plts: 284K/μL

QUESTIONS

1. Initial management with exercise and diet to lower the cholesterol level is not successful. Which of the following is an appropriate choice for initial drug treatment of AL? Select the best answer.

   A. Cholestyramine
   B. Pravastatin
   C. Gemfibrozil
   D. A and B only
   E. A, B, and C

2. Niacin is started as initial therapy. You counsel the patient on the use of this medication. One of the adverse effects you discuss is the flushing that may occur with use of niacin. Which of the following is/are true?

   A. Taking aspirin 325 mg ½ hour before taking niacin may help to avoid or reduce flushing.

   B. Taking ibuprofen ½ hour before taking niacin may help to avoid or reduce flushing.
   C. Avoidance of hot beverages during initiation of niacin therapy may help to reduce the occurrence of this effect.
   D. A and B only
   E. A, B, and C

3. After AL starts drug therapy, when should the initial LDL level be measured to assess efficacy?

   A. 1 week after starting drug therapy
   B. 1 month after starting drug therapy
   C. 3 months after starting drug therapy
   D. 6 months after starting drug therapy
   E. 1 year after starting drug therapy

4. AL stops taking the niacin because she cannot tolerate the adverse effects. The physician prescribes lovastatin. The physician thought he heard something about monitoring the liver function of patients taking lovastatin. You tell him the following:

   A. Liver function test results do not have to be monitored.
   B. Liver function tests should be performed 6 and 12 weeks after initiation of therapy or an increase in dosage and approximately every 6 months thereafter.
   C. Liver function tests should be performed before initiating lovastatin therapy, 6 and 12 weeks after initiation of therapy or an increase in dosage, and approximately every 6 months thereafter.
   D. Liver function tests should be performed before initiation of lovastatin therapy, monthly for the first 3 months, and yearly thereafter.
   E. Liver function tests should be performed before initiating lovastatin therapy and 6 months after therapy is begun.

5. During your counseling session with AL, you are asked about possible side effects of lovastatin. Which of the following side effects may occur with lovastatin?

   A. Muscle aches
   B. Nausea
   C. Headache
   D. A and B only
   E. A, B, and C

PATIENT PROFILE 138
HYPERLIPIDEMIA

PRESENTATION

RF presents to the pharmacist-coordinated lipid clinic at the insistence of his "health crazy" girlfriend. He is a 28-year-old white man. RF recently attended a cholesterol screening at his local community pharmacy. He had just eaten a hot dog and steak tips at the local professional baseball game prior to the screening. His girlfriend recalls that his cholesterol was roughly 200 at that time. Past medical history includes diabetes mellitus type 2. He also broke his left arm last year while playing baseball for his local softball league. A current medication list according to the patient includes lisinopril 10 mg PO qd, metformin 500 mg PO qd, naproxen 500 mg PO bid PRN, and multivitamin 1 PO qd. RF's mother died at age 36 from a myocardial infarction (MI), and his older brother has documented coronary heart disease. He admits to drinking "an occasional beer" with his friends and colleagues.

PHYSICAL EXAMINATION

Blood pressure: 134/82 mm Hg; heart rate: 76 beats per minute; respiratory rate: 18 breaths per minute; temperature: afebrile
General: Alert, oriented, and pleasant patient.
Chest: Heart reveals regular rhythm.
ABD: Soft and nontender without masses.
EXT: No edema

LABORATORY VALUES

Na: 140 mEq/L
Cl: 113 mEq/L
Blood urea nitrogen (BUN): 15 mg/dL
Serum Cr: 0.9 mg/dL

High-density lipoprotein (HDL) cholesterol: 62 mg/dL
Low-density lipoprotein (LDL) cholesterol: 167 mg/dL

K: 3.5 mEq/L
CO_2 content: 28 mEq/L
Glucose: 124 mg/dL

Total cholesterol: 205 mg/dL
Triglycerides: 125 mg/dL

AST: 25 mg/dL
ALT: 22 mg/dL
HbA1c: 8.9%
Uric acid: 5 mg/dL

QUESTIONS

1. According to the National Cholesterol Education Program's (NCEP's) Adult Treatment Panel III (ATP III), how often should low-risk adults over the age of 20 years be screened for hyperlipidemia?

A. Annually
B. Once every 5 years
C. Once every 10 years
D. Once every 15 years
E. With each visit to a physician

2. Based on the NCEP's ATP III, which of the following are RF's positive risk factors for heart disease?

I. Hypertension
II. High HDL cholesterol
III. Family history of premature coronary heart disease

A. I only
B. III only
C. I and III only
D. II and III only
E. I, II, and III

3. What therapeutic lifestyle changes (TLCs) should RF institute?

A. Restrict daily cholesterol to less than 200 mg
B. Exercise 30 minutes per day
C. Increase soluble fiber intake in his diet
D. None of the above
E. All the above

4. A pharmacy student with you on rotation concludes that RF's current LDL cholesterol goal is less than 130 mg/dL. Do you agree or disagree with this assessment?

A. Agree; his LDL cholesterol goal is correct, and follow-up should be in 2 weeks with a lipoprotein profile.
B. Agree; his LDL cholesterol goal is correct, and follow-up should be in 6 weeks with a lipoprotein profile.
C. Disagree; his LDL cholesterol goal is less than 100 mg/dL, and follow-up should be in 6 months with a lipoprotein profile.
D. Disagree; his LDL cholesterol goal is less than 100 mg/dL, and follow-up should be in 12 months with a lipoprotein profile.
E. Disagree; his LDL cholesterol goal is less than 100 mg/dL, and follow-up should be in 18 months with a lipoprotein profile.

5. RF's physician adds fenofibrate to his medication regimen. Which of the following reflects the most appropriate action for this patient at this time?

A. You should approve the prescription. When you dispense the medication, you tell him that he should take it with food to enhance the drug's mechanism.

B. You should approve the prescription. When you dispense the medication, you tell him that he also should make lifestyle modifications.

C. You should approve the prescription. This medication is therapeutically equivalent to metformin and should have a synergistic effect.

D. You should not approve the prescription. With LDL cholesterol being the primary target for this patient, this would not be the best option.

E. You should not approve the prescription. This is a therapeutic duplication with metformin, making it unlikely that there will be any added benefit.

6. How do fibric acid derivatives exert their lipid-lowering effects?

I.   By blocking lipase
II. By binding bile acids
III. By inhibiting the rate-limiting step in cholesterol synthesis

A. I only
B. III only
C. I and II only
D. II and III only
E. I, II, and III

7. Which of the following conditions confers high risk for coronary heart disease (CHD) events (CHD risk equivalent)?

A. Carotid artery disease
B. Peripheral arterial disease
C. Abdominal aortic aneurysm
D. All the above
E. None of the above

8. Given RF's potential compliance issues, the physician is apprehensive regarding drug therapy and wants to know the side effects of the resins. You inform the physician that resins, particularly the older resins, have which of the following side effects?

A. Rash
B. Flatulence
C. Flushing
D. All the above
E. None of the above

9. The physician decides to try cholestyramine as a potential LDL cholesterol–lowering agent. What are some counseling points that you can offer RF to help minimize the adverse effects associated with this medication?

A. Swallow it without engulfing air (administer it through a straw)
B. Minimize intake of fluids
C. Mix the resin in a carbonated juice
D. All the above
E. None of the above

10. In general, what effect do angiotensin-converting enzyme (ACE) inhibitors such as lisinopril have on a lipoprotein profile?

A. Increase total cholesterol
B. Decrease total cholesterol
C. Decrease HDL cholesterol
D. None of the above
E. All the above

PATIENT PROFILE 139

ASTHMA

PRESENTATION

JS is a 4-year-old boy brought to the emergency department by his mother. The child is experiencing dyspnea and coughing that have been getting worse over the past 3 days. Expiratory wheezes, a hyperinflated chest, and accessory muscle breathing are found during the physical examination. Vital signs include increases in both respiratory rate and heart rate. JS is being given no medications.

QUESTIONS

1. Which of the following would be the most appropriate therapy to reverse the acute bronchial obstruction?

A. Oral albuterol
B. Intravenous aminophylline
C. Nebulized albuterol
D. Intravenous hydrocortisone
E. Intravenous terbutaline

2. After acute bronchospasm has resolved, pulmonary function tests are conducted. The results suggest the presence of reversible obstructive airway disease. JS's physician wants to discharge JS with a β_2 agonist and an antiinflammatory agent. The preferred route of administration of antiasthmatic medications to patients in this age group is

A. oral.
B. subcutaneous.
C. intramuscular.
D. through a metered dose inhaler.
E. nebulization.

3. JS's physician is concerned about the side effects of corticosteroids. According to NHLBI guidelines, which of the following agents is the most appropriate alternative to corticosteroids for treatment of JS?

    A. Methotrexate
    B. Theophylline
    C. Ipratropium
    D. Cromolyn
    E. Salmeterol

4. Which of the following side effects is of specific concern with use of corticosteroids to treat children?

A. Dry mouth
B. Growth suppression
C. Oral thrush
D. Fluid retention
E. Irritation of the gastric mucosa

5. You are working with JS's physician to develop an asthma management plan consistent with NHLBI guidelines. The guidelines include all of the following except

    A. environmental control to avoid exposure to allergens or other triggers of asthmatic attacks.
    B. selection of an antiasthmatic drug regimen based on severity of disease.
    C. reservation of inhaled antiinflammatory agents for severe, persistent disease.
    D. a step-down approach once disease is under control.
    E. education on proper use of inhalers and spacer devices.

PATIENT PROFILE 140

ASTHMA

PRESENTATION

RO is a 16-year-old male high school student who is trying out for the varsity hockey team. He generally has been a fairly good player, but he now complains of increased cough and dyspnea when he skates during practices. His coach has had him rest more frequently and has warned RO that he may not make the team if he can't keep up with the rest of the players. He has no significant medical history other than several respiratory infections when he was much younger. He denies smoking or using any recreational drugs. RO is diagnosed with exercise-induced asthma (EIA).

QUESTIONS

1. Which of the following statements concerning EIA is *most correct*?

    A. Most patients with EIA should be encouraged not to exercise.
    B. It may be triggered by cold, dry air.
    C. It may be triggered by warm, humid air.
    D. A and B
    E. A and C

2. Which of the following agents would be *appropriate* for RO to use for prophylaxis of bronchospasm 5 to 15 minutes prior to exercise?

A. Inhaled ipratropium
B. Inhaled albuterol
C. Inhaled fluticasone
D. A and B
E. A, B, and C

3. If RO experiences acute symptoms during practice, which of the following would be *most appropriate* to use for immediate relief of symptoms?

    A. Inhaled ipratropium
    B. Inhaled albuterol
    C. Inhaled fluticasone
    D. A and B
    E. A, B, and C

4. RO is given a salmeterol inhaler to provide a longer period of protection, especially during games. When should RO be advised to use his inhaler?

    A. 5 minutes prior to exercise
    B. 15 minutes prior to exercise
    C. 30 minutes prior to exercise
    D. 2 hours prior to exercise
    E. 8 to 12 hours prior to exercise

5. Which of the following would be an alternative to salmeterol as a long-acting inhaled β-agonist?

    A. Albuterol
    B. Pirbuterol

C. Formoterol
D. A and B
E. B and C

6. Which one of the following side effects is associated with oral administration of β-agonists?

A. Oral thrush
B. Tachycardia
C. Weight gain
D. Hyperkalemia
E. Hyponatremia

7. When advising RO on the use of his metered-dose inhaler, which one of the following steps is *not correct*?

A. Shake canister before use.
B. Exhale slowly.
C. If using open-mouth technique, place mouthpiece between lips.
D. Press down canister as patient starts to inhale.
E. Hold breath for 10 seconds after inhaling.

8. As compared with metered-dose inhalers, when using breath-activated dry-powder inhalers, patients should be advised to do which of the following?

A. Breathe in slowly
B. Breathe in rapidly
C. Do not hold breath
D. A and C
E. B and C

9. Which of the following is an example of a salmeterol breath-activated dry-powder inhaler delivery system?

A. Diskus
B. Aerolizer
C. Rotadisk
D. Turbuhaler
E. None of the above

10. RO asks about possible oral medications for the long-term prevention of EIA. Which of the following oral agents would be *most appropriate* to recommend?

A. Albuterol
B. Montelukast
C. Theophylline
D. Prednisone
E. All the above

P A T I E N T   P R O F I L E   1 4 1

COMPOUNDING CAPSULES

PRESENTATION

A pharmacist is asked to compound 100 capsules, each to contain 5 mg of drug and sufficient diluent to make 200 mg of total powder per capsule. The pharmacist has pure drug powder, calcium carbonate diluent, and commercial tablets that contain as a compounding ingredient 20 mg of drug in tablets of 150 mg total weight.

QUESTIONS

1. How many total milligrams of drug are needed to complete the prescription?

A. 5
B. 20
C. 100
D. 500
E. 5000

2. How many commercial tablets should be used to obtain the desired amount of drug?

A. 1
B. 3⅓
C. 20
D. 25
E. 500

3. How many grams of calcium carbonate diluent should be added to the powder from the crushed tablets to complete the prescription?

A. 0.5
B. 3.75
C. 16.25
D. 20
E. 16,250

4. Rather than using the tablets, the pharmacist uses pure drug powder to compound the prescription. How many grams of calcium carbonate must be mixed with sufficient pure drug powder to complete the prescription?

A. 0.5
B. 19.5
C. 20
D. 500
E. 19,500

5. A number 3 capsule can be used to hold 200 mg aspirin powder. If the density of a powder composed of drug and diluent is less than the density of aspirin powder, which size capsule would you first attempt to use?

A. 00
B. 1
C. 2
D. 4
E. There is insufficient information available to make a decision.

PATIENT PROFILE 142

ACUTE LEUKEMIA

PRESENTATION

CC: Elevated white blood cell count

HPI: LD is a 41-year-old man in his usual state of health until 2 months ago when he felt tired and had constant chest pain. He received a Z-Pack for a presumed bacterial upper respiratory tract infection. The chest pain improved, but he still felt tired. He also had noted easy bruising and frequent nose bleeds over the last 2 to 3 weeks. He has complained of fevers and night sweats over the last 1 to 2 weeks, but he has had no decrease in appetite.

PMH: Hypertension × 3 years, hypercholesterolemia

FH: Father alive with prostate cancer; mother had a myocardial infarction (MI) 3 years ago; no cancer history in siblings

SH: Married, father of 3 sons, works as a school teacher. No tobacco, drinks wine with dinner

Allergies: Bactrim

Medications: Lisinopril 20 mg PO qd, atorvastatin 20 mg PO qd, Advil PRN

VS: Temperature: 99.4°F; blood pressure: 130/80 mm Hg; heart rate: 88 beats per minute; respiratory rate: 20 breaths per minute; O_2 saturation: 95% RA

Height: 5 ft, 10 in; weight: 175 lb

General: Pleasant male in NAD

HEENT: PERRLA, EOMI

Neck: Supple; no LAD

Lungs: CTA bilaterally

Heart: RRR, no MRG

ABD: No HSM, soft, nontender/nondistended, positive bowel sounds

EXT: No C/C/E; several ecchymoses

Neuro: A&O × 3

LABORATORY DATA

Na: 138 mEq/L   K: 4.0 mEq/L
Cl: 108 mEq/L CO_2: 24 mEq/L

Blood urea nitrogen (BUN): 10 mEq/L
Glucose: 111 mg/dL
Mg: 2.4 mg/dL
Total bilirubin: 0.7 mg/dL

Albumin: 3.9 mg/dL
Hct: 26.3%
White blood cell (WBC) count: 291,000/mm³

Serum Cr: 0.6 mg/dL

Ca: 9.5 mg/dL
PO_4: 3.0 mg/dL
Low-density lipoprotein (LDH) cholesterol: 1280 IU/mL
Hgb: 9.3 g/dL
Platelets: 50,000/mm³
10% P, 11% L, 6% M, 1% bands, 72% lymphoblasts

DIAGNOSTIC TESTS

Chest x-ray/CT scan: Negative

Bone marrow aspirate

Differential shows: Blasts 87%; promyelocytes < 1%; myelocytes < 1%; metamyelocytes 2%; bands/neutrophils 3%; plasma cells < 1%; lymphocytes 1%; erythroid 5%

Cellularity: 95%

CD 19+, CD 10+, CD 20+, aberrant expression of CD 33

FISH: Philadelphia chromosome +

Interpretation: Hypercellular marrow consistent with pre B-cell ALL

ASSESSMENT/PLAN

LD is a 41-year-old male with Philadelphia chromosome–positive acute lymphoblastic leukemia (ALL). Plan is to initiate induction chemotherapy using daunorubicin, vincristine, prednisone, and L-asparaginase.

QUESTIONS

1. In this regimen, daunorubicin is dosed at 50 mg/m². What dose of daunorubicin should LD receive today?

A. 50 mg
B. 85.5 mg
C. 98.5 mg
D. 102.5 mg

2. You receive a prescription for this patient for Zyloprim 300 mg PO qd. What is the indication in this patient?

A. Increase the cytotoxicity of the chemotherapy
B. Prevention odvincristine-induced gouty arthritis
C. Prevention of tumor lysis syndrome
D. Prevention of nausea and vomiting

3. Which of the following toxicities is associated with vincristine therapy?

A. Myelosuppression
B. Constipation
C. Pulmonary toxicity
D. Hepatotoxicity

4. During the administration of daunorubicin, LD began to complain of a burning sensation at the infusion site. It was discovered that his IV was partially pulled out and drug was infiltrating the surrounding tissue. What is the *most appropriate* treatment of this extravasation of daunorubicin?

A. Slow the infusion rate.
B. Administer 10 mg IV morphine.
C. Aspirate any drug, consult a plastic surgeon, apply a cold compress, and apply DSMO topical solution.
D. Aspirate any drug, consult a plastic surgeon, apply a warm compress, and apply DSMO topical solution.

5. The patient is to receive intrathecal (IT) chemotherapy after induction chemotherapy. Which of the following agents is *not* appropriate for IT administration?

A. Cytarabine
B. Hydrocortisone
C. Methotrexate
D. Vincristine

6. LD completed induction chemotherapy and is now ready for consolidation. He is to receive a three-part regimen of which one portion is high-dose methotrexate. Which of the following agents will you administer to prevent excess toxicity following high dose methotrexate?

A. Leucovorin
B. Neupogen
C. Epogen
D. Mesna

7. What is the mechanism of action of methotrexate?

A. Inhibits DNA synthesis by intercalation between DNA base pairs
B. Produces DNA strand breaks by inhibiting topoisomerase II
C. Prevents cell division by cross-linking DNA strands
D. Inhibits dihydrofolate reductase

8. On day 14 after the start of chemotherapy, the following laboratory values are reported: WBC count: $100/mm^3$; 20% P, 10% bands, 28% L, 38% M, 0% E, 0% B; Hgb: 8.2 g/dL; Hct: 24.4%; and platelets: $15,000/mm^3$. What is LD's absolute neutrophil count?

A. 30
B. 50
C. 100
D. 1000

9. On day 15 the patient is noted to have an erythematous line site and has a maximum temperature of 39°C. Which antibiotic(s) should the patient be given empirically?

A. Levofloxacin
B. Levofloxacin plus vancomycin
C. Cefepime
D. Cefepime plus vancomycin

10. While receiving L-asparaginase, LD should be monitored for what?

A. Acute pancreatitis
B. Hypersensitivity reactions
C. Bleeding
D. All the above

PATIENT PROFILE 143

SOFT-TISSUE INFECTION

PRESENTATION

CM is a 43-year-old man who visits the clinic in which your pharmacy is located. His chief complaint is pain on his right shin. The story is as follows. In the most recent snowstorm, CM was shoveling snow. When he came to the concrete stairs leading into his house, he slipped on some ice and fell into the stairs banging his shin on the corner of the concrete steps. When he looked at the wound, CM found the skin was broken, and he proceeded to treat the wound superficially. One week has passed, and CM now has a fever and has swelling at the wound site with red lines streaking toward the groin area that suggest infection. CM has no known drug allergies.

QUESTIONS

1. Which type of organism is most likely growing in the leg?

   A. Lactose-fermenting gram-negative enteric bacilli
   B. Atypical pathogens
   C. Gram-positive clusters of cocci
   D. Anaerobes
   E. Non–lactose-fermenting gram-negative rods

2. Which organism would you most commonly find growing in this patient's leg?

   A. *Staphylococcus aureus*
   B. *Escherichia coli*

   C. *Bacteroides fragilis*
   D. *Legionella pneumophila*
   E. *Enterobacter cloacae*

3. Which of the following antibiotics would best control this patient's infection?

   A. Erythromycin
   B. Clindamycin
   C. Cefotaxime
   D. Nafcillin
   E. Metronidazole

4. Which of the following is the most appropriate drug for CM if a rash develops in reaction to penicillin's?

   A. Aztreonam
   B. Cefazolin
   C. Azithromycin
   D. Ceftazidime
   E. Imipenem

5. If CM has an anaphylactic reaction to a β-lactam antibiotic, which of the following drugs would be the most appropriate for managing cellulitis?

   A. Vancomycin
   B. Penicillin
   C. Gentamicin
   D. Rifampin
   E. Ciprofloxacin

PATIENT PROFILE 144

OSTEOARTHRITIS

PRESENTATION

CC: "I have pain in my knees that has been getting worse over the past month."

HPI: MN is an obese 65-year-old year woman who has been experiencing pain in both her knees. This pain has affected her ability to perform activities of daily living such as walking and doing household chores. She associates the pain she experiences with her gardening during the weekends. She describes the pain as a deep, localized ache that is relieved with rest and an ice pack. The stiffness in her knees typically lasts 20 to 30 minutes and then subsides. She denies pain during sleep. During MN's last visit to her primary care physician about 2

months ago, she did not complain of any pain symptoms. MN was sent to a pharmacist-run outpatient clinic for counseling on the nonpharmacologic and pharmacologic options to manage her osteoarthritic pain.

Medications: Ranitidine 150 mg PO bid, Lipitor 10 mg PO qd, Lisinopril 40 mg PO qd, aspirin 81 mg PO qd

PMH: Gastroesophageal reflux disease (GERD) diagnosed 30 years ago, peptic ulcer disease diagnosed 1 month ago, dyslipidemia diagnosed 25 years ago, hypertension diagnosed 15 years ago

PSH: None

FH: Unknown

SH: Widowed. Denies alcohol, tobacco, or illicit drug use.

ALL: Aspirin

PHYSICAL EXAMINATION

General: Obese woman; appearance reflects apparent age.

VS: Blood pressure: 170/96 mm Hg; heart rate: 60 beats per minute; respiratory rate: 22 breaths per minute; temperature: 37°C

Height: 5 ft, 3 in; weight: 100 kg

Skin: Normal skin turgor

HEENT: PERRLA, EOM intact

COR: RRR; no m/r/g

Chest: Lungs CTA

ABD: Soft, nontender, normal bowel sounds

GU: Normal output

RECT: Normal anus

EXT: Normal

NEURO: Normal

ECG: Normal

LABORATORY VALUES

Na: 120 mEq/L

K: 5.1 mEq/L

Cl: 100 mEq/L

HCO_3: 5.3 mEq/L

Blood urea nitrogen (BUN): 18 mg/dL

Serum Cr: 0.7 mg/dL

Glucose: 89 mg/dL (fasting)

Hgb: 14.3 g/dL

Hct: 40.3%

Platelets: 300 (10^3/mm^3

PT: N/A

aPTT: N/A

Triglycerides: 168 mg/dL

Total cholesterol: 204 mg/dL

High-density lipoprotein (HDL) cholesterol: 40 mg/dL

Low-density lipoprotein (LDL): 118 mg/dL

QUESTIONS

1. Which of the following is(are) risk factor(s) for osteoarthritis that MN possesses?

    I.   Overweight
    II. Gardening activity
    III. 65 years old

    A. I only
    B. II only
    C. I and II
    D. II and III
    E. I, II, and III

2. MN decides that she does not want any medications to treat for her osteoarthritis. Which of the following is(are) considered noninvasive, nonpharmacologic therapy used for osteoarthritis?

    I.   Transcutaneous electrical nerve stimulation
    II. Biofeedback
    III. Acupuncture

    A. I only
    B. II only
    C. I and II
    D. II and III
    E. I, II, and III

3. MN would now like to try herbal products for her osteoarthritis. Which of the following is(are) correct counseling points relative to glucosamine?

    I.   Avoid in patients with shellfish allergy.
    II. Improvement is seen after 4 weeks of therapy.
    III. Side effects include prolonged bleeding time.

    A. I only
    B. II only
    C. I and II
    D. II and III
    E. I, II, and III

4. MN would like to try another herbal product for her osteoarthritis. Which of the following is(are) correct counseling points relative to chondroitin?

    I.   Avoid in patients with shellfish allergy.
    II. Improvement is seen after 4 weeks of therapy.
    III. Side effects include prolonged bleeding time.

    A. I only
    B. II only
    C. I and II
    D. II and III
    E. I, II, and III

5. MN's primary care physician would like to initiate a nonsteroidal anti-inflammatory drug (NSAID) for her osteoarthritis. What places MN at a higher risk for gastrointestinal adverse effects from NSAIDs?

    I.   Aspirin use
    II. Peptic ulcer disease
    III. 65 years old

    A. I only
    B. II only
    C. I and II
    D. II and III
    E. I, II, and III

6. Which of the following is(are) strategies to decrease the gastrointestinal (GI) toxicity of nonselective NSAIDs?

    I.   Take with food
    II. Take with a proton pump inhibitor
    III. Take with misoprostol

    A. I only
    B. II only
    C. I and II
    D. II and III
    E. I, II, and III

7. Which of the following is the *most appropriate* action to take in terms of selecting an over-the-counter NSAID to treat MN's osteoarthritic pain?

    A. Recommend naproxen 250 mg PO qd.
    B. Recommend naproxen 250 mg PO bid.
    C. Recommend ibuprofen 800 mg/day in three to four divided doses.
    D. Recommend ibuprofen 1200 mg/day in three to four divided doses.
    E. Do not recommend an NSAID.

8. MN's laboratory report shows that MN had renal dysfunction. Which of the following is an *appropriate* product for MN's osteoarthritis?

    I. Acetaminophen
    II. Nonselective NSAID
    III. COX-2 inhibitor

    A. I only
    B. II only
    C. I and II
    D. II and III
    E. I, II, and III

9. You learn that MN prefers a topical product for her knee pain. You recommend capsaicin cream. Which of the following is a *correct* counseling point?

    A. Capsaicin may be applied on broken skin.
    B. Capsaicin is available only with a prescription.
    C. Capsaicin must be applied at least four times daily.
    D. Capsaicin begins to work after 2 months of continuous use.
    E. Capsaicin should be discontinued if a burning sensation occurs.

10. All over-the-counter therapies prove ineffective in MN. MN's primary care physician would like to initiate hyaluronate injections. How are hyaluronate injections administered?

    A. Intravenously
    B. Intradermally
    C. Intraarticularly
    D. Intramuscularly
    E. Subcutaneously

PATIENT PROFILE 145

PARKINSON'S DISEASE

Patient	BH	
Age	69	
Sex	Male	
Allergies	ASA	
Race	White	
Height	5'8"	
Wt	175 lb	
Diagnosis	Primary	1. Parkinson's disease
		2. Depression
		3. Epilepsy
	Secondary	1. Eczema
		2. Raynaud's phenomenon

	Date	Rx No.	Physician	Drug and Strength	Quantity	Sig	Refills
Medication record (prescription and OTC)	8/21	50034	ZM	Sinemet® (carbidopa-levodopa) 25/250	120	1 po qid	5
	8/21	50035	ZM	Selegiline 2 mg	90	3 po qd	5
	8/21	50036	ZM	HCTZ 25 mg	60	1 po bid	5
	9/13	51078	WS	Dilantin® (phenytoin) 100 mg	90	3 po qd	5
	9/13	51079	WS	Pyridoxine 50 mg	30	1 po qd	5
Dietary considerations	8/21	High-protein diet may compete with levodopa for intestinal absorption					
Pharmacist notes and other patient info	8/21	Decreased levodopa effect from possible drug interactions					

QUESTIONS

1. Which of the following dopamine agonists used to treat patients with Parkinson's disease may exacerbate Raynaud's phenomenon and should not be prescribed for this patient?

   I.   Pergolide
   II. Lisuride
   III. Bromocriptine

   A. I only
   B. III only
   C. I and II only
   D. II and III only
   E. I, II, and III

2. Which of the following options may be used to treat a patient who is experiencing the wearing-off effect?

   I.   Discontinue Sinemet® (carbidopa-levodopa)
   II. Switch Sinemet® to Sinemet® CR formulation
   III. Add an adjunctive agent such as a dopamine agonist or selegiline

   A. I only
   B. III only
   C. I and II only
   D. II and III only
   E. I, II, and III

3. Antidepressants that should not be used to treat patients with Parkinson's disease who are taking levodopa include

   I.   MAOIs
   II. Tricyclic antidepressants
   III. Selective serotonin reuptake inhibitors (SSRIs)

   A. I only
   B. III only
   C. I and II only
   D. II and III only
   E. I, II, and III

4. Why is selegiline not administered at bedtime?

   A. It can cause hypoglycemia.
   B. It can cause leg cramps.
   C. It can cause insomnia.
   D. It can interact with Sinemet® (carbidopa-levodopa).
   E. It can cause nocturia.

5. Which of the following drugs may increase the peripheral decarboxylation of levodopa and lead to a decrease in its effect?

   A. Selegiline
   B. Hydrochlorothiazide
   C. Dilantin® (phenytoin)
   D. Pyridoxine
   E. None of the above

PATIENT PROFILE 146

DERMATOLOGY: ACNE

PRESENTATION

FW is a 25-year-old woman who has comedonal acne. She first tried treating herself with over-the-counter products such as benzoyl peroxide and various acne washes. She has not had appreciable improvement and is frustrated. She comes to your pharmacy to ask your advice. You notice that she has numerous blackheads (open comedones) and whiteheads (closed comedones). You also see inflammatory lesions, including some cysts. You recommend that she go see a dermatologist for a thorough evaluation. FW takes Lo/Ovral® (norgestrel with ethinyl estradiol), a multivitamin daily, and calcium supplements. FW takes your advice and goes to see a dermatologist. The dermatologist carefully evaluates the lesions and recommends tretinoin (Retin-A®), which is efficacious in the management of comedonal acne. FW returns to your pharmacy with a prescription for tretinoin. The dermatologist recommends the combination of tretinoin and benzoyl peroxide.

QUESTIONS

1. Which of the following statement(s) is/are true concerning tretinoin (Retin-A®)?

   A. Tretinoin is a derivative of vitamin A.
   B. Tretinoin is available in various formulations, such as cream, gel, and lotion.

C. Tretinoin increases follicle cell turnover and decreases cohesiveness of cells; this results in extrusion of existing comedones and inhibits formation of new comedones.

D. A and B

E. All of the above

2. Which statement(s) should be included in your counseling session with FW?

A. Tretinoin can cause skin irritation, which ranges from mild to severe and is more common during initiation of therapy.

B. FW may notice an exacerbation of acne at initiation of therapy. This is caused by the mechanism of action of tretinoin. Therapy should be continued, and this flare should resolve in 3 to 6 weeks.

C. FW should be advised to avoid long exposure to UV radiation. If exposure is unavoidable, she should use a sunscreen with an SPF of at least 15.

D. A and B

E. All of the above

3. After an adequate trial of tretinoin and benzoyl peroxide, FW's dermatologist decides to change the therapy. FW appears to have therapy-resistant moderate acne. The dermatologist discusses isotretinoin (Accutane®) as an option for FW. Which statement(s) concerning isotretinoin (Accutane®) is/are true:

A. This agent usually is considered early in the treatment of patients with scars.

B. Unlike other acne therapies, isotretinoin (Accutane®) brings about prolonged remission of acne.

C. Isotretinoin is a synthetic derivative of vitamin A.

D. A and B

E. All of the above

4. The dermatologist has discussed the adverse effects of isotretinoin, particularly effects that occur if this agent is used during pregnancy. Which of the following statement(s) is/are true concerning isotretinoin (Accutane®)?

A. Isotretinoin is pregnancy category X.

B. Sexually active women of childbearing potential should practice contraception 1 month before therapy, during therapy, and for 1 month after therapy is discontinued.

C. Isotretinoin should be avoided in pregnancy because miscarriage and stillbirth are common, and severe congenital anomalies have been associated with use of this agent.

D. A and B

E. All of the above

5. FW asks you to review the adverse effects of isotretinoin with her. You correctly tell her the following:

A. Mucocutaneous side effects, such as dryness of the skin, eyes, nose, and mouth are common.

B. Conjunctivitis and corneal opacities may occur; during this period, patients may not be able to tolerate contact lenses. These effects usually resolve within 6 weeks.

C. Abnormalities in serum triglyceride and cholesterol levels may occur and should be monitored during therapy.

D. A and B

E. All of the above

PATIENT PROFILE 147

MEDICINAL CHEMISTRY

PRESENTATION AND QUESTION

MR is hospitalized because of severe edema related to complex renal problems. Diuretic therapy with furosemide (structure 147.1) 20 mg IV is initiated and followed by 40 and 80 mg oral doses on the second and third days. A check of blood electrolytes reveals normal levels of sodium but severe hypokalemia. The attending physician wants to change the diuretic medication. You are contacted for consultation on the matter.

1. Which drug would you recommend as an alternative to furosemide in this case?

A. Ethacrynic acid (structure 147.2)

B. Hydrochlorothiazide (structure 147.3)

C. Spironolactone (structure 147.4)

D. Indapamide (structure 147.5)

E. B or D

147.1

147.2

147.3

147.4

147.5

PATIENT PROFILE 148

LACTATION

PRESENTATION

A 26-year-old woman G2 P2 is status post NSVD and is breast-feeding her newborn infant. Over the past week, she notes that her right breast has become extremely tender and that she has not felt well overall. She complains of flu-like symptoms.

PMH: Mild hypertension, seasonal allergies, postpartum depression, generalized anxiety disorder

SH: Lives with her husband; drinks occasionally; works as an administrative assistant; planning on returning to work in 6 weeks

FH: Noncontributory

ALL: NKDA

PHYSICAL EXAMINATION

VS: Blood pressure: 150/90 mm Hg; heart rate: 80 beats per minute; respiratory rate: 12 breaths per minute; temperature: 101.2°F

Weight: 70 kg

General: Overall, a well-appearing woman with no significant physical findings

HEENT: PERRLA, EOMI

Heart: NSR; no murmurs, rubs, or gallops

Lungs: CTA

GI: Normal bowel sounds

GU: Trace amounts of blood per vagina, status post episiotomy

EXT: Normal

Pelvic examination: Normal

Last Pap: Approximately 1 year ago, normal

LABORATORY VALUES

Na: 137	CL: 112	Scr: 0.6
K: 3.5	CO$_2$: 38	BUN: 12
	Gluc: 110	

HIV testing: Negative

STD testing: Negative to date

MEDICATIONS

Claritn 10 mg PO qd
Hydrochlorthiaizide 12.5 PO bid (on hold since birth)
Tylenol (for occasional headache)
MVI
Paxil CR 25 mg PO qd
Alprazolam 0.5 mg PO qid

QUESTIONS

1. Factors that determine the passage of drug into breast milk include which of the following?

   A. Molecular weight <200, highly lipid souble, highly protein bound
   A. Molecular weight <200, high lipid soublity, low protein binding
   C. Molecular weight > 600, highly lipid souble, low protein binding
   D. Molecular weight >1000, low lipid soublity, high protein binding

2. Breast pumps are available over the counter (OTC) for what reason?

   A. To help generate additional milk
   B. To ease with feedings
   C. To prevent mastitis
   D. To help excrete drug faster

3. The patient had a problem producing milk after she was restarted on her medication prior to birth. Which of her medications may have caused this problem?

   A. HydroDiurl
   B. Loratidine
   C. Paroxetine
   D. Xanax

4. The patient has been diagnosed with mastitis. What may have contributed to this?

   A. Overfeeding the infant
   B. Tight-fitting clothes
   C. Sleeping on her back
   D. Not giving the baby a pacifier on a regular basis

5. What would be the *most appropriate* treatment option for mastitis in this patient?

   A. Antibiotics
   B. Stopping breast-feeding

   C. Applying heat and gentle massage
   D. Using a breast pump instead of having the baby feeding on the breast

6. When searching for information regarding drugs and breast-feeding, what would be an appropriate source?

   I.   The American Academy of Pediatrics guidelines
   II. Briggs
   III. DiPiro

   A. I
   B. III
   C. I and II
   D. II and III

7. In the event a breast-feeding mother is going to take medication, what are some key points that minimize an infant's drug exposure?

   I.   Using extended-release products
   II. Pumping after the mother takes a dose to help increase excretion of the drug
   III. Time the dose immediately after a feeding

   A. I
   B. III
   C. I and II
   D. II and III

8. On discharge from the hospital, the mother is having some pain from her delivery and is having trouble sleeping. What would the best OTC product to recommend?

   A. Tylenol PM
   B. Unisom
   C. Acetaminophen + discuss good sleep hygiene
   D. Bayer aspirin

9. What would be a good approach to treatment of the patient's depression?

   A. Discontinue the patient's current regimen until she is no longer breast-feeding.
   B. Consider switching to Paxil 20 mg PO qd.
   C. Consider using a monoamine oxidase inhibitor.
   D. Continue the patient on her current regimen, Paxil CR 30 mg PO qd.

10. What should be done regarding the alprazolam therapy?

   A. Should be discontinued
   B. Should be switched to a shorter-acting benzodiazepine PRN
   C. Has been shown to stunt growth in the infant
   D. Causes poor suckling in the infant

ONCOLOGY: ADULT CHRONIC MYELOGENOUS LEUKEMIA

PRESENTATION

BJ is a 55-year-old woman who visits her physician for a routine physical examination. Her only complaints are fatigue, inability to maintain her usual activity schedule, and vague aches and pains. Her medical history includes myocardial infarction 5 years ago and mild congestive heart failure. BJ stopped smoking after the MI (she had smoked 2 packs per day for 20 years). She drinks red wine on holidays. BJ is married and has two children. Her medications include ASA 162 mg qd, atorvastatin 10 mg qd, metoprolol XL 50 mg qd, and ramipril 2.5 mg qd. This medication regimen has not changed over the past 18 months. BJ has no known drug allergies.

PHYSICAL EXAMINATION

BP: 124/70, HR: 62, RR: 16, T: 98°C
Ht: 5'5", Wt: 130 lb
COR: S_1, S_2, + S_3
PULM: No rales or rhonchi
ABD: Mild splenomegaly
NEURO: A/O × 3

LABS

WBC: 80,000
DIFF: Neutrophils 85%, lymphocytes 10%

QUESTIONS

1. Additional lab work and a bone marrow biopsy are performed. Chronic myelogenous leukemia is suspected. Which diagnostic feature would most likely confirm this diagnosis?

   A. Presence of blast cells in the peripheral smear
   B. Presence of thrombocytosis
   C. Presence of the Philadelphia chromosome
   D. Absence of hepatomegaly
   E. Absence of microcytic anemia

2. BJ appears to be in the chronic phase of CML. The primary goal of therapy at this time is

   A. to prevent spread of disease to the CNS.
   B. to prevent progression disease to the blast phase.
   C. patient comfort and palliative care only.
   D. to decrease the number of circulating white blood cells.
   E. to increase the percentage of circulating thrombocytes.

3. Initiating drug therapy with hydroxyurea will most quickly do the following to resolve signs or symptoms of CML?

   A. Decrease fatigue and muscle aches
   B. Decrease WBC count and eliminate the Philadelphia chromosome
   C. Decrease splenomegaly and WBC count
   D. Increase energy level and lymphocyte count
   E. Increase hepatomegaly and muscle aches

4. Bone marrow transplantation is the best chance for cure for BJ. Which marrow donor would provide the best outcome?

   A. HLA-matched sibling
   B. Autologous donor
   C. HLA-mismatched sibling
   D. Donor with blood type match, HLA mismatched
   E. Donor with HLA match, blood type mismatched

5. BJ responds well to the hydroxyurea and bone marrow transplantation. BJ starts interferon therapy. What is the role of interferon in the care of this patient?

   A. Prevent the need for leukapheresis
   B. Allow increased doses of hydroxyurea
   C. Decrease risk of relapse
   D. Prepare BJ for tumor debulking surgery
   E. Minimize need for narcotic analgesic for pain control

PATIENT PROFILE 150

SCHIZOPHRENIA

PRESENTATION

BK is a 37-year-old man with a diagnosis of schizophrenia, paranoid type. He has a fixed belief that the CIA is trying to kill him because of the government secrets he knows. He has become increasingly withdrawn, and his hygiene has deteriorated. The chief complaint is muscle rigidity.

BK was diagnosed with schizophrenia at age 21 while in college studying political science. Over the last few months his delusions regarding the CIA have become stronger and more fixed. In an effort to treat the patient, his psychiatrist increased the haloperidol dose from 10 mg qd to 10 mg bid with little success.

BJ has had schizophrenia for 16 years and a seizure disorder for 26 years. He is allergic to chlorpromazine (neuroleptic malignant syndrome), He takes carbamazepine 200 mg bid, haloperidol 10 mg bid, and lorazepam 1 mg tid prn. His father had diagnosed schizophrenia and died at age 55 of myocardial infarction. BJ is single and lives in a halfway house. He smokes one pack of cigarettes per day. He states he drinks a couple of beers on weekends.

QUESTIONS

1. BK's belief that the CIA wants to kill him because he knows government secrets is an example of

   A. positive symptoms of schizophrenia.
   B. negative symptoms of schizophrenia.
   C. extrapyramidal symptoms.
   D. akathisia.
   E. tardive dyskinesia.

2. What is the best reason for ordering a serum carbamazepine level for this patient?

   A. Haloperidol decreases serum carbamazepine level.
   B. Haloperidol increases serum carbamazepine level.
   C. Persons with schizophrenia have a high rate of medication noncompliance.
   D. Persons with schizophrenia have altered absorption pharmacokinetics.
   E. Carbamazepine chelates with lorazepam causing erratic absorption.

3. What is the most likely cause of the muscle rigidity?

   A. An increase in lorazepam dose
   B. An increase in haloperidol dose
   C. An increase in cigarette smoking
   D. Greater than reported alcohol use
   E. Less than reported carbamazepine use

4. How can BK's social withdrawal and decrease in daily activities be labeled?

   A. Positive symptoms of schizophrenia
   B. Negative symptoms of schizophrenia
   C. Extrapyramidal symptoms
   D. Akathisia
   E. Serotonin syndrome

5. Olanzapine is a potential option for this patient for which reason(s)?

   A. It can lessen the negative symptoms.
   B. It does not lower the seizure threshold.
   C. It has fewer extrapyramidal side effects than butyrophenones.
   D. A and B
   E. A, B, and C

PATIENT PROFILE 151

PEPTIC ULCER MEDICATIONS

PRESENTATION

GG is a 30-year-old woman admitted to the emergency room (ER) complaining of severe stomach pain. The ER physician suspected the presence of an ulcer and immediately referred GG to the gastrointestinal (GI) department for endoscopic examination. The latter revealed a medium-sized ulcer in the pyloric part of the stomach, confirming the initial physician diagnosis. After having her pain treated by analgesic medications, GG was sent home with antiulcer medication prescriptions. Medical history indicates that GG is taking ibuprofen, lisinopril, atorvastatin, and amitriptyline.

QUESTIONS

1. From the list of GG's medications, one can guess that she is probably suffering from what?

   I.   Depression
   II. Arthritis
   III. Hypercholestremia
   IV. Hypertension

   A. I and III
   B. II and IV
   C. I, III, and IV
   D. I and II
   E. All the above

2. If GG's ulcer is suspected to be drug-induced, which of the drugs she is taking may have contributed to the ulcer development?

   A. Ibuprofen
   B. Lisinopril
   C. Atorvastatin

D. Amitriptyline
E. A or D

3. How does the drug you picked in question 2 induce ulcer formation?

   A. By inducing HCl formation
   B. By inducing the synthesis of prostaglandins
   C. By inhibiting the synthesis of prostaglandins
   D. A and B

4. Which of the following is(are) classified as antipeptic ulcer medication(s)?

   I.   Mylanta (Structure 151-1)
   II. Ranitidine (Structure 151-2)
   III. Sucralfate (Structure 151-3)
   IV. Misoprostol (Structure 151-4)
   V.   Omeprazole (Structure 151-5)

   A. I and II
   B. II and III

$Mg(OH)_2$
151.1

$R=SO_3[AL_2(OH)\times(H_2O)]$

151.3

151.2

151.4

151.5

C. I, III, IV, and V
D. I, II, III, and IV
E. All the above

For questions 5 through 7, match each drug with the most appropriate statement that describes the mechanism of action of each drug as an antiulcer agent.

A. Decreases HCl production by blocking histamine binding to its H_2 receptors
B. Decreases HCl production by inhibiting the proton pump
C. Decreases HCl concentration by direct neutralization
D. Decreases gastric irritation by HCl by inducing mucin secretion
E. Decreases gastric irritation by HCl by forming a protective gel on the ulcer

5. Omeprazole

6. Ranitidine

7. Sucralfate

8. If GG is planning to get pregnant, which of the following medications must be contraindicated for her?

A. Mylanta
B. Ranitidine
C. Misoprostol
D. Omeprazole
E. Sucralfate

9. Considering the fact that GG is taking four other medications, what would be the *best* over the counter H_2 blocker that will have no drug interactions with these drugs?

A. Cimetidine
B. Ranitidine
C. Famotidine
D. A or B
E. B or C

10. Considering that GG is taking amitriptyline and that you know that one of its major side effects is high anticholinergic properties, how would that affect GG's ulcer prognosis?

A. It will make it worthwhile.
B. It will help improve it.
C. No basis for judging

PATIENT PROFILE 152

CONGESTIVE HEART FAILURE

PRESENTATION

TT is a 62-year-old man who comes to the clinic with increasing shortness of breath and decreased exercise tolerance. He states that over the past 3 months the distance he can walk before experiencing chest pain has decreased from 8 blocks to 3 or 4 blocks. After further questioning, TT states that he also has had difficulty sleeping while lying flat. The medical history includes CAD (AMI 5 years ago), hyperlipidemia, CHF diagnosed 2 years ago, hypertension, asthma since childhood, and gout.

MEDS

Furosemide 40 mg po qd
KCl 20 mEq po qd
Albuterol inhaler prn
Azmacort® (triamcinolone acetonide) inhaler
Diltiazem 300 mg qd

Isosorbide dinitrate 40 mg po tid
Aspirin 325 mg po qd
Ipratropium inhaler

PHYSICAL EXAMINATION

BP: 125/85, RR: 16, HR: 85
Wt: 80 kg (74 kg 1 month ago)

LABS

Na: 132
Cl: 98
BUN: 15
K: 4.5
HCO_3: 27
SCr: 1.2

QUESTIONS

1. In an effort to alleviate volume overload, the physician increases the furosemide dose to 60, 80, then 100 mg po bid. However, TT is responding minimally to the increased dose of diuretic. Which of the following interventions is the most appropriate in managing the volume overload?

   A. Increase Lasix® (furosemide) to 200 mg po bid
   B. Change Lasix® (furosemide) to 100 mg IV bid
   C. Add metolazone 2.5 mg po qd
   D. Change Lasix® (furosemide) to Bumex® (bumetanide) 3 mg po bid
   E. Change Lasix® (furosemide) to hydrochlorothiazide 25 mg po qd

2. TT starts therapy with IV Lasix® (furosemide), and doses are increased up to 200 mg IV every 8 hours with minimal response. Which of the following interventions is the most appropriate at this time to help resolve volume status?

   A. Add enalapril 5 mg po qd
   B. Add Bumex® (bumetanide) 5 mg po bid
   C. Increase Lasix® (furosemide) to 300 mg IV q8h
   D. Add metolazone 2.5 mg po qd
   E. Add spironolactone 50 mg po qd

3. Volume status is resolved, and TT now receives a standing dose of Lasix® (furosemide) 120 mg po bid. Which of the following interventions would not be appropriate at this time?

   A. Add enalapril 5 mg po bid
   B. Discontinue diltiazem
   C. Add carvedilol 3.125 mg po bid
   D. Add hydralazine 10 mg po qid
   E. Add digoxin 0.125 mg po qd

4. Which of the following diseases can be exacerbated by furosemide?

   A. CAD
   B. CHF
   C. Asthma
   D. Hyperlipidemia
   E. Gout

5. Which of the following would be reasonable to add if TT needed better control of CAD (angina)?

   A. Metoprolol 25 mg po bid
   B. Losartan 50 mg po qd
   C. Amiodarone 200 mg po qd
   D. Felodipine 5 mg po qd
   E. Digoxin 0.125 mg po qd

PATIENT PROFILE 153

CHRONIC RENAL FAILURE

PRESENTATION

CC: Primary care physician (PCP) follow-up office visit

HPI: The patient is a 42-year-old woman with type 1 diabetes mellitus who had an annual physical examination 2 months ago. In the interim, her urine albumin:creatinine test is reported with an elevated value of 200 mg/g, and her serum HgA$_{1C}$ is elevated at 8.5%. The patient is asked to return for a follow-up visit.

PMH: Type 1 diabetes mellitus (DM) since childhood,? gastroparesis

Medications on admission: NPH and regular insulin as directed by PCP

FH: Father and mother (+) hypertension; grandmother (+) colon Ca; grandfather (+) prostate Ca; two siblings (+) type 1 DM

SH: Lives with husband and two sons; works part time as a physical therapist; occasional alcohol use; 10 pack-year tobacco history (stopped smoking 6 months ago); no illicit drug use

ALL: NKDA

PE: Patient is pleasant and sitting comfortably.

ROS: No significant findings

VS: Temperature: 98.2°F; heart rate: 65 beats per minute; blood pressure: 128/75 mm Hg; respiratory rate: 22 breaths per minute

Weight: 145 lb; height: 5 ft, 4 in

LABORATORY VALUES

Na: 138	K: 4.3
Cl: 100	Total CO2: 22
Blood urea nitrogen (BUN): 15	Serum Cr: 0.7
Glucose: 101	Hct: 36.4
Hgb: 13.5	Platelets: 292

U/A: Specific gravity: 1.013; (-) overt protein; spot albumin:creatinine ratio 200 mg/gm

QUESTIONS

1. The medical student who is accompanying you in clinic today asks for your recommendation of an antiproteinuric agent to prevent diabetic nephropathy in this patient. Based on supporting evidence from clinical trials, the class of drugs with proven kidney protective effects in type 1 DM include which of the following?

   A. β-Blockers
   B. Calcium channel blockers (CCBs)
   C. Angiotensin-converting enzyme (ACE) inhibitors
   D. Angiotensin-receptor blockers (ARBs)
   E. Central-acting antihypertensive agents

2. Your recommendation is accepted by the medical team. Two months later when the patient returns for a follow-up visit, her blood pressure is 135/92 mm Hg, and her spot urine albumin:creatinine ratio is moderately lower. Renal laboratory values (serum creatinine and BUN) are WNL. HgA$_{1C}$ is elevated at 7.0%. Three separate blood pressure readings confirm the presence of elevated blood pressure, and the diagnosis of hypertension is confirmed. Based on the guidelines in the most recent JNC-7 and National Kidney Foundation (NKF) report, select your recommendation for optimizing the patient's blood pressure control from the following choices.

   A. Titrate the antihypertensive dose as tolerated; add a thiazide diuretic.
   B. Titrate the antihypertensive dose as tolerated; add a loop diuretic.
   C. Discontinue the antihypertensive; add a thiazide diuretic.
   D. Discontinue the antihypertensive; add a loop diuretic.
   E. Discontinue the antihypertensive; add a thiazide and loop diuretic.

3. What are two other recommendations that are essential in delaying the progression of diabetic nephropathy?

   I. Strict blood pressure control
   II. Strict blood glucose control
   III. Strict cholesterol control

   A. I only
   B. III only
   C. I and II only
   D. II and III only
   E. I, II, and III

4. Owing to medication and dietary nonadherence, the patient develops diabetic nephropathy with overt proteinuria within 3 years. Her serum creatinine and BUN are 1.6 and 28, respectively. She has moderate chronic renal insufficiency (estimated creatinine clearance = 38 mL/min). Her current medications include lisinopril, furosemide, atorvastatin, and insulin as directed by her PCP. She presents to the clinic with a chief complaint of abdominal pain and nausea. The team would like to rule out diabetic gastroparesis, so a CT scan with contrast media is scheduled for tomorrow. Which of the prescribed medications should be temporarily withdrawn 24 hours before and after the imaging study to prevent contrast media nephrotoxicity (CMN)?

   I. Insulin
   II. Lisinopril
   III. Furosemide

   A. I only
   B. III only
   C. I and II only
   D. II and III only
   E. I, II, and III

5. What other interventions should be instituted before the imaging study to prevent CMN in this patient?

   I. Hydration with normal saline IV
   II. N-Acetylcysteine (Mucomyst) PO
   III. Dopamine renal dose

   A. I only
   B. III only
   C. I and II only
   D. II and III only
   E. I, II, and III

6. The patient is also taking calcium carbonate for the management of hyperphosphatemia and hypocalcemia to prevent renal osteodystrophy. She is persistently hypocalcemic. iPTH is tested, and the value is 500 (normal <200). What would be the best initial treatment strategy in this patient to normalize serum calcium in the presence of secondary hyperparathyroidism?

   A. Discontinue calcium carbonate; start calcium acetate (Phos-Lo).
   B. Discontinue calcium carbonate; start sevelamer (Renagel).
   C. Add calcitriol (Rocaltrol).
   D. Add paricalcitol (Zemplar).
   E. Add AlOH/MgOH gel (Mylanta).

7. Which of the following agents may be prescribed to treat uncontrolled secondary hyperparathyroidism in patients who develop persistent hypercalcemia from conventional active vitamin D therapy?

   I. Doxecalciferol (Hectoral)
   II. Paricalcitol (Zemplar)
   III. Cinacalcet (Sensipar)

A. I only
B. III only
C. I and II only
D. II and III only
E. I, II, and III

8. Why should the administration of nonsteroidal anti-inflammatory drugs (NSAIDs) be avoided in this patient?

A. NSAIDs may lead to postrenal azotemia.
B. NSAIDs may lead to acute tubular necrosis (ATN).
C. NSAIDs may lead to glomerulonephritis.
D. NSAIDs may lead to lactic acidosis.
E. NSAIDs may lead to prerenal azotemia.

9. The patient develops end-stage renal disease and is undergoing hemodialysis. Eight weeks ago, erythropoietin (EPO) 2500 mg IV three times weekly after dialysis was begun. She is receiving daily maintenance doses of ferrous sulfate. Blood indices today reveal RBC 2.95, Hct 29.6, and Hgb 9.7. Ferritin and transferrin saturation are greater than 100 ng/mL and greater than 20%, respectively and within target goal. The medical team is concerned that the Hct target goal of 33% to 36% has not been reached despite 2 months of EPO treatment. What is the *most appropriate* recommendation to optimize treatment of anemia in this patient?

A. Administer a transfusion of packed red blood cells.
B. Discontinue EPO; start darbopoeitin (Aranesp).
C. Discontinue EPO and ferrous sulfate; start intravenous iron replacement.
D. Increase the dose of EPO by 25%.
E. Decrease the dose of EPO by 25%.

10. Which of the following pharmacokinetic characteristics may lead to drug dialyzability?

I. $V_d < 1$ L/kg
II. $t\frac{1}{2}$ of 3 to 4 h
III. PPB > 85%

A. I only
B. III only
C. I and II
D. II and III
E. I, II, and III

PATIENT PROFILE 154

THYROID DISEASE

PRESENTATION

HT is a 68-year-old man with a history of hypertension and sinusitis. He arrives in the emergency department with shortness of breath and palpitations that have lasted for 6 days. Almost a week ago he felt short of breath when cleaning the house and "on and off" since that time. He feels his "heart coming through his mouth because it's beating so funny." HT is allergic to penicillin (rash) and takes propranolol 60 mg po qid.

PHYSICAL EXAMINATION

BP: 140/85, HR: 130, RR: 20
HEENT: Extraocular muscles intact, PERRLA
NECK: Neck supple, nonpalpable thyroid
LUNGS: Clear to auscultation
CV: tachycardia, irregular rhythm
ABD: Soft, bowel sounds present
EXT: 1+ pitting edema, normal strength
NEURO: A/O × 3
ECG: Atrial fibrillation, HR 124 beats/min

QUESTIONS

1. Screening for hyperthyroidism was part of the evaluation in determining the cause of atrial fibrillation. Which of the following laboratory results best correlates with hyperthyroidism?

I. FT₄ 6.9 ng/dL (0.6–2.1 ng/dL)
II. FT₄ 0.3 ng/dL
III. TSH 0.2 μU/mL (0.5–5.5 μU/mL)
IV. TSH 8 μU/mL

A. I only
B. I and III only
C. I and IV only
D. II and III only
E. II and IV only

2. Hyperthyroidism is diagnosed. What are the goals of hyperthyroidism therapy?

A. Eliminate excess thyroid hormone
B. Minimize symptoms
C. Minimize long-term consequences

D. A and B only
E. A, B, and C

3. Which of the following medications would be appropriate therapy for HT?

    A. Methimazole
    B. Propylthiouracil
    C. Levothyroxine
    D. A and B only
    E. A, B, and C

4. In HT's case, atrial fibrillation is likely to be secondary to hyperthyroidism. The physician asks you to recommend therapy for immediate control of HT's heart rate. The goal of therapy is to decrease the heart rate to less than 90 beats/min. The best recommendation for HT is to

A. increase propranolol to 80 mg po qid.
B. continue propranolol and add hydrochlorothiazide 25 mg po qd.
C. continue propranolol and add diltiazem 90 mg po qid.
D. continue propranolol and add nifedipine 10 mg po qid.
E. continue propranolol and add amlodipine 5 mg po qd.

5. HT did not have many signs and symptoms of hyperthyroidism; however, many signs and symptoms of hyperthyroidism can occur. Which of the following is/are signs or symptoms of hyperthyroidism?

    A. Tremor
    B. Irritability
    C. Constipation
    D. A and B only
    E. A, B, and C

PATIENT PROFILE 155
BACTEREMIA AND SEPSIS

PRESENTATION

JB is a 74-year-old white woman who received a flu shot 2 weeks before admission who reports progressive weakness. JB is diagnosed with Guillain-Barré syndrome. Despite hospitalization and supportive care, the weakness progresses. Plasmapheresis is considered. Before the first course of plasmapheresis, the muscle weakness is so severe that JB loses control of her glottis and proceeds to aspirate. Now in respiratory distress, JB is taken to the intensive care unit, and an endotracheal tube is inserted.

QUESTIONS

1. Antibiotic therapy was not started immediately. JB had been in the hospital for 5 days before the ICU admission. There are no immediate radiographic changes, and the problem is believed to be chemical pneumonitis. The day after JB is admitted to the ICU, the chest radiograph blossoms with infiltrate in the right middle lobe, suggesting aspiration. A fever spikes to 39°C. Sputum cultures are suctioned deep from the endotracheal tube, blood and urine culture specimens are obtained, a nasogastric tube is placed, and administration is begun of ceftriaxone 1 g IV q24h and metronidazole 500 mg NG q8h for presumed aspiration pneumonia. The preliminary blood cultures are 2 of 2 bottles positive for lactose-fermenting

gram-negative bacilli. Empirical antibiotic therapy should be directed against which of the following organisms?

    A. *Staphylococcus aureus*
    B. *Klebsiella pneumoniae*
    C. *Enterobacter* species
    D. A and B
    E. B and C

2. Which of the following is the *best choice* to cover lactose-fermenting gram negative bacilli?

    A. Ceftizoxime
    B. Cefazolin
    C. Ampicillin
    D. Vancomycin
    E. Penicillin

3. Defervescence occurs over the next 3 days, but JB is producing large amounts of chunky, green, foul-smelling sputum. A temperature spikes again, and the blood pressure begins to drop, necessitating fluid resuscitation and vasopressor support. Cultures of blood, sputum, and urine are obtained and show 3+ non-lactose-fermenting gram-negative bacilli growing from the sputum and blood. The antibiotic coverage should be changed to which of the following?

A. Piperacillin 3 g IV q4h and gentamicin per dosing protocol

B. Vancomycin 1 g IV q12h and gentamicin per dosing protocol

C. Ceftriaxone 1 g IV q24h and tobramycin per dosing protocol

D. Unasyn (ampicillin-sulbactam) 3 g IV q6h and amikacin per dosing protocol

E. Levofloxacin 500 mg IV q24h

4. Culture and sensitivity testing of the organism on sputum and blood showed *Stenotrophomonas maltophilia*. After discontininuing the previously chosen therapy, which antibioitic would be the drug of choice for *S. maltophilia* infection?

A. Clindamycin
B. Vancomycin
C. Trimethoprim-sulfamethoxazole
D. Cefotaxime
E. Penicillin

5. This particular strain of *S. maltophilia* has become resistant very rapidly to the previous choice. What should be the treatment of choice once the primary therapy has failed?

A. Amikacin
B. Trovafloxacin
C. Sparfloxacin
D. Piperacillin-tazobactam
E. Ceftazidime and tobramycin

PATIENT PROFILE 156

CHRONIC OBSTRUCTIVE LUNG DISEASE

PRESENTATION

JH is a 56-year-old man who sees his physician because of increasing shortness of breath and decreasing exercise tolerance. He has a 50-pack year smoking history, and he has been unable to successfully stop. He has experienced several months of a persistent, productive, cough. His medical history is otherwise unremarkable. During the physical examination, JH is found to be somewhat obese and slightly cyanotic. His FEV_i is 65% of predicted and improves only minimally after administration of a β_2 agonist. The preliminary diagnosis is obstructive lung disease.

QUESTIONS

1. The presentation is most consistent with what type of obstructive lung disease?

A. Asthma
B. Acute bronchitis
C. Chronic bronchitis
D. Emphysema
E. α_1-Antitrypsin deficiency

2. JH wants to stop smoking and begins using nicotine gum. In counseling him on the proper use of the gum, what would be the most appropriate advice?

A. Use the gum with food or beverage.
B. Continue chewing a piece of gum until the craving for a cigarette stops.
C. Use no more than 10 pieces of gum per day.

D. Chew the gum slowly to reduce side effects.
E. Once a "tingling" sensation is noticed, the gum should be removed from the mouth.

3. Which of the following transdermal nicotine systems is intended to be left on for 16 rather than 24 hours?

A. Habitrol® (nicotine transdermal)
B. NicoDerm® (nicotine transdermal)
C. Nicotrol® (nicotine transdermal)
D. ProStep™ (nicotine transdermal)
E. All of the above

4. JH starts using a transdermal nicotine system. When counseling him on proper use of the patch, which advice is most appropriate?

A. Remove the patch after 12 hours to have a nicotine-free interval.
B. Rotate sites of administration to minimize skin irritation.
C. Apply as many patches as necessary to reduce the craving for cigarettes.
D. A and B
E. A, B, and C

5. If JH continues to smoke while using a nicotine patch, he may be at risk of what complication?

A. Gastric ulcer
B. Excessive sedation
C. Seizures
D. Cardiac arrhythmias
E. Renal failure

PATIENT PROFILE 157
URINARY TRACT INFECTION

PRESENTATION

PL, a 24-year-old female pharmacy student consults her primary care physician (PCP) with complaints of dysuria, urgency, frequency, and suprapubic pain. She indicates that these symptoms started 1½ days ago. She treated herself with drinking a lot of water and taking Tylenol. However, the symptoms got worse, prompting her to seek medical advice.

CC: The patient is a young woman with previous history of UTIs who presents with a new lower urinary tract infection (uncomplicated cystitis).

PMH: Seasonal allergies

Migraine headaches

Urinary tract infection (UTI) 4 and 7 months ago

Anemia

Med: Allegra® (fexofenadine) 60 mg qd (as needed)

Imitrex® (sumatriptan succinate) 25 mg tablets (take one as directed)

Ferrous sulfate 325 mg tid

ALL: Sulfa (severe rash)

SH: Nonsmoker; no alcohol use; lives with boyfriend; uses diaphragm with spermicide for contraception

PE: Afebrile, BP 120/70 mm Hg, HR 80 beats/min, no CVA tenderness

Labs: Electrolytes within normal limits, glucose 110 mg/dL, Hct 35%, WBC 8.9 K cells/mm3, cloudy urine (a urine dipstick test will be done)

QUESTIONS

1. Which of the following statements regarding the dipstick test is/are correct?

   A. It usually takes several hours for this test to show a result.
   B. It identifies the specific pathogen and allows for directed treatment.
   C. In the presence of a UTI it will most likely be nitrite+, and leukocyte esterase+.
   D. In the presence of a UTI it will most likely be nitrite−, and leukocyte−.
   E. None of the statements is correct.

2. Which of the following is/are the most common microorganism(s) associated with uncomplicated cystitis?

   A. Proteus mirabilis
   B. *Enterobacter* sp.
   C. *Escherichia coli*
   D. Enterococci
   E. *Klebsiella pneumoniae*

3. The PCP asks your advice for treating the patient with a single-dose antibiotic therapy. Which of the following statements about this treatment approach is correct?

   A. Single-dose antibiotic therapy is the currently recommended therapy because it is has been found very effective in uncomplicated cystitis.
   B. Single-dose therapy has been associated with a higher frequency of UTI recurrences, and this may not be appropriate for PL.
   C. Single-dose therapy has been found as effective as multiple-dose therapy in eradicating bacteriuria in numerous clinical studies.
   D. Single-dose therapy includes high doses of cephalosporins.
   E. Single-dose therapy is highly recommended for PL because it is cheap and the likelihood of an adverse reaction is very small.

4. The PCP decides to treat the patient with a multiple-dose regimen. Which of the following options is the *most appropriate* choice for PL?

   A. Fosfomycin 3 g po qd given for 3 days
   B. Bactrim DS po bid given for 3 days
   C. Norfloxacin 400 mg po bid for 3 days
   D. Nitrofurantoin 100 mg po q6H for 3 days
   E. Doxycycline 100 mg po bid for 3 days

5. Which of the following is true regarding the use of trimethoprim-sulfamethoxazole?

   A. It can cause a variety of drug eruptions.
   B. It has been associated with blood dyscrasias.
   C. It should be taken with food.
   D. A and B
   E. A and C

6. If the PCP decided to treat PL with ciprofloxacin PO, which of the following counseling information should she receive?

   I. There may be an interaction with sumatriptan.
   II. She should avoid the use of fexofenadine concurrently.
   III. She should use sunscreen and wear sunglasses while outdoors.
   IV. She should space the intake of ferrous sulfate at least 2 hours apart.

   A. I only
   B. II only

C. III and IV
D. III only
E. I, II, and IV

7. PL is treated appropriately. However, 3 months later she returns to her physician with the same complaints. In managing this patient's fourth episode of recurrent UTI the following issue(s) need to be considered. (Please choose the *most appropriate* answer.)

A. She most likely has a reinfection, and this should initially be treated like a new infection with the antibiotics used effectively in the past.
B. The active infection should be treated and bacterial eradication should be confirmed by a negative culture 1 to 2 weeks after treatment.
C. The recurrent infections may be temporally related to sexual activity and she should consider prophylaxis.
D. Her contraceptive method may be a major risk factor for the frequent UTIs, and she should consider changing them.
E. All of the above parameters need to be considered.

8. Which of the following prophylactic regimens is the *most appropriate* choice for PL?

I. Nitrofurantoin macrocrystals 50 to 100 mg qd postcoital
II. Norfloxacin 200 mg every night
III. Bactrim SS 1 tab postcoital
IV. Trimethoprim 100 mg postcoital
V. Bactrim SS 1 tab every night

A. I and IV
B. II, III, and V
C. IV only

D. II only
E. None is an appropriate choice.

9. Patients who take nitrofurantoin (especially at treatment doses) often complain of nausea and vomiting. Strategies to reduce this problem include which of the following?

A. Potentially lower the dose to less than 7 mg/kg.
B. Take the drug with food or milk.
C. Change to a macrocrystalline preparation.
D. None of the above is a suitable solution.
E. All of the above are suitable strategies.

10. One year later PL has become pregnant, and during a routine check-up asymptomatic bacteriuria is detected. With regard to treating UTIs during pregnancy, which of the following statements is/are correct?

I. Asymptomatic bacteriuria in pregnancy always needs to be treated because symptomatic pyelonephritis may develop, and there is an increased risk of preterm labor and premature delivery.
II. Asymptomatic bacteriuria during pregnancy should not be treated because of the high risk of antibiotic-associated adverse effects to the fetus.
III. Drugs that can be used safely include the quinolones, sulfonamides, and tetracyclines.
IV. Drugs that can be used safely include penicillins and cephalosporins.
V. The duration of treatment is usually 7 to 10 days.

A. II only
B. I and III
C. I and IV
D. I, IV, and V
E. All of the above except II

PATIENT PROFILE 158

PARENTERAL NUTRITION

PRESENTATION

The equation for the resting metabolic equivalent (RME, Harris-Benedict equation, basal metabolic requirement, kcal/day requirement) for men is as follows:

$$RME = 66 + (13.7 \times W) + (5 \times H) - (6.8 \times A)$$

The patient is 5′9″ tall, weighs 200 lb, and is 40 years of age. The patient has been hospitalized for a severe infection and has been categorized by the physician as being under moderate stress (1.6 stress factor according to hospital guidelines). The physician chooses to provide the patient with total parenteral nutrition with 60% of the calories from a lipid source and 0.9 g protein per kg body weight. The pharmacy routinely uses 20% w/v lipid (emulsion) injection, 8.5% w/v amino acid injection, and 50% w/v dextrose injection.

QUESTIONS

1. What is the daily nonstressed kilocalorie requirement for this patient?

   A. 1789
   B. 1848
   C. 1914
   D. 2458
   E. 2879

2. What is the daily stressed kilocalorie requirement for this patient?

   A. 1196
   B. 1912.4
   C. 1914
   D. 1915.6
   E. 3062

3. How many total milliliters of lipid (emulsion) injection should be used daily to provide the allowed kilocalories from fat sources?

   A. 1020
   B. 1063

   C. 1701
   D. 9185
   E. 15310

4. How many total milliliters of amino acid injection should be used daily to provide the allowed amount from protein sources?
   A. 962
   B. 1069
   C. 1188
   D. 2118
   E. 2353

5. How many total milliliters of dextrose injection should be used daily to provide the remaining kilocalories needed from dextrose?

   A. 528
   B. 1273
   C. 1796
   D. 1801
   E. Insufficient information provided

PATIENT PROFILE 1 5 9

SEXUALLY TRANSMITTED DISEASES

PRESENTATION

BT is a 28-year-old woman who arrives in the emergency department with vaginal discharge, mild abdominal pain, and dysuria. Her medical history reveals recurrent gonococcal and nongonococcal urethritis and cervicitis. Gram stain of her vaginal discharge shows gram-negative diplococci and many neutrophils. The culture and susceptibility results are pending. BT has no known drug allergies. When questioned about her medication history, BT admits that she was given an antibiotic, which she does not remember the name of, and did not complete the 7-day course of therapy. The intern consults with you about an appropriate treatment regimen for BT. The pregnancy test result is negative.

QUESTIONS

1. Which of the following regimens is most appropriate for BT?

   A. Ceftriaxone 125 mg IM once and azithromycin 1 g orally once
   B. Cefixime 400 mg orally once and ofloxacin mg orally once

   C. Spectinomycin 2 g IM once and ofloxacin 400 mg orally once
   D. Ceftriaxone 125 mg IM and erythromycin base 500 mg orally qid
   E. Ofloxacin 400 mg once and cefotetan 1 g IM once

2. If BT had been pregnant, which of the following regimens would have been most appropriate?

   A. Ceftriaxone 125 mg IM once and doxycycline 100 mg bid for 7 days
   B. Ceftriaxone 125 mg IM once and erythromycin base 500 mg orally qid for 7 days
   C. Azithromycin 1 g orally once and erythromycin base 500 mg orally qid for 7 days
   D. Azithromycin 1 g oral once and ofloxacin 300 mg orally bid for 7 days
   E. Ceftriaxone 125 mg IM once and ofloxacin 300 mg orally bid for 7 days

3. Which statement concerning doxycycline is true?

   A. Doxycycline is adequate coverage for chlamydia and trichomoniasis.

B. Doxycycline is adequate coverage for chlamydia.
C. Doxycycline is adequate coverage for chlamydia and gonorrhea.
D. Doxycycline is adequate coverage for gonorrhea.
E. Doxycycline is adequate coverage for chlamydia, gonorrhea, and trichomoniasis.

4. Which statement concerning ceftriaxone is true?

A. Ceftriaxone should not be administered intramuscularly.
B. Ceftriaxone is adequate coverage for chlamydia.
C. Ceftriaxone is adequate coverage for chlamydia and gonorrhea.
D. Ceftriaxone is adequate coverage for gonorrhea.
E. Ceftriaxone is adequate coverage for chlamydia, gonorrhea, and trichomoniasis.

5. Which of the following statement(s) is/are true concerning appropriate treatment of BT?

A. BT should be encouraged to refer her sex partner(s) for diagnosis, treatment, and counseling.
B. BT should be offered HIV counseling and testing.
C. BT should be informed of the results of testing at this admission, and prevention strategies should be reinforced.
D. BT should receive education on how to reduce the risk of transmission.
E. All of the above

6. BT is also at risk of other sexually transmitted diseases. If she had been diagnosed with trichomoniasis, which of the following would be the appropriate treatment regimen?

A. Doxycycline 100 mg bid for 7 days
B. Amoxicillin 500 mg tid for 7 days
C. Metronidazole 2 g orally once
D. Azithromycin 1 g orally once
E. Ceftriaxone 125 mg IM once

7. BT drinks alcohol in moderation approximately 3 days a week. Which of the following agents can cause nausea and flushing when taken concomitantly with alcohol?

A. Doxycycline
B. Amoxicillin
C. Metronidazole
D. Azithromycin
E. Ceftriaxone

8. Genital herpes or herpes genitalis is an acute inflammatory sexually transmitted infection cause by the herpes simplex virus (HSV). Which of the following statement(s) is/are true about the antiviral agents listed below?

A. Famciclovir is a prodrug.
B. Valacyclovir is a prodrug.
C. Acyclovir is a prodrug.
D. A and B are prodrugs.
E. All of the above are prodrugs.

9. Which of following agents require(s) careful monitoring in patients with renal impairment?

A. Acyclovir
B. Famciclovir
C. Valacyclovir
D. A and B only
E. All of the above

10. Syphilis is a sexually transmitted disease caused by the spirochete, *Treponema pallidum*. What is the drug of choice for treatment of all stages of syphilis?

A. Tetracycline
B. Ciprofloxacin
C. Parenteral penicillin G
D. Spectinomycin
E. Gentamicin

PATIENT PROFILE 160
SOFT-TISSUE INFECTION

PRESENTATION

DW is a 58-year-old white man who comes to the clinic with fever and chills that have lasted for several days and are unrelieved with acetaminophen. The course over the past couple of days is as follows: Three days ago DW's wife trimmed his toenails, as she has been doing for years. DW put on a new pair of boots and ventured onto his property to prepare it for the coming winter. That night after removing his boots, DW noticed that both feet were a bit discolored from the rubbing of his new boots. The following morning, DW noticed that his wife had trimmed the toenail on his right great toe too close. Clear fluid had begun to drain from that toe. Later that day DW felt feverish and had chills, which eventually led him to the clinic. The medical history includes diabetes mellitus, hypertension, renal insufficiency, and diabetic neuropathy. DW is admitted to the hospital with a diabetic foot infection.

QUESTIONS

1. Choose the best answer regarding the type of organisms found in diabetic foot infections.

   A. Because diabetic foot infections are considered "skin" infections, *Staphylococcus* and *Streptococcus* species are the most common organisms isolated.
   B. On average only one organism is isolated in a diabetic foot infection.
   C. *Proteus mirabilis*, group D streptococci, *Escherichia coli*, *Staphylococcus aureus*, *Bacteroides fragilis*, *Peptococcus*, and *Peptostreptococcus* all are pathogens that can be isolated from a diabetic foot ulcer.
   D. Patients with diabetes typically have a normal immunologic response to infection. This explains why most patients who come to medical attention as DW did receive oral antibiotics for the duration of infection.
   E. The correlation between results of superficial cultures taken from the wound site and deep aspiration of the wound is strong, which rules out the need for deep wound cultures.

2. All of the following about DW's diabetic foot infection are true except:

   A. Today's broad-spectrum antibiotics easily allow us to use antibiotic therapy for osteomyelitis infections, which are infrequent among patients with diabetes.
   B. DW may have had this infection sooner than he reported. Diabetic neuropathy often masks the clinical signs and symptoms of infection.
   C. Foot infections common among persons with diabetes are infection of the soft tissue adjacent to the nail, infection of the middle foot secondary to painless trauma, infection of the toe web space, and infection of the sole over the head of the metatarsals.
   D. Necrotizing skin infections and osteomyelitis are common complications of diabetic foot ulcers.

   E. Specimens for culture and sensitivity testing should be obtained initially for a diabetic patient with a lesion on the foot.

3. Because DW will be admitted to the hospital, antibiotic therapy should be started immediately after cultures are obtained from DW's foot. Which of the following therapies would be the best choice for empiric management of this infection?

   A. Monotherapy with nafcillin lg IV q6h
   B. Monotherapy with aztreonam l g IV q8h
   C. Combination therapy with nafcillin 2 g IV q6h and penicillin 3 million units IV q4h for increased streptococcal coverage
   D. Monotherapy with piperacillin-tazobactam 3.375 g IV q6h
   E. Monotherapy with metronidazole 500 mg po q8h

4. Osteomyelitis is ruled out. Which statement involving DW's therapeutic decisions is most truthful?

   A. Culture and sensitivity results indicate standard diabetic foot flora sensitive to the antibiotic panel against which it was tested. Therapy should continue for 10–12 weeks.
   B. In an attempt at pharmacoeconomic consciousness, 72 hours of IV antibiotic therapy is completed, and you recommend switching to an oral agent in an effort to facilitate this patient's discharge.
   C. Seventy-two hours has passed and not much improvement has occurred. You consider modifying antibiotic therapy to include coverage for *Pseudomonas aeruginosa*.
   D. Right foot amputation is the only alternative available for DW.
   E. You suspect that DW has been colonized with vancomycin-resistant enterococci, and therapy for this infection will resolve the symptoms.

5. Which of the following guideline(s) for foot care of patients with diabetes should be followed?

   A. Inspect feet daily for the presence of cuts, blisters, or scratches. Look between all toes, and examine the bottom of the foot.
   B. Use tepid water to wash feet daily and dry them thoroughly.
   C. Apply lotion to the feet to prevent calluses and cracking.
   D. Wear properly fitting shoes.
   E. All of the above

ASTHMA

PRESENTATION

JJ is a 39-year-old white male who was diagnosed with asthma when he was 11 years old. His asthma has been controlled during this time using only an albuterol inhaler on an "as-needed" basis. About a year ago JJ lost his job, was unable to pay his apartment's rent, and was forced to move into public housing in the inner city. At this time he also lost all of his health insurance benefits. He currently works as a dishwasher in a restaurant to "get by." JJ is divorced with no children. He drinks occasionally and smokes about one pack per day. His parents are in good health and live in Florida. JJ states he has had to use his inhaler more often during this past year, slowly increasing to the point where he needed to seek out medical attention. He states he has been experiencing symptoms a few days a week and has even woken up two nights during this time period. Specifically JJ is complaining about shortness of breath, wheezing, chest pain, and cough. He admits to have tried a number of over-the-counter medications, such as Delsym® and Primatene Mist®, to help with his symptoms. He denies any herbal use with the exception of zinc lozenges to help prevent colds. JJ states he has had a prescription in the past for Protonix®, Zoloft, Zestril®, and Ambien® but can no longer afford these medications. He is concerned about his overall health because of his inability to continue to fill all of his medications. He is also extremely concerned about his blood pressure, which has been elevated at approximately 145/90 over the last month. JJ states that any assistance you can provide would be greatly appreciated because it is all starting to add up and worsen his depression.

MH: Albuterol one to two inhalations by mouth every 2 to 4 hours as needed
Protonix® 40 mg by mouth every day
Zoloft® 50 mg by mouth twice a day
Zestril® 10 mg by mouth every day
Ambien® 5 mg by mouth every night at bedtime
Delsym® 1 tablespoonful by mouth as needed for cough
Primatene Mist® inhale one puff by mouth as needed
MC: Insomnia
Depression
Hypertension
Gastroesophageal reflux disease

QUESTIONS

1. JJ most likely needs education on controlling which of the following asthma triggers?

   I. Indoor mold
   II. Cockroach allergen
   III. House dust mite allergen

   A. I only
   B. III only
   C. I and II
   D. II and III
   E. I, II, and III

2. Which of the following of JJ's disorders can exacerbate asthma symptoms?

   I. Insomnia
   II. Depression
   III. Gastroesophageal reflux disease

   A. I only
   B. III only
   C. I and II
   D. II and III
   E. I, II, and III

3. Based on JJ's information, what classification of asthma is most appropriate?

   A. Step 0: at risk for asthma
   B. Step 1: mild intermittent asthma
   C. Step 2: mild persistent asthma
   D. Step 3: moderate persistent asthma
   E. Step 4: severe persistent asthma

4. Using the stepwise approach, which of the following is the best choice to add to JJ's regimen?

   A. Methylxanthine
   B. Anticholinergic agent
   C. Long-acting $\beta2$ agonist
   D. Low-dose inhaled corticosteroid
   E. Low-dose inhaled corticosteroid and long-acting $\beta2$ agonist

5. What important recommendation might you make about JJ's use of Primatene Mist®?

   A. Counsel JJ about taking the medication on a regular schedule every day to prevent asthma symptoms.
   B. Counsel JJ about taking the medication on a regular schedule every day to alleviate asthma symptoms.
   C. Counsel JJ about taking the medication only as needed to prevent asthma symptoms.
   D. Recommend that JJ discontinue his Primatene Mist® use and obtain a new prescription for his albuterol to use on an as-needed basis.
   E. None of the above

6. Why is theophylline not a good choice of therapy for JJ?

A. His age
B. Smoking one pack per day
C. His alcohol consumption
D. Potential serious drug interactions with his other medications
E. All of the above

7. JJ returns 1 year later on the following medications:
Albuterol inhaler one to two puffs by mouth every 4 to 6 hours as needed
Flovent® 110 µg inhaler one puff by mouth two times a day
Singulair® 10 mg by mouth every night at bedtime
Which of the following is true about the Flovent® that JJ is currently using?

I. Long-term use slows growth rate and reduces adult terminal height.
II. Long-term use increases airway remodeling and decreases the need for rescue therapy.
III. Flovent® improves lung function when used with a long-acting β2-agonist and is usually a first-line agent in the treatment of asthma.

A. I only
B. III only
C. I and II
D. II and III
E. I, II, and III

8. Which of the following is a common adverse effect of Flovent®?

I. Cough
II. Tremor
III. Pharyngitis

A. I only
B. III only
C. I and III
D. II and III
E. I, II, and III

9. Which of the following best describes the mechanism of action of JJ's Singulair®?

A. Methylxanthine
B. Leukotriene modifier
C. Anticholinergic agent
D. Inhaled corticosteroid
E. Long-acting β2 agonist

10. The Singular® that JJ is currently taking is similar in action to which of the following medications?

I. Zileuton
II. Genahist
III. Zafirlukast

A. I only
B. III only
C. I and III
D. II and III
E. I, II, and III

PATIENT PROFILE 162

OSTEOPOROSIS

PRESENTATION

AZ is a slender, 55-year-old woman who comes to your pharmacy with a prescription for estrogen therapy. In your discussion with her, you discover that AZ had recently sustained a fracture and was taken to the emergency department by her son, who witnessed the fall. She fractured her hip and needed surgery. A complete evaluation was performed at the hospital, including bone density testing, which established the diagnosis of osteoporosis. AZ admits that before this fall she was not taking the estrogen that her physician had recommended she start taking at menopause. She states that she was hesitant to take estrogens because she was concerned about some of the side effects. Her medication history is the following: atenolol (Tenormin®) 50 mg/day, simvastatin (Zocor®) 20 mg/day, vitamin C 500 mg/day, vitamin E 400 IU/day, and aspirin 81

mg/day. The medical history includes hypertension, hypercholesterolemia, and ovarian cancer (treatment including hysterectomy was performed as part of the management and a 6-month course of chemotherapy; she is 7 years in remission).

QUESTIONS

1. Which of the following concerning estrogen therapy is/are true?

A. The daily dose of estrogen shown to preserve bone mineral density is equivalent to 0.625 mg conjugated estrogen.
B. Estrogen supplementation at menopause is the single most effective measure for preventing post-menopausal osteoporosis.

C. Estrogen therapy provides benefits other than prevention of osteoporosis, such as relief from vasomotor symptoms associated with menopause, and a reduction in a woman's risk of cardiovascular mortality.
D. A and B
E. All of the above

2. AZ is not receiving progesterone concomitantly with estrogen therapy. The most likely reason is the following:

A. The physician forgot to prescribe progesterone therapy and you will call him to recommend the addition of progesterone with estrogen therapy.
B. Women who have undergone a hysterectomy do not need concomitant progesterone therapy.
C. AZ has a contraindication to progesterone therapy.
D. Concomitant progesterone therapy will cause buildup of endometrial tissue.
E. None of the above

3. In assessing AZ for optimal osteoporosis therapy, which of the following is/are true?

A. It has been demonstrated that the combination of calcium and vitamin D_3 decreases the incidence of hip fractures among elderly women.
B. The National Institutes of Health Consensus Development Conference Statement recommends 1000 mg elemental calcium as optimal daily intake among women older than 50 years who are taking estrogen supplementation.
C. AZ's osteoporosis therapy is already optimal because she is receiving estrogen therapy. No further recommendation is necessary.
D. A and B
E. All of the above

4. Calcitonin-salmon nasal solution (Miacalcin® Nasal Spray) is an alternative therapy for osteoporosis more than 5 years after menopause among women with low bone mass. Which of the following are the recommended daily dosage and proper administration of this medication?

A. One 200-IU spray to one nostril daily (alternate nostrils each day)
B. One 200-IU spray in each nostril daily
C. One 200-IU spray to one nostril weekly (alternate nostrils weekly)
D. One 200-IU spray to each nostril every other day
E. None of the above

5. AZ asks you which factor(s) increase(s) risk of development of osteoporosis. You correctly reply:

A. Cigarette smoking
B. Excessive alcohol intake
C. Excessive caffeine intake
D. A and B only
E. All of the above

PATIENT PROFILE 163
ISOTONIC SOLUTIONS (PHARMACEUTICS)

PRESENTATION

A patient comes to your pharmacy with the following prescription from his ophthalmologist. Presuming this is not a commercially available product, you embark on the compounding process, keeping in mind requirements of ophthalmic preparations. Tonicity is very important for the safety and comfort of the patient. Some of the following questions might be those you consider as you decide how to prepare the prescription.

Rx: Pilocarpine hydrochloride 0.5%
Make isotonic with NaCl
Purified water q.s. a.d. 30 mL
The sodium chloride equivalent for pilocarpine hydrochloride is 0.24.

QUESTIONS

1. How much NaCl is necessary?

A. 0.120 g
B. 0.468 g
C. 0.134 g
D. 0.270 g
E. 0.234 g

2. If using boric acid instead of NaCl, how much is required to make this preparation isotonic? (The sodium chloride equivalent for boric acid is 0.50.)

A. 0.120 g
B. 0.480 g
C. 0.134 g

D.   0.270 g
E.   0.234 g

3. How much NaCl is required to make 120 mL of isotonic NaCl solution?

A.   1.08 g
B.   108 g
C.   10.8 g
D.   108 mg
E.   10.8 mg

4. What is the mole fraction of NaCl in normal saline? Assume the NaCl occupies no volume, and 100 mL of water is used to make the solution. (Molecular weights: O = 16, H = 1, Cl = 35.5, Na = 23; density of water = 1 g/mL)

A.   5.556
B.   0.00276
C.   361.7
D.   0.00175
E.   0.0154

5. How many mEq of Na^+ are there in 120 mL of normal saline?

A.   1080
B.   63,180
C.   18.5
D.   12.7
E.   540

6. How many mOsm theoretically are present in 120 mL of normal saline?

A.   93.9
B.   31.5

C.   18.5
D.   24.8
E.   36.9

7. What is the molarity of NaCl in 120 mL of normal saline?

A.   0.0185
B.   1.85
C.   1.54
D.   0.154
E.   0.59

8. What is the molarity of NaCl in the *preparation?*

A.   0.234
B.   0.154
C.   0.400
D.   0.004
E.   0.133

9. If a tonicity adjuster were not added to a parenteral prescription, which of the following might occur to red blood cells?

A.   Nothing
B.   Crenation
C.   Hemolysis
D.   Equilibration
E.   Shrinking of the cells

10. If the osmotic pressure of a NaCl solution is 250 mOsm/L, then what is its percentage strength?

A.   0.731%
B.   8.55%
C.   0.217%
D.   9.33%
E.   4.21%

PATIENT PROFILE 164

ONCOLOGY: NAUSEA AND VOMITING CONTROL

PRESENTATION

VT is a 42-year-old man receiving chemotherapy for lung cancer. He is scheduled to begin a new chemotherapy regimen containing cyclophosphamide, doxorubicin, and cisplatin administered in a 28-day cycle. The previous chemotherapy regimen consisted of cisplatin and etoposide. VT has no relevant medical history. He had taken no medications before initiating chemotherapy. He has no known drug allergies. He drinks alcohol (scotch 1–2 drinks) 2 or 3 nights per week after work. He still smokes 2 packs per day ("why quit now?"). He is single and works as an engineer for a software company.

QUESTIONS

1. VT had tolerated his previous chemotherapy regimen fairly well. The nausea and vomiting were well

controlled, but VT had frequent bouts of diarrhea. Which antiemetic regimen would most likely be associated with diarrhea?

A. Prochlorperazine 10 mg IM q6h prn
B. Ondansetron 16 mg IV qd before chemotherapy
C. Metoclopramide 120 mg IV before chemotherapy and q4h × 2 doses after chemotherapy
D. Dexamethasone 10 mg IV qd before chemotherapy
E. Marinol® (dronabinol) tabs q3h prn

2. VT agrees to proceed with the new chemotherapy regimen. Which antiemetic regimen would be most appropriate for VT at this time?

A. Methylprednisolone 250 mg IV q6h prn
B. Ondansetron 24 mg IV and dexamethasone 10 mg IV qd before chemotherapy
C. Perphenazine 5 mg IV q4h prn and dexamethasone 10 mg IV before chemotherapy
D. Prochlorperazine 10 mg po q4h prn
E. Lorazepam 1 mg IV before chemotherapy

3. VT had good control of his nausea and vomiting during chemotherapy, but 2 days after treatment is completed, he vomits three times within 12 hours. This pattern of nausea and vomiting is most consistent with

A. psychogenic vomiting.
B. anticipatory vomiting.
C. acute vomiting.
D. chronic vomiting.
E. delayed vomiting.

4. VT spends 30 minutes in the men's room vomiting before his third course of therapy (cyclophosphamide, doxorubicin, and cisplatin). Which agent would be most appropriate to control this vomiting?

A. Lorazepam
B. Prochlorperazine
C. Metoclopramide
D. Ondansetron
E. Granisetron

5. VT is given a prescription for prochlorperazine 10 mg po q6h prn to start the day after he finishes the course of chemotherapy. What is the most important adverse effect to discuss in counseling?

A. Headache
B. GI upset
C. Diarrhea
D. Visual changes
E. Extrapyramidal symptoms

PATIENT PROFILE 165
OPIOID OVERDOSE AND DEPENDENCE

PRESENTATION

JA is a 32-year-old white woman who was brought to the emergency department by ambulance after her roommate found her unresponsive on the bathroom floor. JA was enrolled in an inpatient detoxification program for 5 days and left against medical advice yesterday. Her roommate reports that JA purchased some heroin and has been "shooting-up" for the last 24 hours.

CC: Patient is unresponsive.
PMH: Asthma since childhood
Opioid dependence × 8 years
SH: Tobacco use: smokes one to two packs per day × 15 years
Alcohol use: Drinks occasionally on weekends
Illicit Drug use: heroin dependent × 8 years
FH: Married × 6 years; currently separated from her husband × 6 months. Remaining family history is noncontributory.

ROS: JA is unresponsive upon arrival to the emergency department.
PE: Wt 75 kg
Allergies: PCN, hives
GEN: Groggy, unresponsive woman in some respiratory distress, pinpoint pupils
VS: BP 80/50 mm Hg, HR 49, RR 6, Temp 37.8°C
HEENT: pinpoint pupils and symmetrical
Chest: Decreased respirations, decreased breath sounds on the right, moderate wheezing
Cardiac: Sinus bradycardia
Abd: Decreased bowel sounds
Ext: Skin cool to touch, red marks and scars noted on inside of both arms
Neuro: Responsive to pain, A&O × 0
Laboratory values, urinalysis, and toxicology screen pending.
Methadone (dose unknown) × 5 days at inpatient detoxification center
Ventolin Inhaler two puffs prn

Diagnoses:
1. Opioid (heroin) overdose
2. Opioid dependence × 8 years
3. Asthma since childhood

QUESTIONS

1. Immediate treatment of opioid overdose includes which of the following?

   I.   Airway management and cardiorespiratory support ✓
   II. Opioid reversal with an opioid antagonist ✓
   III. Treatment with a benzodiazepine

   A. I only
   B. III only
   C. I and II only
   D. II and III only
   E. I, II, and III

2. After receiving therapy for opioid overdose, JA developed symptoms of opioid withdrawal. Which of the following symptoms can be attributed to opioid withdrawal?

   I.   Auditory hallucinations
   II. Diaphoresis ✓
   III. Nausea and vomiting ✓

   A. I only
   B. III only
   C. I and II only
   D. II and III only
   E. I, II, and III

3. Which one of the following statements regarding withdrawal from opioids is true?

   A. Opioid withdrawal symptoms are often life threatening.
   B. The onset of opioid withdrawal symptoms is highly variable and dependent on many factors.
   C. Methadone is used to treat withdrawal from heroin because it has no withdrawal symptoms associated with its discontinuation.
   D. The onset of withdrawal symptoms from heroin is similar to that of methadone.
   E. All opioid withdrawal symptoms associated with heroin resolve within 48 to 72 hours.

4. The drug Narcan is also known as which one of the following?

   A. Methadone
   B. Naltrexone
   C. Naloxone
   D. Levomethadyl acetate
   E. Buprenorphine

5. The Drug Addiction Treatment ACT of 2000 allows qualified physicians to prescribe Schedule III, IV, and V medications for treatment of opioid dependence in an office-based setting. Which one of the following medications is currently approved for this indication?

   A. Methadone
   B. Oxycodone
   C. Clonidine
   D. Buprenorphine
   E. Levomethadyl acetate

6. Which of the following medications is a partial opioid agonist?

   I.   Methadone
   II. Naloxone
   III. Buprenorphine

   A. I only
   B. III only
   C. I and II only
   D. II and III only
   E. I, II, and III

7. After treatment of heroin overdose, a pregnancy test performed on JA's admission to the emergency department indicates that she is approximately 3 months pregnant. Which of the following statements about the use of methadone maintenance during pregnancy is/are true?

   I.   Methadone does not appear to be teratogenic.
   II. Methadone crosses the placental barrier.
   III. The infant will display some opioid withdrawal symptoms after birth.

   A. I only
   B. III only
   C. I and II only
   D. II and III only
   E. I, II, and III

8. Clonidine, a nonopioid, can be used in a patient experiencing opioid withdrawal to treat which of the following symptoms?

   A. Anxiety
   B. Musculoskeletal aches and pains
   C. Insomnia
   D. Gastrointestinal hyperactivity
   E. Hypotension

9. Which one of the following statements best describes why naloxone is added to buprenorphine tablets for sublingual use?

   A. To enhance the absorption of the buprenorphine
   B. To speed-up detoxification from opioids

X   To discourage the intravenous abuse of buprenorphine

D.   To prevent the onset of withdrawal symptoms when buprenorphine is discontinued

E.   To decrease the overall total dose of buprenorphine needed to prevent withdrawal symptoms

10. Which of the following statements regarding methadone is/are true?

I.   Methadone is a synthetic, orally acting μ-opioid receptor agonist.

II. Methadone has a duration of action of 12 to 24 hours and can be dosed once daily for detoxification and maintenance therapy for opioid dependence.

III. Methadone is the only medication the FDA has approved as substitution therapy for detoxification and maintenance therapy for opioid dependence.

A.   I only
B.   III only
X   I and II only
D.   II and III only
E.   I, II, and III

PATIENT PROFILE 166

MEDICINAL CHEMISTRY

PRESENTATION

MR, a 55-year-old friend of the family, stops by your house one Sunday morning and chats with you as his preferred pharmacist about the medications he is taking. His medications include carbachol (structure 166.1) for chronic glaucoma and triflupromazine (structure 166.2) for recently diagnosed psychosis. His main complaint is that since he started taking the antipsychotic medication, the glaucoma does not seem to be improving.

QUESTION

1. How do you respond?

A.   There is nothing wrong with taking the two medications together. Your system just needs time to adjust to the medications.

B.   The two medications should not be taken concurrently; take then at different times.

C.   Ask your physician to change the glaucoma medication to atenolol (structure 166.3).

D.   Ask your physician to change the antipsychotic medication to haloperidol (structure 166.4).

E.   C and D

$H_2NCOO-CH_2CH_2-N^+(CH_3)_3Cl^-$

166.1

166.2

166.3

166.4

PATIENT PROFILE 167
HYPERCHOLESTEROLEMIA

PRESENTATION

GK is a 59-year-old white man who was diagnosed with hypercholesterolemia during his last visit. He returns to his primary care physician after a trial of therapeutic lifestyle changes (TLC).

PMH: Hypothyroidism (5 years), eczema
FH: Noncontributory
SH: Married with two children; occasional EtOH use
MH: Levothyroxine 75 μg qd, multivitamin qd, occasional acetaminophen use
Allergy: Amoxicillin
ROS: Noncontributory
PE: BP 128/83, pulse 65, RR 18, Ht 155 cm, Wt 77.5 kg

LABORATORY VALUES

Total cholesterol 270 mg/dL, triglycerides 300 mg/dL, HDL 35 mg/dL, LDL 175 mg/dL, glucose 102mg/dL, TSH 2.6 mU/L, free T4 1.1 ng/dL

QUESTIONS

1. GK was initiated on a trial of TLC by his physician during his last visit. How long should a trial of TLC last before drug therapy is considered?

    A. 18 months
    B. 12 months
    C. 6 months
    D. 3 months
    E. 1 month

2. According to the information in the case expressed above, what is the LDL-cholesterol goal for this patient?

    A. <70 mg/dL
    B. <100 mg/dL
    C. <130 mg/dL
    D. <160 mg/dL
    E. <190 mg/dL

3. Which one of the following is GK's non-HDL cholesterol?

    A. 100 mg/dL
    B. 255 mg/dL
    C. 235 mg/dL
    D. 300 mg/dL
    E. 260 mg/dL

4. What is GK's non-HDL goal?

    A. <190 mg/dL
    B. <300 mg/dL
    C. <100 mg/dL
    D. <130 mg/dL
    E. <160 mg/dL

5. Secondary causes of dyslipidemia should be ruled out before starting lipid-lowering therapy. Which of the following conditions may cause secondary dyslipidemia?

    A. Hypothyroidism
    B. Diabetes
    C. Chronic renal failure
    D. Corticosteroid use
    E. All of the above

6. GK's cholesterol remains elevated after a trial of TLC. The primary care physician decides to initiate drug therapy with simvastatin. What is the usual starting dose of this drug?

    A. 5 mg bid
    B. 10 mg bid
    C. 20 mg qd
    D. 40 mg qd
    E. 80 mg qd

7. GK has heard that vitamin B_3 can lower his cholesterol. Which of the following statements is not true?

    A. Nicotinamide lowers LDL-cholesterol and triglyceride levels and also increases HDL-cholesterol levels.
    B. Nicotinic acid lowers LDL-cholesterol and triglyceride levels and also increases HDL-cholesterol levels.
    C. Niacin lowers LDL-cholesterol and triglyceride levels and also increases HDL-cholesterol levels.
    D. Niaspan® lowers LDL-cholesterol and triglyceride levels and also increases HDL-cholesterol levels.
    E. All of the above statements are true.

8. What is the usual daily dose of Niaspan® when used to treat hyperlipidemia?

    A. 1 to 2 g qd at bedtime
    B. 4.5 g bid
    C. 10 to 20 mg q.a.m.

D. 1.5 to 6 g tid with meals
E. 250 mg qd with meal

9. GK returns to his physician 6 months later for acute bacterial sinusitis and he receives a prescription for a macrolide antibiotic. Which of the following would you recommend to the primary care physician for concomitant use with simvastatin to avoid a drug interaction?

A. Troleandomycin
B. Erythromycin
C. Clarithromycin

D. Azithromycin
E. All of the above would interact with the statin.

10. If GK's statin dose is doubled you can expect his LDL cholesterol to decrease by what percentage for each doubling of the dose?

A. 6%
B. 26%
C. 16%
D. 34%
E. 44%

PATIENT PROFILE 168

OPIATE ABUSE

PRESENTATION

JK is a 33-year-old man recently admitted to a methadone treatment center for maintenance therapy for IV heroin abuse. JK has been using IV heroin for the past 8 years with a six bag a day habit. One week ago he was admitted as an in-patient. He was evaluated and given methadone. He now wants to start methadone maintenance. JK has no known drug allergies. He is taking methadone 60 mg qd. He works as a carpenter, is divorced, and lives alone in an apartment. He smokes 2 packs of cigarettes and drinks a couple of beers a day.

PHYSICAL EXAMINATION

GEN: Casually dressed man who appears stated age
BP sitting R arm: 128/80, HR: 64, RR: 18, T: 98.4°F

LABS

Na: 140 mEq/L
Cl: 104 mEq/L
K: 4.0 mEq/L
Gluc: 120 mg/dL
AST: 41 U/L
ALT: 54 U/L
Alk Phos: 90 U/L
Total bilirubin: 1.6 mg/dL
Conj. bilirubin: 0.8 mg/dL

K: 4.0 mEq/L
CO_2: 22 mEq/L
BUN: 16 mg/dL
SCr: 0.6 mg/dL
WBC: $3.1 \times 10^3/mm^3$
Hct: 46%
Hgb: 16 g/dL
Plts: $325 \times 10^9/L$
INR: 1.1

A/P: JK is a 33-year-old divorced man with a history of IV heroin abuse who is being treated with methadone 60 mg qd and is to start a methadone maintenance treatment program.

QUESTIONS

1. JK's long history of IV heroin use puts him at risk of which disease(s)?

A. AIDS
B. Hepatitis
C. Hypertension
D. A and B
E. A, B, and C

2. How is methadone metabolized?

A. Renal elimination of unchanged drug
B. N demethylation through CYP450 2D6
C. N demethylation through CYP450 3A4
D. Conjugation with glucuronic acid
E. Metabolism through plasma esterases

3. The treatment team wants to start giving the patient nefazodone. What will most likely happen to the patient's serum methadone levels?

A. Increase
B. Decrease
C. Remain the same

D. Increase but without clinical effect
E. Decrease but without clinical effect

4. The patient wants to start LAAM. The best conversion of methadone to an LAAM schedule for this patient would be which regimen?

A. LAAM 72 mg Monday and Wednesday and 80 mg Friday
B. LAAM 72 mg qd
C. LAAM 48 mg Monday and Wednesday and 55 mg Friday

D. LAAM 48 mg qd
E. It is impossible to predict

5. Naltrexone is an option to treat patients who are dependent on opiates. What is the effect of naltrexone on receptors?

A. It is a dopamine-2 antagonist.
B. It is a dopamine-2 agonist.
C. It is an opiate antagonist.
D. It is an opiate agonist.
E. It is a histamine-1 antagonist.

PATIENT PROFILE 169

OSTEOPOROSIS

PRESENTATION

DF is a 68-year-old white woman who comes to clinic for a follow-up visit after a done mineral density test last week. MJ was diagnosed with osteoporosis 2 years ago. Alendronate was prescribed. MJ reports adherence to the regimen. She has not experienced any fractures secondary to osteoporosis.

PMH: Osteoporosis
Osteoarthritis
Two urinary infections (most recent, 1 year ago)
Colon cancer (6 years ago)
Allergies: Questionable reaction to promethazine (no details available)
Current Meds: Alendronate (dose and frequency not recorded)
Celebrex 200 mg po qd
FH: Mother with HTN, osteoporosis, and glaucoma; father died at age 73 s/p myocardial infarction
SH: Denies tobacco, ethanol, and illicit drug use; raising two teenage grandchildren; lives with lifetime partner; exercises three to four times weekly
BP: 114/68, HR 74, RR 14, Temp 98.6°F
Gen: Woman appears younger than age, no apparent distress
HEENT: Normal
Chest: Clear to auscultation
Cor: RRR, no murmurs
Abd: Unremarkable
Ext: Normal range of motion, no edema
Neuro: Unremarkable
Laboratory Values: See Table 169-1.

Table 169-1. Laboratory Values

Region	BMD, Current (g/cm^2)	T-score, Current	BMD, 2 Years Prior (g/cm^2)
Lumbar spine	0.76	−2.6	0.72
Total hip	0.71	−1.9	0.68
Femoral neck	0.65	−1.8	0.66

QUESTIONS

1. Which of the following is a risk factor for osteoporosis in DF?

A. Exercise three to four times per week
B. History of colon cancer
C. History of urinary tract infections
D. White race
E. Use of Celebrex®

2. Which of the following best represents the World Health Organization's definition of osteoporosis based on t-scores?

A. t-score >1
B. t-score −1 to 1
C. t-score −1 to −2.5
D. t-score <−2.5
E. t-score >2.5

3. Which of the following are the recommended daily calcium and vitamin D requirements for DF (according to the Institute of Medicine)?

A. Calcium = 500 mg; vitamin D = 200 IU
B. Calcium = 500 mg; vitamin D = 400 IU
C. Calcium = 1000 mg; vitamin D = 200 IU
D. Calcium = 1200 mg; vitamin D = 400 IU
E. Calcium = 1200 mg; vitamin D = 600 IU

4. Which of the following calcium salts would provide DF with the greatest percentage of elemental calcium?

A. Calcium carbonate
B. Calcium chloride
C. Calcium citrate
D. Calcium gluconate
E. Calcium phosphate tribasic

5. Which of the following doses of calcium is the recommended maximum amount per dose?

A. 50 mg
B. 100 mg
C. 200 mg
D. 400 mg
E. 600 mg

6. Which of the following is an appropriate dosing regimen for alendronate in DF?

A. 5 mg po daily
B. 10 mg po daily
C. 35 mg po weekly
D. A and C only
E. A, B, and C

7. Which of the following is the most appropriate way to instruct DF to take alendronate?

A. Take on an empty stomach. Remain upright for at least 30 minutes.

B. Take with food. Remain upright for at least 30 minutes.
C. Take at least one-half hour before breakfast with 8 oz. of water. Remain upright for at least 30 minutes.
D. Take at least one-half hour before breakfast with 8 oz. of water, juice, or coffee. Remain upright for at least 30 minutes.
E. Take without regard to meals.

8. Which of the following is a contraindication to alendronate therapy?

A. Esophageal stricture
B. Hypocalcemia
C. Hypothyroidism
D. A and B only
E. A, B, and C

9. Which of the following is a potential adverse effect of alendronate?

A. Abdominal pain
B. Dyspepsia
C. Esophagitis
D. A and C only
E. A, B, and C

10. Which of the following medications has been shown to decrease the incidence of hip fractures in prospective controlled trials?

A. Alendronate
B. Calcitonin
C. Calcium
D. Raloxifene
E. Teriparatide

PATIENT PROFILE 170

PARKINSON'S DISEASE

PRESENTATION

Patient	ML
Age	82
Sex	Female
Allergies	NKA
Race	White
Height	5'2"
Wt	110 lb
Diagnosis	Primary

1. Advanced Parkinson's disease
2. Mild CRF

		3. NIDDM	
		4. Depression	
		5. Iron deficiency anemia	
	Secondary	1. Glaucoma	
		2. Mild dementia	
		3. DVT 1994	
	Date	*Test*	
Lab and diagnostic tests	4/15	SCr 1.8 mg/dL and BUN 30 mg/dL	
	4/15	Potassium 4.2 mEq/mL	
	4/15	Blood glucose 170 mg/dL	
	4/15	Ca^{2+} 8.0 mg/dL and Alb 2.8 g/dL	
	4/15	ECG	
	4/15	Vital signs q2h	
	Date	*Drug and Strength*	*Sig*
Medication orders	4/15	Sinemet® CR (carbidopa-levodopa) 25/250	1 po tid
(Prescription and OTC)	4/15	Selegiline 5 mg	1 po qam
	4/15	Fluoxetine 20 mg	1 po qd
	4/15	Mylanta® (magnesium hydroxide–aluminum hydroxide–simethicone)	po prn
	4/16	Famotidine 20 mg	1 po bid
	4/16	Ferrous sulfate 325 mg	1 po tid
Additional orders	4/17	Initiate drug holiday	

QUESTIONS

1. What are some of the complications of a drug holiday for a hospitalized patient?

   A. Serious psychological manifestations
   B. Deep venous thrombosis
   C. Aspiration pneumonia
   D. Decubitus ulcer formation
   E. All of the above

2. What is the rationale for a drug holiday?

   I. Allows dopamine receptors to resensitize
   II. Causes down-regulation of dopamine receptors
   III. Allows patients to tolerate very large doses of levodopa

   A. I only
   B. III only
   C. I and II only
   D. II and III only
   E. I, II, and III

3. Which of the following drugs prescribed to this patient may markedly decrease absorption of levodopa through chelation?

   A. Selegiline
   B. Fluoxetine
   C. Famotidine
   D. Sinemet® (carbidopa-levodopa)
   E. Ferrous sulfate

4. Hypomania may occur when SSRIs such as fluoxetine are taken concomitantly with

   A. selegiline.
   B. famotidine.
   C. bromocriptine.
   D. levodopa.
   E. carbidopa.

5. Which of the following would you recommend next to improve symptomatic control of Parkinson's disease for this patient?

   I. Increase the daily dose of selegiline to 10 mg
   II. Avoid all drug interactions
   III. Maximize the dose of Sinemet® CR (carbidopa-levodopa) or add levodopa immediate-release to the regimen

   A. I only
   B. III only
   C. I and II only
   D. II and III only
   E. I, II, and III

PATIENT PROFILE 171
PARKINSON'S DISEASE

PRESENTATION

BB is a 74-year-old woman who is visiting the physician to-day with her husband for a follow-up on her Parkinson's disease. Her husband states that lately BB has been "acting strange" and wants to know if there is something the physician can give her to prevent this behavior. He states that she has been hallucinating and that it is scaring him. He states that she has struck him a few times because she did not know who he was. He also states that when she is not acting strange she seems a bit depressed. When her children visit she is very quiet and withdrawn, not like she used to be. Her gait symptoms seem to be worsening and she needs to lean on him frequently in order to walk. He states that sometimes she just "freezes" when she is trying to start walking. BB's gait is shuffling and slow and she leans on her husband for stability. She developed Parkinson's disease 6 months ago and has been deteriorating ever since. Previously she was known as a nice lady with a good temperament but now she is having trouble in her interactions with other people.

PMH: Parkinson's disease
Hypertension
Med Hx: Carbidopa/levodopa 25 mg/100 mg qid
2004 Refill history: 3/30/04, 4/29/04, 5/29/04,
    6/30/04, 7/28/04, 8/26/04, 9/26/04
Quinapril 10 mg qd20
2004 Refill history: 1/17/04, 2/18/04, 3/20/04,
    4/22/04, 5/20/04, 6/23/04, 7/21/04, 8/21/04,
    9/18/04
Allergies: NKDA
FH: BB's mother died from a myocardial infarction at age
    75. Her father died from unknown causes at age 65.
SH: BB lives with her husband of 50 years. They were
    happily married until her recent change in behavior.
    She has two sons who are married and a daughter who
    is also married. BB does not smoke or drink alcohol
    and never has.
Labs: Unavailable
PE: BP 135/89, pulse 85, RR 20

PROBLEM LIST

1. Parkinson's disease

2. Psychosis (secondary to Parkinson's disease)

3. Depression (secondary to Parkinson's disease)

4. Hypertension

QUESTIONS

1. BB is experiencing "wearing off" or end of dose deterioration. What change in BB's therapy do you recommend?

    A. Add benztropine 1 mg po tid.
    B. Change to controlled release carbidopa/levodopa.
    C. Add a dopamine agonist.
    D. Do not change therapy.

2. BB's physician decides to change to controlled release carbidopa/levodopa. Of what should the new dosing regimen consist?

    A. The same as before, 25/100 po qid
    B. 50/200 po qid
    C. 50/200 po tid
    D. 25/100 po bid

3. What is carbidopa?

    A. A potent inhibitor of peripheral dopa decarboxylase
    B. A potent inhibitor of MAO-B
    C. A potent inhibitor of COMT
    D. A potent inhibitor of GABA

4. BB is having trouble getting out of bed in the morning because of early morning dystonias. What change to BB's drug therapy do you suggest?

    A. No change
    B. Take the last dose of controlled-release carbidopa/
        levodopa at dinner.
    C. Add a COMT inhibitor.
    D. Take a short-acting carbidopa/levodopa one-half
        hour before arising.

5. BB's physician has considered adding selegiline to BB's drug therapy. What is the mechanism of selegiline in the treatment of Parkinson's disease?

    A. A COMT inhibitor
    B. An MAO-B inhibitor
    C. A dopamine agonist
    D. An anticholinergic

6. What are the important points to stress when counseling BB on her new controlled-release carbidopa/levodopa?

    A. Take on an empty stomach, may cause drowsiness
    B. Take with food, may cause drowsiness/dizziness

C. Take with food, may cause dizziness

D. Take on an empty stomach, may cause dizziness

7. BB's physician would like to initiate therapy for the psychosis. What is an appropriate choice to treat BB's condition?

A. Quetiapine 12.5 mg qhs

B. Haloperidol 0.5 mg qhs

C. Diazepam 5 mg qhs

D. Gabapentin 300 mg qhs

8. A COMT inhibitor, entacapone, was added to BB's drug regimen to further decrease the "wearing off" phenomenon. Which of the following statements is true about entacapone?

A. It can be used as monotherapy.

B. It is dosed every 8 hours.

C. It should be taken with each carbidopa/levodopa dose.

D. It only blocks central COMT from breaking down levodopa.

9. Why is a dopamine agonist not a good choice for therapy in BB?

A. They have a short half-life.

B. Their side-effect profile is prohibitive.

C. They are too expensive.

D. They cannot be used as monotherapy.

10. BB's physician would like to treat her depression. Which of the following is the best therapeutic option for BB?

A. Sertraline 25 mg qd

B. Sertraline 50 mg qd

C. Amitriptyline 50 mg hs

D. Phenelzine 50 mg qd

PATIENT PROFILE 172

ARRHYTHMIAS

PRESENTATION

TC is a 54-year-old man who arrives in the emergency department with a several-day history of progressive shortness of breath, palpitations, and intermittent chest pain, although he is pain free at this time. He also reports that he has nausea and dizziness.

TC has a long history of asthma. He was initially treated with albuterol MDI, but his condition has progressively worsened. He has been admitted to the hospital twice in the last 10 months for management of exacerbations. His last admission was 2 weeks ago. The medical history includes asthma, atrial fibrillation for 3 years with two cardioversions in the last year, coronary artery disease for 8 years, gout, hyperlipidemia, and peptic ulcer disease. He has no known drug allergies. TC smokes one-half pack of cigarettes per day.

MEDS

Albuterol MDI 2 puffs qid and prn

Prednisone tapers, several over the last 9 months

Cimetidine 400 mg po qhs

Digoxin 0.125 mg po qd

Allopurinol 100 mg po qd

Cholestyramine 1 packet qid

Nitroglycerin SL 0.4 mg prn for chest pain

Verapamil 120 mg po qd

PHYSICAL EXAMINATION

GEN: Anxious-appearing man in respiratory distress

BP: 110/60, HR: 120, RR: 30, T: 38.4°C

Wt: 87 kg (ideal 69 kg)

ECG: Irregularly irregular; no ischemic changes

LABS

Na: 130	K: 4.1
Cl: 109	HCO$_3$: 16
BUN: 4.1	SCr: 1.2
Total chol: 190	WBC: 13.2
HDL chol: 40	Hgb: 14
Trig: 140	Hct: 45
Dig: 0.7 mg/dL	Gluc: 124

TC receives prompt treatment for asthma exacerbation with albuterol, ipratropium, and oral steroids (taper). After the symptoms are under control, the medical team begins to address management of the atrial fibrillation. This is the third time TC has gone into atrial fibrillation in the past year. He has stated he became light-headed and felt fatigued with the two previous episodes. At present he reports only palpitations.

QUESTIONS

1. Which of the following would be the most appropriate for TC at this time?

   A. Metoprolol 25 mg po bid
   B. Felodipine 5 mg po qd
   C. Adenosine 6 mg IV push
   D. Quinidine 324 mg po q8h
   E. Diltiazem 30 mg po q6h

2. The medical team decides to try to keep TC in normal sinus rhythm to prevent recurrences because when he has recurrences they usually are symptomatic and to minimize the risk of stroke because he is relatively young. Which of the following is the most appropriate choice to keep TC in normal sinus rhythm?

   A. Sotalol 80 mg po bid
   B. Ibutilide 1 mg IV push
   C. Procainamide 2 mg/min IV infusion
   D. Amiodarone 400 mg po tid then taper
   E. Mexiletine 200 mg po q8h

3. After the addition of amiodarone to TC's medication regimen, which of the following medication combinations does not have the potential for drug-drug interaction?

   A. Digoxin-verapamil
   B. Amiodarone-digoxin
   C. Amiodaorne-allopurinol
   D. Cholestyramine-digoxin
   E. Digoxin-cimetidine

4. TC's physician wants to initiate warfarin to help prevent a stroke. Which of the following statements is true?

   A. Amiodarone decreases the incidence of stroke among patients with atrial fibrillation.
   B. For patients taking warfarin, amiodarone will lower INR values.
   C. Aspirin is adequate to decrease the risk of stroke for TC.
   D. The combination of aspirin and warfarin would be a more appropriate choice than warfarin alone for prophylaxis of stroke.
   E. Because he is taking cimetidine, TC will need a higher dose of warfarin for anticoagulation.

5. Which of the following statements is not true?

   A. The goal INR for TC is 2.5–3.5.
   B. Cholestyramine can decrease the absorption of warfarin.
   C. Increasing TC's digoxin level to 1.5 ng/L may provide greater control of ventricular rhythm.
   D. Amiodarone may cause long-term liver toxicity in TC.
   E. Amiodarone may cause hypothyroidism in TC.

PATIENT PROFILE 173

OSTEOPOROSIS

PRESENTATION

NB is a 58-year-old woman who presents to her primary care physician for her routine yearly physical examination. She states she has been feeling well and has no complaints at this time.

PHM: HTN
Osteoporosis
Hypercholesterolemia
SH: One alcoholic beverage per week, smoked 1 pack of cigarettes per day × 20 years, quit 30 years ago, no illicit drug use; retired, lives with her husband.
FH: Noncontributory
Meds: HCTZ 25 mg po qd
Metoprolol XL 100 mg qd
Alendronate 70 mg qweek on Sundays
Atorvastatin 10 mg po qd

Vitals: BP 130/74, HR 62, RR 12, Temp 97.8°C
Gen: Well-nourished elderly woman in NAD
HEENT: EOMI, PERRLA, MM moist
Cor: nl S1 and S2, RRR, no MRG
Lungs: CTA bilaterally
Abd: Soft, nontender, no masses, + bs
Ext: 2 + pulses bilaterally, no edema
Neuro: A/O×3, no focal deficit

LABORATORY VALUES

Chem 7: 142, 102, 25, 107, 4.2, 24, 1.1
CBC: 7.4, 13, 38, 220
LFTs: ALT 35, AST 40
Lipids: TC 195, LDL 114, TG 205, HDL 40

UA: Negative for RBC, WBC, bacteria, protein, and glucose
EKG: NSR, no ST-T wave abnormalities

QUESTIONS

1. Which of the following results indicates a diagnosis of osteoporosis?

    A. T score <1.0
    B. T score <2.5
    C. Z score <1.0
    D. Z score <2.5
    E. None of the above

2. Which of the following are risk factors for the development of osteoporosis?

    I. Increased age
    II. African-American heritage
    III. Obesity

    A. I only
    B. III only
    C. I and II only
    D. II and III only
    E. I, II, and III

3. Which of the following medications can lead to osteoporotic bone loss?

    I. Corticosteroids
    II. Phenytoin
    III. Heparin

    A. I only
    B. III only
    C. I and II only
    D. II and III only
    E. I, II, and III

4. What is the recommended dose of elemental calcium per day for postmenopausal women not receiving estrogen therapy?

    A. 250 mg daily
    B. 500 mg daily
    C. 1000 mg daily
    D. 1200 mg daily
    E. 1500 mg daily

5. Which of the following calcium salts contains the highest percentage of elemental calcium?

    A. Carbonate
    B. Citrate
    C. Chloride
    D. Lactate
    E. Gluconate

6. Calcium should not be taken concomitantly with which of the following medications because of its ability to decrease their absorption?

    I. Tetracycline
    II. Ciprofloxacin
    III. Vitamin D

    A. I only
    B. III only
    C. I and II only
    D. II and III only
    E. I, II, and III

7. Which of the following best describes the mechanism of action of alendronate?

    I. Inhibition of osteoclasts
    II. Stimulation of osteoblasts
    III. Stimulation of estrogen receptors

    A. I only
    B. III only
    C. I and II only
    D. II and III only
    E. I, II, and III

8. Which of the following are contraindications to the use of alendronate?

    A. History of breast cancer
    B. Liver disease
    C. History of thromboembolic disease
    D. Esophageal stricture
    E. A and C

9. NB was previously treated with hormone replacement therapy but discontinued this treatment on her own when she heard on the news about an increase in the risk of heart disease related to this treatment modality. Which of the following medications has been associated with an increased risk of cardiovascular events?

    A. Prempro®
    B. Miacalcin®
    C. Evista®
    D. Fosamax®
    E. Actonel®

10. Which of the following antihypertensive medications may be beneficial to patients with osteoporosis?

    A. Lisinopril
    B. Terazosin
    C. HCTZ
    D. Diltiazem
    E. Furosemide

PATIENT PROFILE 174

THYROID DISEASE

PRESENTATION

AB is a 54-year-old woman who visits the cardiology clinic for a follow-up appointment. When asked how she is doing, AB states that she has puffy eyes, feels less energetic than usual, feels weak in the legs when climbing stairs, and has been told by two friends that her voice sounds hoarse. Her medical history includes congestive heart failure and atrial fibrillation. She has no known drug allergies, and she weighs 53 kg.

MEDS

Furosemide 20 mg po qd
Enalapril 10 mg po bid
Amiodarone 200 mg po qd
Warfarin 4 mg po qd

LABS

FT_4: 1.1 ng/dL (0.6-2.1 ng/dL)
TSH: 14 μ/mL (0.5-5.5 μU/mL)

QUESTIONS

1. Which of the following is/are true?

   A. The thyroid function test results suggest hypothyroidism caused by amiodarone.
   B. The symptoms reported by AB that suggest hypothyroidism include puffy eyes, less energy, and weak legs when climbing stairs.

C. Amiodarone rarely causes hypothyroidism; therefore baseline thyroid function tests should not be performed before amiodarone therapy is begun.
   D. A and B only
   E. A, B, and C

2. Amiodarone therapy is continued despite the development of hypothyroidism. Which of the following medications would be appropriate for HT?

   A. Methimazole
   B. Propylthiouracil
   C. Levothyroxine
   D. A and B only
   E. A, B, and C

3. Therapy is initiated for AB. When should the TSH level be measured?

   A. 1–2 days after therapy is started
   B. 1–2 weeks after therapy is started
   C. 6–8 weeks after therapy is started
   D. 12 months after therapy is started
   E. 18 months after therapy is started

4. HT had several signs and symptoms of hypothyroidism; however, there are many more signs and symptoms of hypothyroidism. Which of the following is/are signs or symptoms of hypothyroidism?

   A. Cold intolerance
   B. Dry skin
   C. Weight gain
   D. A and B only
   E. A, B, and C

PATIENT PROFILE 175

OBESITY

PRESENTATION

PJ is a 51-year-old woman who presents to her primary care physician seeking advice on her options for weight loss. PJ has been overweight since high school. She has always struggled with her weight. She has attempted "countless" diets over the past 30+ years, but each time she stops the diet, she regains the weight. Her most suc-

cessful weight loss occurred last year when she lost over 100 pounds through the Weight Watchers® program, but the stress of her father's death last winter caused her to gain back all of the weight within 8 months. PJ has suffered with osteoarthritis in both knees for the past 4 years. Given the pain associated with the osteoarthritis, she considers an exercise routine "near impossible." In her attempt to lose weight, PJ has cut down to one meal per day, although she does admit to snacking occasionally.

PMH: Hypertension ×5 years
Osteoarthritis of the knees ×4 years
Hypercholesterolemia ×2 years
PSH: Gallstones 2 years ago treated with lithotripsy
Breast reduction surgery at age 28
FH: Mother had hypertension, heart failure, and type II diabetes, and died of kidney failure at age 76; father had a myocardial infarction at age 68 and died of heart failure at age 83. PJ states that her mother was overweight (but not obese). PJ has two siblings (one sister and one brother), neither of whom is overweight. Brother age 59 has type I diabetes. Sister age 56 has hypothyroidism.
SH: PJ is employed as a secretary. She denies tobacco and illicit drug use; drinks alcohol socially a few times a year.
MH: Atorvastatin 10 mg po qhs
Celecoxib 100 mg bid prn knee pain
Lisinopril 10 mg qd
Allergies: NKDA
ROS: PJ complains of general fatigue, feeling depressed about her weight, and knee pain.
BP 142/88, HR 82, Height 4'11", Wt 253 lbs
Waist circumference estimated at 43"
Gen: Obese white woman in NAD

LABORATORY VALUES (SELF-REPORTED)

T. chol 272 mg/dL
LDL 197 mg/dL
HDL 35 mg/dL
Trig 200 mg/dL
Glu 128 mg/dL

QUESTIONS

1. What is PJ's BMI (body mass index)?

   A. $39.2 \ kg/m^2$
   B. $42.9 \ kg/m^2$
   C. $51.3 \ kg/m^2$
   D. $53.4 \ kg/m^2$
   E. $76.7 \ kg/m^2$

2. How should this BMI be classified?

   A. Normal weight
   B. Overweight
   C. Mild obesity
   D. Moderate obesity
   E. Morbid obesity

3. Which one of the following statements is true about the use of sibutramine for PJ?

   A. It is a good choice for weight loss for PJ.
   B. It should be avoided because it has been associated with elevating blood pressure.
   C. It should be avoided because it may interact with her atorvastatin.
   D. It would not be effective for PJ.
   E. It should be avoided because it may increase her cholesterol.

4. Which one of the following 6-month weight loss goals would you recommend for PJ?

   A. 10 pounds
   B. 25 pounds
   C. 40 pounds
   D. 55 pounds
   E. 70 pounds

5. What rate would you recommend for PJ's weight loss?

   A. 0.5 pounds per week
   B. 2 pound per week
   C. 5 pounds per week
   D. 10 pounds per week
   E. More than 10 pounds per week

6. PJ's physician has prescribed orlistat. Which of the following best describes the mechanism of action of orlistat?

   A. Inhibits the reuptake of dopamine
   B. Inhibits the reuptake of norepinephrine
   C. Inhibits the reuptake of serotonin
   D. Inhibits gastrointestinal lipases
   E. Sympathomimetic activity

7. What is the brand name of orlistat?

   A. Adipex-P®
   B. Didrex®
   C. Fastin®
   D. Meridia®
   E. Xenical®

8. PJ would like to know more about her new medication. Which of the following are important points to cover while counseling PJ on orlistat?

   I. Common side effects include soft stools and flatulence; these symptoms subside with prolonged use.
   II. It may impair your body's ability to absorb vitamin D, you should take a supplement with the orlistat. (Take it at the same time as one dose of the orlistat.)
   III. Diet and exercise are not necessary while taking orlistat.

A. I only
B. III only
C. I and II
D. II and III
E. I, II, and III

D. II and III
E. I, II, and III

9. Which of the following is/are correct components of the dosing regimen for orlistat?

 I.   120 mg tid
 II.   Take during or within 1 hour of each meal.
 III. If a meal is skipped or contains no fat, do not take the orlistat.

 A. I only
 B. III only
 C. I and II

10. PJ asks you about natural products that promote weight loss. Which of the following should be avoided because they may increase PJ's heart rate and blood pressure?

 I.   Citrus aurantii
 II.   Guarana
 III. Green tea

 A. I only
 B. III only
 C. I and II
 D. II and III
 E. I, II, and III

PATIENT PROFILE 176

CHRONIC OBSTRUCTIVE LUNG DISEASE

PRESENTATION

BT is a 60-year-old male lawyer with a 5-year history of chronic bronchitis. For the past 2 years, he has been using a regimen of sustained release theophylline and two bronchodilator inhalers. His most recent theophylline level was "therapeutic." He continues to smoke at least one pack of cigarettes a day. He has an upper respiratory tract infection that necessitates antibiotic therapy.

QUESTIONS

1. Which antibiotic(s) may inhibit the metabolism of theophylline and necessitate a reduction in theophylline dosage?

 A. Ciprofloxacin
 B. Erythromycin
 C. Amoxicillin
 D. A and B
 E. A, B, and C

2. Which side effect(s) of theophylline is/are concentration dependent?

 A. Sleep disturbances
 B. Cardiac arrhythmias
 C. Seizures
 D. A and B
 E. A, B, and C

3. What effect would smoking have on the pharmacokinetics of theophylline?

A. Smoking has no effect.
B. Smoking may increase renal clearance.
C. Smoking may induce hepatic metabolism.
D. Smoking may reduce overall bioavailability.
E. Smoking may reduce the rate of absorption.

4. Which of the following metered dose inhalation agents would be considered the agent of choice for maintenance treatment of BT for COPD?

 A. Ipratropium
 B. Fluticasone
 C. Albuterol
 D. Salmeterol
 E. Cromolyn

5. BT is using both a sympathomimetic and an anticholinergic inhalation agent. Which of the following statements regarding this combination in the treatment of patients with COPD is most correct?

 A. The combination is more effective than monotherapy for short-term use.
 B. The combination is more effective than monotherapy for long-term use.
 C. The sympathomimetic agent should be administered at least 60 minutes before the anticholinergic agent.
 D. The two classes of drugs have similar sites of action.
 E. Before the combination is used, the optimal dose of sympathomimetic agent should be established.

PATIENT PROFILE 177

SMALLPOX

PRESENTATION

AD is a 36-year-old man presenting to the emergency department with his family. He is very ill and thinks he has the chickenpox. AD's wife said his present illness started approximately 5 days ago with a high fever of 103°F, extreme malaise, headache, and a backache. Two days ago he started to develop a rash beginning in his mouth (tiny red spots on his tongue and palate) and they spread to his forehead.

PMH: AD has no past medical problems

SH: AD denies illicit drug use, occasionally drinks two to three beers per week; AD denies smoking and lives with his wife and two children (ages 9 and 12).

FH: Parents are both still alive. Mom has hypertension controlled with medications. Dad has arthritis pain alleviated with NSAIDs.

Gen: Well-nourished man in severe prostration

VS: BP 135/89 mm Hg, HR 90, RR 20, Temp 103°F, Ht 5'10", Wt 185 lb

HEENT: Maculopapular rash on the mucosa of mouth and pharynx

Skin: Small papules on trunk. Vesicles on forehead and upper arms. Lesions are deep, round and hard. Lesions are in varying sizes and are painful to touch. Lesions are at the same stage of development at each site.

Chest: Lungs clear

CV: Normal, no murmurs, rubs, gallops

Abd: Within normal limits

Labs: Lesion specimen was sent to state public health laboratory for confirmation of diagnosis.

Diagnosis: Rule out smallpox. Patient admitted to hospital under virus isolation with initial diagnosis of chickenpox. Diagnosis later changed upon laboratory confirmation of smallpox.

Follow-up notes: Lesions spread to legs, palms of hands, and soles of feet. Initial vesicles have begun to scab.

QUESTIONS

1. The Centers for Disease Control and Prevention (CDC) have categorized smallpox as which category because of its high rate of contagiousness and the need of extra public health preparedness?

   A. Category A
   B. Category B
   C. Category C
   D. Category D

2. Which of the following is the causative organism for smallpox?

   A. Varicella
   B. Variola major
   C. Variola minor
   D. An orthopox virus
   E. B, C, and D are correct.

3. A differential diagnosis must be made between smallpox and chickenpox. Smallpox differs from chickenpox in all except which of the following?

   A. Lesions develop at the same rate.
   B. Lesions are superficial.
   C. Lesions begin on the face.
   D. Lesions can be observed on the palms of hands and soles of feet.

4. What is the average incubation period once exposed to the virus that causes smallpox?

   A. 3 to 5 days
   B. 5 to 10 days
   C. 7 to 17 days
   D. 20 days

5. Smallpox may be spread by which of the following?

   A. Airborne droplets
   B. Aerosols
   C. Fomites
   D. All of the above

6. The last naturally occurring case of smallpox occurred in 1977 and the World Health Organization (WHO) declared the disease eradicated in the 1980s.

   A. True
   B. False

7. Why does administering the smallpox vaccine require extra training?

   A. Routine immunizations ceased over 20 years ago in the United States, so many healthcare workers are unfamiliar with the vaccine.
   B. Vaccine administration requires the knowledge of using a bifurcated needle.
   C. The vaccine requires the vaccinee to learn how to prevent contamination.
   D. All of the above

8. Smallpox Vaccine (Dryvax™) is contraindicated in all except which of the following (assuming no smallpox outbreak)?

   A. Pregnancy
   B. Immunosuppressive conditions
   C. Eczema
   D. Allergy to Neomycin
   E. All of the above

9. Vaccine immune globulin (VIG) is indicated for which of the following?

   A. HIV patients
   B. Accidental implantation (extensive lesions)
   C. Postvaccine encephalitis

   D. Erythema multiforme
   E. Vaccine keratitis

10. Anyone in close contact with a person diagnosed with smallpox should be offered a smallpox vaccine. Which of the following is true about vaccination after exposure?

    A. It can protect against smallpox if administered within 2 to 3 days.
    B. It can protect against a fatal outcome if administered within 4 to 5 days.
    C. It cannot provide any immunization after exposure so is not necessary to immunize.
    D. A and B are correct.
    E. None of the above are correct.

PATIENT PROFILE 178

EYE DROPS

PRESENTATION

An ophthalmic solution is to be manufactured to contain 0.1 g of drug in a 5-mL container. The drug has a sodium chloride equivalent value of 0.2. The usual dose is 2 drops in each eye twice daily. The resultant solution provides 20 drops per milliliter. Solutions containing drug and sodium chloride have been shown to produce some precipitation of the drug.

QUESTIONS

1. How many milligrams of drug can be found in one drop of the solution?

   A. 0.01
   B. 1
   C. 10
   D. 100
   E. 1000

2. How many days will the bottle last?

   A. 5
   B. 12.5
   C. 25
   D. 50
   E. 100

3. What would be the purpose of the addition of sodium chloride to this solution?

   A. Decrease corneal irritation when used
   B. Increase drug solubility
   C. Produce isotonicity of the solution
   D. A and C
   E. All of the above

4. How many grams of sodium chloride should be used to prepare the solution?

   A. 4.9
   B. 0.5
   C. 0.1
   D. 0.045
   E. 0.025

5. If sodium chloride were found to precipitate drug from solution at the desired concentration, how many grams of boric acid (sodium chloride equivalent value of 0.52) would have to be used?

   A. 0.013
   B. 0.048
   C. 0.495
   D. 20.8
   E. Insufficient information is provided to determine an answer.

PATIENT PROFILE 179

GENERALIZED ANXIETY DISORDER

PRESENTATION

LM is a 67-year-old white man with a history of generalized anxiety disorder. He complains of daily anxiety. Prior use of sertraline and paroxetine has led to paresthesias. His mood is bright and his thoughts are logical.

PMH: History of alcohol dependence, abstinent × 7 years
Parkinson's disease
Generalized anxiety disorder
Dysthymia
Cirrhosis, prognosis is 2 to 4 months survival
SH: He is living at a hospice; denies cigarette, drug, or alcohol use.
Meds: Pramipexole 1 mg tid
Labs: All within normal limits except for albumin, 2 g/dL, pt 27 sec, tbili 2.3 mg/dL

QUESTIONS

1. Which of the following benzodiazepines is least impacted by poor liver function?

   A. Lorazepam
   B. Chlordiazepoxide
   C. Diazepam
   D. Alprazolam

2. Which of the following antidepressants could actually worsen this patient's anxiety?

   A. Bupropion
   B. Fluoxetine
   C. Nefazodone
   D. Desipramine

3. Which of the following antidepressants has the highest risk of hepatotoxicity?

   A. Nefazodone
   B. Escitalopram
   C. Mirtazapine
   D. Venlafaxine

4. Which of the following has an onset of action that occurs within hours of initiation?

   A. Lorazepam
   B. Paroxetine
   C. Buspirone
   D. Escitalopram

5. How will this patient's hepatic function affect the pharmacokinetics of citalopram?

   A. It will decrease the elimination half-life.
   B. It will increase the elimination half-life.
   C. It will increase the rate of excretion.
   D. It will have no effect because citalopram is primarily removed via renal excretion.

PATIENT PROFILE 180

SOFT-TISSUE INFECTION

PRESENTATION

AD is a 15-year-old girl who was walking down the street to retrieve the mail when a dog came running out of the woods and bit her hand. The bite punctured the skin. Thinking nothing of the bite, the girl had gone home, cleaned the wound thoroughly, and put antiseptic ointment and a bandage on her hand. The next day AD sought medical attention for pain, purulent discharge, and swelling.

QUESTIONS

1. Which of the listed organisms is of most concern in dog bite wound?

   A. *Pseudomonas aeruginosa*
   B. *Pasteurella multocida*
   C. *Streptococcus pneumoniae*
   D. *Acinetobacter baumannii*
   E. Enterococci

2. It is standard practice to thoroughly irrigate a wound with a sterile saline solution or chlorhexidine scrub solution. In addition to the irrigation, which of the following therapies should routinely be considered for a bite from an animal that has not been captured?

   A. Rabies vaccination
   B. Tetanus vaccination

C. Hepatitis vaccination
D. A and B
E. B and C

3. AD has no known drug allergies. With this in mind, choose the best empiric antibiotic therapy for a mild wound infection from a dog bite.

   A. Metronidazole 500 mg po bid
   B. Vancomycin 125 mg po qid
   C. Amoxicillin–clavulanate 875/125 mg po bid
   D. Cephalexin 500 mg po qid
   E. Piperacillin-tazobactam 3.375 g IV q6h

4. Alternative oral treatment of patients who cannot tolerate β-lactam antibiotics for a mild wound infection from a dog bite might be which of the following?

A. Clindamycin 300 mg po qid and levofloxacin 500 mg po qd
B. Gentamicin 80 mg IV q8h and ceftazidime 1 g IV q8h
C. Vancomycin 1g IV q12h and ciprofloxacin 400 mg IV q12h
D. Cefuroxime axetil 500 mg po bid
E. Loracarbef 400 mg po bid and metronidazole 500 mg po tid

5. Prophylactic antibiotic therapy for bite wounds should be administered for

   A. 7 days.
   B. 10 days.
   C. 14 days.
   D. 3 days.
   E. 5 days.

PATIENT PROFILE 181

DIABETES

PRESENTATION

SN is a 47-year-old African-American man who is concerned about new changes in his visual field he reports as "blurry edges" and "fuzzy vision" that have been persistent and unremitting over the last 6 to 8 weeks.

SN has been lost to follow-up for 9 years. He has been experiencing changes in his visual field since returning from an extended vacation with his family in his native state of Georgia. Many of SN's immediate and extended family have type II diabetes and related complications. After listening carefully to their advice he arrives at the clinic for help with this new visual problem.

PMH: Nine years ago SN met with his family physician and learned he had high blood pressure, was overweight, and was in a prediabetic state where he could develop type II diabetes at any time. SN later admitted to feeling angry about this news, so he decided to stop seeing his physician. He refused to follow-up with additional laboratory tests or keep future appointments.

FH: Mother, alive at 69 years old, suffered recent stroke, lives with diabetes, hypertension, and recent amputation of three toes from left foot. Father, alive at 67 years old, has extensive coronary heart disease (CHD) requiring CABG 5 years ago and PCI in 2002 and in 2004. Uncle, alive at 70, with extensive CHD requiring

CABG 8 years ago and legally blind from diabetic retinopathy. Sister, alive at 45 years old, has type II diabetes diagnosed 20 years after pregnancy complicated with gestational diabetes. Brother, alive at 43 years old, has high blood pressure and a duodenal ulcer.

SH: SN is a local ceramic artisan, painter, and master carpenter. He sells his ceramics and painted works at several local shops and works 40 to 50 hours per week on carpentry jobs. He had a 30 pack-year tobacco history but quit smoking 2 years ago. Drinks 4 to 5 oz. of bourbon or whisky socially with friends one to two times per month and smokes marijuana one to two times per month.

Allergies: None

Meds: None

Gen: Pleasant African-American gentleman, WDWN, somewhat apprehensive, NAD

Vitals: BP 144/92 mm/Hg, pulse 90 beats/min, RR 12 breaths/min, Temp 98.8°F, Ht 6'4", Wt 252 lbs., BMI 30.7 kg/m^2

HEENT: PERRLA, EOMI, + exudates, dot + microhemorrhages

Chest: CTA

Cor: RRR, no MRG

Abd: Nontender, nondistended, + BS

Gu: Deferred

Rect: Deferred

Ext: 3 + pulses throughout, no edema
Neuro: Cranial nerves II to XII intact, no focal deficits

LABORATORY VALUES

Na 140 mEq/L, K 4.3 mEq/L, Cl 101 mEq/L, HCO_3 24 mEq/L, BUN 12 mg/dL, SCr 1.1 mg/dL, fasting glucose 212 mg/dL, WBC 5.1 K cells/mm^3, platelets 325 K cells/mm^3, Hgb 14 g/dL, HCT 42%, HbA1c 9%, LDL 170 mg/dL, HDL 60 mg/dL, TC 280 mg/dL, TG 350 mg/dL, uric acid 7 mg/dL, CRP 9.6 mg/L

QUESTIONS

1. SN has diabetes and hypertension that must be addressed during this visit. SN's provider wants to begin by starting therapy for SN's blood pressure. Which is the most appropriate antihypertensive drug therapy to prescribe for SN?

   A   Felodipine 10 mg po qd
   B. Enalapril 2.5 mg po qd
   C. Hydrochlorothiazide 25 mg po qd
   D. Ramipril 5 mg po qd
   E. Atenolol 50 mg po qd

2. SN's provider wants to begin oral hypoglycemic therapy and lifestyle modification concurrently because diet and lifestyle modification alone will not be sufficient to achieve an HbA1c goal of ≤6.5% in the next 6 months. Which is the most appropriate oral hypoglycemic agent to begin for SN?

   A. Glipizide XL 5 mg po qd
   B. Repaglinide 0.5 mg po taken 15 minutes before each meal
   C. Metformin 500 mg po qd for 2 weeks, then increase to 500 mg po bid
   D. Acarbose 25 mg po tid with the first bite of each meal
   E. Pioglitazone 15 mg po qd

3. SN's provider wants to begin lipid-lowering therapy during this visit. Which of the following is the most appropriate agent for SN?

   A. Atorvastatin 40 mg po qd
   B. Lovastatin 40 mg po qd
   C. Rosuvastatin 40 mg po qd
   D. Pravastatin 40 mg po qd
   E. Fluvastatin 40 mg po qd

4. SN thanks you for advising him on how to use his medication. He returns for follow-up approximately 3 months later. He mentions he saw the ophthalmologist 2 weeks ago who mentioned new cotton wool spots have appeared since his last visit. Blood pressure at this visit is 134/84 mm Hg. He reports that he is tolerating existing therapy without new side effects. What is the most appropriate way to treat SN?

   A. Discontinue ramipril 5 mg po qd and begin amlodipine 10 mg po qd.
   B. Increase ramipril to 10 mg po qd.
   C. Switch ramipril 5mg po qd to lisinopril 10 mg po qd.
   D. Discontinue ramipril and begin valsartan 160 mg po qd.
   E. Add valsartan 80 mg po qd to existing therapy.

5. SN returns in 2 weeks as scheduled. He is unhappy because of a new cough that has developed since the last visit. SN's blood pressure is 122/78 mm Hg. What is the most appropriate strategy to control SN's blood pressure?

   A. Discontinue ramipril 10 mg po qd and begin amlodipine 20 mg po qd.
   B. Continue ramipril 10 mg and advise SN that the cough can be managed with sugar-free lozenges.
   C. Discontinue ramipril 10 mg po qd and begin valsartan 160 mg po qd.
   D. Discontinue ramipril 10 mg po qd and begin hydrochlorothiazide 25 mg po qd.
   E. Switch ramipril 10 mg po qd to lisinopril 20 mg po qd and advise SN that the cough can be managed with sugar-free lozenges.

6. SN returns for follow-up in 3 months. He has not experienced dry cough since this last visit and has no adverse events to report. SN's vitals today are: BP 118/74 mm Hg, pulse 86 beats/min, RR 14 breaths/min, Temp 98.8°F, Ht 6'4", Wt 240 lbs., BMI = 29.2 kg/m^2, fasting glucose 152 mg/dL, SCr 1.0 mg/dL, HbA1c 7.8%. How would you most appropriately maximize SN's drug therapy to improve his glycemic control?

   A. Increase metformin 500 mg po bid to metformin 1000 mg po bid.
   B. Continue metformin 500 mg po bid and add acarbose 25 mg po with each meal.
   C. Increase metformin 500 mg po bid to metformin 850 mg po tid.
   D. Continue metformin 500 mg po bid and add pioglitazone 15 mg po qd.
   E. Increase metformin 500 mg po bid to metformin 1000 mg po bid and add glipizide XR 5 mg.

7. Which of the following is contraindication to metformin therapy in SN?

   A. SCr ≥1.5 mg/dL
   B. Hepatic dysfunction
   C. Metabolic acidosis

D. Dehydration

E. All of the above are contraindications to met-
    formin therapy.

8. SN's lipid profile returns: LDL-C 95 mg/dL, HDL-C
    55 mg/dL, TG 250 mg/dL, TC 200 mg/dL. Which
    of the following should be SN's LDL goal?

    A. LDL-C ≤130 mg/dL
    B. LDL-C ≤110 mg/dL
    C. LDL-C ≤100 mg/dL
    D. LDL-C ≤80 mg/dL
    E. LDL-C ≤70 mg/dL

9. How would you manage SN's lipid profile after re-
    viewing this new lipid panel?

    A. No change in the current management; keep
        atorvastatin 40 mg po qd.

B. Double the dose of atorvastatin from 40 mg po
    qd to atorvastatin 80 mg po qd.

C. Maintain atorvastatin 40 mg po qd and begin
    gemfibrozil 600 mg po bid.

D. Discontinue atorvastatin 40 mg po qd and begin
    gemfibrozil 600 mg po bid.

E. Reduce atorvastatin to 20 mg po qd and begin
    gemfibrozil 600 mg po bid.

10. You review SN's profile and discover that he has never
    received antiplatelet therapy. SN's provider agrees
    that antiplatelet therapy would be appropriate. How
    would you begin antiplatelet therapy in SN?

    A. Aspirin 325 mg po qd
    B. Aspirin 81 mg po qd
    C. Clopidogrel 75 mg po qd
    D. Clopidogrel 150 mg po qd
    E. Ticlopidine 250 mg po bid

OSTEOPOROSIS

PRESENTATION

SR is a 60-year-old woman who is brought by ambulance
to the emergency department because of pain in her right
shoulder and wrist. Earlier that morning she had fallen and
tried to catch herself with her hand. She thought she
would lie down in bed to see whether she would feel better; however, the pain worsened. She took some Advil®
(ibuprofen) in the hope of relieving the pain, but the pain
continued to worsen. SR has a history of diabetes, which
has been managed with careful diet and glipizide (Glu-
cotrol®). She also takes lisinopril (Zestril®) for management of hypertension. She lives at home alone and states
that she has found it difficult to manage things on her own.
She admits that activities of daily living have become over-
whelming for her. A complete examination is performed,
and SR is admitted to the hospital. She is dehydrated, and
her glucose level is elevated at 260 mg/dL. Further evaluation reveals loss of bone density. Before discharge the
medical team decides to initiate therapy with alendronate
(Fosamax®).

QUESTIONS

1. The team asks you to counsel SR on the proper ad-
    ministration of alendronate. Which of the following is
    correct concerning administration of alendronate
    (Fosamax®)?

    A. The patient should take the medication after she
        is up for the day. She should swallow it with a full
        glass (6–8 oz) of orange juice.
    B. The patient should take the medication after she
        is up for the day with a light meal to maximize the
        bioavailability of the drug.
    C. The patient should take the medication after she
        is up for the day. She should swallow it with a full
        glass (6–8 oz) of plain water at least 30 minutes
        before she takes her first food of the day.
    D. The patient should take the medication at bed-
        time and swallow it with a full glass (6–8 oz) of
        plain water.
    E. The patient can take the medication with or with-
        out food and at any time of the day.

2. Which of the following is/are true concerning the
    proper administration of alendronate (Fosamax®)?

    A. The patient should be instructed not to lie down
        for at least 30 minutes after taking the medica-
        tion.
    B. The patient should be instructed to take the med-
        ication lying down for the medication to pass
        through the esophagus quickly.
    C. The patient should be instructed to take the med-
        ication at supper, which will enhance the activity
        of the drug before bedtime.

D. The patient should be instructed to take the medication at lunchtime because insomnia is a common adverse effect of this agent.

E. None of the above

3. The manufacturer does not recommend the use of alendronate (Fosamax®) in the following situation(s):

A. Ulcer disease
B. Severe renal insufficiency
C. Hypertension
D. A and B
E. All of the above

4. The medical team requests drug information concerning one of the newer agents for the prevention of osteoporosis called raloxifene (Evista®). Which statement is true concerning this agent?

A. Raloxifene, like alendronate, is a bisphosphonate and has the same mechanism of action.

B. Raloxifene can be taken with or without food and at any time of the day.

C. Raloxifene is used to manage hot flashes.

D. The most common adverse effect of raloxifene is dyspepsia.

E. Patients should take raloxifene with a full glass of plain water after getting up for the day.

5. Raloxifene (Evista®) belongs to which pregnancy category?

A. Pregnancy category A
B. Pregnancy category X
C. Pregnancy category B
D. Pregnancy category C
E. Pregnancy category D

PATIENT PROFILE 183

HUMAN IMMUNODEFICIENCY VIRUS

PRESENTATION

A 29-year-old man is admitted to the hospital with a chief complaint of fatigue, shortness of breath, fevers, and a dry/nonproductive cough. He has been HIV+ for 5 years. Past opportunistic infections include multiple episodes of oral thrush (two with esophageal involvement) and PCP (*Pneumocystis carinii* pneumonia).

Lopinavir/ritonavir (400 mg/100 mg bid) + lamivudine (150 mg bid) + stavudine (30 mg bid) for the past 10 months
Methadone 40 mg qd
Dapsone 25 mg qd
Mylanta 15 cc q4h for upset stomach
Fluconazole 100 mg qd (ran out 3 weeks ago)
ALL: SMX/TMP (sulfamethoxazole/trimethoprim) (total body rash, erythema, fever)
SH: Cigarette smoker, 1 pack/day × 10 years; occasional alcohol and marijuana; past IVDU
ROS: In addition to the preceding symptoms, he also complains of fever, drenching sweats that require him to change his night clothes, a 10-lb weight loss over the past 2 months, and fatigue
PE:
VS: BP 148/87 mmHg, HR 105, RR 23, Temp 39.0°C, Wt 50 kg, Ht 168 cm

Gen: Ill-appearing cachectic man; looks older than stated age
HEENT: White plaques on tongue, neck supple, injected conjunctiva
Cor: Normal heart sounds
Chest: Bilateral wheezing
Abd: Positive BS, splenomegaly, hepatomegaly
Gu: WNL
Rect: Deferred
Ext: Warm and dry skin, pale nail beds
Neuro: Transient, intermittent tingling in fingers and toes; no numbness
Labs: Na 139 mEq/L, Hct 30%, Glu 130 mg/dL, K 4.5 mEq/L, Hgb 11 g/dL, Cl 103, mEq/L, WBC 2.9K cells/mm^3, HCO$_3$ 21 mEq/L, PLTS 100K cells/mm^3, BUN 15 mg/dL, AST 53 U/L, SCr 1.2 mg/dL, ALT 90 U/L
Arterial oxygen: 65 mm Hg (room air)
Serum cryptococcal antigen titer: 1:128
Toxoplasmosis IgG antibody: Positive
G6PD screen: Negative
CD4: 50 cells/mm^3 (3 months ago) HIV RNA 75,000 copies/mL (3 months ago)
WBC differential: 73% PMN/2% bands/10% lymphocytes/5% monocytes
CXR: Diffuse, bilateral interstitial infiltrates
PPD (1 month ago): Negative

Induced sputum: Positive for *Pneumocystis jiroveci* (previously known as *Pneumocystis carinii*)

QUESTIONS

1. Which of the following options is the best antibiotic treatment for this patient's PCP?

   A. Bactrim IV 15 mg/kg per day (divided into three to four doses per day) × 21 days
   B. Atovaquone po 750 mg bid × 21 days
   C. Dapsone 100 mg po daily × 21 days
   D. Pentamidine IV 4 mg/kg per day daily × 21 days

2. In addition to antimicrobial therapy for the *Pneumocystis*, which of the following pharmacologic interventions also should be considered to treat this patient's PCP?

   A. Leucovorin
   B. Glyburide
   C. Prednisone
   D. Filgrastim

3. Which of the following anti-*Pneumocystis* agents places G6PD patients at risk for hemolytic anemia and methemoglobinemia?

   A. Pentamidine
   B. Trimethoprim
   C. Dapsone
   D. Sulfamethoxazole

4. At the end of this patient's acute PCP treatment, he should receive *Pneumocystis* prophylaxis. Among the following antimicrobial regimens listed, which is considered the most appropriate in this patient to provide prophylaxis for both *Pneumocystis* and *Toxoplasmosis gondii*?

   A. TMP-SMX 1 DS tablet qd
   B. Pyrimethamine 50mg po qd *plus* leucovorin 25 mg po qd *plus* dapsone 50 mg po qd
   C. Atovaquone 1500 mg po qd
   D. Aerosolized pentamidine 300 mg every 4 weeks

5. Which of the following antimicrobial regimens would provide prophylaxis against MAC (*Mycobacterium avium-intracellulare* complex) and have the least potential for drug interactions with this patient's antiretroviral therapy?

   A. Azithromycin po 1200 mg weekly
   B. Clarithromycin po 500 mg bid
   C. Rifabutin po 300 mg qd
   D. Isoniazid po 300 mg qd

6. Which of the following clinical data play a role in determining whether a patient requires prophylaxis against CMV (cytomegalovirus) to prevent CMV retinitis?

   I. CMV antibody serostatus
   II. CD4 cell count
   III. History of opportunistic infections
   IV. Risk factors for anti-CMV drug toxicity

   A. I, II, III, IV
   B. I and II only
   C. I, II, and IV only
   D. III only

7. Which of the following antiretrovirals might be responsible for this patient's neurologic complaints?

   A. d4T
   B. Ritonavir
   C. Lopinavir
   D. 3TC

8. Coformulation of ritonavir with lopinavir takes advantage of "protease-inhibitor boosting." What is "protease-inhibitor boosting" as it applies to this particular formulation?

   A. Lopinavir boosts the virologic activity of ritonavir (i.e., synergy).
   B. Ritonavir boosts the virologic activity of lopinavir (i.e., synergy).
   C. Lopinavir inhibits the hepatic metabolism of ritonavir (boosts its levels).
   D. Ritonavir inhibits the hepatic metabolism of lopinavir (boosts its levels).

9. If this patient were to develop dyslipidemia secondary to his antiretroviral therapy and his physician wished to initiate drug therapy with an HMG-CoA reductase inhibitor, which would have the least significant interaction with his protease inhibitor therapy?

   A. Lovastatin
   B. Simvastatin
   C. Pravastatin
   D. Atorvastatin

10. Patients who have evidence of ongoing viral replication despite their current antiretroviral therapy may be candidates for a regimen containing enfuvirtide and at least two other active antiretrovirals. How does enfuvirtide inhibit HIV replication?

    A. Enfuvirtide inhibits the viral-encoded reverse transcriptase enzyme, thus preventing conversion of the single-stranded viral RNA to double-stranded DNA.
    B. Enfuvirtide binds and causes a conformational change in reverse transcriptase. This alters this

enzyme's target site and inhibits its ability to interact with nucleotides

C. Enfuvirtide inhibits the conformational change of HIV gp41 that is necessary for fusion of the virion to the host cell.

D. Enfuvirtide binds to the active site of HIV protease and prevents it from cleaving the larger viral proteins into important viral enzymes and structural components.

PATIENT PROFILE 184

ONCOLOGY: PAIN CONTROL

PRESENTATION

LB is a retired banker. He is receiving supportive hospice care for metastatic prostate cancer. The sites of metastasis include the hips, lumbar spine, and ribs. The current medication regimen consists of metoprolol 50 mg bid, lisinopril 10 mg qd, simvastatin 20 mg qd, Percocet® (oxycodone-acetaminophen) 2 tabs q3h, and Darvocet-N® 100 (propoxyphene-acetaminophen) 1 tab q6h prn. LB tolerates oral medications and states his pain is about 5 on a 10-point scale. His only complaint is having to take one of his pain medications every 2 to 3 hours. He would like to sleep better during the night. He has previously reported an upset stomach after taking Tylenol® (acetaminophen) with codeine no. 3.

QUESTIONS

1. After reviewing the patient data, one would classify LB's pain most appropriately as

   A. acute.
   B. chronic.
   C. linear.
   D. nonmalignant.
   E. orthopedic.

2. To allow LB better pain control and longer sleeping periods, which of the following regimens would be most appropriate?

   A. Morphine PCA bolus with 6-minute lockout
   B. OxyContin® (oxycodone controlled release) q8h with ibuprofen q8h and oxycodone q3h prn
   C. Percocet® (oxycodone-acetaminophen) 4 tabs q6h with Darvocet® (propoxyphene-acetaminophen) 1 tab q3h prn

   D. Morphine continuous infusion with prn boluses
   E. Ketorolac 30 mg IM q6h and Percocet® (oxycodone-acetaminophen) 4 tabs q6h prn

3. LB continues to have effective pain control with his opiate regimen over the next 2 weeks. To avoid a common side effect of opiates which agent will most likely be added to the medication regimen?

   A. Hydroxyzine
   B. Aluminum-containing antacid
   C. A stimulant laxative
   D. Amphetamine
   E. Trimethobenzamide

4. LB reports a new pain today. This is a shooting pain down the left leg with a burning sensation. He rates the pain 6/10. After other possibilities are ruled out, a diagnosis of neuropathic pain is made. What would be the most appropriate addition to the pain control regimen?

   A. Fentanyl patch applied to the left leg
   B. Dexamethasone
   C. Prochlorperazine
   D. Nortriptyline
   E. Phenobarbital

5. LB has been taking opiates for the past 6 months. His requirement for continued administration of higher doses of opiates would be best characterized as

   A. addiction.
   B. psychological dependence.
   C. tolerance.
   D. physical dependence.
   E. psychosomatic.

PATIENT PROFILE 185
ACUTE OTITIS MEDIA

PRESENTATION

CC: JS is an 11-month-old boy with a diagnosis of acute otitis media. He has no significant past medical history except for a cold that started about 7 days ago.

HPI: According to his mother: JS has a 1-day history of crying, tugging on his left ear, and decreased oral intake. The mother took an oral temperature at 7 AM today (103°F). These symptoms follow a cold that JS developed 1 week ago. No medications were given for cold symptoms. Tylenol drops have been given by the mother to alleviate JS's ear pain and elevated temperature.

PMH: Former 40-week, 3.8-kg healthy infant at birth.
Immunizations are up to date.
Development is normal for age.

FH: Father with mild hypertension; mother in good health; no siblings.

SH: JS lives at home with mother and father. Both parents work outside the home. JS attends day-care 5 days per week (with approximately 10 other children). There is a pet dog in the home.

ALL: NKDA

MH: Tylenol PRN for ear pain and temperature, fluoride drops

PHYSICAL EXAMINATION

Gen: White male infant now crying/screaming

VS: Blood pressure: 100/60 mm Hg; heart rate: 152 beats per minute; respiratory rate: 48 breaths per minute;

Temperature: 100°F; weight: 10.5 kg

HEENT: Both tympanic membranes erythematous (with L > R); both tympanic

membranes bulging and nonmobile; left ear appears to have purulent fluid behind the tympanic membrane; throat is erythematous.

Neck: Supple

Chest: CTA

CV: RRR

Abd: Soft, nontender

Ext: Moves all extremities well; warm, pink, no rashes

Neuro: Responsive to stimulation

LABORATORY STUDIES

None performed

QUESTIONS

1. Select the three organisms that most commonly cause acute otitis media (AOM).

   I. *Staphylococcus aureus*
   II. *Streptococcus pneumoniae*
   III. *Escherichia coli*
   IV. *Hemophilus influenzae*
   V. *Moraxella catarrhalis*
   VI. *Klebsiella pneumoniae*

   A. I, II, and III
   B. II, IV, and V
   C. II, IV, and VI
   D. I, II, and IV
   E. III, IV, and V

2. Which of the following is(are) risk factor(s) for the presence of a bacterial species resistant to amoxicillin?

   A. Age < 2 years
   B. Received antibiotics in last 30 days
   C. Attendance in day care
   D. All the above are risk factors.
   E. B and C only

3. Which of the following would be the *best* initial therapy for JS' AOM?

   A. High-dose amoxicillin
   B. High-dose amoxicillin–clavulanic acid
   C. Clindamycin
   D. Azithromycin
   E. Trimethoprim-sulfamethoxazole

4. If JS has vomiting associated with his AOM and is unable to take his medicine orally, what would be an appropriate intramuscularly administered treatment?

   A. Ampicillin
   B. Cefazolin
   C. Ceftriaxone
   D. Cefuroxime
   E. Penicillin G

5. Which of the following is a possible complication of AOM?

   A. Sinusitis
   B. Tonsillitis
   C. Endocarditis

D. Meningitis
E. Rheumatic heart disease

6. What is the purpose of adding clavulanic acid to amoxicillin?

   A. Decrease the total daily dose
   B. Decrease the incidence of gastrointestinal upset
   C. Decrease the dosing frequency to once daily
   D. Increase the stability of the tablet formulation
   E. Increase the spectrum of activity

7. Which of the following statements is *not true* regarding AOM?

   A. An infant's eustachian tube facilitates better ear drainage than an adults.
   B. Tympanostomy tube placement may be considered in recurrent AOM.
   C. AOM may be associated with hearing loss.
   D. Infants often display nonspecific symptoms of AOM.
   E. Exposure to second-hand smoke is a risk factor for AOM.

8. Appropriate supportive therapy for JS would include

I. Analgesics
II. Antipyretics
III. Decongestants

   A. I only
   B. II only
   C. III only
   D. I and II only
   E. I, II, and III

9. If JS has nasal congestion, what would be the best over-the-counter product to recommend?

   A. Saline nose drops
   B. Oxymetazoline spray
   C. Phenylephrine spray
   D. Pseudoephedrine tabs
   E. Nothing at all

10. How long should JS receive antibiotic treatment?

   A. 2 days
   B. 5 days
   C. 7 days
   D. 10 days
   E. 14 days

PATIENT PROFILE 186

MEDICINAL CHEMISTRY

PRESENTATION AND QUESTION

During a weekly seminar at the hospital where you work, an emergency department physician asks why clonidine (structure 186.1) is not available in the injectable dosage form for the emergency management of hypertension?

1. What would your answer be?

   A. Why bother with clonidine when there are other IV antihypertensive agents, such as diazoxide (structure 186.2) and nitroprusside sodium (structure 186.3)?

   B. Although clonidine is a useful antihypertensive agent, if given by injection it initially may further increase blood pressure.
   C. The chemistry of clonidine does not allow formation of a water-soluble salt for injection; that is why the drug is available only in the oral dosage form.
   D. Clonidine is a prodrug. It has to be given orally to be activated first by the liver.
   E. C and D

186.1

186.2

$-Na_2[Fe(CN)_5NO]$

186.3

IRRITABLE BOWEL SYNDROME

PRESENTATION

DK is a 28-year-old woman who presents to the clinic with complaints of severe abdominal pain, bloating, and the inability to pass stool for 3 days. She states that over the past year she has noticed an increase in her irregular bowel movements. She has gained 30 lb since last year and admits to having "unhealthy" eating habits that include large, fatty meals. Her past medical history includes self-diagnosed "panic attacks." She is not currently taking any medications and has no drug allergies. Her family history includes a maternal grandmother who passed away from colon cancer. She does not drink, smoke, or use illicit drugs. DK appears to be in moderate distress and states that her abdominal pain is 7 on a scale of 10. Her physical examination reveals abdominal distension.

QUESTIONS

1. According to the Rome II criteria, which of the following must be present for the diagnosis of irritable bowel syndrome (IBS)?

   A. Symptoms for > 1 month
   B. Abdominal pain
   C. Pain associated with a change in stool frequency
   D. B and C only
   E. All the above

2. Which neurotransmitter has been identified in the pathophysiology of IBS?

   A. Acetylcholine
   B. Norepinephrine
   C. Serotonin
   D. Dopamine

3. Which of the following factors from DK's history could be attributed to her clinical presentation?

   A. Possible anxiety disorder
   B. Family history of colon cancer
   C. Her eating habits
   D. All the above

4. Which of the following is the *most appropriate* treatment for DK at this time?

   A. Loperamide
   B. Lactulose
   C. Metamucil
   D. Alosetron

5. Which of the following regarding the use of fiber for the management of constipation-predominant IBS is *correct*?

   A. Patients must increase fiber intake gradually to avoid gas and bloating associated with large doses.
   B. Although considered a first-line therapy, long-term data on the benefit of fiber for constipation-predominant IBS are lacking.
   C. Fiber products can alleviate constipation but aggravate abdominal pain by causing bloating.
   D. All the above

6. DK returns 2 months later and states that she has had some success with her current regimen but is still experiencing constipation. She also states that her abdominal bloating has worsened. Which of the following is the *most appropriate* treatment for DK at this time?

   A. Polyethylene glycol
   B. Lactulose
   C. Milk of magnesia
   D. Any of the above would be appropriate to use.

7. Which of the following is(are) side effect(s) associated with the use of osmotic laxatives?

   A. Peripheral edema
   B. Electrolyte abnormalities
   C. Anorexia
   D. None of the above

8. Which of the following is(are) limitation(s) to the chronic use of stimulant laxatives?

   A. High incidence of renal failure
   B. Not a cost-effective therapy
   C. Risk of abuse or dependence
   D. All the above

9. DK has been taking a stimulant laxative now for 6 weeks and reports no improvement in her symptoms. Which of the following is the *most appropriate* treatment for DK at this time?

   A. Tegaserod
   B. Magnesium citrate
   C. Metamucil
   D. Refer her to an IBS specialist because there are no more treatment options available to treat her IBS.

10. DK states that her abdominal pain is still about 7 on a scale of 10. Which of the following medications may help to relieve DK's abdominal pain?

    A. Morphine
    B. Hyoscyamine
    C. Amitriptyline
    D. None of the above

PATIENT PROFILE 188
ALCOHOL ABUSE

PRESENTATION

SB is a 32-year-old man admitted for alcohol detoxification. He had started drinking 3 days ago, when his girlfriend left him. He states that since the breakup he has had a couple of bottles of vodka and some beer. He is disheveled, smells of alcohol, and has slurred speech and an unsteady gait. SB admits to drinking daily for the last year but claims it had never been a problem until 3 days ago. He says he started drinking at age 14. He denies previous hospitalizations for alcohol detox or abuse.

The medical history includes a fracture of the right radius after a fall down stairs 6 months ago. SB is allergic to naproxen (hurts his stomach). He takes famotidine 20 mg bid and Tylenol® no. 3 (acetaminophen) 2 tablets tid prn. His father is an alcoholic. SB smokes 2 packs of cigarettes per day. He is a construction worker who lived with his girlfriend until the recent breakup.

PHYSICAL EXAMINATION

GEN: Disheveled, intoxicated-appearing man
BP sitting R arm: 136/88, HR: 88, RR: 22, T: 99.6°F

LABS

Na: 145 mEq/L
Cl: 106 mEq/L
Ca: 8.8 mg/dL
BUN: 21 mg/dL
Gluc: 90 mg/dL
AST: 95 U/L
ALT: 52 U/L
Alk Phos: 146 U/L
INR: 1.3
Blood alcohol level: 270 mg/dL

K: 5.0 mEq/L
CO_2: 28 mEq/L
PO_4: 3.0 mg/dL
SCr: 1.0 mg/dL
WBC: 9.6×10^3/mm^3
Hct: 39
Hgb: 11 g/dL
Plts: 210×10^9/L
PT: 15 s

A/P: Patient is a 33-year-old alcoholic man who is intoxicated and requesting alcohol detox.

QUESTIONS

1. Which is the most likely lab result after acute alcohol ingestion?

   A. Transient increase in liver function test results (LFTs)
   B. Transient decrease in LFTs
   C. Transient increase in thrombus formation times (TFTs)
   D. Transient decrease in TFTs
   E. Transient decrease in WBC count

2. Benzodiazepines are effective in minimizing alcohol withdrawal symptoms because of which factor(s)?

   A. Alcohol works on the same subunit of the GABA receptor.
   B. Alcohol acts as an antagonist of endogenous benzodiazepines.
   C. Alcohol is metabolized in the same way as chlordiazepoxide.
   D. None of the above
   E. A, B, and C

3. Which pharmacodynamic property can be used to effectively prevent the alcohol withdrawal symptom of tachycardia?

   A. α_1 Antagonists
   B. α_1 Agonists
   C. β_1 Antagonists
   D. β_2 Antagonists
   E. Histamine-1 antagonists

4. Which of the following is most representative of the physiologic sequence of untreated alcohol withdrawal?

   A. Autonomic hyperactivity, hallucinations, seizures, delirium tremens
   B. Hallucinations, autonomic hyperactivity, delirium tremens, seizures
   C. Delirium tremens, seizures, autonomic hyperactivity, hallucinations
   D. Seizures, hallucinations, autonomic hyperactivity, delirium tremens
   E. Seizures, delirium tremens, hallucinations, autonomic hyperactivity

5. Which of the following is the drug of choice for treatment of patients with alcohol withdrawal syndrome?

   A. Ethanol
   B. Neuroleptic agent
   C. Serotonin reuptake inhibitor
   D. Benzodiazepine
   E. Disulfiram

OBESITY

PRESENTATION

CC: HJ is a 40-year-old woman who presents to your clinic with for a routine visit.

HPI: HJ states that she "feels fine" but has been under a lot of stress at work and at home lately and has not been eating very healthy. She was diagnosed with type 2 diabetes 5 years ago and has been coming to see you monthly with her blood glucose log book for evaluation. She has been gaining weight steadily and has expressed her desire to lose weight. She has tried and failed several diets in the past 2 years, including her most recent attempt 6 months ago. She lost 5 lb but gained it back despite the same diet and exercise regimen. She cooks her own food and tries to stick to lean meats and vegetables. She walks two to three times per week for 20 to 30 minutes.

PMH: Hypertension, type 2 diabetes, dyslipidemia, migraines, depression, osteoarthritis, sleep apnea, PSH, status post appendectomy 25 years ago

SH: Married, one child. Smokes (1 pack per day for 20 years). Drinks approximately two drinks per week. Works as an investment banker in Boston.

FH: Mother alive, Alzheimer's disease, emphysema. Father alive and well, status post myocardial infarction (MI) at age 53, dyslipidemia, hypertension, rheumatoid arthritis.

MH: Atorvastatin 20 mg qd, lisinopril 20 mg qd, metformin 500 mg bid, glyburide 5 mg qd, frovatriptan PRN migraines, MVI qd, sertraline 50 mg qd

PHYSICAL EXAMINATION

Gen: Well-dressed, well-nourished female

VS: Blood pressure 162/96 mm Hg; pulse = 76 beats per minute; respiratory rate: 16 breaths per minute; height: 5 ft, 7 in; weight: 192 lb

HEENT: PERRLA, EOMI

CV: RRR, nl S_1, S_2

Pulm: Lungs CTA

Abd: Soft, nontender, nondistended, nl bowel sounds

Ext: No c/c/e

Labs: 137 100 10; 136; 3.7 27 1.2; total cholesterol: 220 mg/dL; low-density lipoprotein (LDL) cholesterol: 154 mg/dL; high-density lipoprotein (HDL) cholesterol: 42 mg/dL; triglycerides: 210 mg/dL

QUESTIONS

1. What is HJ's body mass index (BMI)?

   A. 27
   B. 30
   C. 35
   D. 40

2. According to her BMI, what is HJ's weight classification?

   A. Normal
   B. Overweight
   C. Obese
   D. Morbidly obese

3. According to current guidelines, which of the following are established weight-related diseases in HJ?

   A. Sleep apnea
   B. Osteoarthritis
   C. Migraine headache
   D. Both A and B are correct.

4. Which of the following factors classify HJ as having the metabolic syndrome?

   A. Sleep apnea, migraines, and type 2 diabetes
   B. Osteoarthritis, hypertension, and dyslipidemia
   C. Hypertension, hypertriglyceridemia, type 2 diabetes
   D. Depression, sleep apnea, migraines, and hypertension

5. Is HJ a candidate for drug therapy considering her BMI and the fact that she has failed a 6-month trial of therapeutic lifestyle changes?

   A. No, she would need a BMI of greater than 40.
   B. Yes, she meets the criterion of a BMI of greater than 30.
   C. Yes, her BMI is only 25, but she has multiple risk factors for cardiovascular disease (CVD).
   D. No, her BMI is only 25, and she does not meet the criteria for drug therapy.

6. Based on HJ's history and current drug regimen, which of the following medications would be the *best* first-line agent for HJ?

   A. Orlistat
   B. Topiramate
   C. Sibutramine
   D. Phentermine

7. Which of the following medications should *not* be used in patients with uncontrolled hypertension?

   A. Orlistat
   B. Metformin

C. Topiramate
D. Sibutramine

8. Which of the following weight-loss medications have been studied for long-term use (up to 2 years) for the treatment of obesity?

A. Orlistat
B. Sibutramine
C. Phentermine
D. Both A and B are correct.

9. Which of the following medications has been shown to decrease the absorption of fat-soluble vitamins?

A. Orlistat
B. Metformin
C. Sibutramine
D. Phentermine

10. According to current guidelines, which of the following are *appropriate* cut points for weight-loss surgery?

A. BMI > 35
B. BMI > 35 with comorbid disease
C. BMI > 40 with no comorbid disease
D. Both B and C are correct.

PATIENT PROFILE 190

CONGESTIVE HEART FAILURE AND ARRHYTHMIAS

PRESENTATION

DM is a 71-year-old man who arrives in the emergency department with increased shortness of breath and pleuritic chest pain. He is normally comfortable at home with oxygen at 2.5 L/hour. He states that he has had 2 days of nasal congestion, nausea, no vomiting, and increased temperature. He states that he normally has three to five episodes of angina a day that are relieved with SL nitroglycerin. The pleuritic chest pain is different in character from his usual angina. He also states that in the last few days the number of episodes of anginal pain have increased. He states he has a nonproductive cough and has been using his inhalers with minimal effect. His wife has bronchitis. DM's family history contains no relevant findings. DM is a 70 pack/year smoker and still smokes. He does not drink alcohol.

MEDICAL HISTORY

COPD (O_2 dependent)
Diabetes mellitus type II
Hypertension
Hyperlipidemia
CAD (AMI in 1997, CABG × 4 in 1987)
Degenerative joint disease
DVT 4 months ago
CHF (EF <20% 6 months ago)

MEDS

Aspirin 325 mg po qd
Digoxin 0.125 mg po qod

Lasix® (furosemide) 80 mg po qd
Imdur® (isosorbide mononitrate) 90 mg po bid
Zestril® (lisinopril) 20 mg po qd
Glipizide 2.5 mg po qd
Coumadin® (warfarin sodium) 5 mg po qd
Famotidine 20 mg po bid
Atorvastatin 10 mg po qd
Atrovent® (ipratropium bromide) 2 puffs q6h prn
Nitroglycerin 0.4 mg prn for chest pain
Azmacort® (triamcinolone acetonide) 4 puffs bid

PHYSICAL EXAMINATION

GEN: Elderly man in mild respiratory distress
BP: 143/94, HR: 112, RR: 18, T: 101.2°F
Ht: 69" Wt: 84 kg
O_2 sat: 97% on 2 L
HEENT: Normal
COR: normal S_1 and S_2, no S_3
CHEST: Decreased breath sounds bilaterally, diffuse expiratory wheezes, rales one-third way up
ABD: Normal
GU: Normal
RECTAL: Normal
EXT: 2+ pitting edema up to the knees
NEURO: Normal

LABS

Na: 139   K: 4.6
Cl: 99 CO_2: 27
BUN: 34   Gluc: 219

SCr: 1.7 (baseline 1.5–1.8)
PT: 17.1
PTT: 39.5
INR: 2.0
Total chol: 220
Trig: 180

WBC: 9.2
Hgb: 13.5
Hct: 41.2
Plts: 219,000
HDL chol: 38
LDL chol: 140

A/P: DM is found to have viral pneumonia and myocardial infarction is ruled out. The medical team decides to admit him to the hospital for monitoring of the acute illness.

QUESTIONS

1. Which of the following may be contributing to the increasing frequency of angina?

   A. Lack of a nitrate-free interval
   B. Subtherapeutic INR
   C. Elevated blood sugar levels
   D. Increased total cholesterol
   E. Adverse drug effect of inhaled Atrovent® (ipratropium bromide)

2. Which of the following statements is true?

   A. DM has reached his goal LDL level.
   B. A β-blocker would be contraindicated in the treatment of DM because of COPD.
   C. DM's goal digoxin concentration is 1.5–2.5 mg/L.
   D. Fluvastatin produces a greater decrease in LDL than atorvastatin.

E. DM is within the goal range for his INR (warfarin therapy).

3. Over the course of several months renal failure worsens, necessitating discontinuation of Zestril® (lisinopril). Which of the following is the most appropriate choice to replace Zestril® (lisinopril) in the medication regimen?

   A. Enalapril 10 mg po bid
   B. Losartan 50 mg po qd
   C. Amlodipine 5 mg po qd
   D. Hydralazine 20 mg po qid
   E. Prazosin 1 mg po bid

4. If added, which of the following medications will help decrease the mortality risk of CHF?

   A. Carvedilol
   B. Felodipine
   C. Prazosin
   D. Sotalol
   E. Amlodipine

5. Which of the following is not true regarding CAD risk factor modification (CAD) for DM?

   A. Diabetes is not controlled. Increase glipizide dose.
   B. Hypertension is controlled.
   C. DM should stop smoking.
   D. Atorvastatin should be increased to 20 mg po qd.
   E. Maintain a low fat, low cholesterol diet.

PATIENT PROFILE 191

HEPATIC CIRRHOSIS

PRESENTATION

CC: RH is a 56-year-old woman who presents to the outpatient clinic for a follow-up appointment after transjugular intrahepatic portosystemic shunt (TIPS) placement 2 months ago. She complains of worsening pruritus. In the clinic she is accompanied by her husband, who states that she is becoming more confused and frequently loses her train of thought even in the middle of a sentence.

PMH: RH has primary biliary cirrhosis complicated by ascites, esophageal varices, a gastrointestinal (GI) bleed × 1, and mild encephalopathy. A TIPS was placed 2 months ago for refractory ascites.

SH: Denies alcohol, tobacco, and illicit drug use

FH: Father died 6 years ago (colon cancer). Mother has hypertension and osteoarthritis.

VS: Temperature: 37.6°C; blood pressure: 128/74 mm Hg; heart rate: 82 beats per minute; respiratory rate: 22 breaths per minute

LABORATORY AND DIAGNOSTIC TESTS

Sodium: 138 mEq/L
Chloride: 109 mEq/L
Blood urea nitrogen (BUN): 12 mg/dL
Glucose: 97 mg/dL
Ionized calcium: 4.7 mg/dL

Hematocrit: 32.9%
Total bilirubin: 2.6 mg/dL

Potassium: 3.7 mEq/L
CO_2: 20 mEq/L
Serum creatinine: 0.5 mg/dL
Albumin: 2.8 g/dL
White blood cell (WBC) count: 5000/mm^3
Platelets 109,000/mm^3
AST: 72 IU/L

ALT: 47 IU/L

Prothrombin time: 14.7 s

Alkaline phosphatase:
159 IU/L

International normaliza-
tion ratio (INR): 1.3

CURRENT MEDICATIONS

Furosemide 40 mg PO qd
Lactulose 20 gm PO qid
Pantoprazole 40 mg PO qd
Spironolactone 50 mg PO qd
Ursodiol 300 mg PO tid

QUESTIONS

1. Which of the following medications would be the *best choice* for the treatment of portal hypertension?

   A. Amlodipine
   B. Atenolol
   C. Lisinopril
   D. Propranolol
   E. Verapamil

2. Effective treatment of portal hypertension also will treat or prevent which of the following complications?

   A. Confusion from hepatic encephalopathy
   B. Discomfort from ascites
   C. Bleeding from esophageal varices
   D. Both A and B
   E. All the above

3. Which of the following is the *correct* indication for this patient's lactulose therapy?

   A. Ascites
   B. Esophageal varices
   C. Hepatic encephalopathy
   D. Jaundice
   E. Portal hypertension

4. The dose of lactulose should be titrated according to which of the following parameters?

   A. Development of headache or tremor
   B. Two to three stools per day
   C. Reduction in total bilirubin
   D. Improvement of ascites
   E. Normal AST and ALT

5. Which of the following is a possible cause of RH's pruritus?

   A. Elevated bilirubin
   B. Elevated liver enzymes
   C. Elevated alkaline phosphatase
   D. Decreased albumin
   E. Prolonged partial thromboplastin time (PTT)

6. Which of the following medications would be effective for pruritus associated with liver disease?

   A. Cholestyramine
   B. Chlorpheniramine
   C. Rifampin
   D. Naloxone
   E. All the above

7. The patient may be experiencing ascites owing to which of the following?

   I. Noncompliance. She does not take her spironolactone.
   II. Noncompliance. She does not take her furosemide.
   III. Excessive dietary sodium intake

   A. I only
   B. III only
   C. I and II only
   D. II and III only
   E. I, II, and III

8. Which of the following *most appropriately* describes the use of albumin in the management of ascites?

   A. Albumin attenuates hypovolemia that may occur after aggressive diuretic therapy or large-volume paracentesis.
   B. Albumin is useful to treat hypoalbuminemia, which is commonly associated with chronic liver disease.
   C. Albumin should be prescribed for all patients with fulminant hepatic failure and ascites.
   D. Albumin is useful in treating ascites but may worsen jaundice.
   E. Albumin is not associated with a therapeutic benefit.

9. RH is diagnosed with spontaneous bacterial peritonitis. After acute treatment, which of the following would be the *most appropriate* antibiotic regimen to prevent recurrence?

   A. Amoxicillin 500 mg PO bid
   B. Norfloxacin 400 mg PO qd
   C. Vancomycin 1 g IV q12h
   D. Piperacillin-tazobactam 3.375 mg IV q8h
   E. Metronidazole 500 mg PO tid

10. What of the following *most accurately* describes the side-effect profile of ursodiol?

    A. Ursodiol is associated with significant bone marrow toxicity.
    B. At high doses, ursodiol is associated with renal failure.
    C. Ursodiol is associated with severe hyperlipidemia.
    D. Ursodiol may cause elevations in liver enzymes.
    E. Ursodiol is generally well tolerated.

PATIENT PROFILE 192
THYROID DISEASE

PRESENTATION

CK is a 35-year-old woman who visits her primary care physician for a routine physical examination. She expresses concern regarding increasing irritability and weight loss of 9 pounds over the past 2 months. When asked, she states that she has irregular, scant menses and an increased frequency of bowel movements. The medical history includes a seizure disorder and deep venous thrombosis. CK has no known drug allergies. CK is a married homemaker with three children. There are no relevant findings in her social history.

MEDS

Phenytoin 300 mg po qd
Warfarin 5 mg po M, W, F and 2.5 mg po T, TH, Sat, Sun
Acetaminophen 325 mg po prn

PHYSICAL EXAMINATION

GEN: A nervous woman
BP: 160/90, HR: 72, RR: 24, T: 98.4°F
Wt: 60 kg
HEENT: Minimal proptosis with tearing; enlarged thyroid gland
COR: Regular rate and rhythm
CHEST: clear to ascultation
ABD: Bowel sounds present, soft, nondistended
EXT: Warm moist skin
NEURO: Intact, proximal muscle weakness

LABS

INR: 2.5
TSH: 0.2 μU/mL
T_4: 22 μg/dL

QUESTIONS

1. CK is found to have hyperthyroidism, and therapy with propylthiouracil is started. What is the recommended duration of treatment? Select the best answer.

   A. 2–4 weeks
   B. 1–3 months
   C. 3–6 months
   D. 6–24 months
   E. 24–48 months

2. What side effects may occur with propylthiouracil therapy?

   A. Gastrointestinal intolerance
   B. Agranulocytosis
   C. Benign transient leukopenia
   D. A and B only
   E. A, B, and C

3. CK decides that she does not want to take oral medicine. Propylthiouracil is discontinued, and radioactive iodine (RAI) is used to manage the hyperthyroidism. Seven months after RAI treatment, hypothyroidism develops. Levothyroxine therapy is initiated. CK weighs 62 kg. Recommend an appropriate initial dose. Select the best answer.

   A. Levothyroxine 25 μg po qd
   B. Levothyroxine 50 μg po qd
   C. Levothyroxine 100 μg po qd
   D. Levothyroxine 125 μg po qd
   E. Levothyroxine 150 μg po qd

4. Which of the following medications that CK is currently taking may increase the metabolism of levothyroxine?

   A. Phenytoin 300 mg po qd
   B. Warfarin 5 mg po M, W, F and 2.5 mg po T, TH, Sat, Sun
   C. Acetaminophen 325 mg po prn
   D. A and B only
   E. A, B, and C

P A T I E N T   P R O F I L E   1 9 3

DIABETES MELLITUS

PRESENTATION

GF is a 22-year-old African-American woman seen in the emergency department with swollen lips and a swollen tongue. She is having difficulty breathing. Epinephrine is administered.

According to her medical chart, GF's past medical history includes type 2 diabetes mellitus $\times$ 1 year, hypertension, and obesity. Her current medications are glipizide 10 mg every morning, folic acid 1 mg once daily, a multivitamin once daily, felodipine 10 mg once daily, and lisinopril 10 mg once daily. She also has been taking 325 mg aspirin once daily for 3 years on the advice of her mother who is a nurse. She has been taking the glipizide for 6 months and the felodipine, folic acid, and multivitamin for 1 year. Her endocrinologist prescribed the lisinopril a couple weeks ago.

She is married with one child who is 6 months old. She has been smoking cigarettes since age 25 and smokes 1 pack per day. She started smoking socially when she was in college but did not smoke on a daily basis until about 3 years ago. She tends to smoke more when she is stressed. Her father passed away 2 years ago of lung cancer. The period of time after he was diagnosed was a very difficult time for her because she and her father were very close. During that time, she gained a great deal of weight. She is seriously considering quitting smoking because she knows that it is not good for her. Her mother and her husband have been encouraging her to quit. Her husband quit smoking a year ago. Also, she read recently that kids exposed to second-hand smoke have an increased incidence of ear infections. She does not smoke inside the house but is still concerned about exposure to her infant daughter.

She is a dental hygienist and enjoys her work. She speed walks a half hour every day during her lunch hour. Her husband is the primary person in her household who prepares meals and does the grocery shopping. He is a chef. She says that she has a difficult time watching her meal portion size and tends to overeat at dinner because the meals that her husband prepares are so delicious. She has lost 5 lb since she began exercising regularly 3 months ago. She was told at her last primary care visit that her cholesterol is high, so she has been watching her diet and eating more salmon.

She checks her blood sugar twice daily, once in the morning before breakfast and before she takes her medicine and once in the evening before she eats her evening meal. She states that her morning blood sugars are generally in the 80s, and her evening blood sugars are generally around 110 mg/dL. She denies any recent episodes of hypoglycemia but states that she has experienced cold sweats owing to low blood sugars in the past when she forgot to eat her usual lunchtime meal on a weekend. She reacted appropriately to the low blood sugar reaction by drinking some orange juice. She states that once she drank the orange juice, she felt better within 20 minutes.

She is compliant with her medication regimen. She denies any history of adverse drug reactions or allergic reactions but is extremely concerned that the reaction that she experienced today was due to one of her medications.

GF's height is 5 ft, 5 in, and her weight is 170 lb. Her vital signs are as follows: blood pressure: 160/90 mm Hg; heart rate: 95 beats per minute; respiratory rate: 24 breaths per minute; and temperature: 99.6°F. MB's laboratory values today are as follows: Na: 135 mEq/L; K: 4.0 mEq/L; blood urea nitrogen (BUN): 21 mg/dL; serum Cr: 0.9 mg/dL; and glucose: 120 mg/dL.

You review GF's medical chart and note that at her last primary care visit 3 months ago her vital signs were as follows: blood pressure: 132/86 mm Hg; heart rate: 76 beats per minute; respiratory rate: 18 breaths per minute; and temperature: 98.6°F. Her laboratory values 3 months ago were as follows: A1c: 7.5%; total cholesterol: 200 mg/dL; low-density lipoprotein (LDL) cholesterol: 80 md/dL; high-density lipoprotein (HDL) cholesterol: 80 mg/dL; and triglycerides: 200 mg/dL. All liver function tests were within normal limits.

QUESTIONS

1. Which of the following adverse drug reactions is associated with lisinopril?

    A. Angioedema
    B. Hyperglycemia
    C. Hypokalemia
    D. Gastrointestinal bleed
    E. Tremor

2. Several months later, GF returns to clinic for follow-up. Her A1c is now 8%. Her average glucose meter readings are as follows: fasting AM blood sugars: 100 mg/dL; and pre-evening meal blood sugars: 234 mg/dL. Which of the following medication changes would be the *most appropriate* to recommend?

    A. Increase glipizide to 20 mg every morning.
    B. Increase glipizide to 10 mg twice daily
    C. Add acarbose 200 mg three times daily
    D. Add rosiglitazone 90 mg once daily
    E. Add insulin NPH 10 units at bedtime

3. Two years later, GF is considering having another child. She is currently on glipizide 20 mg bid, and her last A1c was 6.5%. Which of the following medications is *most appropriate* to use for treatment of her type 2 diabetes mellitus during her pregnancy?

   A. Insulin
   B. Glipizide
   C. Metformin
   D. Pioglitazone
   E. Nateglinide

4. Several years later, GF is seen in clinic. Her current medications are as follows: metformin 850 mg twice daily with morning and evening meals, insulin NPH 15 units at bedtime, lisinopril 20 mg once daily, and aspirin 325 mg once daily. Her last A1c about 2 months ago was 7.5%. GF states that since her last clinic visit her morning blood sugars have been much higher than before. Her average glucose meter readings are as follows: fasting AM blood sugar: 180 mg/dL; pre-evening meal blood sugar: 120 mg/dL; and bedtime blood sugar: 140 mg/dL. She denies signs or symptoms of hypoglycemia, and on her mother's advice, she checked a couple 2 AM blood sugars, which were around 180 mg/dL. Which of the following medication changes would be the *most appropriate* to recommend?

   A. Increase metformin to 1000 mg twice daily
   B. Increase metformin to 850 mg three times daily
   C. Decrease metformin to 500 mg twice daily
   D. Decrease insulin NPH to 10 units at bedtime
   E. Increase insulin NPH to 20 units at bedtime

5. GF would like to quit smoking. She is interested in trying the Nicoderm CQ to help her quit. She smokes 1 pack (20 cigarettes) per day. Which of the following doses would be the *most appropriate* to initiate?

   A. 40 mg/24 h patch
   B. 28 mg/24 h patch
   C. 21 mg/24 h patch
   D. 14 mg/24 h patch
   E. 7 mg/24 h patch

6. Which of the following is a side effect associated with using a nicotine patch?

   A. Insomnia
   B. Sedation
   C. Hair loss
   D. Thrombosis
   E. Acute renal failure

7. GF decides to use nicotine gum instead of a nicotine patch. Which of the following statements is *most appropriate* when counseling GF on the nicotine gum?

   A. Chew the gum on a continuous basis for 30 minutes.
   B. Chew the gum until a peppery or minty taste emerges. Then place gum between cheek and gum until taste goes away. Repeat until gum no longer has taste after chewing, which is usually about 30 minutes.
   C. Place the gum between check and gum until a peppery or minty taste emerges. Then chew gum until it no longer has taste, which is usually about 30 minutes.
   D. Chew the gum until a peppery or minty taste emerges. Then swallow the gum.
   E. Place the gum on the tongue until the peppery or minty taste goes away. Chew the gum until the taste emerges. Repeat until the gum no longer has any taste after placing on tongue, which is usually about 30 minutes.

8. GF is seen in the vascular clinic for new symptoms of bilateral leg pain after walking two blocks. She does not have the pain at rest. After a diagnostic workup, she is determined to have intermittent claudication. Which of the following medications is *most appropriate* to use for that indication?

   A. Pletal (cilostazol)
   B. Neurontin (gabapentin)
   C. Percocet (oxycodone-acetaminophen)
   D. Tylenol (acetaminophen)
   E. Coumadin (warfarin)

9. GF's care provider decides to switch her from daily aspirin to Plavix (clopidogrel) 75 mg once daily. Which of the following medications can increase bleeding risk if used in combination with Plavix?

   A. Glipizide
   B. Lisinopril
   C. Felodipine
   D. Ibuprofen
   E. Metformin

10. At the community pharmacy where you work, GF states that her brother-in-law is taking niacin for his cholesterol. You review her medication profile and note that she is on the following medications: metformin 1000 mg twice daily with morning and evening meals, insulin NPH 25 units at bedtime, lisinopril 40 mg once daily, and clopidogrel 75 mg once daily. She has a copy of her most recent lipid profile checked 1 month ago. Her lipid profile values are total cholesterol: 200 mg/dL; LDL: 80 mg/dL; HDL: 80 mg/dL; and triglycerides: 200 mg/dL. She is wondering if niacin would be a good choice for treating her cholesterol. Which of the following responses would be the *most appropriate*?

A. Niacin can increase blood sugar levels. Another cholesterol-lowering agent may be a better choice.

B. Niacin can increase the levels of metformin in your body, which can place you at risk for side effects. Another cholesterol-lowering agent may be a better choice.

C. Niacin can decrease the levels of lisinopril in your body, which could result in poor blood pressure

control. Another cholesterol-lowering agent may be a better choice.

D. Niacin primarily increases triglycerides. Since your triglycerides are low, niacin would be an option for you to discuss with your primary care provider.

E. Niacin primarily decreases LDL and increases HDL. Since your LDL is high and your HDL is low, niacin would be an option for you to discuss with your primary care provider.

P A T I E N T   P R O F I L E   1 9 4

CHRONIC OBSTRUCTIVE LUNG DISEASE

PRESENTATION

CV is a 58-year-old woman who is hospitalized for acute exacerbation of COPD. Her medications on admission include sustained release theophylline, albuterol inhaler, ipratropium inhaler, and prednisone, which she has recently started. She admits not having her theophylline prescription refilled since she ran out 3 weeks ago. Therapy with oxygen, nebulized β_2 agonists, and intravenous aminophylline and hydrocortisone is initiated for immediate control of the condition.

QUESTIONS

1. What would be the most appropriate desired target serum theophylline concentration for management of the COPD?

   A. 5–8 mg/L
   B. 10–15 mg/L
   C. 15–25 mg/L
   D. 25–35 mg/L
   E. >35 mg/L

2. Which of the following would be the most appropriate method to administer the IV aminophylline?

   A. A loading dose followed by intermittent infusion every 6 hours
   B. A loading dose followed by a continuous infusion
   C. An intermittent infusion every 6 hours without a loading dose
   D. A continuous infusion without a loading dose
   E. Total daily dose over 30 minutes

3. After optimizing the serum theophylline concentration with 1000 mg/day IV aminophylline, CV's physician wants to restart oral theophylline. On the basis of the aminophylline dose, what would be the most appropriate daily dose of oral theophylline?

   A. 1200 mg
   B. 1000 mg
   C. 800 mg
   D. 600 mg
   E. 300 mg

4. Which of the following statements most accurately characterizes the role of corticosteroid treatment of patients with COPD such as CV?

   A. Inhaled steroids are more effective in therapy for COPD than therapy for asthma.
   B. Steroid therapy should be maintained indefinitely.
   C. Steroid therapy should be evaluated within 2 weeks of initiation to assess efficacy.
   D. Steroid should be maintained at the maximum effective dose.
   E. The beneficial effects of oral administration are realized almost immediately.

5. The physician asks for a recommendation for an agent to help reduce mucous viscosity. Which of following would be the most appropriate?

   A. α_1-Proteinase inhibitor (Prolastin®)
   B. Acetazolamide (Diamox®)
   C. Acetylcysteine (Mucomyst®)
   D. A and B
   E. A, B, and C

PATIENT PROFILE 195

GOUT

PRESENTATION

RM is a 56-year-old obese man seen in the emergency room who has pain and swelling of his great left toe. RM's pain has escalated since the day prior to admission. He is not wearing a shoe owing to the pain. He is not aware of an injury to the foot and has no history of arthritis or gout. RM has a history of hypertension for 6 years and hyperlipidemia for 4 years. Current medications are hydrochlorothiazide 12.5 mg PO qd, enalapril 20 mg PO qd, atorvastatin 10 mg PO qd, acetaminophen 500 mg PO bid PRN, and multivitamin 1 PO qd. RM's mother died at age 56 of a myocardial infarction (MI), and his father is presently alive and well.

PHYSICAL EXAMINATION

Blood pressure: 152/82 mm Hg; heart rate: 80 beats per minute; respiratory rate: 18 breaths per minute; temperature: afebrile

General: Alert, oriented, and pleasant patient

Chest: Heart reveals regular rhythm.

ABD: Soft and obese without masses

EXT: The first metacarpophalangeal (MTP) joint of the left right foot is acutely swollen, erythematous, warm, and tender. The remaining joints and extremities are normal.

LABORATORY VALUES

Na: 137 mEq/L

K: 3.6 mEq/L

Cl: 107 mEq/L

CO_2 content: 26 mEq/L

Blood urea nitrogen (BUN): 13 mg/dL

Creatinine clearance: 66 mL/min

Total cholesterol: 255 mg/dL

High-density lipoprotein (HDL) cholesterol: 62 mg/dL

Triglycerides: 225 mg/dL

AST: 17 mg/dL

ALT: 10 mg/d

Uric acid: 9.8 mg/dL

Hgb: 11.6 g/dL

Hct: 38%

Platelets: $236,000/mm^3$

QUESTIONS

1. RM's physician suggests that the patient be placed on a probenecid (250 mg PO bid) regimen for the attack. Do you agree or disagree with this suggestion?

   A. Agree; probenecid would be an appropriate suggestion, and the dose is correct for the patient.

   B. Agree; probenecid would be an appropriate suggestion, and the dose should be 500 mg PO bid.

   C. Disagree; probenecid would not be an appropriate suggestion at this time, and the patient should be started on an indomethacin regimen.

   D. Disagree; probenecid would not be an appropriate suggestion at this time, and the patient should be started on an allopurinol regimen.

   E. Disagree; intravenous colchicine would be the most appropriate suggestion at this time.

2. Which of the following diagnostic tests is necessary to make a definitive diagnosis of gout?

   A. Complete blood cell count
   B. Aspiration and analysis of joint synovial fluid
   C. Serum uric acid level
   D. None of the above
   E. All the above

3. Which of RM's medications has been associated with reduced uric acid excretion and precipitation of acute gouty arthritis?

   A. Hydrochlorothizaide
   B. Enalapril
   C. Atorvastatin
   D. Acetaminophen
   E. Multivitamin

4. Based on RM's profile, which of the following are RM's risk factors for acute gouty attacks?

   I. Obesity
   II. Uric acid level
   III. Renal function

   A. III only
   B. II and III only
   C. I and III only
   D. II and III only
   E. I, II, and III

5. Potential complications of gout include which of the following?

   A. Deposition of sodium urate in tissues
   B. Nephropathy caused by deposition of sodium crystals
   C. Progression to osteoporosis
   D. All the above
   E. None of the above

6. Common adverse effects of indomethacin when used for acute attacks of gouty arthritis include which of the following?

   A. Gastrointestinal bleed
   B. Gastrointestinal ulceration
   C. Headache
   D. None of the above
   E. All the above

7. The patient returns to the clinic a month later. The physician concludes after a 24-hour urine collection that the patient is an overproducer and should be placed on a hypouricemic agent. His creatinine clearance is still 66 mL/min. The physician suggests probencid (250 mg PO bid). Do you agree or disagree with this recommendation?

   A. Agree; probenecid would be an appropriate suggestion, and the dose is correct for the patient.
   B. Agree; probenecid would be an appropriate suggestion, and the dose should be 500 mg PO bid.
   C. Disagree; probenecid is not an appropriate suggestion, and the patient should be started on allopurinol 200 mg PO qd.
   D. Disagree; probenecid is not an appropriate suggestion, and the patient should be started on allopurinol 100 mg PO qd.
   E. Disagree; intravenous colchicine would be the most appropriate suggestion at this time.

8. What is the source of uric acid in the human body?

   A. Degradation of hepatocytes
   B. Breakdown of dietary and tissue purines
   C. Release of bile acids
   D. Synthesis from white blood cells
   E. Synthesis in the liver

9. When would corticosteroids be used to treat an acute attack of gouty arthritis?

   A. In patients with severe renal impairment
   B. In patients who are resistant to nonsteroidal anti-inflammatory drugs (NSAIDs) and colchicines
   C. In patients with prior NSAID intolerance
   D. All the above
   E. None of the above

10. Which of the following characteristics are *true* of allopurinol?

    I.   Xanthine oxidase inhibitor
    II. Prevents production of uric acid
    III. Requires a 24-hour urine collection

    A. I only
    B. III only
    C. I and II only
    D. II and III only
    E. I, II, and III

PATIENT PROFILE 196

ARRYTHMIAS

PRESENTATION

TT is a 73-year-old obese woman who reports a recent increase in shortness of breath, two-pillow orthopnea, and nightly paroxysmal dyspnea. She denies any recent cold symptoms, taking any new medications, including any over-the-counter agents, or changes in lifestyle. The medical history includes class II congestive heart failure, hypertension, coronary artery disease (AMI in the past), peripheral vascular disease, stroke, and osteoarthritis.

MEDS

Enalapril 10 mg po bid
Digoxin 0.125 mg po qd
Albuterol inhaler 2 puffs prn
Furosemide 80 mg bid

Verapamil 120 mg po qd
Naproxen 375 mg po bid

PHYSICAL EXAMINATION

BP: 158/98, HR: 94
Wt: 81 kg (dry weight 76 kg)
EXT: 2 + bilateral pitting edema
NECK: Markedly distended neck veins
CHEST: Bibasilar rales and rhonchi
COR: S_3 gallop

LABS

Na: 137
K: 5.1

BUN: 45
SCr: 1.9
Dig: 1.2 mg/L

QUESTIONS

1. Which of the following would provide rapid symptomatic relief to TT?

   A. IV digoxin 0.5 mg
   B. IV furosemide 40 mg
   C. IV enalapril 0.625 mg
   D. Oral metolazone 5 mg
   E. Oral digoxin 0.125 mg

2. After the symptoms are controlled, which one of the following interventions is most appropriate?

   A. Discontinue verapamil
   B. Discontinue verapamil and albuterol
   C. Discontinue verapamil and naproxen
   D. Discontinue verapamil, albuterol, and naproxen
   E. Discontinue albuterol and naproxen

3. Which of the following therapeutic decisions on the use of digoxin to treat this patient should be implemented?

   A. Continue digoxin at 0.125 mg/d
   B. Discontinue digoxin
   C. Increase digoxin to 0.25 mg/d
   D. Lower digoxin dose to 0.0625 mg/d
   E. Change digoxin to 0.125 mg qod

4. TT has an episode of rapid ventricular tachycardia followed by sudden cardiac death from which she is resuscitated. Which of the following is the best choice to help prevent a recurrence of this arrhythmia?

   A. Sotalol
   B. Ibutilide
   C. Adenosine
   D. Procainamide
   E. Amiodarone

5. Which of the following is not true regarding procainamide?

   A. Procainamide can cause a lupus-like syndrome with prolonged administration.
   B. Toxicity is increased among patients with renal failure.
   C. The intravenous form may produce hypotension.
   D. Cimetidine may increase procainamide levels.
   E. Procainamide does not cause any form of proarrhythmia.

PATIENT PROFILE 197

CHRONIC OBSTRUCTIVE PULMONARY DISEASE

PRESENTATION

GG is a 52-year-old man who complains to his physician of increasing shortness of breath and when walking his dog. He has been experiencing several months of persistent, very productive cough that is particularly bothersome when he wakes up in the morning. His medical history generally is unremarkable, except for smoking 2 packs per day of cigarettes for the past 20 years. On physical examination, he is noted to be a moderately obese male who is slightly cyanotic. Coarse breath sounds are noted on auscultation. Spirometry results indicate a forced expiratory capacity at 1 second (FEV_1) that is 65% of predicted, which improves slightly after administration of an inhaled short-acting β-agonist. An initial diagnosis of chronic obstructive pulmonary disease (COPD) is made.

QUESTIONS

1. What is the most appropriate way to interpret this patient's smoking history?

   A. He has a 2 pack-year history of smoking.
   B. He has a 10 pack-year history of smoking.
   C. He has a 20 pack-year history of smoking.
   D. He has a 40 pack-year history of smoking.
   E. He has a 60 pack-year history of smoking.

2. This patient's symptoms are most consistent with what type of obstructive lung disease?

   A. Acute bronchitis
   B. Chronic bronchitis
   C. Asthma

D. Emphysema

E. α_1-Antitrypsin deficiency

3. In addition to relieving symptoms, which of the following agents may alter the natural course of GG's COPD?

A. β-Agonists

B. Glucocorticoids

C. Anticholinergics

D. Expectorants

E. None of the above

4. Which one of the following agents used to treat COPD is considered an anticholinergic?

A. Ipratropium

B. Tiotropium

C. Formoterol

D. A and B

E. A, B, and C

5. For chronic management of COPD, a long-acting β-agonists such as salmeterol should be prescribed how?

A. As needed

B. Once daily

C. Twice daily

D. Every 4 hours

E. Every 6 hours

6. GG is started on a fixed combination of ipratropium and albuterol (Combivent). Which of the following statements about this combination is *most correct*?

A. The onset of action of the ipratopium is much quicker (5 minutes) than that of albuterol (15 minutes).

B. The combination allows for greater flexibility in individualizing dosing.

C. The daily dose should not exceed two inhalations per day.

D. There are few systemic side effects associated with the ipratropium.

E. Only albuterol provides adequate bronchodilation in patients with COPD.

7. After several months, GG has continued to smoke and is now on a regimen that includes scheduled inhaled

fluticasone and oral theophylline therapy. What would be *appropriate* advice to give GG concerning use of his inhaler?

A. He should experience immediate improvement if used for acute symptoms.

B. He may be able to discontinue his albuterol/ipratropium inhaler.

C. He should rinse his mouth out after using.

D. A and B

E. A, B, and C

8. If GG requires antibiotic therapy for the treatment of acute respiratory infection, which of the following agents is *most likely* to inhibit the metabolism of theophylline, resulting in elevated theophylline concentrations?

A. Doxycycline

B. Amoxicillin

C. Trimethoprin-sulfamethoxazole

D. Ciprofloxacin

E. All the above

9. Which of the following side effects of theophylline therapy is a concentration-dependent side effect?

A. Nausea

B. Sleep disturbances

C. Tachycardia

D. Seizures

E. All the above

10. If GG is successful in a smoking-cessation program, what affect could this have on his theophylline dose?

A. None, because smoking does not alter theophylline pharmacokinetics

B. His dose may need to be lowered because smoking increases the hepatic metabolism of theophylline.

C. His dose may need to be increased because smoking decreases the hepatic metabolism of theophylline.

D. His dose may need to be lowered because smoking increases the renal clearance of theophylline.

E. His dose may need to be increased because smoking decreases the renal clearance of theophylline.

PATIENT PROFILE 198
HYPERTENSION

PRESENTATION

LL is a 46-year-old black man who is returning to clinic for a follow-up blood pressure reading.

HPI: LL was started on HCTZ 25 mg po qd 2 months ago for HTN after failing a 3-month trial of non-pharmacologic therapy. He was seen in the clinic approximately 4 weeks ago and his HCTZ was increased to 50 mg po qd because his BP was still uncontrolled.

PMH: Type 2 DM, hypercholesterolemia, HTN, asthma

Drug Allergies: Amoxicillin (rash)

Medication history: Pravastatin 20 mg po qd, beclomethasone 2 puffs BID, albuterol 2 puffs prn, glyburide 10 mg po bid, HCTZ 50 mg po qd

Social history: Smokes half pack of cigarettes per day, drinks 2-3 cups of coffee per day, denies use of alcohol or illicit drugs

Physical examination: BP: sitting R arm-156/96 HR: 60 Wt: 210 lb Ht: 5'7"

A/P: LL is a 46-year-old male who presents for follow-up of his uncontrolled blood pressure.

QUESTIONS

1. LL has several questions about the risks associated with untreated or poorly managed high blood pressure (HBP). Which of the following statement(s) is (are) true regarding these risks?

   A. Patients with isolated systolic HBP are at little to no risk of developing complications secondary to HBP.
   B. Untreated HBP, at any stage, is a significant risk factor for nonfatal and fatal CVD.
   C. Target organs affected by HBP include the brain, heart, kidney, and eyes.
   D. A and B
   E. B and C

2. Which of the following terms best defines LL's current blood pressure reading?

   A. Diastolic high blood pressure
   B. Isolated systolic high blood pressure
   C. High blood pressure
   D. Secondary high blood pressure
   E. Drug-induced high blood pressure

3. In evaluating LL's overall cardiovascular risk, which of the following is (are) considered significant risk factor(s)?

   I. Diabetes
   II. Hypercholesterolemia
   III. Smoking
   IV. Caffeine intake

   A. I and II only
   B. II only
   C. II and III only
   D. I, II, and III only
   E. III and IV only

4. Which of the following electrolyte abnormalities has been reported to occur with HCTZ?

   A. Hyperkalemia
   B. Hypokalemia
   C. Hypernatremia
   D. Hypermagnesemia
   E. Hypocalcemia

5. Which of the following is the next most appropriate step in treating LL's HBP?

   A. Increasing LL's HCTZ to 75 mg po qd
   B. Discontinuing HCTZ and reassessing LL's BP
   C. Discontinuing HCTZ and trying to control LL's BP with lifestyle modifications
   D. Adding lisinopril 10 mg po qd to HCTZ 50 mg po qd
   E. Adding atenolol 100 mg po qd to HCTZ 50 mg po qd

6. When assessing LL's overall treatment plan which of the following would be included in your evaluation of LL?

   A. Assessing LL for compliance with his treatment plan
   B. Assessing LL for any complications secondary to his treatment plan
   C. Assessing LL for any complications secondary to his high blood pressure
   D. Assessing LL for any complications secondary to his other disease states
   E. All of the above are important in evaluating LL's progress

PATIENT PROFILE 199

COLON CANCER

PRESENTATION

CC: "I am here to start my chemotherapy."

HPI: BF is a 67-year-old Italian man with metastatic colon cancer who presents to the clinic today to begin treatment with chemotherapy. BF was diagnosed with stage 2 colon cancer 3 years ago, which was surgically removed. Over the past few months he has developed left lower quadrant pain that radiates down his leg. The pain was originally thought to be sciatic pain, but given the concurrent rise in carcinoembryonic antigen (CEA), the patient underwent restaging. Restaging showed local abdominal disease as well as a liver metastasis. He has been requiring two to three Percocet (regular strength) per day, which is providing adequate pain control.

PMH: Colon cancer (diagnosed 3 years ago), hypertension × 20 years

PSH: Sigmoid colectomy

FH: No family history of cancer

SH: Widowed father of two grown children; lives with oldest son and family; works at local supermarket. No tobacco, alcohol, or illicit drug use.

ALL: latex

MH: Nifedipine XL 60 mg PO qd, lisinopril 40 mg PO qd, HCTZ 12.5 mg PO qd, vitamin E 400 units PO qd, multivitamin 1 tablet PO qd, aspirin 81 mg PO qd, Percocet (regular strength) 1 to 2 tablets PO q4–6h PRN

ROS: No fever, chills, headache; complains of mild abdominal pain that does not radiate.

VS: Temperature: 99°F; blood pressure: 145/90 mm Hg; heart rate: 72 beats per minute; respiratory rate: 18 breaths per minute; O_2 saturation: 98% RA

Height: 5 ft, 7 in; weight: 160 lb

General: Well-appearing male in mild distress

HEENT: PERRLA, EOMI

Neck: Supple: no LAD

Lungs: CTA bilaterally

Heart: RRR, no MRG

ABD: Soft, moderate tenderness, nondistended, positive bowel sounds

EXT: No C/C/E

Neuro: A&O × 3; cranial nerves (CNs) II–XII intact; motor examination is normal with preserved reflexes.

LABORATORY VALUES

Na: 142 mEq/L

Cl: 100 mEq/L

K: 4.4 mEq/L

CO_2: 33 mEq/L

Blood urea nitrogen (BUN): 12 mEq/L

Glucose : 120 mg/dL

AST: 18 units/L

ALP: 98 IU/mL

(LDH) cholesterol: 225 IU/mL Albumin: 4.5 mg/dL

Hct: 36.4%

WBC count: 7100/mm³ 62.7% P, 29.8% L, 4.9% M, 1.4% E, 1.1% B

Serum Cr : 0.6 mg/dL

ALT: 19 units/L

Total bilirubin: 0.2 mg/dL

Low-density lipoprotein

Hgb: 12.2 g/Dl

Platelets: 317,000/mm³

ASSESSMENT/PLAN

BF is a 67-year-old man who presents to the clinic for treatment of metastatic colon cancer. He will begin treatment today with irinotecan, 5-fluorouracil (5-FU), and leucovorin. Continue outpatient antihypertensives and monitor blood pressure. BF may continue his outpatient vitamins and aspirin.

QUESTIONS

1. 5-FU is also known as what?

    A. Fludarabine
    B. Fluorouracil
    C. Carmustine
    D. Lomustine

2. Which dose-limiting toxicity is associated with continuous-infusion 5-FU?

    A. Diarrhea
    B. Myelosuppression
    C. Nephrotoxicity
    D. Cerebellar toxicity

3. What is the role of leucovorin in BF's chemotherapy regimen?

    A. Decrease the toxicity of 5-FU
    B. Increase the cytotoxicity of 5-FU
    C. Decrease the toxicity of irinotecan
    D. Increase the cytotoxicity of irinotecan

4. Which of the following antineoplastics are paired correctly according to mechanism of action?

    A. 5-FU and irinotecan
    B. Methotrexate and irinotecan

C. Irinotecan and topotecan
D. 5-FU and leucovorin

5. In this regimen, irinotecan is dosed at 125 mg/m^2. What dose of irinotecan should BF receive today?

A. 150 mg
B. 230mg
C. 330 mg
D. 350 mg

6. During the infusion of irinotecan, BF begins to experience facial flushing, abdominal cramps, and severe diarrhea. The nurse asks you what should be given to the patient to stop the diarrhea. You recommend what?

A. Loperamide
B. Tincture of opium
C. Atropine
D. No therapy is necessary; the diarrhea will cease when the infusion is complete.

7. How does irinotecan exert its cytotoxicity?

A. Inhibits DNA synthesis by intercalation between base pairs
B. Prevents cell division by cross-linking DNA strands
C. Promotes the assembly of microtubules
D. Prevents DNA resealing by binding to topoisomerase I–DNA complex

8. Fluorouracil is specific to which phase of the cell cycle?

A. G_1 phase
B. G_2 phase
C. M phase
D. S phase

9. Which of the following signs and symptoms are consistent with 5-FU-induced stomatitis?

A. Severe mouth pain
B. Ulceration of the oral mucosa
C. Dysphagia
D. All the above

10. BF was admitted to the hospital for pain control. He is treated initially with morphine sulfate 15 mg PO q4h with good effect. Twenty-four hours later, he is unable to swallow any pills secondary to extreme mouth soreness. The physician wishes to change BF to intravenous hydromorphone to be administered as intermittent boluses. What dose and schedule of hydromorphone do you recommend?

A. Hydromorphone 0.5 mg IV q4h
B. Hydromorphone 1.5 mg IV q4h
C. Hydromorphone 4 mg IV q4h
D. Hydromorphone 8 mg IV q4h

PATIENT PROFILE 200

HYPERTENSION

PRESENTATION

JW is a 62-year-old male who presents to the outpatient clinic for a preoperative evaluation.

HPI: JW presents for preop clearance. He is scheduled to undergo a TURP to treat his BPH but he and his wife are having second thoughts about going ahead with the surgery. He is continuing to have symptoms related to his BPH.
PMH: HTN, BPH
PsurgH: None
Drug Allergies: None
Medication history: HCTZ 50 mg po qd, lisinopril 40 mg po qd, MVI 1 po qd, vitamin E 400 IU po qd
Family history: Noncontributory
Social history: Retired chemical engineer, lifelong non-smoker, drinks a glass of wine with dinner every night, exercises daily

Physical examination: BP: 156/94 HR: 72 Wt: 150 lb Ht: 5'8"
A/P: JW is awaiting surgery and his BP needs to be controlled in order for him to be medically cleared for surgery. He and his wife need additional reassurance in order to proceed with the TURP.

QUESTIONS

1. Which of the following electrolyte abnormalities has been reported to occur with ACEIs?

A. Hyperkalemia
B. Hypokalemia
C. Hypernatremia
D. Hyponatremia
E. Hypercalcemia

2. Which of the following is a rare but potentially fatal adverse effect that has been reported with the use of ACEIs such as JW's lisinopril?

A. Lactic acidosis
B. Hepatotoxicity
C. Pulmonary hypertension
D. Angioedema
E. Stevens-Johnson syndrome

3. Since JW is continuing to have BPH symptoms due to a moderately enlarged prostate gland, his physician has decided to add prazosin to his medication regimen. Why should the initial dose of prazosin not exceed 1mg at bedtime?

A. To minimize the risk of hypersensitivity to the drug
B. To minimize the risk of first-dose syncope
C. To maximize the antihypertensive effects of the drug
D. To minimize the risk of adverse effects
E. To maximize the effectiveness of the drug

4. Of the following adverse effects, which have been reported to occur with prazosin?

A. Drowsiness
B. Headache
C. Weakness
D. Reflex tachycardia
E. All of the above

5. What should JW be instructed to do to help minimize the adverse effect, postural hypotension, which may be seen with prazosin?
A. Drink plenty of fluids
B. Increase his intake of potassium-rich foods
C. Rise more slowly from a seated or supine position
D. Remain seated upright for 30 minutes after taking his prazosin
E. None of the above

6. JW notes that the name on his medication bottle does not match the name of the drug that the physician wrote on his prescription. You inform JW that a genetic drug has been dispensed instead of the brand product which was written on the prescription. What is the brand name for prazosin?

A. Minipress®
B. Hytrin®
C. Plendil®
D. Cardura®
E. Cardene®

7. What other medication may be added to JW's medication regimen to induce atropy of the prostate gland and halt progression of the disease?

A. Testosterone
B. Doxazosin
C. Terazosin
D. Finasteride
E. None of the above

PATIENT   PROFILE   201

ERECTILE DYSFUNCTION

PRESENTATION

CC: "I am having difficulty in maintaining an erection during sexual activity."

HPI: JS is a 38-year-old man who was diagnosed recently with diabetes mellitus type 2. Prior to this diagnosis, JS has consistently reported a healthy sexual lifestyle. Recently, JS has experienced marital problems owing to an inability to maintain an erection. JS denies difficulty in penetrating his partner. JS denies any anxiety in performance. On physical and laboratory examination, JS's blood glucose concentration appears to be in good control. JS was sent to a pharmacist-run outpatient clinic for counseling on general diabetes education and

further assessment of potential drug-induced erectile dysfunction.

Medications: Metformin 500 mg PO bid, lisinopril 20 mg PO qd, benadryl 25 mg PRN, sertraline 50 mg PO qd, cimetidine 200 mg PRN, albuterol metered-dose inhaler (MDI) PRN

PMH: Diabetes type 2 diagnosed 5 year ago, depression diagnosed 7 years ago, seasonal allergies

PSH: None

FH: Father (72 years old) diagnosed with type 2 diabetes; mother (64 years old) healthy

SH: Married 2 years ago; drinks 5 beers per day; quit smoking 10 years ago; denies illicit drug use.

ALL: NKDA

PHYSICAL EXAMINATION

General: Appearance reflects apparent age.

VS: Blood pressure: 128/72 mm Hg; heart rate: 60 beats per minute; respiratory rate: 20 breaths per minute; temperature: 37°C

Height: 5 ft, 9 in; weight: 80 kg

HEENT: PERRLA, EOMI

COR: RRR; no murmur, rubs, or gallops; posterior tibial and dorsalis pedis pulses normal.

Chest: Lungs CTA

ABD: Soft, nontender, normal bowel sounds

GU: Normal scrotum; penis without curvature/discharge

RECT: Normal anus

EXT: No edema; no calluses or ulcers on foot

NEURO: Cranial nerves (CNs) II–XII intact.

ECG: Normal

LABORATORY VALUES

Na: 135 mEq/L
K: 4.2 mEq/L
Cl: 98 mEq/L
HCO_3: 6.0 mEq/L
Blood urea nitrogen (BUN): 15 mg/dL
Serum Cr: 0.7 mg/dL
Glucose: 175 mg/dL (nonfasting)
Hgb: 15.0 g/dL
Hct: 47%
Platelets: $300 \times 10^3/mm^3$
PT: N/A
aPTT: N/A
Triglycerides: 140 mg/dL
Total cholesterol: 188 mg/dL
High-density lipoprotein (HDL) cholesterol: 60 mg/dL
Low-density lipoprotein (LDL) cholesterol: 89 mg/dL
Testosterone: Normal (500 ng/dL)

QUESTIONS

1. Which of the following is a current risk factor for JS's reported erectile dysfunction?

   A. Age
   B. Hypertension
   C. Hypogonadism
   D. Diabetes mellitus
   E. Cigarette smoking

2. Which of the following drugs may have contributed to JS's erectile dysfunction?

   I. Benadryl
   II. Cimetidine
   III. Lisinopril

   A. I only
   B. II only
   C. I and II

   D. II and III
   E. I, II, and III

3. Which of the following is the *best* action to take with regard to JS's depression therapy in order to decrease drug-induced erectile dysfunction?

   A. Change JS's sertraline therapy to paroxetine.
   B. Change JS's sertraline therapy to citaolpram.
   C. Change JS's sertraline therapy to buproprion.
   D. Change JS's sertraline therapy to amitryptiline.
   E. Do make any changes to JS's sertraline therapy.

4. JS's primary care physician believes that JS's erectile dysfunction may be drug-induced. Which of the following action(s) may you recommend?

   I. Wait for remission or tolerance of symptoms of erectile dysfunction
   II. Reduce dose of drug causing erectile dysfunction
   III. Add on a medication to treat erectile dysfunction

   A. I only
   B. II only
   C. I and II
   D. II and III
   E. I, II, and III

5. JS's primary care physician is considering the initiation of a phosphodiesterase inhibitor for JS's erectile dysfunction. Which of the following would be a contraindication to such therapy?

   A. History of retinopathy
   B. History of unstable angina
   C. Resting moderate hypertension
   D. History of a stroke within the past year
   E. History of myocardial infarction with the past year

6. After a recent conversation with JS, his primary care physician is considering the initiation of androgen therapy in JS. Which of the following should be considered prior to initiating such therapy?

   I. Testosterone levels
   II. History of prostate cancer
   III. History of benign prostatic hyperplasia

   A. I only
   B. II only
   C. I and II
   D. II and III
   E. I, II, and III

7. JS's primary care physician wants to initiate Striant, a testosterone administered via the buccal route. What would be an important counseling point for JS?

   A. Avoid taking Striant for 2 hours after meals.
   B. Avoid chewing gum while taking Striant.

C. Avoid taking Striant for 4 hours after alcohol comsumption.

D. Remove Striant if it does not dissolve after 12 hours.

E. Chew and swallow Striant if it does not dissolve after 12 hours.

8. JS does not like the buccal formulation of testosterone. JS's primary care physician asks you what other formulation(s) are available? How do you respond?

I. Patch
II. Gel
III. Intramuscular injection

A. I only
B. II only
C. I and II
D. II and III
E. I, II, and III

9. JS chooses the pellet formulation of testosterone because of its convenience. What is(are) disadvantage(s) of such a formulation?

I. Inflammation at pellet site
II. Difficult dose adjustment
III. Fluctuation in testosterone levels

A. I only
B. II only
C. I and II
D. II and III
E. I, II, and III

10. JS's testosterone levels have returned to and have been maintained at normal levels after 8 weeks of therapy. JS would now like to try noninvasive therapies for erectile dysfunction. What would you recommend?

A. Alprostadil
B. Vacuum device
C. Vascular surgery
D. Penile prosthesis
E. Phentolamine/papaverine

PATIENT PROFILE 202

ANTICOAGULATION

PRESENTATION

AQ is a 30-year-old female who has undergone heart valve replacement.

HPI: AQ underwent placement of a mechanical prosthetic heart valve in the aortic position this morning.

PMH: Structural abnormality of the aortic valve

PsurgH: None

Drug Allergies: Penicillin (bronchospasm and rash)

Medication history: None

Family history: Non-contributory

Social history: Denies smoking and alcohol or illicit drug use

Physical examination: BP: 120/76 HR: 75 Wt: 176 lb Ht: 5'7"

Labs: aPTT 30 seconds, INR 1.2

A/P: AQ needs anticoagulant therapy and the medical team asks for your assistance in initiating AQ's heparin therapy.

QUESTIONS

1. What additional labs would you request prior to initiating AQ's heparin?

A. Complete blood count
B. Liver function tests
C. Renal function tests
D. Antithrombin III levels
E. Protein C levels

2. Which of the following is the most appropriate initial bolus dose for AQ?

A. Heparin 1500 units IVB
B. Heparin 3200 units IVB
C. Heparin 5000 units IVB
D. Heparin 6400 units IVB
E. Heparin 10,000 units IVB

3. Which of the following is the most appropriate initial infusion rate for AQ's heparin drip?

A. Heparin infusion at 500 units/hr
B. Heparin infusion at 700 units/hr
C. Heparin infusion at 1000 units/hr

D. Heparin infusion at 1400 units/hr
E. Heparin infusion at 2000 units/hr

4. Once AQ receives her heparin bolus and is placed on the heparin infusion, when would you recommend checking her first aPTT?

A. 2 hours after the heparin bolus
B. 4 hours after the heparin bolus
C. 6 hours after the heparin bolus
D. 12 hours after the heparin bolus
E. 24 hours after the heparin bolus

5. AQ's first aPTT is 60 seconds with a control aPTT of 30 seconds. What would you recommend now?

A. Rebolus with 5000 units and increase the rate of the infusion
B. Increase the rate of the heparin infusion
C. Keep the heparin infusion at the same rate
D. Decrease the rate of the heparin infusion
E. Hold the heparin infusion for 1 hour and restart at a lower rate

6. AQ should be monitored for which of the following blood dyscrasias that has been reported to occur with heparin?

A. Neutropenia
B. Pancytopenia
C. Agranulocytosis
D. Thrombocytopenia
E. Reticulocytosis

PATIENT PROFILE 203

MENOPAUSE

PRESENTATION

A 57-year-old woman presents with complaints of "hot flashes." She explains that these episodes last about 5 to 10 minutes and have been occurring about two times a day for the past month or so. She sometimes will awake from her sleep at night in a sweat.

PMH: Deep venous thrombosis (12 years ago), seasonal allergies, migraine headaches
SH: Lives with her husband; has three children, all attending college; her oldest daughter is getting married next month; she is employed as a nurse; nonsmoker; drinks occasionally
FH: Mother: diabetes, coronary artery disease (CAD); sister: breast cancer; father: CAD, chronic obstructive pulmonary disease (COPD)
ALL: PCN (rash)

PHYSICAL EXAMINATION

VS: Blood pressure: 150/90 mm Hg; heart rate: 89 beats per minute; respiratory rate: 12 breaths per minute; temperature: 98.6°F
Weight: 90 kg
General: Overall, a well-appearing women with no significant physical findings
HEENT: PERRLA, EOMI
Heart: NSR, no murmurs
Lungs: CTA

GU: Weak bladder tone, vaginal dryness
GI: normal BS
EXT: Normal

LABORATORY VALUES

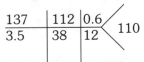

Total cholesterol: 260 mg/dL
Low-density lipoprotein (LDL) cholesterol: 160 mg/dL
High-density lipoprotein (HDL) cholesterol: 35 mg/dL
Triglycerides: 120 mg/dL
Follicle-stimulating hormone (FSH): > 20

Pap smear 6 months ago: Normal
Mammogram 1 year ago: Normal
Perform self breast exams once a month
Last menstrual period 8 months ago

MEDICATIONS

Tenomrin 50 mg PO qd
Atorvastatin 10 mg PO qd
Aspirin 81 mg PO qd
Imitrex 25 mg PO PRN at headache onset

QUESTIONS

1. All the following are symptoms of menopause *except*

    A. Amenorhhea for less than 6 months
    B. Hot flashes
    C. Vaginal dryness
    D. Urinary incontinence

2. An over-the-counter (OTC) menopause test kit such as the Estroven menopause monitor detects which of the following?

    A. Level of human chorionic gonadotropin (HCG) in the urine
    B. Level of follicle-stimulating hormone (FSH)
    C. Level of estrogen
    D. Level of progesterone

3. This patient has which of the following contraindications to using hormone-replacement therapy (HRT)?

    A. Coronary artery disease (CAD) risk factor
    B. History of DVT
    C. Family history of breast cancer
    D. All the above

4. Who are candidates for estrogen-alone therapy?

    A. Women who have contraindications to combination estrogen-progestin
    B. Women who have had a hysterectomy
    C. Women who experience hot flashes only
    D. Women who experience vaginal atrophy only

5. Premarin vaginal cream is most effective for what symptom?

    A. Hot flashes
    B. Emotional instability
    C. Vaginal atrophy
    D. Bone loss

6. What is the *most significant* difference between Prempro and Premphase?

    A. Prempo is associated more with increased risk of CAD and stroke.
    B. Premphase is associated more with increased risk of CAD and stoke.
    C. Prempro is associated with a brief period of spotting, followed by amenorrhea.
    D. The products contain different amounts of estrogen.

7. According to the Women's Health Initiative, published in July 2002, HRT is *not* associated with causing which of the following?

    A. Stroke
    B. CAD
    C. DVT
    D. Colon cancer

8. Assuming that this patient is not a candidate for HRT, what would be an option to manage her hot flashes?

    A. OTC herbal products that contain soy
    B. Esclim patches
    C. Increase her aspirin dose to help with flushing
    D. Raloxifine

9. Vaginal dryness can be managed by which of the following?

    A. Douching regularly
    B. OTC vagninal moisturizer (Gyne-Moistrin)
    C. HRT
    D. Kegal exercises

10. HRT benefits include which of the following?

    I. Prevention of bone loss
    II. Management of hot flashes and genitourinary atrophy
    III. Prevention of CAD

    A. I
    B. III
    C. I and II
    D. II and III

PATIENT PROFILE 204
ANGINA AND BLOOD CLOTTING

PRESENTATION

LW is a 55-year-old man who recently suffered from sudden fainting and sever chest pain. LW was admitted to the emergency room (ER), where an ECG was recorded immediately and an IV drip of nitroglycerin was administered. The ECG revealed some abnormalities and confirmed the occurrence of an acute anginal attack, but it has not progressed to myocardial infarction (MI). Blood tests indicated alarming signs of fast blood coagulation. After stabilizing

LW's condition with the nitroglycerin infusion, the physician sent LW home with several prescription medications to safeguard against future anginal attacks. The medications are aimed toward keeping his coronary arteries dilated, reducing the potential of blood clotting, and preventing long-term lipid deposition in the coronary arteries.

QUESTIONS

1. Why is nitroglycerin the drug of choice to alleviate sudden anginal attacks?

   A. It is a fast-acting coronary vasodilator.
   B. It decreases both preload and afterload.
   C. Nitroglycerin is a very stable drug, so it acts for a prolonged period.
   D. A and B
   E. A, B, and C

2. Considering the acid-base properties of nitroglycerin (structure 204.1), how do you think it is solubilized for IV infusion?

   A. As a sodium salt
   B. As a hydrochloride salt
   C. As is because it is water soluble
   D. As a solution in a mixture of water and propylene glycol
   E. None of the above

$$CH_2-ONO_2$$
$$CH\ ONO_2$$
$$CH_2-ONO_2$$
204.1

3. Which of the following list of drugs is(are) expected to target the blood coagulation aspect of LW?

   A. Aspirin (Structure 204.2)
   B. Clopedogril (Structure 204.3)
   C. Warfarin (Structure 204.4)
   D. A or B
   E. A, B, or C

204.2

204.3

204.4

4. Assuming that all the preceding drugs are useful to decrease the chances of internal blood clotting, which of the three medications is expected to act by inhibiting platelet aggregation?

   A. Aspirin
   B. Clopedogril
   C. Warfarin
   D. A and B
   E. A, B, and C

5. Which of the preceding medications is expected to show its blood-thinning action by an enzyme-inhibitory mechanism?

   A. Aspirin
   B. Clopedogril
   C. Warfarin
   D. A or B
   E. A, B, or C

6. What is the enzyme that is expected to be the target for decreasing blood clotting called?

   A. Dihydrofolate reductase
   B. Vitamin K reductase
   C. HMG-CoA reductase
   D. N-Acetyl transeferase
   E. None of the above

7. Which of the following drugs is(are) expected to decrease lipid deposition in the coronary arteries?

   A. Clofibrate (Structure 204.5)
   B. Atorvastatin (Structure 204.6)
   C. Clopedogril
   D. A or B
   E. A, B, or C

204.5

204.6

8. Which of the preceding drugs lowers cholesterol levels by enzyme inhibitory mechanism?

   A. Clofibrate
   B. Atorvastatin
   C. Clopedogril

D. A and B

E. A, B, and C

9. The enzyme that is expected to be the target for decreasing plasma cholesterol is called what?

A. Dihydrofolate reductase

B. Vitamin K reductase

C. HMG-CoA reductase

D. *N*-Acetyl transeferase

E. None of the above

10. Which of the following statements is(are) *true* about plasma cholesterol levels?

A. Total cholesterol of less than 200 mg/dL is desirable.

B. Low-density lipoprotein (LDL) cholesterol of less 130 mg/dL is desirable.

C. LDL:high-density lipoprotein (HDL) ratio under 3 is desirable

D. A and B

E. A, B, and C

PATIENT PROFILE 205
PARKINSON'S DISEASE

PRESENTATION

CC: Primary care physician (PCP) referral

HPI: The patient is a 74-year-old man who is referred to the neurology clinic because of progressive stiffness and difficulty walking and going down stairs, as reported by his family. He was discharged from the rehabilitation center 2 weeks ago and is recovering from a fractured shoulder. On examination, he is noted with expressionless face, staring gaze with limitation of gaze in all directions, and bradykinesia. Examination reveals tremor in his hands and arms, rigidity and stiffness of the limbs and trunk, bradykinesia, postural instability, and impaired coordination of gait.

PMH: Parkinson's disease (PD) × 5 years, hypertension × 10 years, benign prostatic hypertrophy (BPH) × 1 year, depression × 5 years, anemia, insomnia

Medications on admission: Sinemet (carbidopa-levodopa) 25/250 mg tid, selegiline (Eldepryl) 5 mg qd, trihexyphenidyl (Artane) 5 mg bid, fluoxetine (Prozac) 20 mg qd, lisinopril (Zestril) 5 mg qd, ferrous sulfate 325 mg tid, acetaminophen (Tylenol) 650 mg 2 tablets q4h PRN

ALL: Codeine

FH: Noncontributory

SH: Lives at home with wife; supportive family members (sons, daughters-in-laws, grandchildren involved with his care); retired radio broadcaster; no alcohol use; no tobacco use

PE: Pleasant, well-nourished man, notably distressed because he is unable to get up from his chair and ambulate.

HEENT: PERRLA, EOMI, MMM

Neck: Supple, (−) LAD

COR: RRR, (−) M/R/G

PULM: CTA

ABD: Soft, nontender, nondistended

EXT: Mild resting tremor; (+) DP

VS: Temperature: 99°F; blood pressure: 140/87 mm Hg; heart rate: 72 beats per minute; respiratory rate: 20 breaths per minute

Height: 5 ft, 8 in; weight: 165 lb

U/A: No bacteria, no sediment

LABORATORY VALUES (CHEM-7)

Na: 143	K: 4.7
Cl: 99	Total CO_2: XX
Blood ures nitrogen (BUN): 17	Serum Cr: 1.2
Glucose: 125	

QUESTIONS

1. Which of the following agents is used as a first-line agent to extend the time to levodopa treatment in the early stages of PD (<65 years-old)?

A. Dopamine replacement such as levodopa

B. catechol-*O*-methyltransferase (COMT) inhibitors such as entacapone (Comtan)

C. Dopamine agonists such as pramipexole (Mirapex)

D. Monoamine oxidase B inhibitor such as (Selegiline)

E. Anticholinergics such as trihexiphenidyl (Artane)

2. The initial response to levodopa is quite favorable and is termed the *honeymoon period*. How long does this usually last?

   A. 6 months
   B. 1 year
   C. 2 years
   D. 5 years
   E. 10 years

3. The "wearing off" effect from levodopa in this case may be *best managed* with the addition of which one of the following agents?

   A. COMT inhibitor
   B. Amantidine
   C. Dopamine agonist
   D. Vitamin E
   E. Coenzyme Q10

4. Why are anticholinergics such as trihexyphenidyl prescribed in the early stage of PD?

   A. To control insomnia
   B. To control tremor
   C. To control forgetfulness
   D. To control constipation
   E. All the above

5. Why should trihexyphenidyl be avoided in this patient with BPH?

   A. It may cause urinary retention.
   B. It may interact with sertraline.
   C. It may cause hyponatremia.
   D. It may cause insomnia.
   E. It may increase uric acid concentrations.

6. In advanced, late stages of PD, which of the following drugs would be expected to produce the *best* results?

   A. Levodopa-carbidopa (Sinemet)
   B. Tolcapone (Tasmar)
   C. Selegiline (Eldepryl)
   D. Amantidine (Symmetrel)
   E. Ropinirole (Requip)

7. Which of the following is *not* expected to be a side effect of levodopa therapy?

   A. Hypotension
   B. Tachycardia
   C. Hallucinations
   D. Mania/paranoid psychosis
   E. Nausea/vomiting

8. Dose-limiting side effects of levodopa are minimized when the drug is used in combination with a dopa de-carboxylase inhibitor, e.g., carbidopa. Which of the following statement(s) is(are) *true*?

   I. Carbidopa inhibits the peripheral conversion of levodopa to dopamine.
   II. Carbidopa does not penetrate the blood-brain barrier but increases the amount of dopamine to the brain.
   III. Carbidopa doses of 75 to 100 mg are needed to saturate peripheral dopa decarboxylase.

   A. I only
   B. III only
   C. I and II only
   D. II and III only
   E. I, II, and III

9. Which of the following is(are) consideration(s) when converting a patient from Sinemet to Sinemet CR?

   A. "Wearing off" effect
   B. Compliance
   C. Cost
   D. Bioavailability
   E. All the above

10. Which of the following drugs may markedly decrease absorption of levodopa through chelation?

    A. Selegiline
    B. Fluoxetine
    C. Trihexyphenidyl
    D. Ferrous sulfate
    E. Lisinopril

ANTICOAGULATION

CASE PRESENTATION

JF is a 66-year-old male who was recently hospitalized for pneumonia and developed a DVT during his hospital stay.

HPI:	During JF's hospitalization, he developed a DVT that was initially treated with heparin, then he was switched to warfarin. At discharge, his INR was 2.5. JR reports that he has been compliant with his medications since discharge 1 week ago.
PMH:	HTN, hyperlipidemia, DVT
PsurgH:	None
Drug Allergies:	IV contrast dye (rash)
Medication history:	Lisinopril 20 mg po qd, verapamil SR 240 mg po qd, lovastatin 40 mg po qd, warfarin 4 mg po qd
ROS:	JR denies any signs and symptoms of bleeding complications
Physical examination:	BP: 130/85 HR: 70 T: 98.2°F
A/P:	JR presents to the Anticoagulation Clinic 7 days after discharge with an INR of 5.

QUESTIONS

1. Which of the following statements may help explain JF's increased INR since discharge?

   A. JF's estimated maintenance dose was too high.
   B. JF's dietary intake of vitamin K has increased.
   C. Lovastatin could be increasing his INR.
   D. A and B
   E. A and C

2. What course(s) of action should be undertaken to initially treat JF's supratherapeutic INR?

   A. Administer vitamin K 10 mg IV × 1
   B. Hold the next dose and recheck INR
   C. Administer vitamin K 5 mg SQ × 1
   D. A and B
   E. B and C

3. When establishing a new warfarin maintenance dose and follow-up treatment plan for JF, what would you recommend?

   I. Decreasing the total weekly dose by 10–15%
   II. Decreasing the total weekly dose by 33%
   III. Rechecking the INR in 4 weeks
   IV. Rechecking the INR in 1-2 weeks

   A. I only
   B. I and III only
   C. I and IV only
   D. II and III only
   E. II and IV only

4. Based on JF's indication for anticoagulation, what is his INR goal?

   A. 1
   B. 1–2
   C. 2–3
   D. 2.5–3.5
   E. 3–4

5. Based on JF's indication how long should he be treated with warfarin?

   A. 1 month
   B. 3 months
   C. 9 months
   D. 12 months
   E. Lifelong

PARENTERAL NUTRITION

PRESENTATION

The equation for the resting metabolic equivalent (RME, Harris-Benedict equation, basal metabolic requirement, kcal/day requirement) for men is as follows:

$$RME = 66 + (13.7 \times weight) + (5 \times height) - (6.8 \times age)$$

The patient is 5 ft, 9 in tall, weighs 200 lb, and is 40 years of age. The patient has been hospitalized for a severe infection and has been categorized by the physician as being under moderate stress (1.6 stress factor according to hospital guidelines). The physician chooses to provide the patient with total parenteral nutrition with 60 percent of the calories from a lipid source and 0.9 g protein per kilogram of body weight. The pharmacy routinely uses 20% w/v lipid (emulsion) injection, 8.5% w/v amino acid injection, and 50% w/v dextrose injection.

QUESTIONS

1. What is the daily nonstressed kilocalorie requirement for this patient?

   A. 1789
   B. 1848
   C. 1914
   D. 2458
   E. 2879

2. What is the daily stressed kilocalorie requirement for this patient?

   A. 1196
   B. 1912.4
   C. 1914
   D. 1915.6
   E. 3062

3. How many total milliliters of lipid (emulsion) injection should be used daily to provide the allowed kilocalories from fat sources?

   A. 1020
   B. 1063
   C. 1701
   D. 9185
   E. 15,310

4. How many total milliliters of amino acid injection should be used daily to provide the allowed amount from protein sources?

   A. 962
   B. 1069
   C. 1188
   D. 2118
   E. 2353

5. How many total milliliters of dextrose injection should be used daily to provide the remaining kilocalories needed from dextrose?

   A. 528
   B. 1273
   C. 1796
   D. 1801
   E. Insufficient information provided

PATIENT PROFILE 208

GASTROINTESTINAL INFECTIONS

PRESENTATION

MM is a 75- year-old man who presents to the emergency department with a 1-day history of severe abdominal cramps, severe nausea, vomiting, chills, and several episodes of nonbloody diarrhea. He indicates that he usually never has diarrhea and has no real explanation for this. Upon further questioning he mentions that he celebrated his seventy-fifth birthday 2 days ago, and he had invited his family to a restaurant for a festive turkey dinner. Coincidently, just before coming to the emergency department his grandson and his wife called and told him of similar gastrointestinal symptoms, so he became concerned about a possible foodborne infection.

PMH: Hypertension
Hyperlipidemia
Colon cancer (finished radiation therapy 3 weeks ago)
s/p Gastrectomy
Coronary artery disease
Medications: Lisinopril 20 mg po qd
Hydrochlorothiazide 25 mg po qd

Aspirin 325 mg qd
Metoprolol 100 mg po qd
Pantoprazole 40 mg po qd
Allergies: NKDA
PE: BP 145/95 mm Hg, HR 75 beats/min, Temp 37.8°C; dry skin and mucous membranes
Labs: Na 134 mEq/L, K 3.2 mEq/L, Cl 99 mEq/L, bicarbonate 18 mEq/L, BUN 30 mg/dL, Scr 1.2 mg/dL, Glu 115 mg/dL, Hct 34%, WBC 4.0 K cells/mm^3, Plt 150/μL
A stool culture shows: fecal leukocytes, *Salmonella* sp.

QUESTIONS

1. All except which of the following statements about salmonella gastroenteritis are true?

   A. Salmonella usually causes a noninflammatory infection with watery diarrhea.
   B. The diagnosis of fecal leukocytes in the stool suggests inflammatory diarrhea associated with *Salmonella* sp.

C. Salmonella is an invasive pathogen.
D. Salmonella is commonly associated with contaminated poultry, poultry products (i.e., eggs), or water.
E. Salmonella gastroenteritis can cause both an uncomplicated gastroenteritis and a severe systemic infection called enteric fever.

2. The patient MM should be treated with which of the following?

A. Oral rehydration solutions containing 45 to 75 mEq of sodium (e.g., Pedialyte®)
B. Oral rehydration solutions (see A) and antibiotics
C. IV fluids (i.e., Ringer's lactate or NS) plus potassium and bicarbonate
D. IV fluids (see C) and antibiotics
E. Diluted fruit juices or other flavored soft drinks

3. MM is at risk for developing gastrointestinal infections and complications (e.g., bacteremia and extraintestinal infections) from *Salmonella* because of which of the following?

I. His underlying malignancy
II. Use of pantoprazole
III. History of gastrectomy
IV. Age

A. I only
B. I and IV
C. II and III
D. IV only
E. All of the above

4. Antibiotics that are effective for the treatment of *Salmonella* infections include all except which of the following?

I. Third-generation cephalosporins (i.e., ceftriaxone)
II. First-generation cephalosporins
III. Fluoroquinolones
IV. Aminopenicillins
V. Bactrim

A. I and II
B. III only
C. IV only
D. V only
E. All except II

5. Eleven months later MM sustains a severe fall and is admitted to the hospital with skin lacerations in his face accompanied by erythema and periorbital swelling. In addition to his regular medications, he receives IV clindamycin for the cellulitis as well as SQ heparin for DVT prevention. One week after admission he complains of watery diarrhea with greenish, foul-smelling stools and fever. His stool shows fecal leukocytes, and a rapid EIA test indicates Toxin A and B produced by *Clostridium difficile*. The patient is suspected to have *Clostridium difficile*-associated diarrhea (C-DAD). This infection most likely results from which of the following?

A. His previous antibiotic use for the Salmonella infection
B. His recent treatment with clindamycin
C. His treatment with SQ heparin
D. His history of gastrectomy
E. His history of colon cancer

6. Which of the following is the drug of choice for the treatment of *C. difficile*–associated diarrhea?

A. IV vancomycin 500 mg bid × 7 to 10 days
B. IV metronidazole 500 mg IV tid × 7 to 10 days
C. PO Metronidazole 500 mg tid × 7 to 10 days
D. PO Vancomycin 125 mg qid × 7 to 10 days
E. PO Bacitracin 80,000 U/day

7. Which of the following should the patient be counseled about in case he had received metronidazole?

I. The drug causes an unpleasant metallic taste.
II. Abstain from alcohol use while taking the drug.
III. The drug may cause central nervous system symptoms.
IV. Avoid antacids while taking the drug.

A. I only
B. II only
C. I, II, and III
D. IV only
E. I, II, and IV

8. MM's grandson and his wife (see Presentation) decide to go to South America for a 2-week vacation. Based on the unpleasant experience with their recent gastrointestinal infection (which subsided with nonpharmacologic measures) they ask for advice about prophylaxis for traveler's diarrhea (TD). Which of the following is the most appropriate measure?

I. Strictly adhere to nonpharmacologic prevention measures.
II. Take bismuth subsalicylate 2 tablets with meals and at bedtime (8 tab/day) for 2 weeks.
III. Take Bactrim DS qd for 2 weeks.
IV. Prophylax with levofloxacin 500 mg QD for 2 weeks.
V. Prophylax with loperamide.

A. All are excellent choices
B. I and II only

C. I and III only
D. I and IV only
E. I and V only

9. The use of bismuth subsalicylate (524 mg/dose) for prophylaxis (8 tab/day) may be associated with complications in which patients?

A. Those who take aspirin concurrently
B. Those who are elderly
C. Those who have renal disease
D. Those who have bleeding disorders
E. All of the above

10. Which of the following is not a correct treatment of traveler's diarrhea?

A. It is usually a self-limiting disease, and antibiotics are not necessary for patients with milder disease.
B. Loperamide with or without a single dose of fluoroquinolones is effective in mild to moderate illness.
C. Quinolones are the drug of choice.
D. Bactrim is the drug of choice.
E. A 1- to 3-day antibiotic course usually is sufficient.

PATIENT PROFILE 209

ANTICOAGULATION

PRESENTATION

MS is a 60-year-old obese white female who underwent elective abdominal surgery for hernia repair this morning.

PMH:	HTN, hypercholesterolemia, CHF
PsurgH:	None
Drug Allergies:	None
Medication history:	Losartan 50 mg po qd, digoxin 0.125 mg po qd, simvastatin 10 mg po qd
Physical examination:	BP: 130/80 HR: 68 T: 97.8°F Ht: 5'4" Wt: 198 lb
A/P:	After surgery, MS will be transferred to the general surgical floor of the hospital. The medical team anticipates that MS will be immobilized during her recovery and will need prophylactic anticoagulation.

QUESTIONS

1. What positive risk factor(s) does MS have which could lead to the development of post-surgical DVT?

A. Immobility
B. Age
C. Obesity
D. A and C
E. All of the above

2. What therapeutic interventions might decrease MS's risk of developing a post-surgical DVT?

A. Warfarin 10 mg IV q 12 hours
B. Warfarin dosed to an INR goal of 2.5–3.5
C. Heparin 5,000 units IM q 12 hours
D. Heparin 5,000 units SQ q 12 hours
E. ECASA 325 mg po qd

3. What laboratory monitoring parameter would you monitor to evaluate the effectiveness of MS's prophylactic anticoagulation?

A. aPTT
B. PT/INR
C. Bleeding time
D. Hematocrit
E. None of the above

4. What clinical signs and symptoms would you monitor for to evaluate the effectiveness of MS's prophylactic anticoagulation?

A. Chest pain and SOB
B. Redness and swelling of a lower extremity
C. Nausea, vomiting, and halovision
D. A and B
E. A and C

PATIENT PROFILE 210
TUBERCULOSIS

PRESENTATION

AS is a 25-year-old woman who arrives in the emergency department with fever, chills, night sweats, fatigue, weight loss, and a productive cough. These symptoms have persisted for a few weeks. She is a full-time pharmacy student and works on weekends in a hospital. Her medical history is significant for a seizure disorder. She was HIV-negative when tested 1 year ago. Medications on admission are phenytoin 300 mg/day, ibuprofen PRN, multivitamins daily, and Os-Cal® (calcium carbonate) 1000 mg/day. The purified protein derivative (PPD) skin test result is positive, and three sputum specimens contain acid-fast bacilli. Culture and susceptibility results are pending. A chest x-ray reveals extensive pulmonary consolidation. Lab data on admission include AST 22 IU/L, serum creatinine 0.8 mg/dL, BUN 7 mg/dL, and albumin 3.8 mg/dL. The phenytoin serum level at admission is 15 mg/L.

QUESTIONS

1. Tuberculosis is spread mainly by which of the following?

   A. Contact with items touched by an infected patient
   B. Inhaling infectious airborne particles coughed by an infected patient
   C. Contact with animals with tuberculosis
   D. Skin contact with an infected patient
   E. None of the above

2. Which of the following statement(s) is/are true regarding the proper administration and interpretation of the purified protein derivative (PPD) skin test for this patient?

   A. Administer an intradermal injection of 5 tuberculin units (5 TU) of PPD of killed tubercle bacilli on the inner forearm.
   B. The delayed-type hypersensitivity response to the PPD skin test should be examined and interpreted by a trained healthcare provider 48 to 72 hours after the injection.
   C. The delayed-type hypersensitivity response to the PPD skin test should be examined and interpreted by a trained health care provider 6 to 12 hours after the injection.
   D. A and B
   E. A and C

3. Which of the following statement(s) concerning isoniazid therapy is/are true?

A. AS should receive pyridoxine (vitamin B_6) with isoniazid.
B. AS should be counseled that isoniazid may impart an orange discoloration to urine, stool, sputum, saliva, tears, and sweat and that soft contact lenses may be permanently discolored.
C. AS should receive baseline examination of visual acuity before initiation of isoniazid therapy, followed by monthly eye examinations.
D. A and B
E. All of the above

4. The most toxic effect of ethambutol is which of the following?

   A. Hepatotoxicity
   B. Nephrotoxicity
   C. Ototoxicity
   D. Optic neuritis
   E. Tinnitus

5. Which of the following antituberculosis agents is appropriately listed with its class and potential adverse effect?

   A. Capreomycin; macrolide; hepatotoxicity
   B. Kanamycin; fluoroquinolone; central nervous system effects
   C. Paraaminosalicylic acid; pyrazine analogue of nicotinamide; hepatitis
   D. Rifabutin; synthetic derivative of rifamycin B; hematologic toxicity
   E. Cycloserine; analogue of amino acid D-alanine; aplastic anemia

6. The addition of rifampin therapy to a patient taking phenytoin may _____ phenytoin serum concentrations because of the _____ effect of rifampin.

   A. Increase, inhibitory
   B. Decrease, induction
   C. Decrease, inhibitory
   D. Increase, induction
   E. None of the above

7. Which of the following is the most toxic effect of pyrazinamide?

   A. Hepatotoxicity
   B. Optic neuritis

C. Nephrolithiasis
D. Peripheral neuropathy
E. Ototoxicity

8. Which of the following is a potentially life-threatening adverse effect of isoniazid?

A. Congestive heart failure
B. Hepatotoxicity
C. Aplastic anemia
D. Stroke
E. Pulmonary embolism

9. Which of the following toxicities is/are associated with streptomycin?

A. Nephrotoxicity
B. Ototoxicity
C. Anemia

D. A and B
E. All of the above

10. Which of the following statement(s) concerning rifampin therapy is/are true?

A. Patients receiving rifampin should be counseled to use alternative forms of birth control while taking this agent.
B. Patients should be counseled that rifampin may impart an orange discoloration to urine, stool, sputum, saliva, tears, and sweat and that soft contact lenses may be permanently discolored.
C. Rifampin is primarily eliminated through the kidneys. The dose must be adjusted if renal impairment occurs to prevent accumulation of the drug.
D. A and B
E. All of the above

PATIENT PROFILE 211

CHRONIC OBSTRUCTIVE PULMONARY DISEASE

PRESENTATION

AP is a 54-year-old obese man who presents to you complaining of increased productive cough, wheezing, and shortness of breath. AP is 5'10" and weighs 230 lbs. You have been evaluating AP for the past few years for his blood pressure and diabetes. This is the first time you have seen AP in a while, which he states is because of his busy schedule. AP informs you that he has had a new job for the last 2 years that requires him to work nights, limiting his ability to keep his normal daily routine. His current job is as security personnel at a nearby college. Before this change in profession he worked in a textile mill for 33 years. He states he has been compliant with his medications and feels good with the exception of his breathing problems. He does admit to not being compliant with the exercise and diet that was originally developed for him. AP still has not quit smoking and has a history of smoking 1 pack a day for the past 30 years. He also drinks occasionally, usually a "few mixed drinks" on the weekend. His parents are both deceased. They died in a car accident a few years ago and at that time both were diagnosed with bronchitis. AP is single and lives alone in his condominium in the middle of the city. He states he enjoys having the ability to go out in the city whenever he desires. His current medications are Zestril® every day for blood pressure, metformin every day for his diabetes, and a once-a-day multivitamin. This is the

first time you have seen AP in 2 years. His current fasting blood glucose is 140 and his HbA1c is 9%. AP's blood pressure is currently 145/90. Upon questioning, AP admits that his symptoms have progressed over this time, especially from September to December. His FEV_1/FVC is <70% and FEV_1 is 75% of personal best.

MH:
Zestril® 10 mg by mouth once a day
Metformin 500 mg by mouth twice a day
Daily multivitamin
Med History:
Diabetes for 3 years
Hypertension for 5 years

QUESTIONS

1. Based on AP's information, what classification is most appropriate?

A. Stage 0, at risk for COPD (chronic obstructive pulmonary disease)
B. Stage I, mild COPD
C. Stage II, moderate COPD
D. Stage III, severe COPD
E. Stage IV, very severe COPD

2. What is the best option for first-line chronic therapy for AP?

   A. Albuterol as needed and rehabilitation
   B. Albuterol as needed, theophylline 200 mg twice a day, and rehabilitation
   C. Albuterol as needed, salmeterol discus two puffs by mouth two times a day, and rehabilitation
   D. Albuterol as needed, flunisolide inhaler two puffs by mouth two times a day, and rehabilitation
   E. Albuterol as needed, Ipratropium inhaler two puffs by mouth three times a day, and rehabilitation

3. What is true concerning oxygen therapy in AP?

   I. Should be initiated once AP is placed in stage III.
   II. The decision to be initiated is based on AP's evening PaO_2.
   III. AP's goal of therapy is to attain an SaO_2 of at least 90%.

   A. I only
   B. III only
   C. I and III
   D. II and III
   E. I, II, and III

4. Which of the following classes of medications are contraindicated in AP?

   I. Antitussives
   II. Antioxidants
   III. Mucolytic agents

   A. I only
   B. III only
   C. I and III
   D. II and III
   E. I, II, and III

5. If AP had a documented anaphylactic allergy to peanuts, which of the following medications would he not be able to take?

   A. Albuterol
   B. Salmeterol
   C. Fluticasone
   D. Ipratropium
   E. Methylprednisolone

6. Which of the following is true concerning the use of antibiotics for AP?

   I. Daily prophylactic antibiotic therapy is not justified.
   II. Seasonal prophylactic antibiotic therapy is justified.
   III. When exacerbations are numerous, prophylaxis is justified in most clinical situations.

   A. I only
   B. III only

   C. I and III
   D. II and III
   E. I, II, and III

7. Which of the following is true concerning the use of inhaled corticosteroids in AP?

   I. Regular treatment with inhaled corticosteroids is appropriate when AP's FEV1 <50% predicted.
   II. The inflammation present in COPD is greatly suppressed by inhaled or oral corticosteroids.
   III. Long-term treatment with oral corticosteroids is recommended because of documented improvement in symptoms.

   A. I only
   B. III only
   C. I and III
   D. II and III
   E. I, II, and III

8. If AP was placed on an inhaled corticosteroid, which of the following is the most appropriate regimen?

   A. Triamcinolone inhaler one puff by mouth daily
   B. Beclomethasone inhaler two puffs by mouth daily
   C. Flunisolide inhaler two puffs by mouth two times a day
   D. Fluticasone inhaler two puffs by mouth three times a day
   E. Budesonide inhaler two puffs by mouth four times a day

9. Which of the following nicotine replacement products is available for over-the-counter purchase to assist AP in his attempt to quit smoking?

   I. Nicotine inhaler
   II. Nicotine lozenge
   III. Nicotine sublingual tablet

   A. I only
   B. III only
   C. I and II
   D. II and III
   E. I, II, and III

10. Which of the following prescription medications may be used to assist AP in his attempt to quit smoking?

   I. Zyban®
   II. Nortriptyline
   III. Clonidine

   A. I only
   B. III only
   C. I and II
   D. II and III
   E. I, II, and III

HYPERCHOLESTEROLEMIA

PRESENTATION

HH is a 50-year-old female who presents to her PCP for routine follow-up.

PMH:	PUD, TAH/BSO 5 years ago
PsurgH:	TAH/BSO
Drug Allergies:	None
Medication history:	Omeprazole 20 mg po qd, ibuprofen 200 mg q 6 hours prn, estrogen 0.625 mg po qd, calcium 500 mg po tid, MVI 1 tablet po qd, and an unidentified blue pill with markings for occasional headaches
Family history:	Negative for cardiac disease, hypertension, and diabetes; no family history of breast cancer
Social history:	Negative for smoking and alcohol; exercises daily—walking, swimming, mountain biking, etc.; avid reader
Physical examination:	BP: 120/80 HR: 60 Wt: 130 lb Ht: 5'5"
Labs:	Total cholesterol 250 mg/dL HDL: 48 mg/dL
A/P:	HH is a healthy, active 50-year-old female who presents with no complaints and is found to have an elevated total cholesterol.

QUESTIONS

1. To evaluate HH's medication history you would like to identify the "unknown" blue pill she takes for headaches. What reference would be most useful in identifying this product?

   A. Facts & Comparisons
   B. Identidex
   C. AHFS
   D. Medline
   E. Martindale

2. How many cardiovascular risk factors, besides hypercholesterolemia, does HH have?

   A. 0
   B. 1
   C. 2
   D. 3
   E. 4

3. Based on HH's presentation what is her LDL goal?

   A. <100 mg/dL
   B. <130 mg/dL
   C. <160 mg/dL
   D. <190 mg/dL
   E. None of the above

4. If HH were to be initiated on drug therapy, which of the following would be contraindicated?

   A. Lovastatin
   B. Niacin
   C. Gemfibrozil
   D. Cholestyramine
   E. Cholestipol

5. What benefit does estrogen have on HH's lipid profile?

   A. Increases her HDL
   B. Decreases her HDL
   C. Increases her LDL
   D. Increases her triglycerides
   E. Decreases her triglycerides

6. Although HH has been on estrogen replacement since her TAH, she would like to discontinue the estrogen because she is concerned about the potential risk of cancer. What would you recommend to HH?

   A. Discontinue the estrogen because she is at a high risk of developing breast cancer from the estrogen.
   B. Continue the estrogen because it offers numerous benefits such as prevention of osteoporosis and relief of menopausal symptoms.
   C. Switch to a synthetic estrogen product in order to decrease the risk of developing breast cancer related to the estrogen itself.
   D. Add cyclic progesterone to HH's regimen to decrease her risk of developing endometrial cancer.
   E. Add continuous progesterone to HH's regimen to decrease her risk of developing endometrial cancer.

P A T I E N T   P R O F I L E   2 1 3
^{99m}Tc-MAA CONSIDERATIONS

PRESENTATION

A nuclear pharmacist comes to the pharmacy every morning and prepares many kits for use in the nuclear medicine clinic that day. Among the radiopharmaceuticals she prepares is ^{99m}Tc-MAA. Four 10-mL kits normally are sufficient for the number of procedures performed by area nuclear medicine units each day.

QUESTIONS

1. Four 10-mL kits of ^{99m}Tc-MAA need to be prepared and made available by 9:30 AM, and the manufacturer recommends that no more than 60 mCi of activity be added to each kit. How many 4-mCi doses would be available at 9:30 AM if the ^{99m}Tc activity is added at 6:25 AM? Assume 100% radiochemical purity. The half-life of ^{99m}Tc is 6.02 hours.

   A. 42
   B. 22
   C. 62
   D. 12
   E. 52

2. When assaying radiochemical purity of the labeled MAA, which of the following is *correct* about thin-layer silica gel chromatography strips?

   A. Free ^{99m}TcO$_4^-$ will remain at the origin when acetone is the solvent.
   B. Free ^{99m}TcO$_4^-$ will remain at the origin when saline is the solvent.
   C. ^{99m}Tc-MAA will remain at the origin when acetone is the solvent.
   D. Hydrolyzed ^{99m}Tc will move with the solvent front when acetone is the solvent.
   E. ^{99m}Tc-MAA will move with the solvent front when saline is the solvent.

3. ^{99m}Tc-MAA containing particles larger than what size in diameter should be discarded?

   A. 90 μm
   B. 8 μm
   C. 75 μm
   D. 10 μm
   E. 150 μm

4. Which camera system is most useful for ^{99m}Tc imaging?

   A. SPECT
   B. PET
   C. CT
   D. RIA
   E. x-ray film

5. The emission of ^{99m}Tc is which of the following?

   A. α
   B. β$^-$
   C. β$^+$
   D. γ
   E. x-ray

6. ^{99m}Tc is in which oxidation state when it is first eluted from the generator?

   A. +1
   B. +4
   C. +5
   D. +6
   E. +7

7. At what time would all the MAA doses (above) have decayed such that a syringe that contained 4 mCi at 6:25 AM would now contain 1.5 mCi?

   A. 9:45 AM
   B. 6:25 PM
   C. 2:55 PM
   D. 12:05 PM
   E. 11:35 AM

8. The most common and economical shielding material for ^{99m}Tc-labeled radiopharmaceuticals is which of the following?

   A. Lead
   B. Lucite
   C. Steel
   D. Gold
   E. Titanium

9. ^{99m}Tc-MAA is used for which of the following?

   A. Thyroid imaging
   B. Liver and spleen imaging
   C. Renal imaging
   D. Lung imaging
   E. Cardiac imaging

10. "MAA" stands for which of the following?

    A. Myocardial administered antibody
    B. Macroaggregated albumin
    C. Myosin-active antibody
    D. Myoclonic-active actin
    E. Medulla affinity albumin

POST-TRAUMATIC STRESS DISORDER

PRESENTATION

GN is a 35-year-old man who presents to his primary care physician's office complaining of feeling afraid, depressed, and angry. He cannot sleep or eat. GN is in the Army Reserve and returned from a 10-month tour of duty in Iraq 2 months ago. He is a computer software engineer and has found returning to his job to be very stressful. He has had a hard time concentrating and is concerned about being fired. He and his wife have been arguing "more than usual" and he gets mad a lot. GN complains of recurrent nightmares of his time in Iraq, where he witnessed what he describes as "some pretty scary stuff." He notes that he often thinks about what he and his buddies experienced and he avoids situations (watching television or visiting with friends) that might trigger a flashback. GN's wife states that he has isolated himself from others and seems depressed and irritable most of the time.

Tobacco: One pack per day, started 9 months ago
Alcohol: Describes himself as a "moderate drinker" and acknowledges drinking one six-pack per day, noting that "it is the only way I can get any sleep lately."
Illicit drugs: Denies
Caffeine: Two to three cups per day in the morning to "get going"
FH: Married 7 years; two children (girl age 5, boy age 3). His wife is concerned about his drinking, which has increased since his return 2 months age. She is willing to participate in GN's treatment plan.
ROS: GN denies recent weight loss, fever, chills, shortness of breath, chest pain, seizures, nausea, vomiting, diaphoresis, constipation, or urinary incontinence. He complains of dull headaches that are made worse by stress and chronic insomnia.
Gen: Alert, cooperative, overweight man in no acute distress
VS: BP 150/100, HR 106, RR 16, Temp 98.8°F, Ht 6′ 3″, Wt 250 lbs
Allergies: NKDA
HEENT: Within normal limits
Cardiac: Tachycardia, NL rate and rhythm
Abd: Mild epigastric pain
Ext: Tinea pedis associated with onychomycosis; fine hand tremor
Neuro: A&O × 3; fine tremor, mild hyperreflexia in both hands; somewhat exaggerated startle when door slammed in office next door
Laboratory and Diagnostic Tests: None available at this time
Diagnosis: Post-traumatic stress disorder (PTSD)

QUESTIONS

1. Which of the following statements about post-traumatic stress disorder are true?

    I.   Everyone exposed to a traumatic event develops symptoms of PTSD.
    II. PTSD is characterized by symptoms of intrusive re-experiencing of the event and intense distress associated with the traumatic event.
    III. Symptoms of PTSD can cause significant impairment in social and occupational functioning.

    A I only
    B. III only
    C. I and II only
    D. II and III only
    E. I, II, and III

2. Why is GN at higher risk for developing PTSD?

    A. He is male.
    B. His trauma involves personal assault through combat.
    C. He is obese and has a sedentary job.
    D. He drinks more than two cups of coffee per day.
    E. He experienced his trauma in a foreign country.

3. Which of the following statements about the pharmacologic treatment of PTSD are true?

    I.   First-line medications in the treatment of PTSD are the selective serotonin reuptake inhibitors (SSRIs).
    II. Chronic use of benzodiazepines is generally ineffective in treating PTSD.
    III. Atypical antipsychotics do not appear to be useful in treating core PTSD symptoms.

    A. I only
    B. III only
    C. I and II only
    D. II and III only
    E. I, II, and III

4. The physician has decided to start sertraline for the treatment of PTSD symptoms in GN. Why is sertraline an appropriate choice?

    A. Sertraline is Food and Drug Administration (FDA) approved for the treatment of PTSD.
    B. Sertraline has no side effects when used to treat patients with PTSD.
    C. Sertraline is the only medication shown to be effective in the treatment of PTSD associated with combat.

D. Sertraline will also help to reduce symptoms of alcohol withdrawal when GN stops drinking.
E. Sertraline will also help reduce symptoms of nicotine withdrawal when GN stops smoking.

5. Which of the following is the most appropriate starting dose of sertraline for GN?

A. 25 mg per day
B. 50 mg per day
C. 75 mg per day
D. 100 mg per day
E. 150 mg per day

6. A prescription for sertraline can be filled with which one of the following?

A. Prozac
B. Celexa
C. Geodon
D. Zoloft
E. Effexor

7. Which one of the following medications would be the least helpful in the treatment of GN's PTSD symptoms?

A. Sertraline
B. Paroxetine
C. Citalopram
D. Fluvoxamine
E. Diazepam

8. GN returns for a follow-up visit 3 weeks later. He is experiencing no side effects to the sertraline but complains that his PTSD symptoms have not significantly improved. Which one of the following is the most appropriate physician response?

A. Discontinue the sertraline and start another SSRI.
B. Discontinue the sertraline and start an atypical antipsychotic.
C. Continue the sertraline at the current dose and add an atypical antipsychotic.

D. Continue the sertraline at the current dose because response to pharmacotherapy occurs gradually over 8 to 12 weeks or longer.
E. Continue the sertraline at the current dose for 2 more weeks and switch to another SSRI if complete response is not seen.

9. Which of the following statements about cognitive behavioral therapy (CBT) in the treatment of PTSD is/are true?

I. CBT alone is useful for the treatment of mild, moderate, and severe symptoms of PTSD.
II. CBT alone may be appropriate for initial treatment of mild symptoms of PTSD.
III. CBT should be combined with pharmacotherapy for the treatment of moderate to severe symptoms of PTSD.

A. I only
B. III only
C. I and II only
D. II and III only
E. I, II, and III

10. GN experiences a response in his PTSD symptoms after 3 months of sertraline. He wants to know when he can discontinue the sertraline. Which one of the following is the most appropriate response?

A. He can begin to taper his dose of sertraline immediately and discontinue it in 1 to 2 weeks.
B. He can decrease his dose of sertraline by 50% and if his symptoms do not return in 1 to 2 weeks he can discontinue the sertraline.
C. He can discontinue the sertraline immediately because sertraline does not cause dependence.
D. He should continue the sertraline at the current dose for an additional 8 to 12 weeks just to be sure that his symptoms have resolved.
E. He should continue the sertraline at the current dose for an additional 6 to 12 months to prevent relapse of his symptoms.

PATIENT PROFILE 215

HYPERCHOLESTEROLEMIA

PRESENTATION

TA is a 60-year-old male who presents to the Lipid Clinic for follow-up.

PMH: Post-MI × 2 years, hypercholesterolemia × 10 years, BPH × 2 years, osteoarthritis × 5 years, hypertension × 5 years, COPD × 10 years

Psurg Hx: Left knee replacement 4 years ago
Drug Allergies: ASA (bronchospasm)
Medication history: Lovastatin 40 mg po bid, terazosin

5 mg po qd, metoprolol 25 mg po bid, albuterol 2 puffs prn, ipratropium bromide 2 puffs tid, and a product his brother sends to him from France to treat his BPH

Family history: Father died of an MI at 65, mother is alive at the age of 82 with history of HTN and CHF

Social history: Positive for smoking 1 ppd for 40 years and negative for alcohol

Physical examination: BP: 136/88 HR: 74 Wt: 170 lb Ht: 5'7"

Labs: Cholesterol 230 mg/dL LDL 140 mg/dL HDL 36 mg/dL

A/P: TA is a 60-year-old male with several cardiovascular risk factors, including a history of a prior MI, whose hypercholesterolemia is still uncontrolled.

QUESTIONS

1. To completely evaluate TA's medication history, you would like to know the name of the product that he is using from France. He does not recall the name of the product but he is willing to call you back with its name. Once you have this information, what resource would you use to identify this product?

   A. Facts & Comparsions
   B. AHFS
   C. Martindale
   D. Drug Information Handbook
   E. PDR

2. What is TA's LDL goal?

   A. <100 mg/dL
   B. <130 mg/dL
   C. <160 mg/dL
   D. <190 mg/dL
   E. None of the above

3. How does smoking affect TA's lipid profile?

   A. Decreases his LDL
   B. Decreases his HDL
   C. Increases his HDL
   D. Decreases his triglycerides
   E. Increases his triglycerides

4. In general, what effects do alpha blockers such as terazosin have on lipids?

   A. Increases LDL
   B. Decreases LDL
   C. Increases total cholesterol
   D. Decreases total cholesterol
   E. Increases triglycerides

5. How often do you check the CPK in a patient such as TA who is maintained on lovastatin?

   A. Every 2–4 weeks during the first 3 months of therapy
   B. Four to 8 weeks after a dosage change
   C. Every 6–8 weeks during the first year
   D. Only when the patient has unexplained symptoms of myopathy
   E. Only when the patient has unexplained symptoms of abdominal pain

6. What laboratory parameters are routinely checked in patients receiving a "statin" for hypercholesterolemia?

   A. Liver function tests
   B. Thyroid function tests
   C. Renal function tests
   D. Complete blood counts
   E. Red blood cell indicies

7. With respect to TA's current lipid profile, what would you recommend?

   A. Discontinue atenolol
   B. Increase lovastatin
   C. Add cholestyramine
   D. Add gemfibrozil
   E. Add probucol

8. Once you make the above modification in TA's therapy, when would you recommend rechecking TA's lipid profile?

   A. 2 weeks
   B. 4 weeks
   C. 3 months
   D. 6 months
   E. 1 year

9. Although you have discussed smoking cessation with TA numerous times, you want to readdress this issue with him. What would you stress as the benefit(s) of smoking cessation?

   A. The risk of various forms of cancer decreases with smoking cessation.
   B. The risk of myocardial infarction decreases with smoking cessation.
   C. The risk of stroke decreases with smoking cessation.
   D. The risk of chronic obstructive airways disease decreases with smoking cessation.
   E. All of the above

10. TA is willing to make an attempt at smoking cessation. He wants you to recommend an OTC transdermal nicotine product for him. What factor(s) should be considered when making your recommendation?

   A. TA's past medical history
   B. TA's hepatic function
   C. TA's renal function
   D. A and B
   E. A and C

11. After selecting an appropriate transdermal product for TA, you counsel him in regard to what to expect and how to use the product. Which of the following statements would be included in your counseling session?

   A. Transdermal products have caused some local irritation at the site of application; therefore, site rotation is very important.
   B. Gastrointestinal effects such as diarrhea or nausea have been reported with transdermal nicotine products although more commonly reported with other delivery systems.
   C. TA should also seek out a behavioral modification program in order to increase his chance of success with smoking cessation.
   D. Since weight gain is a common deterrent to successful nicotine cessation, TA should be advised to modify his diet and exercise program accordingly.
   E. All of the above

PATIENT PROFILE 216

METABOLIC SYNDROME

PRESENTATION

MJ is a 58-year-old black man who was noted to have elevated total cholesterol (220 mg/dL) during a community screening program 2 months ago. Follow-up lipid levels performed at his physician's office revealed the following.

Labs: TC 203 mg/dL, TG 185 mg/dL, HDL 35 mg/dL, LDL 131 mg/dL
PMH: Hypertension for 9 years; newly diagnosed type 2 diabetes
SH: Smokes one pack per day; retired school teacher; EtOH (12 oz/month).
FH: Father died of a heart attack at 52 years of age; mother died at 78 years of age from unknown causes; 59-year-old sister who is alive and a type 2 diabetic
MH: HZTC 25 mg po qd for 5 years; no pertinent over-the-counter drug use; NKDA
ROS: Noncontributory
PE: BP 156/86 right arm, seated (average of three readings); BMI 32 kg/m^2; waist circumference 42 inches; Rest of examination unremarkable
Laboratory Values: Fasting glucose 130 mg/dL; Na$^+$ 137 mEq/L; Cl$^-$ 95 mEq/L; BUN 16 mg/dL; serum creatinine 1.4 mg/dL; albumin 3.1 mg/dL; PT 13.9; AST 25: ALT 19

QUESTIONS

1. What is MJ's target LDL level?

   A. <100 mg/dL
   B. <130 mg/dL
   C. <160 mg/dL
   D. <140 mg/dL
   E. <70 mg/dL

2. How many of the risk factors does MJ have for metabolic syndrome?

   A. 1
   B. 2
   C. 3
   D. 4
   E. 5

3. How many risk factors for metabolic syndrome must a patient exhibit to be diagnosed as having metabolic syndrome?

   A. 1
   B. 2
   C. 3
   D. 4
   E. 5

4. The physician has initiated therapeutic lifestyle changes but wants to initiated drug therapy. Which of the following statins has the greatest potential to lower MJ's LDL enough and elevate MJ's HDL enough when given alone?

   A. Lovastatin
   B. Fluvastatin
   C. Simvastatin
   D. Rosuvastatin
   E. Pravastatin

5. Which of the following lipid lowering medications may make it more difficult to control MJ's diabetes?

   A. Cholestyramine
   B. Pravastatin
   C. Fenofibrate
   D. Atorvastatin
   E. Niacin

6. Which of the following medications would be most beneficial to add to MJ's statin therapy?

   A. Fenofibrate
   B. Colesevelam
   C. Colestipol
   D. Fluvastatin
   E. Ezetimibe

7. What is the maximum daily dose of fenofibrate?

   A. 1200 mg daily
   B. 600 mg daily
   C. 1000 mg daily
   D. 200 mg daily
   E. 300 mg daily

8. When combining a fibrate and statin to treat a dyslipidemia there may be an increased risk of developing which of the following adverse reactions?

   A. Myopathy
   B. Gall stones
   C. Renal dysfunction
   D. Arrhythmias
   E. Heart failure

9. On what other medication should JW be initiated?

   A. Metoprolol
   B. Warfarin
   C. Aspirin
   D. Fish oil
   E. Atorvastatin

10. Which of the following statins is known to lower serum LDL levels by the least amount?

    A. Atorvastatin
    B. Fluvastatin
    C. Simvastatin
    D. Rosuvastatin
    E. Pravastatin

PATIENT PROFILE 217

OSTEOPOROSIS

PRESENTATION

TH is a 74-year-old white woman who presents to the Family Health Center for a follow-up visit for her hypertension (HTN) and osteoporosis. She has been experiencing episodes of nausea since she began taking Os-Cal 500® after her last clinic visit.

PMH: HTN (× 30 years)
Hypothyroidism
Osteoporosis
Esophageal stricture
Breast cancer (at 46 years old)
Menopause (at 52 years old)
PSH: Left breast mastectomy
Allergies: None
Meds: Amlodipine (Norvasc®) 10 mg po qd
Atenolol 50 mg po qd
Levothyroxine (Synthroid®) 75 μg po qd
Calcium carbonate (Os-Cal 500®) po tid × 3 months
FH: Mother has osteoporosis and DM; father has HTN, hypercholesterolemia
SH: Widowed, no children/no pregnancies

ROS: Chronic back pain; height has decreased by 2" since she was 45 years old
PE: BP 158/84, pulse 68, RR 14, Temp 99.6°F, Ht 5'3", Wt 65.8 kg
Gen: WDWN white woman in NAD
Skin: Normal
HEENT: Funduscopic examination reveals mild arteriolar narrowing
Neck: Normal
Chest: Normal
CV: Normal
Abd: Normal
Ext: Normal
Neuro: Normal
Labs: TSH 3.5 μIU/mL
Other: Bone mineral density measured 4 months ago

L 2–4 = 0.780 g/cm² (t-score − 3.5 SD)
R femoral neck = 0.615 g/cm² (t-score − 3 SD)

QUESTIONS

1. Which of the following is considered the "gold standard" bone mineral density test for osteoporosis diagnosis?

   A. Dual energy x-ray absorptiometry
   B. Magnetic resonance imaging
   C. Quantitative computed tomography
   D. Single energy x-ray absorptiometry
   E. Ultrasound

2. Which of the following is a factor that places TH at risk for development of osteoporosis?

   A. Age
   B. Family history
   C. Thyroid replacement therapy
   D. A and C only
   E. A, B, and C

3. Which of the following indicates the presence or severity of TH's osteoporosis?

   A. Chronic back pain
   B. DEXA (dual energy x-ray absorptiometry) results
   C. Loss of height
   D. A and C only
   E. A, B, and C

4. Which of the following is a goal of pharmacotherapy for osteoporosis in TH?

   A. Increase bone mass
   B. Prevent falls
   C. Prevent fractures (and maintain height)
   D. A and C only
   E. A, B, and C

5. Which of the following best represents the daily calcium requirement of TH (according to the Institute of Medicine)?

   A. 210 mg
   B. 500 mg
   C. 800 mg
   D. 1000 mg
   E. 1200 mg

6. Which of the following best represents the daily vitamin D requirement of TH (according to the Institute of Medicine)?

   A. 50 IU
   B. 100 IU
   C. 200 IU
   D. 400 IU
   E. 600 IU

7. Which of the following medications is the most appropriate choice for the management of osteoporosis in TH?

   A. Alendronate
   B. Calcitonin (nasal)
   C. Estrogen
   D. Raloxifene
   E. Teriparatide

8. Which of the following food allergies is a contraindication to calcitonin use?

   A. Eggs
   B. Milk
   C. Peanut
   D. Salmon
   E. Wheat

9. Which of the following is a potential adverse effect of raloxifene?

   A. Endometrial cancer
   B. Esophagitis
   C. Seizures
   D. Thromboembolism
   E. Tremor

10. Which of the following best represents when TH should have a follow-up bone mineral density measurement to monitor therapy?

   A. 2 days
   B. 1 to 2 weeks
   C. 2 to 6 months
   D. 1 to 2 years
   E. 5 to 10 years

PATIENT PROFILE 218

ALZHEIMER'S DISEASE

PRESENTATION

MS is a 91-year-old woman who presents to the pharmacy with her daughter for monthly refills and with a new prescription for donepezil (Aricept®). According to her daughter, MS is newly diagnosed with Alzheimer's disease. Her daughter noticed that MS was getting excessively forgetful. She states that she cannot rely on her mother to care for herself; MS has forgotten at times that the stove is on. She also forgets people's names and where she has put things. MS has been confusing her medications lately and sometimes takes either two of one medication or none at all. MS's blood pressure is not under control and she has experienced urinary incontinence. Her daughter has insisted that MS move in with her even though MS does not think that anything is wrong.

PMH: Urinary incontinence
GERD
Hypertension
Med Hx: Oxybutynin 5 mg bid
2004 Refill History: 1/5/04, 4/5/04, 7/2/04,
    8/21/04, 9/19/04
Pantoprazole 40 mg po qd
1/5/04, 3/7/04, 4/5/04, 5/8/04, 7/2/04, 7/30/04,
    9/5/04
Furosemide 20 mg
1/5/04, 2/2/04, 3/7/04, 4/5/04, 5/8/04, 6/7/04,
    7/2/04, 8/21/04, 9/19/04
OTC/ Herbal use is unknown
Allergies: NKDA
FH: MS has one daughter age 65 with hypertension. Her husband died of a heart attack in 2002 at age 88.
SH: MS currently is moving in with her 65-year-old daughter. She has lived alone since her husband died but now requires constant monitoring so she does not harm herself.
Labs: Unavailable
PE: BP 145/95 mm Hg, taken by the pharmacist

PROBLEM LIST

1. Alzheimer's disease
2. Hypertension
3. GERD
4. Urinary incontinence

QUESTIONS

1. Which of the following is considered diagnostic criteria for Alzheimer's disease?

   A. Impaired memory
   B. Aphasia
   C. Agnosia
   D. All of the above

2. Alzheimer's disease involves a neurochemical imbalance of which of the following neurotransmitters?

   A. Dopamine
   B. Acetylcholine
   C. Serotonin
   D. Norepinephrine

3. MS's physician would like to initiate therapy with donepezil (Aricept®). Which of the following is the appropriate starting dose for MS?

   A. 5 mg po qam
   B. 10 mg po qhs
   C. 5 mg po bid
   D. 10 mg po bid

4. What is the mechanism of action of donepezil (Aricept®)?

   A. Reversible inhibition of dopamine
   B. Irreversible inhibition of dopamine
   C. Irreversible inhibition of acetylcholine
   D. Reversible inhibition of acetylcholine

5. Which of the following is a side effect of donepezil (Aricept®)?

   A. Diarrhea
   B. Urinary incontinence
   C. Constipation
   D. Dry mouth

6. What is the probable cause of MS's high blood pressure reading?

   A. Inadequate drug therapy
   B. Inadvertent noncompliance
   C. Alzheimer's disease
   D. The need to change to an ACE inhibitor

7. Which of the following constitute the goals of therapy for Alzheimer's patients?

   A. Slow progression of the disease
   B. Provide a cure
   C. Maintain a level of independence
   D. A and C only

8. At what point should therapy with donepezil (Aricept®) be discontinued and switched to another drug therapy because of lack of efficacy?

   A. 2 weeks
   B. 1 month
   C. 3 months
   D. 6 months

9. MS's physician wants to add Namenda® to the current regimen. What is the mechanism of action of Namenda®?

   A. MAO-B inhibition
   B. Antioxidant
   C. Serotonin reuptake inhibitor
   D. NMDA receptor antagonist

10. MS's daughter is interested in adding gingko biloba to MS's drug therapy. What is the proposed mechanism of action for gingko biloba in Alzheimer's disease?

    A. Cytotoxic
    B. Antioxidant
    C. MAO-B inhibition
    D. Antipsychotic

PATIENT PROFILE 219

TYPE 1 DIABETES

PRESENTATION

SS is a 17-year-old high school student who presents to the family medicine clinic for follow-up with her primary care physician after being discharged from the hospital for dehydration and ketoacidosis. A fasting and random plasma glucose were ordered subsequently and revealed levels of 200 and 265 mg/dL, respectively. SS has been under a lot of stress lately applying to colleges, studying for the SATs, and running for senior class president. Upon further questioning, she states that she has had mild symptoms of polydipsia, nocturia, fatigue, and a 15-lb weight loss, which she attributed to stress.

PMH: Recurrent upper respiratory infections
FH: Noncontributory
Meds: Ortho TriCyclen 1 tab po qd
NPH Insulin 12 U SC bid (started in hospital)
Regular insulin by sliding scale (started in hospital)
Allergies: Penicillin rash
Vitals: BP 120/78, HR 62, RR 14, Temp 98.4°C,
    Ht 5′4″, Wt 50 kg
HEENT: PERRLA, MMM
Cor: RRR, no MRG
Chest: Clear bilaterally
Abd: No mass, NT/ND, +BS
Ext: No edema, +DTR's
Neuro: Cranial nerves II to XII intact
Labs: FPG 280 mg/dL, HgbA1c 14%, urine glucose 2+,
    urine ketones: trace

QUESTIONS

1. An apparent remission of diabetes resulting in a decrease in blood glucose and a decrease in insulin requirements in newly diagnosed patients is called which of the following?

    A. Somogyi effect
    B. Dawn phenomenon
    C. Honeymoon phase
    D. Gluconeogenesis
    E. Hypoglycemic unawareness

2. Which of the following are needed to make a diagnosis of diabetes mellitus according to the diagnostic criteria set by the American Diabetes Association?

    A. A fasting blood glucose >110 mg/dL
    B. Classic symptoms of diabetes and a random BG >200 mg/dL

    C. HgbA1C >7%
    D. A blood glucose of >140 mg/dL 2 hours after an oral glucose tolerance test
    E. All of the above

3. In what situations should patients with type 1 diabetes test their urine for the presence of ketones?

    I.   When their blood glucose is >300 mg/dL
    II. When their blood glucose is <60 mg/dL
    III. Every 3 months

    A. I only
    B. III only
    C. I and II only
    D. II and III only
    E. I, II, and III

4. Which of the following statements is true about the pharmacokinetic properties of insulin?

    A. The dose may need to be reduced in patients with renal failure.
    B. The rate-limiting step of insulin action is degradation of insulin by the liver.
    C. Absorption rates are easy to predict because of small levels of inter-patient variability.
    D. Human insulin is the most immunogenic form of insulin available.
    E. All of the above

5. Which is the best match of insulin type and pharmacokinetic characteristics?

    A. Regular: onset 15 to 30 min, peak 1 to 3 hours, duration 3 to 4 hours
    B. Glargine: onset 6 hours, peak 18 to 24 hours, duration 24+ hours
    C. Lispro: onset 15 to 30 minutes, peak 30 to 90 minutes, duration 3 to 4 hours
    D. NPH: onset 1 to 3 hours, peak 18 to 20 hours, duration 36+ hours
    E. None of the above

6. Which of the following statements best describes insulin glargine?

    A. Its activity closely resembles the physiologic release of insulin from the pancreas in response to food.
    B. It is a formulation in which insulin is co-crystallized with protamine to make an intermediate-acting insulin.

C. It has a lower pH, which causes precipitate formation on injection.

D. It can be mixed safely with other insulin types.

E. All of the above

7. Which of the following statements about insulin pumps is/are true?

A. Allow patients to test their blood glucose less frequently than those on intensive insulin injection regimens.

B. Regimens include a basal rate and meal time boluses.

C. They are more efficacious at controlling blood glucose than intensive split regimens involving insulin injections.

D. All of the above

8. Which of the following is a valid counseling point about the administration of insulin?

A. You must clean injection site with alcohol before injecting insulin.

B. Inject air equaling the amount of insulin that will be withdrawn into the insulin vial to prevent the creation of a vacuum.

C. Be sure to rotate injections sites among the arms, thighs, abdomen, and buttock.

D. B and C

E. All of the above

9. Which of the following is the most common side effect associated with insulin therapy?

A. Hypotension

B. Rash

C. Hypoglycemia

D. Hypernatremia

E. Anemia

10. Which of the following is/are reasonable treatments for a patient experiencing acute hypoglycemia?

I. Glyburide

II. Dextrose

III. Glucagon

A. I only

B. III only

C. I and II only

D. II and III only

E. I, II, and III

PATIENT PROFILE 220

OBESITY

PRESENTATION

EL is a 56-year-old obese man who presents to the diabetes clinic for evaluation. EL states that he has diabetes and he has come to the clinic to check on his overall health. EL was diagnosed with type 2 diabetes 9 months ago, GERD 2 years ago, hypercholesterolemia 5+ years ago, and hypertension 10+ years ago. EL also has osteoarthritis in both knees; he ambulates slowly with a limp and uses a cane for support. He has been feeling very depressed about his declining health; at his last check-up his primary care physician initiated treatment with paroxetine.

PMH: Osteoarthritis (both knees) × 1 year
Depression × 2 months
Type 2 diabetes × 9 months
GERD × 2 years
Hypertension × 10+ years
Hypercholesterolemia × 5+ years
FH: Both mother and father had hypertension and type 2 diabetes. Two sons, ages 22 and 19, are healthy with no known disorders.

SH: EL works as a mortgage broker. He states that this is a very busy and high-stress job. He admits that he rarely has time to prepare or even to eat a "good" meal at work so he often eats fast food. He also admits to minimal physical activity; he sits behind a desk all day, then is too tired to exercise when he gets home.
MedHx: Paroxetine 20 mg qd
Lansoprazole 30 mg qd
Atorvastatin 10 mg po qhs
Lisinopril 10 mg qd
Novolin® 70/30 32 units SQ q.a.m. and 18 units q.p.m.
APAP 1000 mg q6 prn knee pain
Denies current use of any other over-the-counter and herbal drugs
Allergies: NKDA
ROS:
GI: Heartburn two to three times per week, managed with lansoprazole
Ext: Complains of constant pain in both knees
Gen: Obese male, walks with notable discomfort

VS: BP 134/84; HR 72 bpm, Ht 5′10″, Wt 160 kg (352 lbs), BMI 50.6 kg/m^2

Labs: Plasma blood glucose 131 mg/dL (nonfasting), Tchol 198 mg/dL, HDL 42 mg/dL

QUESTIONS

1. What is EL's ideal body weight?

   A. 68.5 kg
   B. 78.6 kg
   C. 150.7 lbs
   D. 160.6 lbs
   E. 317.3 lbs

2. What is a reasonable 6-month goal weight for EL?

   A. 68.5 kg
   B. 78.6 kg
   C. 150.7 lbs
   D. 160.6 lbs
   E. 317.3 lbs

3. Which of EL's conditions may be associated with his obesity?

   I. Depression
   II. GERD
   III. Hypertension

   A. I only
   B. III only
   C. I and II
   D. II and III
   E. I, II, and III

4. EL would like to start "dieting." Which of the following diet plans would you recommend?

   A. A low-carbohydrate plan such as the South Beach diet
   B. A high-fat, low-carbohydrate plan such as the Atkins diet
   C. A low-fat diet such as the Pritikin or Ornish diet
   D. A diet that offers group support such as Weight Watchers
   E. A balanced plan such as the Zone diet

5. Which of the following is/are appropriate recommendations for EL about his caloric intake?

   I. Only a reduction of dietary fat is necessary because fat is highest in calories.
   II. Consume less than 800 calories per day.
   III. Reduce caloric intake by 500 to 1000 calories per day.

   A. I only
   B. III only

C. I and II
D. II and III
E. I, II, and III

6. Which of the following statements about obesity and weight loss is/are true?

   I. Obesity is a chronic condition that requires lifelong effort.
   II. Weight loss should be achieved rapidly to ensure success.
   III. Once a patient achieves the goal weight, his or her obesity is considered cured.

   A. I only
   B. III only
   C. I and II
   D. II and III
   E. I, II, and III

7. EL's cardiologist thinks that bupropion is a more appropriate antidepressant for EL. Do you agree?

   A. No, the most suitable antidepressant for EL is escitalopram.
   B. No, there is no reason to alter EL's antidepressant therapy.
   C. No, the most suitable antidepressant for EL is mirtazapine.
   D. Yes, bupropion has been associated with weight loss.
   E. Yes, paroxetine is an inappropriate choice given that it may interact with EL's lisinopril.

8. What is the brand name of sibutramine?

   A. Bontril®
   B. Didrex®
   C. Meridia®
   D. Tenuate®
   E. Xenical®

9. Which of the following statements about sibutramine is/are true?

   I. Sibutramine is approved for weight loss and weight maintenance.
   II. The starting dose sibutramine is 10 mg daily.
   III. Concurrent use of sibutramine with dextromethorphan may cause serotonin syndrome.

   A. I only
   B. III only
   C. I and II
   D. II and III
   E. I, II, and III

10. Which of the following statements about phentermine is/are true?

I.   Phentermine is approved for weight loss and weight maintenance.
II. Phentermine is DEA schedule IV.
III. Phentermine is contraindicated in patients with hypertension.

A. I only
B. III only
C. I and II
D. II and III
E. I, II, and III

PATIENT PROFILE 221

PLAGUE

PRESENTATION

DA is a 54-year-old man visiting from Arizona who presents to the emergency department complaining of extreme fatigue and swelling on one side of his groin for 2 days. He contacted his primary care physician at home and was instructed to go to the emergency department. He has had a fever of 103°F and inguinal swelling for 2 days.

PMH: DA has hypertension that he says is controlled with medication and has seasonal allergies.

SH: Patient denies tobacco use. He says he drinks at least two cups of coffee each day and one or two beers a week. He lives with his wife. He is retired from the military.

FH: Both of DA's parents are deceased; mother at age 70 and father at age 76. Not sure of cause.

Gen: Well-nourished middle-age man, very ill, diaphoretic, rigors and lower extremity cyanosis.

VS: BP 78/50 mm Hg, pulse 50 ppm, Ht 5'8", Wt 185 lbs, Temp 104°F.

HEENT: Cervical lymph nodes tender and slightly swollen with mild edema in surrounding area

Chest: Apparent diaphoresis, rigors

CV: No murmurs, gallops, or rubs

Abd: Tender swollen unilateral inguinal swelling surrounded with edema

Ext: Lower extremities showing signs of cyanosis, small pustule on leg

Labs: White blood cell count 23,000/mm^3 (5000 to 10,000/mm^3)

Blood culture: Gram-negative rods with a "safety pin" appearance

Medications:

HCTZ 25 mg po qd

Allegra 180 mg po qd prn seasonal allergies

Diagnosis:

Bubonic plague

QUESTIONS

1. Which of the following is the causative organism of plague?

A. Variola
B. *Bacillus anthracis*
C. *Yersinia pestis*
D. *Francisella tularensis*

2. What is the most common natural form of plague?

A. Bubonic
B. Pneumonic
C. Septicemic
D. All of the above

3. Which of the following is the typical incubation period of bubonic plague?

A. 2 to 10 days
B. 2 to 10 days
C. 1 to 6 days
D. 2 to 14 days

4. Treatment for pneumonic plague must occur within 24 hours to be effective. What is the recommended treatment per the Centers for Disease Control and Prevention (CDC) guidelines?

A. Ciprofloxacin 500 mg po q12 hours
B. Doxycycline 100 mg po q12 hours
C. Streptomycin 1 g intramuscularly q12 hours
D. Gentamicin 1 to 1.7 mg/kg intravenously q8 hours
E. C or D

5. How long should the treatment be administered?

A. 5 days
B. 7 days
C. 10 days
D. 20 days
E. 60 days

6. To what class of antibiotic do streptomycin and gentamicin belong?

A. Fluoroquinolones
B. Aminoglycosides

C. Penicillins
D. Macrolides

7. What adverse reaction is a concern with this class of drugs?

A. Discoloration of teeth
B. Nephrotoxicity
C. Ototoxicity
D. Gastrointestinal upset
E. B and C only

8. Chloramphenicol can be used as an adjunct therapy for plague meningitis. What dose-dependent adverse reaction has been associated with this drug?

A. Ataxia
B. Blood dyscrasia

C. Alopecia
D. Xerostomia

9. Prophylaxis treatment for exposure to plague includes which of the following?

A. Doxycycline 100 mg po bid
B. Tetracycline 500 mg po bid
C. Erythromycin 250 mg po bid
D. Amoxicillin 500 mg po bid

10. Outdated or degraded tetracycline has been associated with what syndrome?

A. Stevens-Johnson
B. Red man
C. Fanconi's
D. Raynaud's

PATIENT PROFILE 222

SCHIZOPHRENIA

PRESENTATION

BD is a 47-year-old black man with paranoid schizophrenia. He has been treated in the past with chlorpromazine 200 mg tid with fair efficacy but poor compliance. Currently he is not taking anything for schizophrenia.

PMH: Diabetes mellitus type 2
Osteoarthritis in left knee
Alcohol dependence (sober × 2 years)
Hypertriglyceridemia
Meds: Acetaminophen 650 mg qid prn, Glyburide 10 mg q.a.m.
SH: Smokes 2 ppd of cigarettes
PE: He is obese, Wt 235 lbs, Ht 5'8", bp 126/78, HR 72

QUESTIONS

1. Which of the following atypical antipsychotics is likely to promote the best compliance?

A. Quetiapine
B. Ziprasidone
C. Olanzapine dissolvable tablet
D. Risperidone long-acting injection

2. Which atypical antipsychotic has the greatest risk of causing weight increase?

A. Clozapine
B. Olanzapine

C. Quetiapine
D. Ziprasidone

3. Which of the following is a true statement about switching the patient from chlorpromazine to aripiprazole?

A. Chlorpromazine and aripiprazole have the same mechanism of action.
B. Chlorpromazine has a higher risk of tardive dyskinesia.
C. Aripiprazole has a higher rate of sedation.
D. Aripiprazole has a higher rate of efficacy on positive symptoms.

4. Which of the following antipsychotics has the highest risk of prolonging the QT interval?

A. Olanzapine
B. Haloperidol
C. Ziprasidone
D. Thioridazine

5. Which of the following antipsychotic medications will have an increase in serum levels if the patient stops smoking cigarettes?

A. Quetiapine
B. Aripiprazole
C. Risperidone
D. Olanzapine

PATIENT PROFILE 223
DIABETES

PRESENTATION

RG is a 67-year-old Hispanic woman who presents to the disease state management clinic with a new 6-lb weight gain. She is concerned about the new weight gain and shortness of breath over the last 2 weeks while trying to keep up with her grandchildren. RG has a 10-year history of hypertension and diabetes that have not been optimally managed. She recently experienced new-onset congestive heart failure requiring 2-day hospitalization 6 months ago. She began metoprolol XL, furosemide, lisinopril, and K-Dur during hospitalization for new-onset CHF. She has been NYHA class II heart-failure since she was discharged. After hospitalization her primary care physician increased her glimeperide slowly to 8 mg qd.

FH: Rg's mother died at 82 years old because of a stroke. Her father died at age 56 from trauma after an industrial accident.

SH: Rg has been married 41 years. They have two sons, ages 37 and 40, both with hypertension. They have five grandchildren.

Allergies: NKDA

Meds: HCTZ 12.5 mg po qd
Glimepiride 8 mg po qd
Pioglitazone 15 mg po qd
Metoprolol XL 25 mg po qd
Lisinopril 10 mg po qd
Furosemide 20 mg po qd
K-Dur 20 mEq po qd
Fluvastatin 40 mg po qd

Gen: Pleasant, WDWN older woman with NYHA functional class II in NAD

Vitals: BP 140/90 mm Hg, pulse 68 beats/min, RR 14 breaths/min, Temp 99°F, Ht 5'1", Wt 178 lbs, BMI 33.6 kg/m^2

HEENT: PERRLA, EOMI

Chest: CTA

COR: RRR, +S$_3$

Abd: Nontender, nondistended, +BS

GU: Deferred

EXT: 3+ Pitting edema BL in both lower extremities

Neuro: Cranial nerves II to XII intact

Labs: Na 137 mEq/L, K 4.9 mEq/L, Cl 98 mEq/L, HCO$_3$ 25 mEq/L, BUN 13 mg/dL, SCr 0.9 mg/dL, fasting glucose 235 mg/dL, WBC 8.9 K cells/mm^3, platelets 289 K cells/mm^3, Hgb 12 g/dL, HCT 36%, HbA1c 8.7%, LDL 135 mg/dL, HDL 52 mg/dL, TC 215 mg/dL, TG 210 mg/dL, EF 35%

QUESTIONS

1. Which of RG's medications may be contributing to her new weight gain, shortness of breath, and 3+ edema in her extremities?

   A. Fluvastatin 40 mg po qd
   B. Glimepiride 8 mg po qd
   C. Pioglitazone 15 mg po qd
   D. Metoprolol XL 25 mg po qd
   E. Furosemide 20 mg po qd

2. After reviewing this drug-induced problem with RG's physician a decision is made to discontinue the offending agent. What is the most appropriate strategy to manage RG considering the severity of her symptoms?

   A. Discontinue the offending agent and hold any additional changes unless symptoms worsen.
   B. Discontinue the offending agent and double the dose of oral furosemide for 3 days.
   C. Discontinue the offending agent and begin intravenous furosemide for 3 days.
   D. Discontinue the offending agent and furosemide and begin torsemide.
   E. Discontinue the offending agent and admit to urgent care for diuresis with nesiritide.

3. What is RG's HbA1c goal according to the American Diabetes Association?

   A. ≤4.5%
   B. ≤5%
   C. ≤5.5%
   D. ≤6%
   E. ≤7%

4. RG's physician wants to consider additional therapy to improve glycemic control. Before initiating therapy, a Chem-7 is drawn and the following information is obtained: Na 138 mEq/L, K 4.5 mEq/L, Cl 100 mEq/L, HCO$_3$ 24 mEq/L, BUN 12 mg/dL, SrCr 1.0 mg/dL. RG is still in NYHA functional class II heart failure. Recommend an appropriate strategy for glucose control considering RG's health status and laboratory values.

   A. Nateglinide 120 mg po tid with the first bite of each meal
   B. Metformin 1000 mg po bid
   C. Insulin NPH 20 units sq at bedtime

D. Insulin NPH 54 units in the morning and 28 units in the evening

E. Insulin glargine 10 units sq at bedtime

5. RG has been receiving therapy over the last 3 months and appears to be tolerating it well. During her routine follow-up appointment the following data are collected: BP 138/84 mm Hg, P 70 beats/min, RR 15 breaths/min, Wt 170 lb, BMI 32.1 kg/m^2, Na 140 mEq/L, K 4.9 mEq/L, Cl 101 mEq/L, HCO$_3$ 23 mEq/L, BUN 12 mg/dL, SrCr 1.4 mg/dL, HbA1c 8.0%. Which medication is contraindicated after reviewing these findings?

A. Glimepiride
B. Lisinopril
C. Fluvastatin
D. Metformin
E. K-Dur

6. After discontinuing this newly contraindicated agent the physician asks you to consider adding insulin therapy to RG's therapy. RG is hesitant initially but agrees to begin insulin after several extended counseling sessions. Which of the following is not a reasonable goal of therapy when beginning insulin?

A. Reduce HbA1c to ≤7%.
B. Minimize hypoglycemic episodes.
C. Prevent microvascular complications.
D. Educate and empower the patient.
E. Use minimal doses of insulin.

7. RG feels she will be more successful with an insulin strategy that is easy to administer and requires few adjustments. RG's physician agrees with this initial approach to insulin strategy. Which insulin regimen is associated with greatest patient satisfaction, fewest instances of nocturnal hypoglycemia, and less weight gain?

A. Insulin regular
B. Insulin NPH
C. Insulin lispro
D. Insulin glargine
E. Insulin ultralente

8. Recommend an appropriate starting dose of insulin glargine for RG. At the last visit: Wt 170 lbs, Ht 5'1", BMI 32.1 kg/m^2.

A. Insulin glargine 15 U sq at bedtime
B. Insulin glargine 6 U sq every 12 hours
C. Insulin glargine 15 U sq before each meal
D. Insulin glargine 6 U sq 15 minutes before each meal
E. Insulin glargine 32 U sq at bedtime

9. RG tolerates her insulin-glimeperide combination well without any new side effects of hypoglycemia or weight gain over the last 3 months. Her HbA1c is 7.4% at this visit. A review of her glucometer readings of the last 2 weeks reveals her morning glucose ranges between 150 mg/dL and 180 mg/dL. How would you begin to adjust her insulin glargine to reduce her morning glucose?

A. Increase her insulin glargine by 7.5 U.
B. Increase her insulin glargine by 35%.
C. Increase her insulin glargine by 4 U.
D. Increase her insulin glargine by 15%.
E. Increase her insulin glargine by 2 U.

10. RG needs a new prescription for her insulin glargine. Her daily insulin requirement is determined to be 20 U/day. How long will a vial of insulin glargine last using this dosage?

A. 60 days
B. 50 days
C. 40 days
D. 30 days
E. 20 days

PATIENT PROFILE 224

HUMAN IMMUNODEFICIENCY VIRUS

PRESENTATION

FA is a 31-year-old woman who was admitted to the hospital recently. She was sent by her primary care physician after being seen in the office for complaints of nausea and vomiting. Three days before presentation, FA became nauseous and eventually started to vomit bilious material. Over the last

month, she has also had temporal headaches and neck stiffness, which she has been attributing to her sleep position.

PMH: Ulcerative colitis (diagnosed 10 years ago)
Diabetes mellitus, type II
Hypertension
GERD

HIV infection (diagnosed 8 years ago). She thinks she acquired the HIV virus from unprotected sex during a premarital relationship.

Past opportunistic infections: PCP, CMV retinitis, oral and esophageal candidal infections. No current antiretroviral therapy. FA has experienced several virologic and toxicity-related failures and is currently refusing salvage therapy.

SH: Married, works as a cashier in a pet shop. She does not take care of the animals. HIV-positive husband (she is considered to be the source).

FH: Mother and father are alive. Both have a history of coronary artery disease. Father has type II diabetes mellitus.

All: Codeine (rash)

MH: Dipentum 500 mg bid

Fluconazole 100 mg qd

Nexium 40 mg qd

Glyburide 5 mg qd

HCTZ 50 mg qd

Atovaquone 1500 mg qd

Valganciclovir 900 mg po qd

ROS: Progressively lethargic over the last week. She describes one episode of blurred vision in her left eye, but no photophobia.

PE: VS: BP 135/75 mm Hg, HR 100, RR 22, Temp 39.3°C, Ht 158 cm, Wt 55 kg

Gen: Lethargic, in moderate distress

HEENT: PEERLA, EOMI, pale conjunctiva, neck supple

Cor: Normal heart sounds

Chest: Lungs CTA

Abd: Nontender, no HSM

Ext: Trace edema in lower extremities

Neuro: Negative Kerning's sign, cranial nerves intact, oriented × 3

Labs: Na 137 mEq/L, Hct 33%, Glu 150 mg/dL, K 3.9 mEq/L, Hgb 12 g/dL, Cl 107 mEq/L, WBC 3.0K cells/mm^3, HCO$_3$ 19 mEq/L, PLTS 90K cells/mm^3, BUN 10 mg/dL, AST 45 U/L, SCr 0.7 mg/dL, ALT 30 U/L, serum cryptococcal antigen titer: 1:2048, toxoplasmosis IgG antibody: negative, CD4: 55 cells/mm^3 (3 months ago), HIV RNA 55,000 copies/mL (3 months ago)

CSF: Protein 74 mg/dL, glucose 6 mg/dL, WBC 15 cells/mm^3 (PMN 10%/lymphocytes 51%/monocytes 21%), cryptococcus antigen positive, high opening pressure

QUESTIONS

1. What is considered the induction therapy of choice for cryptococcal meningitis in an HIV-positive patient?

    A. Fluconazole 800 mg IV qd plus flucytosine po 100 mg/kg per day (in four divided doses)

    B. Amphotericin B IV 1 mg/kg per day plus flucytosine po 100 mg/kg per day (in four divided doses)

    C. Flucytosine po 150 mg/kg per day (in four divided doses)

    D. Itraconazole 200 mg bid plus flucytosine po 100 mg/kg per day (in four divided doses)

2. Which of the following is considered the maintenance therapy of choice for preventing future episodes of cryptococcal meningitis (secondary prophylaxis)?

    A. Itraconazole po 200 mg qd

    B. Fluconazole po 200 mg qd

    C. Amphotericin B IV 1 mg/kg weekly

    D. Ketoconazole po 100 mg qd

3. Which of the following is considered a common and significant therapy-limiting side effect of amphotericin B therapy?

    A. Hypercalcemia

    B. Hepatotoxicity

    C. Agranulocytosis

    D. Nephrotoxicity

4. Which of the following is considered a therapy-limiting side effect of flucytosine therapy?

    A. Bone marrow suppression

    B. Nephrotoxicity

    C. Hyperkalemia

    D. Ventricular arrhythmias

5. Which of the following interventions is most likely to reduce the nephrotoxicity associated with amphotericin B therapy?

    A. Predose ibuprofen

    B. Normal saline boluses before and after amphotericin administration

    C. Predose diphenhydramine

    D. Predose hydrocortisone

6. If FA is to be restarted on antiretroviral therapy, which class of antiretrovirals is most likely to alter her glycemic control?

    A. Protease inhibitors

    B. Nucleoside reverse transcriptase inhibitors

    C. Nonnucleoside reverse transcriptase inhibitors

    D. Fusion inhibitors

After drawing blood from LB in the laboratory, the technician sticks himself with the needle. His injury consists of a deep puncture wound on the fleshy part of his palm. He notes that the needle did have noticeable blood on it before the needle stick injury.

7. After occupational exposure to blood, initiation of postexposure prophylaxis (PEP) and the decision to

start two or three antiretroviral medications depends on which of the following factors?

I. The type of exposure (percutaneous versus mucous membrane/skin)
II. The degree of exposure (severity of injury and volume of exposure)
III. The HIV status of the source patient
IV. The clinical status and viral load of the source patient

A. I and II only
B. I, II, and III only
C. I and III only
D. I, II, III, and IV

8. By how much is the risk of HIV transmission reduced with PEP administration after percutaneous HIV exposure?

A. 10%
B. 50%
C. 80%
D. This has not been well defined with currently recommended PEP regimens.

9. The recommended basic PEP regimen includes administration of two nucleoside reverse-transcriptase inhibitors. What is the mechanism of action for this class of antiretrovirals?

A. They exert their antiviral effect in the cytoplasm of the host cell by inhibiting the viral-encoded reverse transcriptase enzyme, thus preventing conversion of the single-stranded viral RNA to double-stranded DNA.
B. They bind to reverse transcriptase and cause a conformational change in its structure, thus altering its target site and inhibiting its ability to interact with nucleotides.
C. They bind to the active site of HIV protease, thus preventing it from cleaving the large viral proteins into important viral enzymes and structural components.
D. They inhibit the conformational change of gp41 that is necessary for fusion of virion to the host cell.

10. An expanded three-drug PEP regimen is used for high-risk exposures. Which of the following PEP agents is the most likely to cause a rash when used as a component of this three-drug PEP?

A. Zidovudine
B. Lamivudine
C. Abacavir
D. Nelfinavir

PATIENT PROFILE 225

SEROTONIN SYNDROME

PRESENTATION

CC: LD is a 47-year-ols woman who presents to the emergency room with altered mental status (agitation and confusion), diaphoresis, diarrhea, mydriasis, and tachycardia.

HPI: On questioning, you find out that LD was just given Zyban to help her quit smoking, which she started 3 days prior to her visit to the ED. Her signs and symptoms started shortly after her first dose of Zyban and have become worse with the most recent doses.

PMH: Parkinson's disease × 3 years, diabetes mellitus type 2 × 17 years, hyperlipidemia × 2 years, depression, insomnia

MH: Atorvastatin 10 mg PO qhs; trazodone 50 mg PO qhs; carbidopa/levodopa 25/100 mg PO tid; buspirone 15 mg PO bid; fluoxetine 40 mg PO qam; rosiglitazone 4 mg PO qd; Glipizide ER 5 mg PO qd; Zolpidem 5 mg PO qhs PRN

Allergies: Penicillin (hives)

SH: Smokes 1.5 ppd × 26 years; drinks alcohol occasionally on weekends; divorced; has 2 children; drinks 2 to 3 cups of coffee daily
Works as an underwriter for a large insurance company

FH: Father died of acute myocardial infarction (MI) at age 73. Mother is alive, status post breast cancer. Older brother diagnosed with bipolar disorder at age 33. Younger sister suffers from depression.

PHYSICAL EXAMINATION

Gen: Well-nourished Caucasian female in slight distress

VS: Blood pressure: 131/81 mm Hg; heart rate:103 beats per minute; respiratory rate: 24 breaths per minute; temperature: 99°F; height: 6 ft, 3 in; weight: 137 lb

HEENT: Eyes dilated, forehead cold

CV: Normal S_1 and S_2; (−) MRG; slight tachycardia

Pulm: Clear bilaterally; rapid, shallow breath sounds

Abd: Normal
Ext: Skin cold and clammy to palpation
Neuro: Confused and agitated

LABORATORY STUDIES

Na$^+$: 138 mEq/L
Cl$^-$: 101 mEq/L
Blood urea nitrogen (BUN):
    13 mg /dL
Glucose (fasting):
    98 mg/dL
Hemoglobin: 14 g/dL
Plt: 310/mm^3

K$^+$: 4.1 mEq/L
CO$_2$: 30mEq/L
Serum creatinine:
    0.8 mg/dL
White blood cell (WBC)
    count: 12,000/mm^3
Hematocrit: 43%
ECG: Sinus tachycardia

QUESTIONS

1. Which of LD's medications would *not* contribute to her signs and symptoms of serotonin syndrome?

    A. Trazodone
    B. Buspirone
    C. Fluoxetine
    D. Rosiglitazone
    E. Zyban

2. Which mechanism is *most likely* responsible for causing serotonin syndrome in LD?

    A. Inhibition of serotonin synthesis and release
    B. Acute overstimulation of 5-HT$_{1A}$ receptors
    C. Activation of β_1 and β_2 adrenergic receptors
    D. Overdose or excessive use of anticholinergics
    E. Noncompliance with her diabetic medication

3. Which drug, when given with fluvoxamine, might precipitate serotonin syndrome?

    A. Zaleplon
    B. Ondansetron
    C. Scopolamine
    D. Tamsulosin
    E. Phenelzine

4. Which of the following antidepressants has a clinically important active metabolite?

    A. Mirtazapine
    B. Fluoxetine
    C. Fluvoxamine
    D. Protriptyline
    E. Paroxetine

5. Which of the following drug combinations is *least likely* to result in serotonin syndrome?

    A. Lexapro and clomiphene
    B. Venlafaxine and trazodone

    C. Nardil and Cymbalta
    D. Tofranil and sertraline
    E. Buspirone and paroxetine

6. A physician decides to take LD off of fluoxetine and start her on a new drug, Wellbutrin XL. Why might this new regimen cause even worse problems for LD?

    A. This new drug regimen is suitable for LD.
    B. Zyban and Wellbutrin XL both have the same mechanism of action.
    C. Zyban and Wellbutrin XL both contain buspirone.
    D. Both B and C are correct.
    E. None of the above are correct.

7. LD presents to her primary care physician with severe pain. Considering LD's current medications, which analgesic would *not* be a good choice to add to her drug regimen?

    A. Morphine
    B. Percocet 5/325
    C. Norco
    D. Vicoprofen
    E. Ultracet

8. LD's physician sends her to a psychiatrist. Her new doctor decides to start over with her medications for depression and anxiety. He prescribes Celexa 10 mg PO qam and clonazepam 0.5 mg PO bid PRN for anxiety. In 3 months, she returns to her new doctor, and he adds Wellbutrin XL 150 mg PO bid. What adjustments could be made to this regimen to make it correct?

    I. Change Wellbutrin XL to Wellbutrin SR 150 mg bid because the SR formulation is dosed twice daily.
    II. Change to Wellbutrin XL 300 mg qd because the XL version is long-acting for once-daily dosing.
    II. Change the Wellbutrin XL to nefazodone to decrease the risk of liver toxicity.

    A. I only
    B. II only
    C. I and II
    D. II and II
    E. I, II, and III

9. LD is diagnosed with high blood pressure, and the Celexa has not worked for her depression despite increased doses. Which of the following antidepressants would *not* be a good option for LD owing to her elevated blood pressure?

    A. Lexapro
    B. Effexor
    C. Zoloft

D. Remeron
E. Desyrel

10. Which of the following metals used commonly in practice could lead to serotonin syndrome?

A. Gold
B. Calcium
C. Iron
D. Lithium
E. Magnesium

PATIENT PROFILE 226

CHRONIC HEPATITIS C

PRESENTATION

JM is a 36-year-old Hispanic man who presents to the clinic with increasing complaints of fatigue and abdominal pain. He was diagnosed with hepatitis C (genotype 2b) in 1994 prior to donating blood. He has been asymptomatic since that time. He states that he has been unable to get up for work in the morning and has no appetite. He reports a 10-lb weight loss over the past 3 weeks.

JM has no other chronic diseases and is currently not taking any medications. He uses acetaminophen when needed for pain relief. He has no allergies to medications. He is a previous intravenous (IV) drug user, smokes two packs of cigarettes per day, and does not drink alcohol. He lives alone and denies any sexual partners. He has no living relatives.

JM appears to be in moderate distress. His vital signs are blood pressure = 137/77 mm Hg; heart rate = 69 beats per minute; temperature = 37°C; and a pain score of 6. His physical examination reveals abdominal pain and tenderness in the right upper quadrant (RUQ). There is presence of scleral icterus and ascites.

JM has tested negative for HIV. His laboratory values are AST = 270 units/L; ALT = 300 units/L; total bilirubin = 3.5 ng/mL; and direct bilirubin = 1.9 ng/mL. He is serum anti-HCV positive with an HCV RNA level of 7000 viral equivalents/mL. Results from a liver biopsy are pending.

QUESTIONS

1. Which of the following are modes of transmission for the hepatitis C virus?

   A. IV drug use
   B. Unprotected sex
   C. Body piercing
   D. All the above

2. JM's liver biopsy reveals inflammation and fibrosis. His physician is considering initiating treatment of his chronic hepatitis C infection. What additional information from JM's history makes him a candidate for therapy?

A. Presence of ascites
B. HCV RNA level >50
C. Total bilirubin >3 ng/mL
D. Abdominal pain and tenderness

3. Which of the following is considered a goal of therapy in the management of chronic hepatitis C?

   A. Eradicate the virus
   B. Normalize biochemical markers
   C. Reduce morbidity and mortality
   D. All the above

4. The physician would like to initiate interferon therapy. Which subtype of interferon has been shown to be effective in the treatment of chronic hepatitis C?

   A. Interferon-β-1A
   B. Interferon-β-1B
   C. Interferon-α-2B
   D. Interferon-γ

5. Which of the following is(are) common side effect(s) associated with the use of interferon?

   A. Flulike symptoms
   B. Neutropenia
   C. Alopecia
   D. All the above

6. Which of the following statements about the use of interferon is *correct*?

   A. Interferon is administered as an injection, and a new needle and syringe should be used for each dose.
   B. Interferon should be stored at room temperature.
   C. Interferon should be shaken prior to use.
   D. All the above are correct.

7. The physician also would like to start ribavirin. Which of the following is(are) side effect(s) to the use of ribavirin?

   A. Anemia
   B. Hypothyroidism

C. Retinal hemorrhage
D. All the above

8. JM has received 6 weeks of interferon/ribavirin therapy. He is considered to be a partial responder. The physician considers the use of a pegylated interferon. Which of the following best describes the advantage of using pegylated interferon as an alternative to interferon?

A. Longer half-life
B. Quicker onset of action
C. Less incidence of side effects
D. All the above

9. Pegylated interferon causes similar side effects to interferon, but it has been associated with a higher incidence of _____ and _____.

A. Cytopenias, depression
B. Cytopenias, injection-site reactions
C. Injection-site reactions, depression
D. Injection-site reactions, renal failure

10. JM is 3 weeks into his new therapy, and he states that he feels depressed. After a more thorough evaluation, his physician believes that JM may be experiencing depression from the interferon. Which of the following has been effective in the management of depression induced by interferon therapy?

A. Notriptyline
B. Paroxetine
C. A or B
D. None of the above

PATIENT PROFILE 227

HYPERTENSION

PRESENTATION

CC: FD is a 53-year-old man who presents to your pharmacy weekly for a blood pressure reading.

HPI: FD has been checking his blood pressure regularly at your pharmacy for the past 6 months, and his blood pressure has been increasing steadily. His blood pressure medication was increased 2 months ago, and his blood pressure has stabilized, although he is still not at goal. FD walks every day and reports a low-salt diet, many fruits and vegetables, and lean meats. He feels fine, although his blood pressure is consistently high. He has an overactive bladder and has attempted to treat this condition in the past but has not tolerated medical treatment. He was treated with chlorthalidone "years ago" but did not tolerate this medication because of his overactive bladder.

PMH: Hypertension, anxiety, overactive bladder, alcohol abuse, substance-free for 10 years

ALL: NKDA

MH: Atenolol 100 mg PO qd, diazepam 2 mg PO qd PRN

FH: Father alive, status post myocardial infarction (MI) at age 50. Mother alive and well, rheumatoid arthritis.

SH: Denies smoking or alcohol use

VS: Blood pressure: 168/102 mm Hg; height: 6ft, 1 in; weight: 180 lb

Labs: 138 102 11; total cholesterol: 170 mg/dL; low-density lipoprotein (LDL) cholesterol: 118 mg/dL; 92; high-density lipoprotein (HDL) cholesterol: 40 mg/dL; triglycerides: 140 mg/dL; 3.5 28 0.9

VISIT NOTES

FD is considerably uptight when he comes to see you in the pharmacy. He is pleasant and talkative, although visibly frustrated about his blood pressure before it is even tested. At each visit he mentions his overactive bladder and is upset that it cannot be treated. He walks to the beach daily and has to stop several times along the way to go to the bathroom. You have tried to encourage him to purchase an ambulatory blood pressure monitor, but he prefers to come to the pharmacy. His systolic blood pressure usually drops by 5 to 10 mm Hg on the second reading, after he has been sitting for 15 minutes, although the diastolic blood pressure usually remains the same.

QUESTIONS

1. According to the JNC VII guidelines, what is FD's goal blood pressure?

A. <130/80 mm Hg
B. <130/85 mm Hg
C. <140/80 mm Hg
D. <140/90 mm Hg

2. According to the JNC VII guidelines, which of the following blood pressure ranges reflects a new category called *prehypertension*?

A. 110–120 mm Hg SBP and/or 80–89 mm Hg DBP

    B. 115–130 mm Hg SBP and/or 70–80 mm Hg DBP

    C. 120–139 mm Hg SBP and/or 80–89 mm Hg DBP

    D. 130–139 mm Hg SBP and/or 80–89 mm Hg DBP

3. According to the JNV VII guidelines, please classify FD's blood pressure.

    A. Prehypertension
    B. Stage 1 hypertension
    C. Stage 2 hypertension
    D. Stage 3 hypertension

4. Which of the following patient-specific characteristics is considered a cardiovascular risk factor in FD?

    A. Age
    B. Anxiety
    C. Diabetes
    D. Family history of premature cardiovascular disease

5. According to ALLHAT, which of the following medications is considered first-line treatment for hypertension in otherwise healthy adults?

    A. Atenolol
    B. Doxazosin
    C. Furosemide
    D. Hydrochlorothiazide

6. Which of the following action steps is the *most appropriate* option to help manage FD's hypertension at this point?

    A. Increase the atenolol dose to 150 mg PO qd.
    B. Discontinue the atenolol and start doxazosin.
    C. Keep the atenolol dose as is and begin lisinopril.
    D. Keep the atenolol dose as is and begin hydrochlorothiazide.

7. FD mentions that he sometimes gets dizzy when he gets up in the morning and after his nap in the afternoon. You suspect that he is suffering from orthostatic hypotension. Which of the following definitions is the *most appropriate* to define orthostatic hypotension?

    A. Decrease in diastolic blood pressure of greater than 10 mm Hg
    B. Decrease in diastolic blood pressure of greater than 20 mm Hg
    C. Decrease in systolic blood pressure of greater than 10 mm Hg
    D. Decrease in systolic blood pressure of greater than 20 mm Hg

8. Which of the following medical conditions may be contributing to FD's orthostatic hypotension?

    A. Anxiety
    B. Hypertension
    C. History of alcohol use
    D. Overactive bladder (causing dehydration)

9. Which of the following antihypertensive agents may be helpful in patients who also suffer from benign prostatic hypertrophy (BPH)?

    A. Angiotensin-converting enzyme (ACE) inhibitor
    B. ARBs
    C. β-Blockers
    D. α-Blockers

10. Which of the following adverse effects is an important counseling point for patients beginning therapy with ACE inhibitors?

    A. Lactic acidosis
    B. Rhabdomyolysis
    C. Visual disturbances
    D. Persistent dry cough

PATIENT PROFILE 228

LIVER TRANSPLANTATION

PRESENTATION

CC: BU is a 56-year-old man who was admitted to the hospital 4 days ago for a cadaveric liver transplant. He has no current complaints and is ambulating well.

PMH: Chronic active hepatitis C (genotype 1); failed interferon (IFN) therapy owing to medication side effects; hepatocellular carcinoma

SH: History of heavy alcohol use; has been abstinent for 1 year. Denies tobacco and illicit drug use. Has two tattoos.

FH: Noncontributory

VS: Temperature: 38.2°C; blood pressure: 136/82 mm Hg; heart rate: 78 beats per minute; respiratory rate: 18 breaths per minute

LABORATORY AND DIAGNOSTIC TESTS

Sodium: 133 mEq/L   Potassium: 4.6 mEq/L

Chloride: 100 mEq/L CO_2: 27 mEq/L

Blood urea nitrogen   Serum creatinine: 0.8 mg/dL
(BUN): 20 mg/dL

Glucose: 163 mg/dL   Albumin 2.0 g/dL

Calcium: 8.1 mg/dL   White blood cell (WBC) count:
                     10,500/mm^3

Hematocrit: 28%   Platelets 77,000/mm^3

Total bilirubin: 2.1 mg/dL   AST: 90 IU/L

ALT: 284 IU/L   Tacrolimus trough: 5.5 ng/mL

One month ago:

Hepatitis A antibodies: nonreactive

Hepatitis B surface antigen, surface antibody, and core
    antibody: nonreactive

Hepatitis C antibodies: reactive

Cytomegalovirus (CMV) IgG: positive

Herpes simplex virus (HSV) type 1 IgG: positive

CURRENT MEDICATIONS

Bactrim DS PO qd

Famotidine 20 mg PO bid

Ganciclovir 1000 mg PO tid

Methylprednisolone 20 mg IV q6h (tapering dose)

Metoprolol 50 mg PO bid

Mycophenolate mofetil 1000 mg PO bid

Nystatin 500,000 units swish and swallow qid

Percocet 5/325 mg PO as needed for pain

Tacrolimus 3 mg PO bid

Ursodiol 300 mg PO tid

QUESTIONS

1. Which medications comprise BU's current immuno-suppressive regimen?

   A. Methylprednisolone and tacrolimus
   B. Methylprednisolone and mycophenolate mofetil
   C. Methylprednisolone, tacrolimus, and mycophenolate mofetil
   D. Tacrolimus and mycophenolate mofetil
   E. Tacrolimus, mycophenolate mofetil, and ursodiol

2. Which of the following best describes mycophenolate mofetil's mechanism of action?

   A. Inhibits production of interleukin 1 (IL-1) and IL-2
   B. Inhibits calcineurin
   C. Prevents T cells from recognizing the allograft
   D. Prevents proliferation of T cells
   E. Induces apoptosis of activated T cells

3. The immunosuppressive activity of mycophenolate mofetil is most similar to which of the following medications?

   A. Sirolimus
   B. Cyclosporine
   C. Daclizumab
   D. Azathioprine
   E. Thymoglobulin

4. Which of the following most appropriately describes BU's current serum calcium concentration?

   A. 7.3 mg/dL
   B. 8.1 mg/dL
   C. 8.9 mg/dL
   D. 10.1 mg/dL
   E. 12.1 mg/dL

5. What is the indication for ganciclovir therapy in this patient?
   A. Prophylaxis for cytomegalovirus
   B. Treatment of CMV
   C. Prophylaxis for herpes
   D. Treatment of herpes
   E. Treatment of hepatitis C (HCV)

6. Which of the following medications require(s) a dose adjustment in renal insufficiency?
   A. Sirolimus
   B. Ursodiol
   C. Ganciclovir
   D. Methylprednisolone
   E. All the above

7. Which of the following statements is true regarding recurrent hepatitis C in liver transplantation?

   A. Hepatitis C does not recur after liver transplantation.
   B. Hepatitis C does not recur after liver transplantation if the HCV viral load is low at the time of transplant.
   C. Recurrent hepatitis C after transplant progresses to advanced disease at a faster rate than the original progression to cirrhosis.
   D. Genotype 1 responds better to treatment than other HCV genotypes.
   E. Immunosuppressive medications do not affect recurrence rates.

8. Which of the following medications is(are) associated with an increased rate of recurrent HCV infection after liver transplantation?

   A. Methylprednisolone IV pulse therapy to treat rejection
   B. Prednisone PO for chronic maintenance immunosuppression
   C. OKT3 IV for induction immunosuppression
   D. A and B
   E. A and C

9. Which of the following would be the *treatment of choice* for recurrent HCV infection in this patient?

    A. Interferon-alfa monotherapy
    B. Pegylated interferon-alfa monotherapy
    C. Ribavirin monotherapy
    D. Interferon-alfa and ribavirin combination therapy
    E. Pegylated interferon-alfa and ribavirin combination therapy

10. Which of the following *best describes* common severe side effects associated with pegylated interferon-alfa and ribavirin combination therapy?

    A. Elevated transaminases and thrombocytopenia
    B. Bone marrow toxicity and depression
    C. Renal insufficiency and hyperkalemia
    D. Decreased seizure threshold and tremors
    E. Gastrointestinal intolerance and pulmonary fibrosis

PATIENT PROFILE 229
DIABETES MELLITUS

PRESENTATION

JH is a 30-year-old Caucasian man seen in the primary care clinic for the first time. He states that his vision is sometimes blurry and that he has been very tired lately, so he is concerned. He also purchased a new pair of shoes for a wedding recently and developed a blister on the bottom of his right foot that does not seem to be healing well and is very painful. He states that this morning he was feeling like he was getting a fever, so he took some Tylenol a couple hours ago. He did not check his temperature prior to taking the Tylenol. He has not seen a primary care provider for over 10 years. He is followed by a neurologist on an annual basis ever since he experienced several seizures 4 years ago.

His past medical history includes obesity and epilepsy. His current medications are valproic acid 500 mg twice daily, folic acid 1 mg once daily, and thiamine 100 mg once daily.

JH smokes 2 packs of cigarettes per day. He started smoking at age 14. He drinks 1 oz of vodka mixed with cranberry juice every day. On the weekends, he occasionally will drink an entire 20-oz bottle of vodka. The only illicit drug he uses is marijuana, which he smokes several times a month when he gets together with his friends on the weekends. He is a cook at a local Chinese restaurant.

JH states that he drinks a lot of water and coffee on a daily basis. He drinks about 10 eight-ounce glasses of water every day and about 9 eight-ounce cups of coffee every day. He is frequently thirsty. Because he drinks a lot of water, he also urinates frequently. He states he has to use the bathroom at least once every hour while he is awake. He also wakes up several times during the night to use the bathroom.

He is constantly hungry and has been eating a lot of fruit because he knows that it is healthier than junk food. He has gained 30 lb over the past 4 years. He states that the valproic acid has been effective in preventing his tonic-clonic seizures and that he is makes sure that he takes the medication every single day so that he does not lose his driver's license. He states that two other medications had been tried for his seizures before valproic acid that did not work and made him feel terrible. He does not remember the names of the medications.

JH states that he has never had an allergic reaction. He has experienced adverse reactions to a couple of seizure medications. One seizure medication made him really dizzy. Another medication gave him severe headaches.

JH lives by himself. He eats dinner at fast-food restaurants frequently but regularly eats his breakfast at home. He generally eats lunch at the Chinese restaurant where he works. He likes to go dancing at local salsa clubs with his friends almost every weekend. He does not exercise during the week.

JH's height is 5 ft, 11 in, and his weight is 280 lb. JH's vital signs are as follows: blood pressure: 180/98 mm Hg; heart rate: 78 beats per minute; respiratory rate: 18 breath per minute; and temperature: 99.6°F. JH's laboratory values are as follows: Na: 134 mEq/L; K: 5.0 mEq/L; blood urea nitrogen (BUN): 30 mg/dL; serum Cr: 2.1 mg/dL; glucose: 434 mg/dL; thyroid-stimulating hormone (TSH): 3.4; total cholesterol: 313 mg/dL; and high-density lipoprotein (HDL) cholesterol: 30 mg/dL. JH ate breakfast this morning before his blood was drawn.

Visual inspection of JH's right foot reveals a large open wound about 3 inches in diameter oozing pus indicative of infection. All other physical examination findings are normal, with the exception of very dry mucous membranes.

QUESTIONS

1. JH is diagnosed with diabetes mellitus. He has a diabetic foot infection. Which of the following antibiotics would be the *most appropriate* to use?

    A. Topical triple-antibiotic ointment
    B. Oral Augmentin (amoxicillin–clavulanic acid)
    C. Oral dicloxacillin

D. Oral vancomycin

E. Intravenous vancomycin

2. JH is placed on clindamycin plus ciprofloxacin for the treatment of his diabetic foot infection. Which of the following is a side effect that is associated with clindamycin?

A. Photosensitivity

B. Kidney stones

C. Diarrhea

D. Vision changes

E. Elevated blood pressure

3. Which of the following is known to cause weight gain, which may have contributed to the onset of diabetes mellitus in JH?

A. Ethanol

B. Acetaminophen

C. Folic acid

D. Thiamine

E. Valproic acid

4. JH is placed on insulin therapy. Several weeks later he is seen in primary care clinic for a follow-up appointment. He is currently on Lantus (insulin glargine) 30 units at bedtime and 10 units of Humalog (insulin lispro) before each meal. He eats three meals a day. His average blood sugar concentrations from his home glucose meter are as follows: fasting AM blood sugar: 120 mg/dL; prelunch: 180 mg/dL; predinner 100 mg/dL; and prebedtime: 120 md/dL. Which of the following insulin regimen changes would be the *most appropriate* to recommend?

A. Discontinue Lantus

B. Decrease Lantus to 10 units at bedtime

C. Increase prebreakfast Humalog to 14 units

D. Increase prelunch Humalog to 14 units

E. Increase prebedtime Humalog to 14 units

5. One of the lifestyle modifications that JH's primary care provider has recommended is decreasing his alcohol intake. Why is binge drinking hazardous for someone on insulin for treatment of diabetes mellitus?

A. Binge drinking increases blood sugar levels, which increases the risk of developing complications.

B. Binge drinking inhibits hepatic gluconeogenesis, which increases the risk of developing diabetic coma secondary to hypoglycemia.

C. Binge drinking increases urinary frequency, which can lead to severe dehydration.

D. Binge drinking decreases intraocular pressure, which increases the risk of developing narrow-angle glaucoma.

E. Binge drinking increases glucose utilization by the muscles, which increases the risk of rhabdomyolysis.

6. JH's fasting lipid profile is checked. The results are as follows: total cholesterol: 300 mg/dL; LDL: 180 mg/dL; HDL: 30 mg/dL; and triglycerides: 450 mg/dL. Which of the following medications would have the most effect on lowering JH's triglycerides?

A. Simvastatin

B. Cholestyramine

C. Ezetimibe

D. Niacin

E. Gemfibrozil

7. JH's primary care provider decides to initiate atorvastatin 20 mg daily. In addition to JH's lipid profile, which of the following objective parameters needs to be monitored?

A. Creatinine

B. Liver function tests

C. Albumin

D. Calcium

E. Potassium

8. Several months later, JH brings a prescription for gemfibrozil 600 mg twice daily to your pharmacy. He confirms that he is also taking atorvastatin 20 mg once daily. Which of the following adverse effects is it important to counsel JH on, particularly since he is on combination therapy?

A. Photosensitivity

B. Urinary retention

C. Orthostatic hypotension

D. Gastrointestinal bleeding

E. Muscle weakness or pain

9. Several years later, JH is hospitalized owing to a myocardial infarction. During the hospitalization, he lost 20 lb. On discharge, his medications are as follows: metformin 500 mg twice daily with morning and evening meals, aspirin 325 mg once daily, atenolol 25 mg once daily, lisinopril 40 mg once daily, atorvastatin 20 mg once daily, valproic acid 500 mg twice daily, folic acid 1 mg once daily, and thiamine 100 mg once daily. He is seen in the primary care clinic for a follow-up visit after discharge from the hospital. According to JH's home glucose meter, his average fasting blood sugar is 180 mg/dL, and his average pre-evening meal blood sugar is 180 mg/dL. He still eats three meals a day. His serum creatinine today is 1.4 mg/dL and his liver function tests are within normal limits. His left ventricular ejection fraction when he was in the hospital was 50%. Which of the following medication

changes would be the *most appropriate* to recommend based on JH's home blood glucose readings?

A. Add Lantus (insulin glargine) 10 units at bedtime
B. Add Novolog (insulin lispro) 10 units before noon-time meal
C. Add Novolog (insulin lispro) 10 units before bedtime
D. Decrease metformin dose to 250 mg twice daily
E. Increase metformin dose to 1000 mg twice daily

10. JH develops chronic renal insufficiency secondary to his diabetes mellitus and anemia secondary to his renal insufficiency. The decision is made to initiate epoetin injections and oral iron therapy. Which of the following is a side effect of epoetin therapy?

A. Elevated blood pressure
B. Damage to veins due to extravasation
C. Diarrhea
D. Nosebleeds
E. Increased infections owing to immunosuppression

PATIENT PROFILE 230

GOUT

PRESENTATION

LF is a 38-year-old woman who presents to the clinic with a chief complaint of a history of gouty attacks that are re-occurring too frequently in her opinion. LF has been experiencing acute flare-ups of gout in her toes and hands for the past 2 years. She notices a correlation with acute ingestion of alcohol and during very cold weather. She takes indomethacin for these flare-ups. LF's past medical history is significant for acute gouty arthritis. LF's medication regimen includes indomethacin 25 mg 1 PO bid-tid PRN and a multivitamin 1 PO qd. LF's family history is negative for gout. Both her parents are alive and healthy with no significant disease states.

PHYSICAL EXAMINATION

VS: Blood pressure: 120/78 mm Hg; heart rate: 60 beats per minute; respiratory rate: 16 breaths per minute; temperature: 37°C
General: Alert, oriented, and pleasant patient
Skin: Warm and dry
Chest: Heart reveals regular rhythm.
ABD: Soft and obese without masses
EXT: Some swelling and redness on her left foot, but not painful. The remaining joints and extremities are normal.

LABORATORY VALUES

Na: 134 mEq/L
Cl: 107 mEq/L
Glucose: 92 mg/dL
Total cholesterol: 155 mg/dL

K: 3.3 mEq/L
Blood urea nitrogen (BUN): 13 mg/dL
Serum Cr: 1.2 mg/dL
High-density lipoprotein (HDL) cholesterol: 52 mg/dL

Triglycerides: 125 mg/dL
ALT: 16 mg/dL
Hgb: 15.6 g/dL
Platelets: 236,000/mm^3

AST: 18 mg/dL
Uric acid: 9.3 mg/dL
Hct: 46%
White blood cell (WBC) count: 10.0×102/mm^3

A 24-hour urine collection for uric acid revealed a urine volume of 1500 mL with a uric acid concentration of 67.6 mg/dL.

QUESTIONS

1. Which of the following characteristics is(are) *true* of probenecid?

   I. Uricosuric
   II. Decreases uric acid reabsorption
   III. Requires a 24-hour urine collection

   A. I only
   B. III only
   C. I and II only
   D. II and III only
   E. I, II, and III

2. LF's physician decides to start her on probenecid therapy. Which of the following should you recommend to prevent uric acid stone formation?

   A. Acidify the urine
   B. Increase fluid intake
   C. Initiate therapy at a high dose
   D. None of the above
   E. All the above

3. Which of the following statements about colchicines is *true*?

   A. Colchicine should *never* be administered intravenously.

B. Colchicine is effective if symptoms have been present for 7 days.

C. Colchicine is a useful option in patients that are fluid restricted.

D. Colchicine enhances renal clearance of uric acid.

E. All the above

4. LF has taken a "fluid pill," but there is no record of this on her medication profile. What reference would be most useful in identifying this product when she brings it in for identification?

A. *Drug Topics*
B. *Fact & Comparison*
C. Identidex
D. Yahoo
E. All the above

5. Which of the following medications is *appropriate* for treatment of patients who are classified as overproducers of uric acid?

A. Allopurinol
B. Probenecid
C. Naproxen
D. All the above
E. None of the above

6. Which of the following medications can be an *appropriate* treatment(s) for patients who are classified as having decreased renal clearance of uric acid?

A. Prednisone
B. Allopurinol
C. Probenecid
D. B and C only
E. A, B, and C

7. In a case such as LF's, where there is a history of chronic attacks of gout, prophylactic therapy may be initiated in which of the following?

A. Patients with a serum uric acid level greater than 10 mg/dL
B. Very severe attacks
C. Patents with hyperuricemia from medications that are essential to treatment
D. None of the above
E. All the above

8. Based on LF's 24-hour urine collection for uric acid, she may be put into what category?

A. An underexcretor of uric acid
B. An overproducer of uric acid
C. Both an overproducer and an underexcretor of uric acid
D. A normal production and excretion of uric acid
E. Not enough information

9. Probenecid's brand name (trademark name) is which of the following?

A. Zyloprim
B. Purinethol
C. Zetia
D. Benemid
E. Vytorin

10. When initiating probenecid therapy in LF, which of the following is *true*?

A. No additional treatment is necessary for LF.
B. Allopurinol should be added to LF's regimen.
C. Prednisone should be added to LF's regimen.
D. An opioid should be added to LF's regimen.
E. Colchicine should be added to LF's regimen.

PATIENT PROFILE 231

SEIZURES

PRESENTATION

NM is a 16-year-old male high school student with a 3-year history of complex partial seizures and secondary generalized seizures. He has not been able to tolerate previous therapy with either phenytoin or valproate owing to significant side effects. Currently, he is on carbamazepine 600 mg three times a day but still has experienced four complex partial seizures and two generalized seizures over the previous 2 months. While this represents some improvement in seizure frequency, higher doses of carbamazepine cause gastrointestinal distress and makes him "feel out of it." His current carbamazepine level is 12 mg/L (8–12 mg/L). His other most current laboratory tests are unavailable. His medical history is significant for an allergy to sulfonamides and penicillin (rash).

QUESTIONS

1. NM's physician is considering adjunctive therapy with another antiepileptic drug (AED). Which one of the following AEDs is contraindicated in someone who is allergic to sulfonamides?

   A. Topiramate
   B. Levetiracetam
   C. Lamotrigine
   D. Zonisamide
   E. Tiagabine

2. What serum electrolyte abnormality may be observed in patients receiving carbamazepine?

   A. Hyponatremia
   B. Hypokalemia
   C. Hypophosphatemia
   D. Hypomagnesimia
   E. Hypocalcemia

3. How does oxcarbazepine compare with carbamazepine as an AED?

   A. It is a prodrug of carbamazepine.
   B. It lacks the autoinduction properties of carbamazepine.
   C. It may be better tolerated than carbamazepine.
   D. A and B
   E. A, B and C

4. Although phenobarbital is considered effective against the type of seizure disorder NM has, his physician is reluctant to prescribe it because of its side-effect profile. What particular side effect limits the use of phenobarbital as an AED?

   A. Nephrolithiasis
   B. Leukopenia
   C. Hypersensitivity reactions
   D. Cognitive impairment
   E. Thrombocytopenia

5. Which of the following AEDs is metabolized to phenobarbital?

   A. Topiramate
   B. Primidone
   C. Tiagabine
   D. Gabapentin
   E. Lamotrigine

6. NM is not on valproate because of side effects. Which of the following side effects is *most likely* associated with valproate therapy?

   A. Nephrotoxicity
   B. Leukopenia
   C. Skin rash
   D. Hepatotoxicity
   E. Hypokalemia

7. NM's physician requests information about extended-release carbamazepine preparations (Tegretol XR, Carbatrol) in order to simplify his regimen given that he will be taking a second AED. Which of the following statements concerning these two preparations is *most correct*?

   A. Both may be dosed twice daily.
   B. The empty tablet shell for the Tegretol XR does not dissolve in the gastrointestinal tact and may be visible in the stool.
   C. Carbatrol beads may be sprinkled on food.
   D. A and B
   E. A, B, and C

8. A paradoxical increase in seizures observed with high serum concentrations of carbamazepine is thought to be secondary to accumulation of what product(s)?

   A. The parent compound
   B. Oxcarbazepine
   C. The epoxide metabolite
   D. A and B
   E. B and C

9. NM develops a respiratory track infection and is started on erythromycin therapy. What effect would erthyromycin have on serum carbazmazepine levels?

   A. No effect because there is no drug-drug interaction
   B. Increased levels owing to decreased renal clearance of carbamzepine
   C. Increased levels owing to decreased hepatic metabolism of carbamazepine
   D. Decreased levels owing to increased renal clearance of carbamzepine
   E. Decreased levels owing to increased hepatic metabolism of carbamzepine

10. Of the following AEDs NM has ever received, which one is characterized by dose-dependent (Michaelis-Menton) pharmacokinetics?

    A. Phenytoin
    B. Valproate
    C. Carbamazepine
    D. All the above
    E. None of the above

LUNG CANCER

PRESENTATION

CC: "I am beginning new chemotherapy."

HPI: LM is a 70-year-old woman with newly diagnosed non-small cell lung carcinoma. Approximately 6 weeks ago LM began feeling fatigued and developed a productive cough that subsequently became dry. She felt that she had a cold and did not see her physician. A week later she presented to the emergency department with a syncopal episode and was admitted to the hospital and was worked up and ruled out for myocardial infarction and arrhythmia. At that time, a chest x-ray showed a right upper lobe infiltrate. The patient was given antibiotics for possible right upper lobe pneumonia. On a follow-up CT scan, LM was found to have a 2.0 × 4.0 cm mass in the right upper lobe with linear opacities extending to the pleura. The patient also had an enlarged right hilar lymph node and precarinal adenopathy. An abdominal CT showed bilateral adrenal masses. Biopsy of the lung mass showed evidence of malignant cells consistent with non-small cell lung carcinoma.

PMH: Excessive uterine bleeding (20 years ago), hypertension

PSH: Hysterectomy (20 years ago)

FH: No family history of cancer; history of hypertension in both parents

SH: Smoked 1 pack of cigarettes per day for the past 50 years; quit 2 months ago; no alcohol or drugs; married with five children; retired school teacher.

ALL: NKDA

MH: Status post 14-day course of levofloxacin, atenolol 50 mg PO qd

ROS: No weight loss, fever, chills, or night sweats; no significant shortness of breath and no hemoptysis

VS: Temperature: 98.9°F; blood pressure: 118/68 mm Hg; heart rate: 70 beats per minute; respiratory rate: 16 breaths per minute; O_2 saturation: 96% RA

Height: 5 ft, 0 in; weight: 120 lb

HEENT: PERRLA, EOMI, no other oral lesions

Neck: No cervical, supraclavicular, axillary, or inguinal lymphadenopathy

Lungs: CTA bilaterally

Heart: RRR, no MRG

ABD: Soft, nontender/nondistended, positive bowel sounds

EXT: No C/C/E

Neuro: A&O × 3, cranial nerves (CNs) II–XII intact

LABORATORY VALUES

Na: 139 mEq/L

Cl: 102 mEq/L

K: 4.6 mEq/L

CO_2: 28 mEq/L

Blood urea nitrogen (BUN): 9 mEq/L

Glucose : 120 mg/dL

Mg: 3.3 mg/dL

ALT: 12 units/L

Total bilirubin: 0.4 mg/dL

Low-density lipoprotein (LDH) cholesterol: 147 IU/mL

Hgb: 12.1 g/dL

Platelets: 360,000/mm^3

Serum Cr : 0.6 mg/dL

Ca: 9.5 mg/dL

PO_4: 1.8 mg/dL

AST: 15 units/L

ALP: 131 IU/mL

White blood cell (WBC) count: 8800/mm^3

Hct: 36.6%

ASSESSMENT/PLAN

LM is a 70-year-old woman with newly diagnosed non-small cell lung carcinoma. She will begin initial treatment today with cisplatin and etoposide.

QUESTIONS

1. Cisplatin belongs to which class of antineoplastic agents?

   A. Alkylating agents
   B. Antimetabolites
   C. Plant alkaloids
   D. Topoisomerase II inhibitors

2. Cisplatin is associated with which of the following adverse event(s)?

   A. Nephrotoxicity
   B. Ototoxicity
   C. Delayed emesis
   D. All the above

3. Which of the following agents is *most appropriate* for the prevention of delayed emesis from cisplatin?

   A. Ondansetron
   B. Diphenoxylate/atropine
   C. Dexamethasone
   D. Proclorperazine

4. Which of the following chemotherapeutic agents are paired correctly according to their mechanism of action?
   A. Cyclophosphamide, cisplatin
   B. Dacarbazine, methotrexate
   C. Doxorubicin, irinotecan
   D. Mitoxantrone, mercaptopurine

5. In this regimen, etoposide is dosed at 100 mg/m^2. What dose of etoposide should LM receive today?

A. 100 mg
B. 150 mg
C. 200 mg
D. 250 mg

6. LM's physician wishes to switch LM to oral etoposide capsules. Since etoposide has an oral bioavailability of 50%, what dose of oral etoposide do you recommend?

A. 200 mg/day
B. 300 mg/day
C. 400 mg/day
D. 500 mg/day

7. Which of the following adverse reactions is more common with oral etoposide than with intravenous etoposide?

A. Myelosuppression
B. Fever
C. Nausea and vomiting
D. Alopecia

8. Which of the following agents can be used to prevent cisplatin-induced nephrotoxicity?

A. Mesna
B. Amifostine
C. Sargramostim
D. Dexrazoxane

9. LM's oncologist wishes to begin amifostine. After reviewing LM's history, you make what recommendation?

A. Hold atenolol becaise amifostine can cause significant hypotension.
B. Increase atenolol to 100 mg PO qd because amifostine can cause significant hypertension.
C. Add furosemide because diuretic therapy is best for amifostine-induced hypertension.
D. No changes are necessary; amifostine is a benign medication.

10. Etoposide exerts its cytotoxicity how?
A. By inhibiting DNA synthesis by intercalation between DNA base pairs
B. By producing DNA strand breaks by inhibiting topoisomerase II
C. By preventing cell division by cross-linking DNA strands
D. By inhibiting dihydrofolate reductase

PATIENT PROFILE 233

ERECTILE DYSFUNCTION

PRESENTATION

CC: "I am having problems with penetrating my partner during sexual intercourse."

HPI: PK is a 55-year-old man who was laid off recently from his job of 20 years. With concerns of the stability of his company over the past 2 years, he has been experiencing episodes of stress and anxiety over the past 2 years. Such occurrences have affected his marital life; he has been married for 30 years. After 2 years of sexual difficulties, JS is now seeking care for his sexual dysfunction. The cause of PK's erectile dysfunction has been evaluated, and drug-induced causes have been ruled out. PK is appropriately treated with behavioral therapy for his stress and anxiety. PK is looking to initiate medication therapy to "cure" his erectile dysfunction to help salvage his marriage. PK was sent to a pharmacist-run outpatient clinic for counseling on general erectile dysfunction and therapeutic options.

Medications: Claritin 10 mg PO qd, lipitor 40 mg PO qd, aspirin 81 mg PO qd

PMH: Depression diagnosed 2 years ago, erectile dysfunction (initiated 2 years ago; reported recently), seasonal allergies (2 years ago only)

PSH: None

FH: Not available

SH: Married 30 years ago; denies alcohol use; unemployed.

ALL: NKDA

PHYSICAL EXAMINATION

General: Appearance reflects apparent age.

VS: Blood pressure: 120/82 mm Hg; heart rate: 60 beats per minute; respiratory rate: 22 breaths per minute; temperature: 37°C

Height: 5 ft, 7 in; weight: 75 kg

HEENT: PERRLA, EOMI

COR: RRR; no m/r/g; normal S_1 and S_2

Chest: Lungs CTA

ABD: Soft, nontender, normal bowel sounds

GU: Normal scrotum; penis without curvature/discharge.

RECT: Normal anus
EXT: Normal
NEURO: Carnial nerves (CNs) II–XII intact.
ECG: Normal

LABORATORY VALUES

Na: 132 mEq/L   K: 4.0 mEq/L
Cl: 100 mEq/L HCO_3: 5.8 mEq/L
Blood urea nitrogen Serum Cr: 1.0 mg/dL
  (BUN): 14 mg/dL
Glucose: N/A   Hgb: 15.0 g/dL
Hct: 47%   Platelets: $300 \times 10_3$/mm3
PT: N/A   aPTT: N/A
Triglycerides: 130 mg/dL   Total cholesterol: 172 mg/dL
High-density lipoprotein (HDL) cholesterol: 50 mg/dL
Low-density lipoprotein (LDL) cholesterol: 91 mg/dL
Testosterone: Normal (700 ng/dL)

QUESTIONS

1. Which of the following is(are) risk factor(s) that PK has for erectile dysfunction?

   I.   Anxiety
   II. Depression
   III. Hyperlipidemia

   A. I only
   B. II only
   C. I and II
   D. II and III
   E. I, II, and III

2. Which of the following need(s) to be considered to address other potential risk factors prior to initiating a medication in PK for erectile dysfunction?

   I.   History of diabetes
   II. Smoking history
   III. Over-the-counter medication use

   A. I only
   B. II only
   C. I and II
   D. II and III
   E. I, II, and III

3. A phosphodiesterase inhibitor is effective in which of the following erectile dysfunction–related conditions?

   A. Hypogonadism
   B. Performance anxiety
   C. Psychological distress
   D. Vascular erectile dysfunction
   E. Dysfunction owing to a lack of an intact neurologic pathway

4. If PK is initiated on Viagra, which of the following is(are) correct counseling point(s)?

   I.   Take 15 minutes prior to sexual activity.
   II. Duration is 4 to 6 hours.
   III. Take on an empty stomach.

   A. I only
   B. II only
   C. I and II
   D. II and III
   E. I, II, and III

5. If PK is initiated on Cialis, which of the following is(are) correct counseling point(s)?

   I.   Take 15 minutes prior to sexual activity.
   II. Duration is 4 to 6 hours.
   III. Take on an empty stomach.

   A. I only
   B. II only
   C. I and II
   D. II and III
   E. I, II, and III

6. If PK is initiated on Levitra, which of the following is(are) correct counseling point(s)?

   I.   Take 15 minutes prior to sexual activity.
   II. Duration is 4 to 6 hours.
   III. Take on an empty stomach.

   A. I only
   B. II only
   C. I and II
   D. II and III
   E. I, II, and III

7. In order to determine the appropriate dose reduction of the phosphodiesterase inhibitor for PK, which of the following conditions must be considered?

   I.   Renal dysfunction
   II. Hepatic dysfunction
   III. Cytochrome P450 3A4 inhibitor use

   A. I only
   B. II only
   C. I and II
   D. II and III
   E. I, II, and III

8. Which of the following medications used for erectile dysfunction may cause priapism?

   I.   Yohimbine
   II. Sildenafil
   III. Trazodone

   A. I only
   B. II only

C. I and II
D. II and III
E. I, II, and III

9. If PK is initiated on Caverject, which of the following is(are) correct counseling point(s)?

A. Inject penis at 3 o'clock and 9 o'clock angles.
B. Inject penis at 12 o'clock and 6 o'clock angles.
C. Inject penis at 2 o'clock and 10 o'clock angles.
D. Wait 12 hours between injections.

E. Applying pressure at site of injection is not necessary.

10. If PK is initiated on Muse, which of the following is(are) correct counseling point(s)?

A. Insert applicator ¼ in into urethra.
B. Insert applicator ¾ in into urethra.
C. Insert applicator 1 in into urethra.
D. Apply pressure at site of insertion after administration.
E. Massage penis for 10 seconds after administration.

PATIENT PROFILE 234

PREGNANCY

PRESENTATION

A 30-year-old woman G3 P4 presents with amenorrhea of 1 month's duration and daily episodes of nausea and overall fatigue.

PMH: Mild hypertension (usually resolves after pregnancy), asthma, depression (with a suicide attempt at 19 years of age)
SH: Former drug abuser (has been clean for 15 years); smokes and drinks occasionally; not married
FH: Noncontributory
ALL: NKDA

PHYSICAL EXAMINATION

VS: Blood pressure: 140/90 mm Hg; heart rate: 89 beats per minute; respiratory rate: 12 breaths per minute; temperature: 98.6°F
Weight: 80 kg
General: Over~~ll~~ well-appearing women with no signifi-
~~   ~~dings
~~   ~~EOMI
~~   ~~murs, rubs, or gallops

~~   ~~nds
~~   ~~a
~~   ~~rmal.
~~   ~~y 1 year ago): Normal
~~   ~~eriod: 5 weeks ago

LABORATORY VALUES

Na: 135   Cl: 112   Scr: 0.8
K: 4.0   CO$_2$: 38   BUN: 10
                 Gluc: 120

HCG (+)
HIV testing: CD4 < 500, HIV RNA > 10,000 copies
STD testing: Negative to date
Radiology: Ultrasound results: The fetus and associated pelvic structures are normal in appearance and appropriate for the gestational age.
Pulmonary function test: Peak flowmeter readings have been >80% of personal best

MEDICATIONS

Adviar 2 puffs bid
Advil (for occasionally headache)
MVI
Prozac 40 mg PO qd

QUESTIONS

1. In the case, what does G3 P4 mean?

A. The patient has had a total of seven pregnancies.
B. The patient has experienced four miscarriages.
C. The patient has been pregnant three times.
D. The patient has three living children.

2. What do over-the-counter (OTC) pregnancy tests detect?

   A. The amount of human chorionic gonadotropin (HCG) in the urine
   B. Gestational age of the fetus
   C. The amount of follicle-stimulating hormone (FSH) in the urine
   D. The luteinizing hormone (LH) surge in the menstrual cycle

3. Folic acid has been shown to decrease the risk of neural tube defects. What is considered a sufficient amount per day of folic acid according to the U.S. Public Health Service?

   A. 4000 μg
   B. 400 μg
   C. 4 mg
   D. 40 μg

4. The patient currently has a blood pressure of 140/90 mm Hg. What would be the *best choice* to manage her hypertension?

   A. Lisinopril
   B. Metoprolol
   C. Avapro
   D. Methyldopa

5. Studies in animals or humans have demonstrated fetal abnormalities or there is evidence of fetal risk based on human experience best describes which Food and Drug Administration (FDA) pregnancy category?

   A. B
   B. C
   C. X
   D. D

6. Based on the patient's recent HIV status, which would be the *best* treatment option?

   I. Patient should be stated on HAART.
   II. No treatment can be recommended because the patient is pregnant.
   III. Start zidovudine monotherapy

   A. I
   B. III

   C. I and II
   D. II and III

7. In HIV-infected women who did not receive therapy, based on Centers for Disease Control and Prevention (CDC) recommendations, what would the be best option for the infant?

   I. No treatment; the baby should be fine because it is not infected with the virus.
   II. The baby should receive zidovudine therapy for 2 weeks.
   III. The baby should receive zidovidine therapy for 6 weeks.

   A. I
   B. III
   C. I and II
   D. II and III

8. What should the management of the patient's asthma be given her pregnancy?

   A. Unchanged; continue taking salmetrol/fluticasone.
   B. Patient should just use albuterol PRN.
   C. Patient should be put on a course of systemic corticosteroids.
   D. Patient should be switched from Advair to plain Flovent.

9. How should the patient's depression be treated?

   A. Discontinue the patient's current regimen until birth.
   B. Consider switching to a tricyclic antidepressant.
   D. Consider using a a monoamine oxidase inhibitor.
   E. Continue the patient on her current regimen, fluoxetine 40 mg qd.

10. The patient should be advised to avoid alcohol for the duration of her pregnancy because of which of the following concerns?

   A. Moon face defect on the infant
   B. Micrognathia
   C. Deformation of the limbs
   D. Neural tube defects

PATIENT PROFILE 235

ANTI-PARKINSON MEDICATIONS

PRESENTATION

GB is a 70-year-old man suffering from Parkinson's disease. Medical history indicates that he has been on levodopa therapy for over 10 years. GB is not suffering from any other medical problems and taking no other medications.

QUESTIONS

1. What is Parkinson's disease?

   I.   A neurodegenerative disease
   II. A disease manifested with high EPS
   III. A disease associated with hypercholinergic activity in the brain
   IV. A disease that mostly affect geriatrics

   A. I and II
   B. II, III, and IV
   C. I, II, and IV
   D. III and IV
   E. All the above

2. Parkinson's disease is associated with low brain activity of the neurotransmitter dopamine (Structure 235.1). Why is dopamine not a suitable drug to treat the disease?

   A. Dopamine has a lot of unwanted side effects.
   B. It is a very polar molecule.
   C. It has a very poor absorption kinetic.
   D. A and B
   E. B and C

3. Why is levodopa (Structure 235.2) superior to dopamine in the treatment of Parkinson's disease?

   A. It is more lipophilic than dopamine, so it has better passive diffusion to the brain.
   B. It is selectively transported to the brain by active transport mechanisms.
   C. It is more potent than dopamine as a direct agonist at the dopamine receptors.
   D. A and B
   E. B and C

4. Which of the following statements about levodopa is(are) *true?*

   A. It is a substrate for the enzyme dopa decarboxylase.
   B. It is a chiral molecule.
   C. It acts as a prodrug.
   D. A and B
   E. A, B, and C

5. Levodopa is combined with carbidopa (Structure 235.3) in a medication called *sinemet.* What is the rationale of such combination ?

   A. To decrease levodopa metabolism both in the periphery and the in the brain
   B. To enhance levodopa metabolism into its active form, dopamine
   C. To inhibit levodopa peripheral metabolism only without affecting the central one
   D. A and B
   E. A and C

6. Why does carbidopa not cross the blood-brain barrier?

   A. It is very lipophilic.
   B. It is very polar.
   C. It is not an amino acid.
   D. A and C
   E. B and C

7. Among the newer antiparkinsonian agents are the drugs ropinirole (Structure 235.4) and pramixole (Structure 235.5). What is the mechanism of action of these drugs?

   A. Act as prodrugs to generate dopamine in vivo
   B. Enhance dopamine transport through the CNS
   C. Act as direct dopaminergic agents in the CNS
   D. Inhibit dopa metabolism
   E. None of the above

235.3

235.1

235.2

235.4

235.5

8. The drug tolcapone (Structure 235.6) is a new anti-Parkinson agent that acts through enzyme inhibitory mechanism. Which of the following enzymes does tolcapone target?

   A. Serum estrases
   B. Monoamine oxidase (MAO)
   C. COMT
   D. Dopa decarboxylase
   E. None of the above

9. Anticholinergic drugs are useful in alleviating Parkinson's symptoms.
   A. True
   B. False

235-6

10. Which of the following agents is considered the drug of choice to suppress the cholinergic symptoms of Parkinson's disease?

    A. Atropine (Structure 235.7)
    B. Carbachol (Structure 235.8)
    C. Benzotropine (Structure 235.9)
    D. A or B
    E. None of the above

235-7

235-8

235-9

PATIENT PROFILE 236
BACTEREMIA AND SEPSIS

PRESENTATION

DL is a 40-year-old man with a history of rheumatic heart disease. DL visited his dental hygienist for a routine cleaning approximately 1 week prior to his hospital admission. DL's usual practice had been to take erythromycin before having his teeth cleaned; however, he lost his prescription and didn't think much of it. DL was healthy until 2 days ago, when he spiked a fever to 39.5°C, which was unrelieved with acetaminophen. On the morning of admission, the fever persists, and DL reports abnormalities of his hands (Janeway lesions). At admission, two specimens for blood cultures are drawn from peripheral sites, and a transthoracic echocardiogram reveals a valvular vegetation consistent with endocarditis.

QUESTIONS

1. Choose an empirical antibiotic regimen for DL?

   A. Nafcillin 2 g IV q4h and gentamicin 1 mg/kg IV q12h
   B. Ceftazidime 2 g IV q8 hours and ciprofloxacin 400 mg IV q8h
   C. Trovafloxacin 300 mg PO q24h
   D. Aztreonam 1 g IV q8h and gentamicin 1 mg/kg IV q8h
   E. Cefoxitin 1 g IV q6h

2. If culture results show methicillin-resistant *Staphylococcus aureusI* (MRSA), the drug of choice becomes IV vancomycin. What additional drug from the following list can be added for synergy?

   A. Isoniazid
   B. Ciprofloxacin
   C. Azithromycin
   D. Clindamycin
   E. Rifampin

3. Nafcillin is the mainstay for *S. aureus* infections. Which of the following can be attributed to nafcillin?

   A. Pain and irritation with IV infusion
   B. Hypokalemia with doses of 200 to 300 mg/kg/d
   C. Reversible neutropenia with more than 3 weeks of treatment

D. Interstitial nephritis

E. All the above

4. DL had been taking erythromycin for endocarditis prophylaxis for years. Knowing that DL is not allergic to β-lactam antibiotics and is capable of taking oral therapy, which would be the *best* regimen for DL?

A. Amoxicillin 2 g PO 1 hour before dental procedures

B. Ampicillin 2 g IM or IV 30 minutes before dental procedures

C. Cephalexin 2 g PO 1 hour before dental procedures

D. Azithromycin 500 mg PO 1 hour before dental procedures

E. Clindamycin 600 mg IV within 30 minutes before procedures

5. All the following statements are *true* regarding penicillin-resistant strains of *Streptococus* in endocarditis except

A. Penicillin can be used to manage infection with penicillin-resistant strains of *Streptococcus*.

B. There are no differences in dosing of penicillin for patients who have penicillin-susceptible strains of *Streptococcus* and those with penicillin-resistant strains.

C. Ampicillin in combination with gentamicin can be used to control streptococci with a high level of penicillin resistance.

D. Cefazolin may be used to treat patients who are allergic to penicillins.

E. Vancomycin may be used to treat patients with high-level penicillin resistance.

PATIENT PROFILE 237

NOSOCOMIAL URINARY TRACT INFECTIONS

PRESENTATION

WA is an 80-year-old woman who is transferred from a nursing home with severe chest pain, dyspnea, and shortness of breath. She has been hospitalized three times within the past 3 months with similar complaints, and each time a myocardial infarct was ruled out.

PMH: Unstable angina

Hypertension

s/p Breast cancer

Atrial fibrillation

Epilepsy

Nosocomial urinary tract infections (UTIs)

Medications: Lisinopril 10 mg po qd

Isosorbide dinitrate 10 mg po tid

Diltiazem CD 240 mg po qd

Warfarin 5 mg po qd

Phenytoin 200 mg po qd

Allergies: NKDA

PE: BP 150/95 mm Hg, HR 90 beats/min, O_2 sat 95%, Ht 5'5", Wt 68 kg, Temp 37.2°C

Labs: Na 140 mEq/mL, K 4.7 mEq/mL, BUN 23 mg/dL, SCr 1.4 mg/dL, WBC 9.5×10^3 cells/mm³, INR 2.5, phenytoin level 11.5 μg/mL

Urine analysis: Multiple organisms but no pyuria

EKG: Pending

The patient was initially treated with aspirin, nitroglycerin, metoprolol and oxygen, and her symptoms quickly decreased. CPK and troponin levels were not diagnostic for myocardial infarction. As part of her care, the patient also was catheterized.

QUESTIONS

1. The physician is concerned about WA's asymptomatic bacteriuria on admission and asks the team pharmacist if this should be treated with antibiotics.

    Asymptomatic bacteriuria in elderly patients should not be treated because the drug therapy may be associated with adverse reactions, risk of resistant organisms, and high costs that outweigh potential benefits.

    A. True statement

    B. False statement

2. Three days after admission WA complains of severe burning on urination, urgency, and abdominal pain. The diagnosis of hospital-acquired UTI is made, and a urine C&S is ordered. Which of the following is/are true regarding hospital-acquired (nosocomial) UTI?

    I.   The sensitivity of hospital-acquired urinary pathogens to antibiotics may be different than that of community-acquired urinary pathogens.

    II. Organisms frequently associated with nosocomial UTIs include E. coli, other gram-negative organisms such as *Proteus* and *Pseudomonas* sp., and gram-positive organisms such as staphylococci and enterococci as well as yeast.

III. Antibiotic-resistant organisms are more frequently seen in nosocomial infections.

A. I only
B. III only
C. I and III
D. I , II, and III
E. II and III

3. Based on a urine gram stain showing gram-positive cocci, it is decided to treat the patient empirically for enterococci. Which of the following regimens is suitable?

I. Vancomycin IV ± gentamicin IV
II. Penicillin IV
III. Nafcillin IV ± gentamicin IV
IV. Ampicillin IV ± gentamicin IV
V. Ciprofloxacin IV

A. I only
B. II only
C. III or IV
D. V only
E. I or IV

4. If the patient were to receive gentamicin IV (2 mg/kg), which of the doses indicated below would be an appropriate *loading dose* for her?

A. 60 mg
B. 120 mg
C. 160 mg
D. 70 mg
E. 140 mg

5. The loading dose calculated in Question 4 is continued in the patient (given q12h). A trough level taken after the fourth dose shows a gentamicin concentration of 3.1 μg/mL. What conclusion should be drawn from this result?

A. This level is too high because the therapeutic maintenance dose was not adjusted according to the patient's renal function.
B. This level is too low, and the patient should receive a higher dose.
C. This level cannot be interpreted because the trough level always should be taken after the loading dose.
D. The next dose should be increased and the interval shortened to q8h.
E. The next dose should be decreased and the interval should be decreased.

6. Elevated gentamicin trough levels should be avoided because of potential toxic effects of the drug. These include which of the following?

A. Rash and tinnitus
B. Hyperlipidemia and hepatotoxicity
C. Arrhythmias and cardiac arrest
D. Nephrotoxicity and ototoxicity
E. Stevens-Johnson syndrome and hyperuricemia

7. The physician treating WA is curious about once-daily gentamicin dosing (5 to 7 mg/kg per day) and wants more information on that. Which answer(s) is/are correct?

I. qd Dosing of gentamicin is based on the drug's time-dependent killing.
II. qd Dosing of gentamicin is based on the drug's postantibiotic effect.
III. qd Dosing of gentamicin is based on the drug's concentration-dependent killing.
IV. qd Dosing is recommended for all infections that need treatment with aminoglycoside because it is more cost effective and less toxic.
V. qd Dosing is not recommended for a patient with renal impairment.

A. I and II
B. I, II and IV
C. II and III
D. II, III and V
E. I and IV

8. The physician wants to know which of the following drugs have a similar spectrum as gentamicin with respect to gram-negative coverage (including *Pseudomonas aeruginosa*).

A. Piperacillin-tazobactam
B. Amoxicillin
C. Cefazolin
D. Quinupristin-dalfopristin
E. Oxacillin

9. Soon after WA's successful treatment of her bacterial nosocomial UTI, she again complains of urinary burning and lower abdominal pain. Her urine analysis shows pyuria and yeast, which are later identified as *Candida* sp. What is an appropriate oral antifungal treatment for her urinary candidiasis?

A. Metronidazole 500 mg po qid
B. Nystatin 4 MU oral suspension swish and swallow qid
C. Clotrimazole troches 80 mg po tid
D. Fluconazole 200 mg po qd
E. Amphotericin B 1 mg/kg per day po

10. If the patient were to receive fluconazole, which of the following needs to be closely monitored?

I. Her INR level
II. Her phenytoin level

III. Her blood pressure
IV. Her renal function

A. I only

B. I and II
C. III only
D. IV only
E. I, II, and IV

PATIENT PROFILE 238

DERMATOLOGY

PRESENTATION

CR is a 20-year-old-woman who comes to your pharmacy with a prescription for benzoyl peroxide gel (Benzac® AC 2.5%). You notice several whiteheads on her forehead, and she has a few blackheads on her nose. No inflamed papules, pustules, or nodular lesions are apparent. CR states that she went to see a dermatologist and he prescribed a form of benzoyl peroxide for 2 weeks and had little success. Her medical history includes recurrent sinusitis and she was treated for the last episode with amoxicillin-clavulanate (Augmentin®). She also takes ibuprofen for menstrual cramps and norgestrel with ethinyl estradiol (Lo/Ovral®).

QUESTIONS

1. Which of the following should be emphasized to CR concerning the initiation of benzoyl peroxide therapy?

   A. Initial treatments should be applied once daily to decrease irritation.
   B. The gel should be applied sparingly, and the periorbital, perinasal, and perioral skin should be avoided.
   C. Mild erythema, burning, or stinging may occur with the initial application. If the medication is applied at bedtime, the erythema should be minimal by the next morning.
   D. A and B
   E. All of the above

2. What other information should be included in your counseling session with CR?

   A. Tolerance to adverse effects should occur as therapy continues.
   B. Because benzoyl peroxide can bleach hair and clothes, the preparation should be allowed to dry before coming into contact with fabrics.
   C. The full therapeutic effect occurs in 1 to 2 weeks and CR should be told to expect optimal results during this period.
   D. A and B
   E. All of the above

3. CR responds fairly well to the benzoyl peroxide therapy and continues the therapy for approximately 7 months. At that time, however, CR notices worsening of her acne and inflamed lesions. The dermatologist decides to add systemic therapy with minocycline while continuing the benzoyl peroxide therapy. CR comes to your pharmacy with a prescription for minocycline. Which of the following statement(s) concerning minocycline is/are true?

   A. Minocycline should be avoided in pregnancy.
   B. Vestibular side effects, such as dizziness, vertigo, and light-headedness, can occur with minocycline use, particularly at higher doses.
   C. Minocycline is a macrolide antibiotic that blocks the translocation step of protein synthesis by targeting the 23S rRNA of the 50S subunit.
   D. A and B
   E. All of the above

4. Tetracycline is another systemic antibiotic that could have been prescribed for CR. Which of the following statement(s) is/are true concerning this agent?

   A. Photosensitivity can occur, and patients should be counseled to wear sunscreen with an SPF of at least 15 if planning to spend time in the sun.
   B. Vaginal yeast infection is a potential side effect of tetracycline.
   C. Coadministration with dairy products, antacids, bismuth salts, sucralfate, and iron can decrease absorption of tetracycline, and administration should be separated.
   D. A and B
   E. All of the above

5. Tretinoin (Retin-A®) is another option for treatment of acne. Which of the following statement(s) is/are true regarding this agent?

   A. Tretinoin is a derivative of vitamin A.
   B. Tretinoin is available in various formulations, such as cream, gel, and lotion.

C. Tretinoin increases follicle cell turnover and decreases cohesiveness of cells; this results in extrusion of existing comedones and inhibits formation of new comedones.
D. A and B
E. All of the above

6. Which statement(s) should be included in your counseling session with a patient beginning treatment with tretinoin?

A. Tretinoin can cause skin irritation, which ranges from mild to severe and is more common during initiation of therapy.
B. Patients may notice an exacerbation of acne at initiation of therapy. This is caused by the mechanism of action of tretinoin. Therapy should be continued, and this flare should resolve in 3 to 6 weeks.
C. Patients should be advised to avoid long exposure to UV radiation. If exposure is unavoidable, she should use sunscreen with an SPF of at least 15.
D. A and B
E. All of the above

7. Isotretinoin (Accutane®) is available as an option for management of acne. Which statement(s) concerning isotretinoin (Accutane®) is/are true?

A. This agent usually is considered for patients with mild acne as a first option for acne treatment.
B. Unlike other acne therapies, isotretinoin (Accutane®) brings out prolonged remission of acne.
C. Isotretinoin is a synthetic derivative of vitamin D.
D. A and B
E. All of the above

8. The dermatologist has discussed the adverse effects of isotretinoin, particularly effects that occur if this agent is used during pregnancy. Which of the following statement(s) is/are true concerning isotretinoin (Accutane®)?

A. Isotretinoin is pregnancy category B.
B. Isotretinoin is considered to be safe to use during the second and third trimesters of pregnancy.
C. Isotretinoin should be avoided in pregnancy because miscarriage and stillbirth are common, and severe congenital anomalies have been associated with use of this agent.
D. A and B
E. All of the above

9. Patient receiving isotretinoin for treatment of acne should be counseled regarding potential adverse effects. Your counseling should include which of the following?

A. Mucocutaneous side effects, such as dryness of the skin, eyes, nose, and mouth are common.
B. Conjunctivitis and corneal opacities may occur; during this period, patients may not be able to tolerate contact lenses. These effects usually resolve within 6 weeks.
C. Abnormalities in serum triglyceride and cholesterol levels may occur and should be monitored during therapy.
D. A and B
E. All of the above

10. What baseline and period monitoring parameters should be followed in patients receiving isotretinoin?

A. Lipid panel
B. Serum liver transaminases
C. Serum uric acid level
D. A and B
E. All of the above.

PATIENT PROFILE 239

CHRONIC OBSTRUCTIVE PULMONARY DISEASE

PRESENTATION

MR is a 47-year-old woman whom you have seen for a number of years. Her medical history is significant for a diagnosis of chronic obstructive pulmonary disease (COPD), which has been controlled with albuterol (for symptom management) for the past 2 years. Today she presents to you with the complaint of difficult breathing, shortness of breath, and productive cough. She states that she has felt these symptoms slowly worsening over the past few months but also mentions that she does not suffer from any nocturnal symptoms. Today she has an FEV_1 of 45% of predicted. MR states she has not been able to completely quit smoking but has decreased her smoking from two packs to one pack daily. Since attempting to quit, she does admit to drinking alcohol a little more often to help her get by without smoking. MR states she currently drinks about two glasses of wine with dinner. Because of this increase in alcohol consumption MR would like to try bupropion to help her quit smoking. She mentions that she had a friend who used it and said it worked great. Both of MR's parents are alive and living in Florida; neither has any significant medical conditions. She has one brother who lives in Wyoming who is also healthy. MR lives with her husband and only son, for whom she is trying to quite smoking. Both husband and son are very healthy. She informs you that she is also taking Vicodin® for back pain resulting from an accident she was in last year, as well as Allegra® for allergies. MR mentions that the symptoms have progressed so much that she has had to miss days from work and at times even go to the hospital. She is currently working as an accountant for a private school and is concerned that her health is starting to affect her job.

Albuterol inhaler one to two puffs by mouth every 4 to 6 hours as needed
Vicodin® one tablet by mouth four times a day as needed
Allegra® 60 mg one tablet by mouth twice a day
Medical Conditions:
COPD
Back pain
Seasonal allergies

QUESTIONS

1. In which of the following stages would MR most likely be currently classified?

   A. Stage 0, at risk for COPD
   B. Stage I, mild COPD
   C. Stage II, moderate COPD
   D. Stage III, severe COPD
   E. Stage IV, very severe COPD

2. What is the best option for first-line chronic therapy for MR?

   A. Albuterol as needed, Ipratropium inhaler two puffs by mouth three times a day, and rehabilitation
   B. Albuterol as needed, Ipratropium inhaler two puffs by mouth three times a day, rehabilitation, and theophylline 200 mg twice a day
   C. Albuterol as needed, Ipratropium inhaler two puffs by mouth three times a day, rehabilitation and salmeterol diskus two puffs by mouth two times a day
   D. Albuterol as needed, Ipratropium inhaler two puffs by mouth three times a day, rehabilitation, and fluticasone inhaler two puffs by mouth two times a day

   E. Albuterol as needed, Ipratropium inhaler two puffs by mouth three times a day, rehabilitation, and prednisone 10-mg tablets by mouth every day for 10 days

3. Which of the following is true concerning the medication ipratropium on which MR will be placed?

   A. Dry mouth is a side effect.
   B. Rarely used in the treatment of severe COPD
   C. Will reverse the inflammation associated with COPD
   D. Available in a combination product with fluticasone
   E. Available in both tablet and metered dose inhaler form

4. MR inquires under which class of medication Ipratropium falls. Which of the following is your reply?

   A. A xanthine
   B. An antioxidant
   C. An anticholinergic
   D. An inhaled corticosteroid
   E. A long-acting β_2-agonist

5. MR inquires what the difference is between ipratropium and tiotropium. Which of the following is your reply?

   I. Dosage form
   II. Duration of action
   III. Side-effect profile

   A. I only
   B. III only
   C. I and II
   D. II and III
   E. I, II, and III

6. Which of the following is the appropriate dosing of tiotropium if MR is placed on the medication?

   A. One inhalation once a day
   B. One inhalation twice a day
   C. One inhalation three times a day
   D. One inhalation four times a day
   E. One inhalation every 4 to 6 hours

7. Which of the following is the most appropriate maintenance dose of bupropion for MR?

   A. One tablet once a day
   B. Two tablets once a day
   C. One tablet twice a day
   D. Two tablets twice a day
   E. One tablet three times a day

8. Which of the following should MR be counseled on concerning the use of bupropion?

I. It may cause drowsiness.
II. It may cause hypotension.
III. It should be initiated 1 week before the patient stops smoking.

A. I only
B. III only
C. I and II
D. II and III
E. I, II, and III

9. MR returns 3 months later to discuss her current therapy. At this time you are informed that her FEV$_1$ is 80% and she is having minimal daily symptoms. In which of the following stages would MR most likely be currently classified?

A. Stage 0, at risk for COPD
B. Stage I, mild COPD

C. Stage II, moderate COPD
D. Stage III, severe COPD
E. Stage IV, very severe COPD

10. At this time MR is currently on the following medications: prednisone tablets, albuterol inhaler, tiotropium inhaler, and flunisolide inhaler. Which of her current medications are most likely to be discontinued at this time?

I. Albuterol inhaler
II. Tiotropium inhaler
III. Prednisone tablets

A. I only
B. III only
C. I and II
D. II and III
E. I, II, and III

PATIENT PROFILE 240
^{18}F-FDG

PRESENTATION

LD is a 75-year-old woman who was admitted with a suspected brain tumor. It was determined that an ^{18}F-FDG study would be performed. Images showed focal uptake indicating a glioblastoma.

QUESTIONS

1. ^{18}F is best imaged using which of the following imaging systems?

A. PET
B. SPECT
C. CT
D. X-ray film
E. RIA

2. The emission of ^{18}F is which of the following?

A. α
B. β$^-$
C. β$^+$
D. γ
E. X-ray

3. FDG is an abbreviation for which of the following?

A. Fasting deacylated guanine
B. Fast-degrading glycogen

C. Fluorodeltaguanine
D. Freeze-dried glycerin
E. Fluorodeoxyglucose

4. ^{18}F-FDG shows increased uptake in areas of increased metabolism because it mimics which of the following?

A. DNA
B. Glucose
C. Adenosine triphosphate
D. Liposomes
E. Water

5. Which of the following is the proper dose of ^{18}F-FDG to be given to the patient?

A. 500 to 1000 μCi
B. 1 to 5 mCi
C. 5 to 10 mCi
D. 10 to 50 mCi
E. 50 to 100 mCi

6. Which of the following is the *end* result of an ^{18}F decay?

A. α
B. β$^-$
C. X-rays
D. γ
E. β$^+$

7. The half-life of ^{18}F is 110 minutes. Calculate its decay constant (λ).

    A. 0.00630 hr
    B. 0.1578^{-1} hr
    C. 158.7 min
    D. 0.00630 min^{-1}
    E. 0.630 min

8. Approximately how long would it take for 48 μCi of ^{18}F to decay to 1.5 μCi?

    A. 10 hours, 12 minutes
    B. 8 hours, 50 minutes
    C. 8 hours, 35 minutes
    D. 14 hours, 18 minutes
    E. 9 hours, 10 minutes

9. At 6:30 AM you have available 45 mCi of ^{18}F-FDG. Approximately what is the *latest* time this can be given to a patient and still provide a 5-mCi dose?

    A. 2:30 PM
    B. 12:20 PM
    C. 9:45 AM
    D. 3:40 PM
    E. 8:15 AM

10. ^{18}F is acquired from which of the following?

    A. A cyclotron
    B. Naturally occurring sources that are enriched
    C. A linear particle accelerator
    D. A reactor
    E. Any of the above

PATIENT PROFILE 241

SMOKING CESSATION

PRESENTATION

TS is a 55-year-old white woman who presents to her community pharmacy for a refill on her Atrovent inhaler. She states that it has been getting harder to breathe. She does not exercise on a regular basis because walking often leaves her "out-of-breath."

She is interested in quitting smoking. TS has tried to quit before but continues to smoke because she feels "jittery" and cannot sleep if she does not smoke. She currently smokes two packs of cigarettes per day. The patient states that her first cigarette of the day is upon wakening, before her morning shower. She admits to smoking more in the afternoon and evening while watching television. Her smoking has increased since her husband's death 5 years ago.

Her breathing difficulties have become increasingly worse during the past week. However, she has continued to smoke as usual but has not been able to use her inhaler because she "ran out" 2 weeks ago and has not had the time to refill her prescription. She is at the pharmacy to have her prescription for her inhaler refilled and would also like some information on smoking cessation.

Hypothyroidism diagnosed at age 39
Menopause at age 42
COPD diagnosed at age 45
Osteoporosis diagnosed at age 53
Tobacco use: One to two packs per day ($\times$ 40 years); currently two packs per day for the past 5 years

Alcohol use: One to two glasses of wine each night (to help her sleep)
Denies use of illicit or recreational drugs
Caffeine use: One to two cups of tea each morning; (–) coffee, soda
FH: TS lives alone since her husband's death 5 years ago. She is a retired homemaker with two sons ages 30 and 32. Her father died of a heart attack at age 52 and her mother age 80 is alive and suffers from diabetes and arthritis. TS is the second child of four siblings. All close family members are cigarette smokers.
ROS: TS denies headache, dizziness, chest pain, seizures, nausea, diarrhea, constipation, or urinary incontinence. She complains of shortness of breath after walking two flights of stairs or walking to her brother's home (approximately 1/2 mile). This has worsened over the past 2 weeks because of the lack of an Atrovent inhaler.
Gen: Well-groomed, thin woman who looks her stated age with a flushed face and in obvious respiratory distress. She sits through the interview with chest forward and hands resting on her knees; breathing through pursed lips. She is slightly nervous about quitting smoking.
VS: BP 120/70 mm Hg, HR 74 beats/min, RR 17 rpm, Ht 5'5"
HEENT: WNL; wears dentures
Chest: Expiratory bilateral wheezes
Cardiac: Normal rate and rhythm; no murmurs or gallop
Skin: Marked "crow's feet" around eyes and wrinkling around mouth

Table 241-1.   Medication Record

Date	Drug/Dosage	Quantity	Sig	Refills
8/20	Atrovent MDI	1	2 puffs qid	6
8/20	Synthroid 75 μg	30	1 tab po qd	3
9/1	Fosamax 10 mg	30	1 tab po qd	5
9/1	Theophylline 300 mg	60	1 tab po q 12h	5

Neuro: A&O × 3
Allergies: PCN (rash)
Laboratory and Diagnostic Tests: **None available at this time**

PHARMACIST NOTES/ADDITIONAL PATIENT INFORMATION

11/22/03: Smoking cessation discussed with patient. TS continues to be unwilling to quit at this time.

5/20/03: Metered dose inhaler technique reassessed and patient re-educated about proper technique.

4/1/03: Smoking cessation discussed with patient. She seemed interested, yet unwilling to quit at this time.

8/1/02: TS discontinued estrogen/progestin replacement therapy for menopause. Started herbal therapy containing black cohosh and soy.

DIAGNOSIS

1. Tobacco dependence (40 to 80 pack-years)
2. Hypothyroidism × 16 years
3. COPD × 10 years
4. Osteoporosis × 2 years
5. Post-menopausal × 13 years

QUESTIONS

1. Which one of the following is an assessment tool used in research and clinical practice to assess nicotine dependence?

   A. DSM-IV
   B. PANSS
   C. BRPS
   D. FTND
   E. CAGE

2. Polycyclic aromatic hydrocarbons (PAHs) in cigarette smoke are responsible for most drug interactions associated with smoking. Polycyclic aromatic hydrocarbons are potent inducers of which one of the following hepatic cytochrome P450 microsomal enzymes?

   A. CYP 3A4
   B. CYP 1A2
   C. CYP 1C3
   D. CYP 2D6
   E. CYP 2C19

3. The clearance of which one of the following medications may be altered when TS quits smoking?

   A. Atrovent
   B. Synthroid
   C. Fosamax
   D. Theophylline
   E. Black cohosh

4. Which of the following statements about smoking cessation is true?

   I. Screening of tobacco use should be a routine component of clinical care.
   II. All tobacco users should be advised to quit and patient-specific health problems should be linked to cigarette smoking.
   III. The patient's ability to quit smoking is dependent only on the use of nicotine replacement therapy; follow-up counseling interactions are not needed.

   A. I only
   B. III only
   C. I and II only
   D. II and III only
   E. I, II, and III

5. TS is concerned about withdrawal symptoms after she quits smoking. Which one of the following is a common symptom of nicotine withdrawal that she may experience if she abruptly stops smoking?

   A. Diarrhea
   B. Difficulty concentrating
   C. Anorexia

D. Palpitations
E. Hypersomnia

6. TS would like to use nicotine replacement therapy (NRT) to help her quit smoking. Which of the following statements regarding the use of NRT is true?

I.   The nicotine nasal spray reaches peak nicotine plasma concentrations more rapidly than other forms of NRT.
II. The nicotine transdermal patch has the slowest onset of the NRT products, but provides more consistent plasma nicotine concentrations.
III. The FDA classifies nicotine as pregnancy risk category D.

A. I only
B. III only
C. I and I only
D. II and III only
E. I, II, and III

7. TS has decided to use a nicotine transdermal patch to help her quit smoking. Which of the following is the most important information to provide the patient about the patch?

A. To provide consistent nicotine absorption, apply the patch to the same clean, dry, hairless area of the skin at approximately the same time each day.
B. To ensure patch adherence, advise the patient not to bathe, shower, swim, or exercise while wearing the patch.
C. The most common side effects associated with the nicotine patch are erythema, burning, and pruritus at the skin application site.
D. No over-the-counter nicotine transdermal patch products are available; the patient should be advised to see her physician for a prescription.
E. The patient should use only the 24-hour nicotine transdermal patch in achieving smoking cessation because it offers many advantages over the 16-hour patch.

8. TS returns to your pharmacy 6 months later and tells you that she was successful in smoking cessation for the 8 weeks that she used the nicotine-replacement therapy. Now she is feeling very down about her health and because she has relapsed to smoking again. She states that when she was not smoking she had a strong craving to smoke. Her physician has prescribed Zyban to help her in her current attempt to quit smoking. Which of the following statements regarding Zyban is true?

I.   Zyban is an oral form on nicotine replacement therapy that helps reduce cravings for cigarettes and symptoms of nicotine withdrawal.
II. Treatment with Zyban should be initiated while the patient is still smoking, approximately 1 week before the quit date.
III. Zyban can be used safely in conjunction with a nicotine transdermal patch.

A. I only
B. III only
C. I and II only
D. II and III only
E. I, II, and III

9. TS is interested in a short-acting NRT product. Which of the following NRT products is the least appropriate for TS?

A. Nicotine polacrilex gum
B. Nicotine lozenge
C. Nicotine nasal spray
D. Nicotine oral inhaler
E. Nicotine transdermal patch

10. Although not approved by the Food and Drug Administration (FDA) specifically for smoking cessation, which one of the following is recommended as a second-line agent?

A. Amitriptyline
B. Nortriptyline
C. Bupropion SR
D. Sertraline
E. Fluoxetine

PATIENT PROFILE 242

HYPERCHOLESTEROLEMIA

PRESENTATION

JW is a 57-year-old white woman, with a history of hypercholesterolemia, who reports to her primary care physician to follow up on her elevated LDL level.

PMH: Mild asthma (4 years), hypertension (12 years), hypercholesterolemia (3 years), postmenopausal
FH: Noncontributory
SH: Smokes 1/2 pack per day; married with two children; occasional EtOH use

MH: Metoprolol 50 mg bid, Albuterol inhaler two puffs prn (three times per week), 40 mg atorvastatin qd, occasional ibuprofen use; NKDA

ROS: Noncontributory

PE: BP 132/88, P 67, RR 14, Temp 37.0°C, Wt 61.6 kg, Ht 168 cm

Labs: TC 185 mg/dL, TG 165 mg/dL, HDL 35 mg/dL, LDL 120 mg/dL; glucose 98 mg/dL.

QUESTIONS

1. How many independent coronary heart disease risk factors, other than LDL, does JW have?

   A. 5
   B. 4
   C. 3
   D. 2
   E. 1

2. The physician wants JW's LDL to be below 100 mg/dL. He wants to start her on a bile acid sequestrants. You choose to start her on colesevelam. What is the usual daily dose of colesevelam?

   A. 4 to 16 g/day
   B. 5 to 20 g/day
   C. 2.6 to 3.8 g/day
   D. 2.6 to 3.8 mg/day
   E. 400 to 1600 mg/day

3. When do you obtain lipid serum levels to monitor for the efficacy of the statins when they are first initiated or there is a dosage change?

   A. 4 weeks
   B. 4 months
   C. 6 weeks
   D. 6 months
   E. 2 weeks

4. When are bile acid sequestrants absolutely contraindicated for therapy?

   A. When triglycerides are >200 mg/dL
   B. When triglycerides are >100 mg/dL
   C. When triglycerides are >300 mg/dL
   D. When triglycerides are >400 mg/dL
   E. Elevated triglycerides are not a contraindication for therapy

5. How do you best avoid drug interactions with bile acid sequestrants?

   A. Take medications 1 hour before or 4 hours after the sequestrants.
   B. Take the medication 2 hours after the sequestrant.
   C. Take the medication 4 hours before the sequestrant.
   D. Take the medication 6 hours after the sequestrant.
   E. Take the medication 6 hours before the sequestrant.

6. Which of the following is not a major side effect of bile acid sequestrants?

   A. Flatulence
   B. Constipation
   C. Bloating
   D. Elevated liver function tests
   E. Abdominal pain

7. What is the mechanism of action for bile acid sequestrants?

   A. They inhibit the secretion of bile acids.
   B. They decrease the metabolism of triglycerides in the liver.
   C. They increase the metabolism of cholesterol in the liver.
   D. They bind bile acids in the intestine through anionic exchange.
   E. They bind cholesterol in the intestine through anionic exchange.

8. The physician has heard of a new drug, ezetimibe, and he would like JW to use it instead of a bile acid sequestrant. What is the initial starting dose for ezetimibe?

   A. 20 mg po qd
   B. 10 mg po qd
   C. 10 mg po twice daily
   D. 5 mg po qd
   E. 20 mg po twice daily

9. When used in combination with statins there is an increased risk of elevating which of the following laboratory values?

   A. Serum creatinine
   B. White blood count
   C. Serum sodium
   D. Bilirubin
   E. Liver function tests

10. What is ezetimibe's mechanism of action?

   A. It inhibits the metabolisms of cholesterol in the liver.
   B. It increases the metabolism of cholesterol on the liver.
   C. It decreases the absorption of cholesterol in the intestines.
   D. It binds with cholesterol in the stomach.
   E. It increases the metabolism of triglycerides in the liver.

PATIENT PROFILE 243
BACTERIAL VAGINOSIS

PRESENTATION

FM presents to clinic requesting another prescription for metronidazole to treat recurrent bacterial vaginosis. FM is a 21-year-old woman who experiences recurrent episodes of bacterial vaginosis, which occurs approximately 2 weeks after the onset of menses. It does not occur with every cycle. Since the last visit, MS has had unprotected intercourse with one partner. They do not use condoms because of pain and vaginal irritation. The last course of treatment was 2½ months ago, metronidazole 500 mg po bid.

PMH: None
Allergies: None
Current Meds: None
FH: Mother is alive and well, 55 years old; father died at age 57 with DM complications, heart disease, and kidney disease; one sister with obesity.
SH: Denies use of tobacco, caffeine, ethanol, and recreational drugs; moved to the United States from Puerto Rico 5 years ago; works in a factory assembly line; currently lives with her boyfriend.
BP: 100/60, HR 64, RR not available, T afebrile, Wt 48 kg, Ht 5'4"
Gen: Well-appearing woman in no apparent distress
HEENT: PERRLA, EOMI
Chest: Clear to auscultation
Cor: RRR
Abd: Nontender, nondistended
Ext: Alert and oriented ×3; CN II to XII intact
Labs:
Wet mount: (−) Yeast
(−) Trichomonas
(+) Clue cells
(+) Whiff test

QUESTIONS

1. Which of the following organisms is associated with bacterial vaginosis?

   A. Candida albicans
   B. *Gardnerella vaginalis*
   C. *Trichomonas vaginalis*
   D. A and C only
   E. A, B, and C

2. With which of the following is bacterial vaginosis associated?

   A. Douching
   B. Lack of vaginal lactobacilli
   C. Multiple sex partners
   D. A and C only
   E. A, B, and C

3. Which of the following is a goal of therapy of bacterial vaginosis in FM?

   A. Minimize the risk for infectious complications.
   B. Prevent transmission to her partner.
   C. Relieve vaginal symptoms and signs of infection.
   D. A and C only
   E. A, B, and C

4. Which of the following would be the drug of choice for the management of bacterial vaginosis if FM were allergic to oral metronidazole?

   A. Clindamycin (oral)
   B. Erythromycin (oral)
   C. Metronidazole gel (intravaginal)
   D. Ofloxacin (oral)
   E. Tetracycline (oral)

5. Which of the following is a potential adverse effect of metronidazole?

   A. Dizziness
   B. Metallic taste
   C. Nausea
   D. A and C only
   E. A, B, and C

6. Which of the following is a possible effect of metronidazole?

   A. Arthropathy
   B. Disulfiram reaction with alcohol ingestion
   C. Kernicterus
   D. Permanent discoloration of the teeth
   E. Red man syndrome

7. Which of the following is accurate patient counseling information for metronidazole?

   A. Do not consume alcoholic beverages during therapy and for at least 24 hours after the last dose.
   B. Your urine may appear dark or reddish-brown during therapy.
   C. You may take it with food if it upsets your stomach.
   D. A and C only
   E. A, B, and C

8. FM asks if her partner needs to be treated. Which of the following is the best response?

   A. No, it is never necessary for your partner to be treated.
   B. Treatment for the partner is not routinely recommended.
   C. Yes, your partner should be treated with oral therapy.
   D. Yes, your partner should be treated with topical therapy.
   E. Yes, your partner should be treated with oral and topical therapy.

9. Which of the following is an alternative treatment to oral metronidazole in the management of bacterial vaginosis?

   A. Clindamycin cream
   B. Levofloxacin
   C. Metronidazole gel
   D. A and C only
   E. A, B, and C

10. How many days of metronidazole gel 0.75%, one (5-g) application intravaginally once a day, is recommended when used to treat bacterial vaginosis?

    A. 1
    B. 5
    C. 10
    D. 14
    E. 21

PATIENT PROFILE 244
ALZHEIMER'S DISEASE

PRESENTATION

JB is a 72-year-old woman who presents to her physician's office for an assessment of her "forgetfulness" and delusional behavior. She is accompanied by her husband, who has reported this issue to the physician. JB states that it is Monday even though it is Friday. She does not remember her physician's name. JB states that she lives with many people and has conversations with them. She cannot understand why her husband does not see these people and does not know why her husband brought her to the doctor today. JB's husband states that he has to watch JB closely now since she has left the stove on and puts food that belongs in the refrigerator in the cabinet. He states that he frequently hears her talking to the "people" that she claims live in the house with them. He is very concerned about her behavior and is afraid that she will "injure herself" or "burn the house down" someday. When he goes out he makes sure that one of their sons comes over to watch their mother. He believes that she is taking her medications as prescribed and obtained the following refill history from the local pharmacy. He also reports that she seems thinner than she used to be.

PMH: Hypertension diagnosed in January, 2004
Hypothyroidism diagnosed in January, 2004
Med Hx: Lisinopril 10 mg qd
2004 Refill history: 1/17/04, 2/18/04, 3/20/04, 4/22/04, 5/20/04, 6/23/04, 8/21/04, 10/18/04
Metoprolol 100 mg bid
2004 Refill history: 1/17/04, 2/18/04, 3/20/04, 4/22/04, 5/20/04, 6/23/04, 8/21/04, 10/18/04
Levothyroxine 25 µg qd
2004 Refill history: 1/17/04, 2/18/04, 3/20/04, 4/22/04, 5/20/04, 6/23/04, 8/21/04, 9/18/04
ASA 81 mg qd #100 purchased a bottle in April 2004
Allergies: NKDA
FH: Husband is alive and has hypertension, three sons alive and healthy, mother died at age 81 with symptoms of senility
SH: JB lives with her husband of 40 years. Her three sons live nearby and visit regularly.
Labs: BP 140/95 mm Hg, HR 85 bpm, Ht 5'6", Wt 49 kg
PE: Thin, pleasant woman in NAD, slightly confused

PROBLEM LIST

1. Alzheimer's disease (AD)
2. Hypertension
3. Hypothyroidism

QUESTIONS

1. Which of JB's symptoms are consistent with a diagnosis of Alzheimer's disease?

   A. Loss of memory
   B. Loss of weight
   C. Medication nonadherence
   D. All of the above

2. Which of the following is a complication associated with Alzheimer's disease?

   A. Malnutrition
   B. Thyroid dysfunction

C. Hypertension

D. Insomnia

3. JB's physician would like to prescribe galantamine. What is the difference between galantamine and the other cholinesterase inhibitors?

A. Once-daily dosing

B. Faster onset of action

C. Action at the nicotinic receptors

D. Inhibits butylcholinesterase

4. What is the initial dosing schedule for galantamine?

A. 10 mg po qhs

B. 10 mg po q.a.m.

C. 5 mg po q.a.m.

D. 4 mg po bid

5. What is the most common adverse effect of galantamine?

A. Nausea

B. Diarrhea

C. Headache

D. Agitation

6. JB's physician would like to treat JB with an antipsychotic to help alleviate the hallucinations. Which of the following would you recommend?

A. Oxazepam

B. Lithium

C. Olanzapine

D. Citalopram

7. After a few weeks of galantamine therapy JB has shown signs of depression such as crying spells. Which of the following would you recommend to treat the depression?

A. Trazodone

B. Fluoxetine

C. Amitriptyline

D. Phenelzine

8. JB has been experiencing "sundowning." Which of the following best describes that phenomenon?

A. Sleeping early in the evening

B. Late afternoon irritability

C. Wandering at midday

D. Early morning delusions

9. Which of the following nonpharmacologic treatments would you suggest for JB?

A. Perform complex tasks to keep brain stimulated

B. Argue with patient

C. Use orientation cues

D. Let patient wander

10. What are the benefits of vitamin E for JB?

A. It is an antioxidant.

B. It has minimal side effects.

C. It is an over-the-counter preparation and does not cost much.

D. All of the above

P A T I E N T   P R O F I L E   2 4 5

TYPE 2 DIABETES MELLITUS

PRESENTATION

DM is a 40-year-old woman who presents to the family medicine clinic for her yearly physical and to get a new prescription for her oral hypoglycemic medication. She has not been seen in the clinic since last year at this time.

PHM: Hypertension × 8 years

Hyperlipidemia × 5 years

Diabetes mellitus (DM) type 2 × 3 years

FH: Mother DM, died of stroke at age 60; father died of a myocardial infarction at age 48; two siblings alive and well

SH: Married 15 years with four children, works full-time as a bank teller, smokes two packs per day since age 14, drinks two beers per day, no recreational drug use, rarely exercises, admits to trying fad diets for weight loss with little success

Meds: Propranolol LA 80 mg po qd

Multivitamin 1 po qd

Glyburide 2.5 mg po qd

Allergies: Penicillin

ROS: Occasional polydipsia, polyphagia, fatigue, weakness, and blurred vision. Denies CP, dyspnea, tachycardia, dizziness, or lightheadedness upon standing, tingling or numbness in extremities, leg cramps, peripheral edema, changes in bowel movements, gastrointestinal bloating, nausea or vomiting, urinary incontinence, sexual dysfunction, or presence of skin lesions.

Gen: Pleasant, obese, African-American woman who is in
no acute distress
VS: BP 150/96, pulse 80, RR 16, Ht 5'5", Wt 100 kg
Skin: Normal
HEENT: PERRLA, EOMI, TMs intact, no hemorrhages or
exudates on funduscopic examination, mucous mem-
branes normal, nose and throat clear without exudates
Neck: Supple, no lymphadenopathy, thyromegaly, or JVD
CV: RRR, normal S1 and S2, no MRG
Lungs: CTA bilaterally
Breasts: Normal, no masses
Abd: Soft, NT, obese, + BS, no organomegaly or distention
Ext: Normal range of motion and sensation, peripheral
pulses 2+, no lesions, ulcers, or edema
Neuro: A&O × 3, CN II to XII intact, DTRs 2+ through-
out, feet with normal vibratory and pinprick sensation
Labs: HgbA1C 9.4, TC 256, LDL 165, TG 280, HDL 35

QUESTIONS

1. Which clinical trial compared intensive therapy using
an oral agent to conventional therapy in type 2 diabetics and found that the risk of developing microvascular complications was decreased by 25% in the
intensively treated patients?

   A. DCCT
   B. ALLHAT
   C. UKPDS
   D. HOPE
   E. MERIT

2. Which of the following is the most common side effect
of glyburide?

   A. Hypoglycemia
   B. Increased LFTs
   C. Diarrhea
   D. Edema
   E. DKA

3. Which of the following best describes glyburide's
mechanism of action?

   A. Inhibits intestinal enzymes to prevent the absorp-
tion of carbohydrates
   B. Decreases hepatic glucose production
   C. Activates the PPAR-γ receptor
   D. Increases the secretion of insulin from pancreatic
β cells
   E. None of the above

4. Liver function tests should be monitored routinely in
patients on which of the following oral hypoglycemic
agents?

   A. Metformin
   B. Rosiglitazone
   C. Glimepiride
   D. Miglitol
   E. Nateglinide

5. Which of the following is an appropriate starting dose
of metformin?

   A. 25 mg tid
   B. 4 mg qd
   C. 500 mg bid
   D. 2.5 mg qd
   E. 120 mg tid

6. Which of the following oral agents has a delayed onset of action?

   A. Glucophage®
   B. Actos®
   C. Glucotrol®
   D. Precose®
   E. Prandin®

7. The use of which drug(s) is contraindicated in patients
with renal insufficiency?

   I. Metformin
   II. Rosiglitazone
   III. Acarbose

   A. I only
   B. III only
   C. I and II only
   D. II and III only
   E. I, II, and III

8. Which of the following drugs can mask the signs and
symptoms of hypoglycemia?

   A. Pentamidine
   B. Prednisone
   C. HCTZ
   D. Bisoprolol
   E. Diltiazem

9. Which of the following agents is considered a first-line
instrument for the treatment of hypertension in diabetic patients?

   A. Dihydropyridine CCB
   B. β-Blocker
   C. Thiazide
   D. ACE inhibitor
   E. Loop diuretic

10. Based on her history, what is the LDL goal for DM?

    A. <130 mg/dL
    B. <100 mg/dL
    C. <200 mg/dL
    D. <250 mg/dL
    E. >60 mg/dL

PATIENT PROFILE 246

MIGRAINE

PRESENTATION

AL is a 36-year-old woman who presents to the pharmacy to refill her oral contraceptives and purchase a 240-count bottle of ibuprofen 200 mg. During the course of the transaction, AL states, "I wish there was something I could do to get rid of these migraines." She would like more information about the "triptans," because her primary care physician keeps trying to persuade her to try zolmitriptan.

AL complains of monthly migraines that begin on the first day of her menstrual cycle and continue for 24 to 48 hours. AL states that the migraines began about 15 years ago, coinciding with the start of oral contraceptives. The migraines occur almost every month on awakening and are associated with a debilitating throbbing unilateral headache, nausea, vomiting, photophobia, and phonophobia. (AL states that lights and sounds make the headache worse.) AL tries to take 600 mg ibuprofen every 6 hours on the day before menstruation. This seems to "helps some" with the pain, but does not prevent the migraine from occurring. She continues the ibuprofen throughout the headache and states that eventually after two or three doses it somewhat "kicks in." She states that the only thing that really works is lying in bed with the blinds closed for the whole day, but she is not able to miss 1 to 2 days of work each month. AL usually is able to work through the pain, but says she is miserable throughout those days, and her work is not her best.

Med Hx: Tri-Norinyl 1 tab qd
Ibuprofen 600 mg (3 × 200 mg) q6 prn headache
Levothyroxine 100 µg qd
Lansoprazole 30 mg qd
PMH: Migraines × 15 years
Hypothyroidism × 10 years
GERD × 2 years
FH: Mother and father alive and well. Mother has hypothyroidism, hypertension, and hyperlipidemia. Father has hypertension and asthma.
SH: Married, lives with husband, no children, professional, has both a full-time and part-time job, and is a graduate student.
Tobacco use: Denies
ETOH: One or two glasses of wine per month
Caffeine: Two large cups of coffee each morning and two to three cans of caffeine-containing diet soda each day
Diet: Too busy to eat three scheduled meals, eats "when she can." Tends to eat a lot of chocolate, especially when she has symptoms of premenstrual syndrome
Allergies: Penicillin, rash

BP: 128/76 (per store automated machine), HR 74, est Ht 5′4″, est Wt 140 lbs

QUESTIONS

1. Which of the following factors may precipitate AL's migraines?

   I. Caffeine
   II. Alcohol
   III. Chocolate

   A. I only
   B. III only
   C. I and II
   D. II and III
   E. I, II, and III

2. Oral contraceptives have been associated with inducing or exacerbating migraine headaches. Which of the following is the best choice for AL?

   A. Estrostep®
   B. Modicon®
   C. Necon 1/35®
   D. Ovcon 35®
   E. Ovral®

3. Triptans are described as serotonin agonists. Which serotonin receptor(s) do the triptans affect?

   I. 5-HT_3
   II. 5-HT_{1B}
   III. 5-HT_{1D}

   A. I only
   B. III only
   C. I and II
   D. II and III
   E. I, II, and III

4. AL has heard that the triptans may cause a heart attack. How would you counsel AL about potential cardiovascular side effects of the triptan?

   A. Triptans have no cardiovascular side effects. Don't believe everything you hear.
   B. A potential side effect of triptan therapy is chest tightness associated with cardiac ischemia.
   C. Symptoms of chest pressure are associated with triptan therapy and may persist all day.
   D. Triptans have been linked to myocardial infarction, but it is very unlikely to occur in healthy patients without coronary artery disease or risk factors.

E. Chances of vascular events are rare with triptans. Patients with coronary artery disease can safely take triptan therapy

5. AL's physician is finally able to persuade her to try abortive therapy with a triptan, but does not want an oral formulation because her migraines cause significant nausea and vomiting. Which of the following is an appropriate agent and would accommodate AL's request?

A. Amerge® 1 mg IN (intranasally)
B. Frova® 10 mg subcutaneously (SQ)
C. Imitrex® 25 mg SQ
D. Maxalt® 15 mg IN
E. Zomig® 5 mg IN

6. Which of the following ß antagonists is/are effective for migraine prophylaxis?

I.   Atenolol
II. Propranolol
III. Acebutolol

A. I only
B. III only
C. I and II
D. II and III
E. I, II, and III

7. Which of the following may interact with rizatriptan?

I.   DHE
II. Fluoxetine
III. Propranolol

A. I only
B. III only

C. I and II
D. II and III
E. I, II, and III

8. Which of the following statements is/are true about butorphanol?

I.   Butorphanol is available as a nasal spray.
II. Butorphanol is a schedule IV narcotic analgesic.
III. The brand name of butorphanol is Stadol®.

A. I only
B. III only
C. I and II
D. II and III
E. I, II, and III

9. What is the brand name of DHE?

A. Axert®
B. Cafergot®
C. Fioricet®
D. Migranal®
E. Relpax®

10. Midrin® is a combination product containing which of the following ingredients?

I.   APAP
II. Dichloralphenazone
III. Isometheptene

A. I only
B. III only
C. I and II
D. II and III
E. I, II, and III

PATIENT PROFILE 2 4 7

TULAREMIA

PRESENTATION

AB is a 40-year-old woman who presents to the emergency department with nonspecific flulike symptoms. She said her symptoms started abruptly 2 days ago with a high fever of 104°F, headache, chills, and muscle aches throughout her body. She claims she has had a sore throat and occasional tightness in her chest. She also states that her cough is somewhat productive.

PMH: Insignificant
SH: Patient denies smoking and illicit drug use. She claims she drinks at least two cups of caffeinated cups of

coffee or cola a day. She may drink one or two alcoholic drinks per week. AB is a teacher, married, with no children.
FH: Both parents are alive. Mother is a non–insulin-dependent diabetic; father is hypertensive. They live in another state.
Gen: Well-nourished middle-aged woman, very ill and having difficulty breathing
VS: BP 140/85, pulse 95, RR 25, Temp 104°F, Wt 130 lbs
HEENT: Within normal limits

Chest: Diminished breath sounds, rales
Diagnosis: Rule out community acquired pneumonia.

LABORATORY VALUES

Chest x-ray: Infiltrates on left lower lung, pleural effusions
   and enlarged hilar nodes, widened mediastinum
Sputum gram stain: Gram-negative coccobacilli present
Electrolytes: Within normal limits
 WBC: 25,000/mm^3
Platelets: 378,000/mm^3

MEDICAL NOTE

AB is the tenth patient with similar symptoms in this emergency department today. Twenty patients in other emergency departments have reported similar signs and symptoms. AB's diagnosis was changed to tularemia after blood cultures (after 12 hours of growth) were positive for a tularemia diagnosis.

QUESTIONS

1. The gram-negative coccobacilli seen on the sputum gram stain are most likely which of the following?

    A. *Yersinia pestis*
    B. *Rickettsia rickettsii*
    C. *Francisella tularensis*
    D. *Bunyaviridae*

2. The typical incubation period for tularemia is which of the following?

    A. 1 to 2 days
    B. 2 to 5 days
    C. 5 to 7 days
    D. 1 to 14 days

3. Tularemia is a naturally occurring disease that may be transmitted by which of the following?

    A. Rodents
    B. Arthropods
    C. Woodchucks
    D. All of the above

4. The drug of choice in the treatment of tularemia per the Centers for Disease Control and Prevention (CDC) guidelines is which of the following?

    A. Streptomycin
    B. Amikacin
    C. Amoxicillin
    D. Clarithromycin

5. The typical length of treatment for AB is which of the following?

    A. 5 days
    B. 10 days
    C. 20 days
    D. 60 days

6. What laboratory tests should be performed to reduce or avoid adverse drug reactions to the above drug?

    A. Blood urea nitrogen (BUN)
    B. Blood drug concentrations
    C. Creatinine clearance
    D. All of the above

7. Exposure prophylaxis is required for those in close contact with AB. The drug of choice per CDC guidelines is which of the following?

    A. Ciprofloxacin 250 mg po q24 hours
    B. Doxycycline 100 mg po q12 hours
    C. Clarithromycin 250 mg po qid
    D. Amoxicillin 500 mg po qid

8. In reference to the preceding question, what class of anti-infective is that antibiotic?

    A. Tetracycline
    B. Penicillin
    C. Quinolone
    D. Macrolide

9. All except which of the following are important counseling for the preceding drug?

    A. It may cause photosensitivity.
    B. Finish all medications.
    C. Take it with a full glass of water.
    D. Antacids may decrease absorption of this drug.
    E. None of the above. They are all important counseling points.

10. What might be an indicator that a possible biological attack occurred?

    A. Surveillance data suggest a point-source of an outbreak.
    B. Unusual disease entities in the same patient population
    C. Reports of a disease that is not common or does not naturally occur in a specific geographic location
    D. All of the above

GERIATRIC MENTAL ILLNESS TREATMENT

PRESENTATION

AY is a 75-year-old man who has been referred to the geriatric consult service for assessment. Recently he has had worsening memory. Family members express that the patient displays agitation and anxiety with worse sleep.

CC: Patient and family state he has had worsening memory.
PMH: Schizophrenia
Hypertension
Chronic obstructive pulmonary disease
Generalized anxiety disorder
Dementia
Transient ischemic attacks in past
Meds:
Theophylline 300 mg tid
Fluphenazine decanoate 18.75 mg q 2 weeks IM
Amitriptyline 150 mg qhs
Diltiazem SA 240 mg qd
Albuterol 90 μg inh 2p qid prn
Flunisolide 250 μg inh 2p bid
Acetaminophen 500 mg 2 tabs qid prn

QUESTIONS

1. Which of the following patient's medications could worsen cognition?

   A. Albuterol
   B. Amitriptyline
   C. Theophylline
   D. Acetaminophen

2. On which receptor is there an additive effect between amitriptyline and fluphenazine?

   A. Postsynaptic dopamine receptors
   B. Serotonin reuptake pump
   C. Postsynaptic GABA receptor
   D. Postsynaptic muscarinic receptor

3. Which of the following could worsen this patient's anxiety?

   A. Albuterol
   B. Fluphenazine
   C. Diltiazem
   D. Acetaminophen

4. Which of the following antipsychotics would have least impact on worsening this patient's cognitive dysfunction?

   A. Chlorpromazine
   B. Haloperidol
   C. Ziprasidone
   D. Perphenazine

5. Which of the following statements best describes the drug interaction between fluphenazine and donepezil?

   A. Donepezil increases the amount of available acetylcholine, and fluphenazine blocks cholinergic receptors.
   B. Donepezil increases the amount of dopamine, and fluphenazine blocks dopamine receptors.
   C. Donepezil increases histamine, and fluphenazine blocks histamine receptors.
   D. Donepezil increases norepinephrine, and fluphenazine blocks alpha adrenergic receptors.

DIABETES

PRESENTATION

IV is a 48-year-old Hispanic woman who returns for follow-up about her recent blood glucose readings. IV has been diagnosed with type 2 diabetes since she was 45 years old. After about 2 months of therapy with metformin 1000 mg bid, she refused to continue with the medication because of gastrointestinal (GI) side effects, and changed to glyburide 20 mg po qd. After 8 months of therapy initial HbA_{1C} of 8.8 was brought down to 6.6. Patient became noncompliant after her daughter moved out, and her HbA_{1C} went up to >15. Her glucometer shows an average for the last month is 330 mg/dL. This morning the patient admits to having a cup of coffee with milk and sugar and a glass of Koolaid®. She describes a filmlike distortion in her field of vision, which makes objects a couple of feet from her very blurry. She has severe calluses developing on the heels, and she admits to wearing sandals as soon as she arrives home.

PMH: IV was diagnosed with type 2 diabetes and hypertension 3 years ago. She received 2 months of metformin 1000 mg bid and began to experience troubling gastrointestinal side effects and refused to continue with metformin. She then received glyburide 20 mg po qd. After 8 months of lifestyle modification and glyburide her initial HbA_{1C} of 8.8% was reduced to 6.6%. Shortly after reaching her personal HbA_{1c} goal, IV's youngest daughter moved away from home and IV self-discontinued all of her medication for several months. During this time IV's HbA_{1C} reached 15% and she began to experience polyuria, polydipsia, and polyphagia, and gained 25 lbs. She recently restarted all her medications 3 months ago.

FH: IV's parents are deceased. Her mother had diabetes and colorectal cancer, and her father had colorectal cancer as well. IV has no siblings.

SH: IV is currently unemployed. She denies alcohol and illicit drugs. She quit smoking 3 years ago with a previous 10-pack year smoking history.

Allergies: NKDA

Meds:

Glyburide 10 mg po bid

Atenolol 100 mg po qd

Ranitidine 150 mg po qd

Gabapentin 300 mg po tid

Lisinopril 10 mg po qd

HCTZ 25 mg po qd

Gen: Obese woman in no acute distress, AO × 3

VS: BP 128/76, pulse 62 beats/min, RR 15 breaths/min, Ht 5′3″, Wt 177 lbs, IBW 115 lb, BMI 31.4

HEENT: PERRLA, EOMI

Chest: CTA

Cor: RRR

Abd: Nontender, nondistended, +BS

GU: Deferred

Ext: 2+ pulses, normal perfusion, no CEE

Neuro: Cranial nerves II to XII intact

Labs: Na 139 mEq/L, K 4.7 mEq/L, Cl 103 mEq/L, HCO_3 24 mEq/L, BUN 10 mg/dL, SCr 0.8 mg/dL, fasting glucose 251 mg/dL, HbA1c 10.2%, WBC 8.9 K cells/mm^3, platelets 289 K cells/mm^3, Hgb 11 g/dL, HCT 33%, TC 190 mg/dL, HDL 43.3 mg/dL, LDL 102 mg/dL, TG 220 mg/dL

QUESTIONS

1. All except which of the following lab values suggest that IV may have metabolic syndrome? (Fasting glucose = 251 mg/dL)

   A. HDL = 43.3 mg/dL
   B. TG = 220 mg/dL
   C. TC = 190 mg/dL
   D. HCO_3 = 24 mEq/L

2. You explain the importance of daily ASA therapy in patients with diabetes and recommend that IV begin taking daily ASA. She agrees and begins taking 81 mg of ASA daily for primary prevention against cardiovascular events. How does ASA exert antiplatelet effects and prevent myocardial infarction?

   A. ASA inhibits platelet activation by inhibiting PGI_2.
   B. ASA inhibits platelets by inhibiting TxA_2.
   C. ASA inhibits ADP-mediated platelet activation.
   D. ASA inhibits platelets by antagonizing fibrin.
   E. ASA inhibits platelet GP IIb/IIIa receptor expression.

3. Which medication has been associated with a reduction in diabetes-related complications in a randomized controlled trial?

   A. Glyburide
   B. Atenolol
   C. Lisinopril
   D. Metformin
   E. All of the above

4. Which of the following is not a beneficial effect of angiotensin-enzyme inhibitors in patients with diabetes?

   A. ACE-inhibitor therapy reduces the risk of unstable angina.
   B. ACE-inhibitor therapy reduces the risk of myocardial infarction.
   C. ACE-inhibitor therapy reduces the risk of stroke.
   D. ACE-inhibitor therapy reduces the risk of cardiovascular death.
   E. ACE-inhibitor therapy reduces the risk of revascularization.

5. IV uses glyburide as the main intervention for glycemic control. Sulfonylureas can cause hypoglycemia if IV forgets to have a meal. Which of the following is not a typical symptom of drug-induced hypoglycemia?

   A. Tachycardia
   B. Sweating
   C. Tremor
   D. Thirst
   E. Confusion

6. IV is using atenolol to keep her blood pressure under control. Which symptom of hypoglycemia is not masked by ß-blockers?

   A. Tachycardia
   B. Sweating
   C. Tremor
   D. Increased systolic and diastolic pressure
   E. Palpitations

7. Which of the following is the primary mechanism of action for the HCTZ that IV uses to control her blood pressure?

   A. Inhibition of the Na^+-K^+-$2Cl^-$ symport in the loop of Henle
   B. Inhibition of the Na^+H^+ antiporter in the proximal convoluted tubule
   C. Inhibition of the Na^+Cl^- transport in the proximal convoluted tubule
   D. Inhibition of the Na^+Cl^- transport in the distal convoluted tubule
   E. Inhibition of the Na^+-K^+-$2Cl^-$ symport in the distal convoluted tubule

8. IV is receiving gabapentin for diabetic polyneuropathy. What is the maximum effective daily dose of gabapentin that has been studied for diabetic neuropathy?

   A. 3600 mg/day
   B. 2700 mg/day
   C. 2100 mg/day
   D. 1800 mg/day
   E. 900 mg/day

9. What should be IV's LDL goal?

   A. LDL-C ≤130 mg/dL
   B. LDL-C ≤110 mg/dL
   C. LDL-C ≤100 mg/dL
   D. LDL-C ≤80 mg/dL
   E. LDL-C ≤70 mg/dL

10. IV's primary care physician wants to begin simvastatin 40 mg qd for cholesterol reduction. How much LDL-C reduction can be expected using this dose of simvastatin?

    A. 80 mg/dL
    B. 70 mg/dL
    C. 60 mg/dL
    D. 50 mg/dL
    E. 40 mg/dL

PATIENT PROFILE 250

GASTROENTERITIS

PRESENTATION

GI is a 65-year-old woman who is admitted to the hospital today by her primary care physician. Two weeks before admission, GI suffered a laceration to her right hand during a vacation trip to Cancun, Mexico. She sought medical attention, receiving local wound care and several sutures. Four days later, the wound was noted to be tender, swollen, and red. She again sought local medical care and was prescribed a 10-day course of an oral antibiotic. Although the wound infection responded to treatment, she developed diarrhea and abdominal cramping on day 6 of therapy (2 days after returning to the United States). When these symptoms failed to abate and she started to feel dizzy and lightheaded, she called her primary care physician, who subsequently admitted her after seeing her in the office. While on vacation, she tried to avoid ingesting unbottled water, ice cubes, and fresh vegetables; she has been eating a normal diet since arriving home.

PMH: GERD, postmenopausal, HTN, DM type II, osteoarthritis
MH: Esomeprazole 20 mg qd, HCTZ 25 mg qd, metoprolol 50 mg bid, metformin 850 mg BID, alendronate 70 mg once weekly, vitamin D, prn ibuprofen
ALL: NKDA

SH: Lives alone, does not smoke, drinks socially
PE: VS: 130/75 mm Hg (lying) 120/55 mm Hg (standing), RR 25, HR 75, Temp 37.2°C,
Ht 160 cm, Wt 88 kg
Gen: Obese, pale woman in moderate distress
HEENT: Dry mucous membranes
Skin: Dry, pale, cool skin; dry axillae
Chest: Clear
COR: Normal S1 and S2, no extra heart sounds
Abd: Diffuse tenderness in the lower abdomen, no rebound, increased bowel sounds. Stools are guaiac negative.
Neuro: Fatigued but alert and oriented. Neurologic examination is normal.
Labs: Glu 160 mg/dL, Na 129 mEq/L, K 3.1 mEq/L, Cl 110 mEq/L, HCO_3 20 mEq/L, BUN 40 mg/dL, SCr 1.9 mg/dL, WBC 9.0K cells/mm³, PLTS 150K cells/mm³, Hct 32 g/dL, Hgb 10%
Fecal leukocytes: Negative
C. difficile toxin: Pending

QUESTIONS

1. Assuming GI's symptoms result from a case of traveler's diarrhea, which of the following is the most likely causative organism?

A. *Campylobacter jejuni*
B. Enterotoxigenic *E. coli* (ETEC)
C. A gastrointestinal virus
D. *Salmonella* species

2. Which of the following antibiotics provides the broadest coverage against enteric pathogens implicated in traveler's diarrhea?

   A. Erythromycin
   B. Clindamycin
   C. Ciprofloxacin
   D. TMP/SMX

3. Rifaximin (Xifaxan) might be a treatment option to treat this patient's traveler's diarrhea. How does this product work for this indication?

   A. It kills noninvasive strains of *E. coli* (i.e., ETEC).
   B. It absorbs the toxin produced by *E. coli*.
   C. It acts as an antimotility agent to help with symptom resolution.
   D. It absorbs fluid to help reduce the volume of diarrhea.

4. If GI would like to ensure that she does not have another episode of traveler's diarrhea, what prophylactic regimen would provide her with the most effective protection during her next vacation?

   A. Bismuth subsalicylate, two tablets chewed with meals and at bedtime
   B. Levofloxacin, 500 mg PO qd
   C. TMP/SMX, one DS tablet qd
   D. Loperamide 4 mg PO with meals and at bedtime

5. Which of the following place GI at greater risk for a symptomatic gastrointestinal infection after ingestion of a contaminated food source?

   I.   She is taking alendronate.
   II. She is 65 years of age.
   III. She is taking esomeprazole.
   III. She was taking antibiotic therapy while on vacation.

   A. I, II, and III
   B. I, III, and IV
   C. III and IV
   D. I, II, and V

6. If GI's symptoms resulted from a *C. difficile* infection that required specific antimicrobial therapy, which of the following would be considered first-line treatment?

   A. Vancomycin IV
   B. Vancomycin PO
   C. Metronidazole IV
   D. Metronidazole PO

7. If GI's *C. difficile* toxin study was positive and she was prescribed metronidazole, you would expect to observe an interaction between this drug and which of the following after her discharge from the hospital?

   A. The wine she consumes during social events
   B. Her metoprolol therapy
   C. Her esomeprazole therapy
   D. Her metformin therapy

8. Loperamide could be safely used to treat an enteric infection for which of the following organisms?

   A. *C. difficile*
   B. ET *E. coli*
   C. *Salmonella typhi*
   D. *Shigella*

9. Which of the following antibiotics are most commonly implicated as a cause of *C. difficile* diarrhea?

   A. Vancomycin, metronidazole, and cephalosporins
   B. Macrolides, fluoroquinolones, and TMP/SMX
   C. Aminoglycosides, carbapenems, and clindamycin
   D. Clindamycin, cephalosporins, and aminopenicillins

10. If GI's presentation included fever, fecal leukocytes, and blood in her stool, it is likely that she is suffering from infection with a more invasive pathogen such as *Salmonella*. If she were infected with a nontyphoidal *Salmonella* sp., then which of the following factors would prompt initiation of antimicrobial therapy for this organism?

    A. She is taking alendronate.
    B. She is 65 years of age.
    C. She is taking esomeprazole.
    D. She was taking antibiotic therapy while on vacation.

UNITED STATES PHARMACY LAW AND DRUG REGULATION REVIEW

INTRODUCTION

In the United States, all food, drugs, cosmetics, and medical devices, for both humans and animals, are regulated under the authority of the Food and Drug Administration (FDA). The Food and Drug Administration and all of its regulations were created by the government in response to the pressing need to address the safety of the public with respect to its foods and medicinals. The purpose of this review is to describe and explain the nature and extent of these regulations as they apply to drugs in the United States. This review discusses the FDA's regulatory oversight and that of other agencies, the drug approval and development process, the mechanisms used to regulate manufacturing and marketing, as well as various violation and enforcement schema.

PHARMACEUTICALS

The primary responsibility for the regulation and oversight of pharmaceuticals and the pharmaceutical industry lies with United States Food and Drug Administration (FDA). The FDA was created in 1931 and is one of several branches within the US Department of Health and Human Services (HHS). The FDA's counterparts within HHS include agencies such as the Centers for Disease Control and Prevention (CDC), National Institutes of Health (NIH), and Healthcare Financing Administration (HCFA).

The FDA is organized into a number of offices and centers headed by a commissioner who is appointed by the president with consent of the senate. It is a scientifically based law enforcement agency whose mission is to safeguard the public health and ensure honesty and fairness between health-regulated industries (i.e., pharmaceutical, device, biological, and the consumer).[1] It licenses and inspects manufacturing facilities; tests products; evaluates claims and prescription drug advertising; monitors research; and creates regulations, guidelines, standards, and policies. It does all of this through its Office of Operations, which contains component offices and centers such as the Center for Drug Evaluation and Research (CDER), the Center for Biologics Evaluation and Research (CBER), the Center for Devices and Radiological Health (CDRH), the Center for Food Safety and Applied Nutrition (CFSAN), the Center for Veterinary Medicine (CVM), the Office of Orphan Products Development, the Office of Biotechnology, the Office of Regulatory Affairs, and the National Center for Toxicological Research. Each of these entities has a defined role, although sometimes their authorities overlap. For example, if a pharmaceutical company submits a drug that is contained and delivered to a patient during therapy by a device not comparable to any other, then the CDER and CDRH may need to coordinate that product's approval. Although most prescription drugs are evaluated by the CDER, any other center or office may become involved with its review. One of the most significant resources to industry and consumers is the FDA's web site *www.fda.gov*. Easily accessible and navigable, each center and office has its own HTML within the site.

The FDA is not the only agency within the US government with a stake in pharmaceutical issues. The Federal Trade Commission (FTC) has authority over general business practices in general, such as deceptive and anticompetitive practices (i.e., false advertising). In addition, the FTC regulates the advertising of over-the-counter (OTC) drugs, medical devices, and cosmetics.

NEW DRUG APPROVAL AND DEVELOPMENT

A drug is a substance that exerts an action on the structure or function of the body by chemical action or metabolism and is intended for use in the diagnosis, cure, mitigation, treatment, or prevention of disease.[2] A new drug is defined as one that is not generally recognized as safe and effective for the indications proposed. However, this definition has much greater reach than simply a new chemical entity. The term new drug also refers to a drug product already in existence, although never approved by the FDA for marketing in the United States; new therapeutic indications; a new dosage form; a new route of administration; a new dosing schedule; or any other significant clinical differences than those approved.[3] Therefore, any chemical substance intended for use in humans or animals for medicinal purposes, or any existing chemical substance that has some significant change associated with it, is considered not safe or effective and a new drug until proper testing and FDA approval are met.

PRECLINICAL INVESTIGATION

Human testing of new drugs cannot begin until there is solid evidence that the drug product can be used with reasonable safety in humans. This phase is called preclinical investigation. The basic goal of preclinical investigation is to assess potential therapeutic effects of the substance on living organisms and to gather sufficient data to determine the reasonable safety of the substance in humans through laboratory experimentation and animal investigation.[4] The

FDA requires no prior approval for investigators or pharmaceutical industry sponsors to begin a preclinical investigation on a potential drug substance. However, investigators and sponsors are required to follow Good Laboratory Practices (GLP) regulations.[5] GLPs govern laboratory facilities, personnel, equipment, and operations. Compliance with GLPs requires procedures and documentation of training, study schedules, processes, and status reports that are submitted to facility management and included in the final study report to the FDA. Preclinical investigation usually takes 1 to 3 years to complete. If at that time enough data are gathered to reach the goal of potential therapeutic effect and reasonable safety, the product sponsor must formally notify the FDA of their wish to test the potential new drug on humans.

INVESTIGATIONAL NEW DRUG APPLICATION

Unlike the preclinical investigation stage, the Investigational New Drug Application (INDA) phase has much more direct FDA activity throughout. Because a preclinical investigation is designed to gather significant evidence of reasonable safety and efficacy of the compound in live organisms, the INDA phase is the clinical phase in which all activity is used to gather significant evidence of reasonable safety and efficacy data about the potential drug compound in humans. Clinical trials in humans are carefully scrutinized and regulated by the FDA to protect the health and safety of human test subjects and ensure the integrity and usefulness of the clinical study data.[6] Numerous meetings between both the agency and sponsor occur during this time. As a result, the clinical investigation phase may take as many as 12 years to complete. Only one in five compounds tested may actually demonstrate clinical effectiveness and safety and reach the US marketplace.

The sponsor submits the INDA to the FDA. The INDA must contain information on the compound itself and information of the study. All INDAs must have the same basis components: a detailed cover sheet, a table of contents, an introductory statement and basic investigative plan, an investigator's brochure, comprehensive investigation protocols, the compound's actual or proposed chemistry, manufacturing and controls, any pharmacology and toxicology information, any previous human experience with the compound, and any other pertinent information the FDA deems necessary. After submission, the sponsor company must wait 30 days to commence clinical trials. If the FDA does not object within that period, the trials may begin.

Before the actual commencement of the clinical investigations, however, a few ground rules must be established. For example, a clinical study protocol must be developed, proposed by the sponsor, and reviewed by an Institutional Review Board (IRB). An IRB is required by regulation[7] and is a committee of medical and ethical experts designated by an institution such as a university medical center in which the clinical trial will take place. The charge of the IRB is to oversee the research to ensure that the rights of human test subjects are protected and rigorous medical and scientific standards are maintained.[8] An IRB must approve the proposed clinical study and monitor the research as it progresses. It must develop written procedures of its own regarding its study review process and its reporting of any changes to the ongoing study as they occur. In addition, an IRB must review and approve documents for informed consent before commencement of the proposed clinical study. Regulations require that potential participants are informed adequately about the risks, benefits, and treatment alternatives before participating in experimental research.[9] An IRB's membership must be sufficiently diverse in order to review the study in terms of the specific research issue; community, legal, and professional standards; and conduct and practice norms. All of its activities must be well documented and open to FDA inspection at any time.

The proposed trial begins once the IRB is satisfied that it is ethical and proper. The clinical trial phase has three steps or phases. Each has a purpose, requires numerous patients, and can take more than 1 year to complete.

PHASE I

A Phase I study is relatively small (<100 subjects) and brief (1 year or less). Its purpose is to determine toxicology, metabolism, pharmacologic actions, and if possible any early evidence of effectiveness. The results of the Phase I study are used to develop the next step.

PHASE II

Phase II studies are the first controlled clinical studies using several hundred subjects who are afflicted with the disease or condition being studied. The purpose of Phase II is to determine the compound's possible effectiveness against the targeted disease or condition and its safety in humans. Phase II may be divided into two subparts: Phase IIa is a pilot study that is used to determine initial efficacy, and Phase IIb uses controlled studies on several hundred patients. At the end of the Phase II studies, the sponsor and FDA will usually confer to discuss the data and plans for Phase III.

PHASE III

Phase III studies are considered "pivotal" trials that are designed to collect all of the necessary data to meet the safety and efficacy standards the FDA requires to approve the compound for the US marketplace. Phase III studies usually are very large, consisting of several thousand patients in numerous study centers with a large number of investigators who conduct long-term trials over several months or years.

Also, Phase III studies establish final formulation, marketing claims and product stability, packaging, and storage conditions. On completion of Phase III, all clinical studies are complete, all safety and efficacy data have been analyzed, and the sponsor is ready to submit the compound to the FDA for market approval. This process begins with submission of a New Drug Application (NDA).

NEW DRUG APPLICATION

An NDA is a regulatory mechanism that is designed to give the FDA sufficient information to make a meaningful evaluation of a new drug.[10] All NDAs must contain the following information: preclinical laboratory and animal data; human pharmacokinetic and bioavailability data; clinical data; methods of manufacturing, processing, and packaging; a description of the drug product and substance; a list of relevant patents for the drug; its manufacture or claims; and any proposed labeling. In addition, an NDA must provide a summary of the application's contents and a presentation of the risks and benefits of the new drug.[11] Traditionally, NDAs consisted of hundreds of volumes of information, in triplicate, all cross referenced. Since 1999, the FDA has issued final guidance documents that allow sponsors to submit NDAs electronically in a standardized format. These electronic submissions facilitate ease of review and possible approval.[12]

The NDA must be submitted complete, in the proper form and with all critical data. If accepted, the FDA then determines the application's completeness. If complete, the agency considers the application filed and begins the review process within 60 days.[13] The purpose of an NDA from the FDA's perspective is to ensure that the new drug meets the criteria to be "safe and effective." Safety and effectiveness are determined through the Phase III pivotal studies based on "substantial evidence" gained from a well-controlled clinical study. Because the FDA realizes that there are no absolutely safe drugs, it looks to the new drug's efficacy as a measure of its safety. It weighs the risks versus benefits of approving the drug for use in the US market.

Also, the NDA must be very clear about the manufacture and marketing of the proposed drug product. The application must define and describe manufacturing processes, validate Current Good Manufacturing Practices (CGMPs), provide evidence of quality, purity, strength, identity, and bioavailability (a preinspection of the manufacturing facility is conducted by the FDA). Finally, the FDA reviews all product packaging and labeling for content and clarity. Statements on a product's package label, package insert, media advertising, or professional literature must be reviewed. Of note, "labeling" refers to all of the above and not just the label on the product container.

The FDA is required to review the application within 180 days of filing. At the end of that time, the agency is required to respond with an "action letter." There are three

kinds of action letters. An Approval Letter signifies that all substantive requirements for approval are met and that the sponsor company can begin marketing the drug as of the date on the letter.

An Approvable Letter signifies that the application substantially complies with the requirements but has some minor deficiencies that must be addressed before an approval letter is sent. Generally, these deficiencies are minor in nature and the product sponsor must respond within 10 days of receipt. At this point, the sponsor may amend the application and address the agency's concerns, request a hearing with the agency, or withdraw the application entirely.

A Non-Approvable Letter signifies that the FDA has major concerns with the application and will not approve the proposed drug product for marketing as submitted. The available remedies a sponsor can take for this type of action letter are similar to those in the "Approvable Letter."

PRESCRIPTION DRUG USER FEE ACT/FOOD AND DRUG ADMINISTRATION MODERNIZATION ACT EFFECTS

New drug application review has been significantly affected by both the Prescription Drug User Fee Act (PDUFA) and FDA Modernization Act (FDAMA) legislation. The PDUFA allows the FDA to collect fees from sponsor companies who submit applications for review. The fees are used to update facilities and hire and train reviewers. The fees only apply to NDA drug submissions, biologic drug submissions, and any supplement thereto. The fees do not apply to generic drugs or medical devices. The results of the PDUFA legislation were significant; approval rates have increased from approximately 50% to near 80% and the review times have decreased to less than 15 months for most applications.[14]

In 1997, the FDAMA reauthorized PDUFA till the year 2002. It waives the user fee to small companies who have fewer than 500 employees and are submitting their first application. It allows payment of the fee in stages and permits some percentage of refund if the application is refused. Also, it exempts applications for drugs used in rare conditions (orphan drugs), supplemental applications for pediatric indications, and applications for biologicals used as precursors for other biologics manufacture. In addition, the FDMA permits a "fast-track" approval of compounds that demonstrate significant benefit to critically ill patients, such as those who suffer from AIDS.[15]

BIOLOGICS

Biologics are defined as substances derived from or made with the aid of living organisms, which include vaccines, antitoxins, serums, blood, blood products, therapeutic protein drugs derived from natural sources (i.e., anti-thrombin III), or biotechnology (i.e., recombinantly derived proteins), or gene or somatic cell therapies.[16] As with the more traditionally derived drug products, biologics follow virtually the same regulatory and clinical testing schema with regard to safety and efficacy. A Biologics License Application (BLA) is used rather than an NDA, although the official FDA Form is designated the 356h and is one and the same. The sponsor merely indicated in check box if the application is for a drug or a biologic. Compounds characterized as biologics are reviewed by CBER.[17]

ORPHAN DRUGS

Orphan drugs are approved using many of the same processes as any other application. However, there are several significant differences. An orphan drug as defined under the Orphan Drug Act of 1993 is a drug used to treat a "rare disease" that would not normally be of interest to commercial manufactures in the ordinary course of business. A rare disease is defined in the law as any disease that affects fewer than 200,000 persons in the United States or one in which a manufacturer has no reasonable expectation of recovering the cost of its development and availability in the United States. The Act creates a series of financial incentives that manufacturers can take advantage of. For example, the Act permits grant assistance for clinical research, tax credits for research and development, and a 7-year market exclusivity to the first applicant who obtains market approval for a drug designated as an orphan. This means that if a sponsor gains approval for an orphan drug, the FDA will not approve any application by any other sponsor for the same drug for the same disease or condition for 7 years from the date from the first applicant's approval provided certain conditions are met, such as an assurance of sufficient availability of drug to those in need or a revocation of the drug's orphan status.[18,19]

ABBREVIATED NEW DRUG APPLICATIONS

Abbreviated New Drug Applications (ANDAs) are used when a patent has expired for a product that has been on the US market and a company wishes to market a copy. In the United States, a drug patent is 20 years. After that time, a manufacturer is able to submit an abbreviated application for that product provided that they certify that the product patent in question has already expired, is invalid, or will not be infringed.

The generic copy must meet certain other criteria as well. The drug's active ingredient must already have been approved for the conditions of use proposed in the ANDA, and nothing has changed to call into question the basis for approval of the original drug's NDA.[20] Sponsors of ANDAs are required to prove that their version meets with standards of bioethical and pharmaceutical equivalence. The FDA

publishes a list of all approved drugs called, *Approved Drug Products with Therapeutic Equivalence Evaluations,* also known as the "Orange Book" because of its orange cover. It lists marketed drug products that are considered by the FDA to be safe and effective and provides information on therapeutic equivalence evaluations for approved multi-source prescription drug products[21] monthly. The Orange Book rates drugs based on their therapeutic equivalence. For a product to be considered therapeutically equivalent, it must be both *pharmaceutically equivalent* (i.e., the same dose, dosage form, strength), and *bioequivalent* (i.e., the rate and extent of its absorption is not significantly different than the rate and extent of absorption of the drug with which it is to be interchanged).

Realizing that there may be some degree of variability in patients, the FDA allows pharmaceuticals to be considered bioequivalent in either of two methods. The first method studies the rate and extent of absorption of a test drug that may or may not be a generic variation, and a reference or brand name drug under similar experimental conditions and in similar dosing schedules where the test results do not show significant differences. The second approach uses the same method and from which the results determine that there is a difference in the test drug's rate and extent of absorption, except that the difference is considered to be medically insignificant for the proper clinical outcome of that drug.

Bioequivalence of different formulations of the same drug substance involves equivalence with respect to the rate and extent of drug absorption. Two formulations whose rate and extent of absorption differ by 20% or less are generally considered bioequivalent. The use of the 20% rule is based on a medical decision that, for most drugs, a 20% difference in the concentration of the active ingredient in blood will not be clinically significant.[22]

The FDA's Orange Book uses a two-letter coding system that is helpful in determining which drug products are considered therapeutically equivalent. The fist letter, either an A or a B, indicates a drug product's therapeutic equivalence rating. The second letter describes dose forms and can be any one of a number of different letters.

The A codes are described in the Orange Book as drug products that the FDA considers to be therapeutically equivalent to other pharmaceutically equivalent products (i.e., drug products for which):

1. There are no known or suspected bioequivalence problems. These are designated AA, AN, AO, AP, or AT, depending on the dose form; or
2. Actual or potential bioequivalence problems have been resolved with adequate in vivo and/or in vitro evidence supporting bioequivalence. These are designated AB.[23]

The B codes are a much less desirable rating when compared to a rating of A. Products that are rated B still may be commercially marketed; however, they may not be considered therapeutically equivalent. The Orange Book describes B codes as follows:

> Drug products that FDA at this time does not consider to be therapeutically equivalent to other pharmaceutically equivalent products, i.e., drug products for which actual or potential bioequivalence problems have not been resolved by adequate evidence of bioequivalence. Often the problem is with specific dosage forms rather than with the active ingredients. These are designated BC, BD, BE, BN, BP, BR, BS, BT, or BX.[24]

The FDA has adopted an additional subcategory of B codes. The designation, B* is assigned to former A-rated drugs "if FDA receives new information that raises a significant question regarding therapeutic equivalence."[25] Not all drugs are listed in the Orange Book. Drugs obtainable only from a single manufacturing source, drugs listed as Drug Efficacy Study Implementation (DESI) drugs or drugs manufactured before 1938 are not included. Those that do appear are listed by generic name.

PHASE IV AND POST-MARKETING SURVEILLANCE

Pharmaceutical companies that successfully gain marketing approval for their products are *not* exempt from further regulatory requirements. Many products are approved for market on the basis of a continued submission of clinical research data to the FDA. These data may be required to further validate efficacy or safety, detect new uses or abuses for the product, or determine the effectiveness of labeled indications under conditions of widespread usage.[26] The FDA also may require a Phase IV study for drugs approved under FDAMA's "fast-track" provisions.

Any changes to the approved product's indications, active ingredients, manufacture, or labeling require the manufacturer to submit a supplemental NDA (SNDA) for agency approval. Also, adverse drug reports are required to be reported to the agency. All reports must be reviewed by the manufacturer promptly, and if found to be serious, life-threatening, or unexpected (not listed in the product's labeling), the manufacturer is required to submit an alert report within 15 days working days of receipt of the information. All adverse reaction thought not to be serious or unexpected must be reported quarterly for 3 years after the application is approved, and annually thereafter.[27]

OVER-THE-COUNTER REGULATIONS

The 1951 Durham-Humphrey Amendments of the FDCA specified three criteria to justify prescription-only status. If the compound is habit forming, requires a prescriber's supervision, or has an NDA prescription-only limitation, it requires a prescription. The principles used to establish

OTC status (no prescription required) are a wide margin of safety, method of use, benefit-to-risk ratio, and adequacy of labeling for self-medication. For example, injectable drugs may not be used OTC with certain exceptions such as insulin. Over-the-counter market entry is less restrictive than that for prescription drugs and do not require premarket clearance. Pose many fewer safety hazards than prescription drugs because they are designed to alleviate symptoms rather than disease. Easier access far outweighs the risks of side effects, which can be addressed adequately through proper labeling.

As discussed, OTC products underwent a review in 1972. Although reviewing the 300,000 + OTC drug products in existence at the time would be virtually impossible, the FDA created OTC Advisory Panels to review data based on some 26 therapeutic categories. Over-the-counter drugs are only examined by active ingredient within a therapeutic category. Inactive ingredients are only examined if they are shown to be safe and suitable for the product and not interfering with effectiveness and quality.

This review of active ingredients results in the promulgation of a regulation or a "monograph," which is a "recipe" or set of guidelines applicable to all OTC products within a therapeutic category. Over-the-counter monographs are general and require that OTC products show "general recognition of the safety and effectiveness of the active ingredient." Over-the-counter products do not fall under prescription status if their active ingredients (or combinations) are deemed by the FDA to be "generally recognized as safe and effective" (GRASE). The monograph system is public, with a public comment component included after each phase of the process. Any products for which a final monograph has not been established may remain on the market until one is determined.

There are four phases in the OTC monograph system. In Phase I an expert panel is selected to review data for each active ingredient in each therapeutic category for safety, efficacy, and labeling. Their recommendations are made in the federal register. A public comment period of 30 to 60 days is permitted and supporting or contesting data are accepted for review. Then the panel re-evaluates the data and publishes a "Proposed Monograph" in the federal register, which publicly announces the conditions for which the panel believes that OTC products in a particular therapeutic class are GRASE and not misbranded. A "Tentative Final Monograph" is then developed and published stating the FDA's position on safety and efficacy of a particular ingredient within a therapeutic category and acceptable labeling for indications, warnings, and directions for use. Active ingredients are deemed: Category I (GRASE for claimed therapeutic indications and not misbranded), Category II (not GRASE and/or misbranded), or Category III (insufficient data for determination).

After public comment, the final monograph is established and published with the FDA's final criteria for which all drug products in a therapeutic class become GRASE and not misbranded. Following the effective date of the final monograph, all covered drug products that fail to conform to its requirements are considered misbranded and or an unapproved new drug.[28]

However, because the monograph panels are no longer convened, many current products are switched from prescription status. A company who wishes to make this switch and offer a product to the US marketplace can submit an amendment to a monograph to the FDA, who acts as the sole reviewer. They may also file an SNDA provided that they have 3 years of marketing experience as a prescription product, can demonstrate a relatively high use during that period, and can validate that the product has a mild profile of adverse reactions. The last method involves a "Citizens' Petition," which is rarely used.[29]

REGULATING MARKETING

The FDA has jurisdiction over prescription drug advertising and promotion. The basis for these regulations lies within the 1962 Kefauver-Harris Amendments. Essentially, any promotional information, in any form, must be truthful, fairly balanced, and fully disclosed. The FDA views this information as either "advertising" or "labeling." Advertising includes all traditional outlets in which a company places an ad. Labeling includes everything else, including brochures, booklets, lectures, slide kits, letters to physicians, company-sponsored magazine articles, and so on. All information must be truthful and not misleading. All material facts must be disclosed in a manner that is fairly balanced and accurate. If any of these requirements are violated, the product is considered "misbranded" for the indications in which it was approved under its NDA. The FDA is also sensitive to the promotion of a product for "off-label" use. Off-label use occurs when a product is in some way presented in a manner that does not agree with or is not addressed in its approved labeling. Also, provisions of the Prescription Drug Marketing Act (PDMA) of 1987 apply. The Act prohibits company representatives from directly distributing or reselling prescription drug samples. Companies are required to establish a closed system of record keeping that can track a sample from their control to that of a prescriber in order to prevent diversion. Prescribers are required to receive these samples and record and store them appropriately.[30]

VIOLATIONS AND ENFORCEMENT

The FDA has the power to enforce the regulations for any product as defined under the FDCA. It has the jurisdiction to inspect a manufacturer's premises and records. After a facilities inspection, an agency inspector issues an FDA Form 483s, which describes observable violations. Response to the finding as described on this form must be made promptly. A warning letter may be used when the agency determines that one or more of a company's practices, products, or procedures are in violation of the FDCA. The FDA district has 15 days to issue a warning letter after an inspection. The company has 15 days in which to respond. If the company response is satisfactory to the agency, no other action is warranted. If the response is not, the agency may request a recall of the violated products. The FDA has no authority to force a company to recall a product, but it may force removal of a product through the initiation of a seizure.

Recalls can fall into one of three classes. A Class I recall exists when there is a reasonable possibility that the use of a product will cause either serious adverse effects on health or death. Class II recall exists when the use of a product may cause temporary or medically reversible adverse effects on health or when the probability of serious adverse effects on health is remote. A Class III recall exists when the use of a product is not likely to cause adverse health consequences. Recalls are also categorized as consumer level, in which the product is requested to be recalled for the consumer's homes or control; a retail level, in which the product is to be removed from retail shelves or control; and a wholesale level, in which the product is to be removed from wholesale distribution. Companies who conduct a recall of their products are required to conduct effectiveness checks to determine the effectiveness of recalling the product from the marketplace.

If a company refuses to recall the product, the FDA will seek an injunction against the company.[31] An injunction is recommended to the Department of Justice (DOJ) by the FDA. The DOJ takes the request to federal court, which issues an order that forbids a company from carrying out a particular illegal act, such as marketing a product that the FDA considers a violation of the FDCA. Companies can comply with the order and sign a consent agreement, which specifies changes required by the FDA in order for the company to continue operations, or litigate.

The FDA also may initiate a seizure of violative products.[32] A seizure is ordered by the federal court in the district where the products are located. The seizure order specifies products, their batch numbers, and any records determined by the FDA as violative. United States Marshals carry out this action. The FDA institutes a seizure to prevent a company from selling, distributing, moving, or otherwise tampering with the product.

The FDA also may debar individuals or firms from assisting or submitting an ANDA, or directly providing services to any firm with an existing or pending drug product application. Debarment may last for up to 10 years.[33]

However, one of the more powerful deterrents that the FDA uses is adverse publicity. Although the agency has no authority to require a company to advertise adverse publicity, it does publish administrative actions against a company in any number of federal publications, such as the *Federal Register,* the *FDA Enforcement Report,* the *FDA Medical Bulletin,* and the *FDA Consumer.*[34]

FEDERAL LAWS AND REGULATIONS GOVERNING PHARMACIES, PHARMACISTS, AND PRESCRIPTIONS

The basis for all practice-oriented drug law and regulation stems from the Federal Controlled Substances Act (CSA) of 1970 (21 U.S.C. 801, et seq). The Act, also known as Title II, was part of a much larger piece of legislation, the Comprehensive Drug Abuse Prevention and Control Act of 1970 (PL91-513). The CSA was enacted to regulate the manufacturing, distribution, dispensing, and delivery of drugs or substances that are subject to, or have the potential for, abuse or physical or psychological dependence. These drugs are designated as "controlled substances" because they are "controlled" under the CSA.[35]

The CSA falls under the regulatory authority of the Drug Enforcement Administration (DEA), which controls access to regulated substances. This control is achieved through the federal registration of all persons in the legitimate chain of manufacture, distribution, or dispensing of controlled substances, except the ultimate user.[36] The "ultimate user" is defined as (a) the patient who is competent to use these drugs as prescribed by a practitioner, or (b) the patient's caregiver who administers them to the incompetent patient (i.e., the parent of a sick child).[37] All healthcare providers who deal with the issues of pain management through the use of controlled substances are subject to the CSA as well as those drug control laws of the state in which they are licensed and practicing unless such practice is exclusively in a federal facility (e.g., a Veterans Administration [VA] Hospital).[38]

The CSA empowers the DEA to register all persons, businesses, and institutions that would conduct any activity that would involve controlled substances by issuing them a registration number, the DEA number. A DEA registration must be renewed triennially.[39] In addition, the CSA establishes a closed system of record keeping provisions that control and track the flow of controlled substances through the healthcare system. For example, if a registrant, one who has been issued a DEA registration, wishes to order a controlled substance from a wholesaler or manufacturer, some very specific record keeping provisions exist depending on how the drugs ordered are categorized or "scheduled."[40] All registrants who order, fulfill an order, store, distribute, or dispense a controlled substance must report this activity to DEA as well as maintain their own records for a period of 2 years.

The CSA places medicinal substances in schedules (or classes) in descending order based on their potential for abuse, psychological or physiologic dependence, and medical use. These substances include narcotics, amphetamines, and barbiturates and are denoted by a C and a roman numeral in the regulations and literature and on manufacturers' containers. Scheduling provisions also include prescription dispensing limitations. Five schedules of drugs are described by the CSA.

Much of what appears in the federal act also appears in the state acts and regulations with some additional and more stringent modification. For example, in Massachusetts, prescriptions issued for medications listed in Schedule II must be filled by a pharmacy within 5 days after the date in which it was issued.[41] Also, drugs listed in Schedule II or III are only fillable for a 30-day supply on any single filling.[42,43] In addition, Massachusetts considers any prescription drug product not included in a federal schedule to be designated as Schedule VI.[44] Therefore, in Massachusetts, a patient's antihypertensive medication or prescription eye drops are considered to be controlled substances.

DRUG ENFORCEMENT ADMINISTRATION REGISTRATION

A DEA registration may be issued to certain qualified healthcare and non-healthcare professionals as needed to treat patients, dispense controlled substances, conduct research, manufacture, repackage, wholesale, or teach. A DEA registration may be issued to physicians, dentists, podiatrists, veterinarians, mid-level practitioners, or other registered practitioners who are authorized to prescribe controlled substances by the jurisdiction in which he or she is licensed to practice and who are registered with the DEA or exempted from registration, such as those who practice for the US Public Health Service and/or Bureau of Prison physicians.[45] These registrations must be renewed every 3 years.

A DEA registration number for a practitioner begins with the letter A or B. Registration numbers issued to mid-level practitioners begin with the letter M. The first letter of the registration number is followed by the first letter of the registrant's last name (e.g., J for Jones or S for Smith), and then a computer-generated sequence of seven numbers (such as MJ3614511).[46] It is interesting that the computer-generated sequence of seven numbers may be of benefit to pharmacists in their efforts to deter prescription fraud. The computer randomly generates the first six numbers and calculates the final number according to the following formula. Add the sum of the numbers in the "odd" position to the sum of the numbers in the "even" position multiplied by 2. The second number in the final sum is called the "check digit" and is the last number in the sequence.

For example, take the following MJ3614511. The letter M represents the practitioner as a mid-level prescriber. The letter J represents the first letter of the last name Jones. The numbers are randomly generated and the final check digit is the number 1. The formula is as follows:

1st	2nd	3rd	4th	5th	6th	7th
odd	even	odd	even	odd	even	check
3	6	1	4	5	1	1

Odd position: $3 + 1 + 5 = 9$
Even position: $6 + 4 + 1 = 11 \times 2 = 22$
$22 + 9 = 31$ "1" is the seventh or check digit

Pharmacies seeking to become registered for the first time must request a DEA Form 224. Any pharmacy engaged in cooperative buying of controlled substances also must register as a distributor with the DEA. To obtain this registration, a pharmacy must meet distributor (wholesaler) security and record keeping requirements. An affidavit system for expediting pharmacy applications may be used to obtain a DEA registration number for a new pharmacy or for transferring ownership of an existing pharmacy. Any time a pharmacy moves to a new physical location or the postal address changes at the same location, a new DEA certificate reflecting the new address must be obtained. It is the pharmacy's responsibility to notify the DEA about a change of address before the effective date of the move. A written request for modification of registration should be sent to the DEA Registration Field Office responsible for the state. If the modification is approved, the DEA issues a new certificate of registration and, if requested, new Schedule II order form (DEA Form 222). A Renewal Application for Registration (DEA Form 224a) is only sent to the registered address on file with the DEA. It cannot be forwarded.[47]

TRANSFERRING A PHARMACY BUSINESS

A registrant transferring a pharmacy business to another registrant[48] shall notify the nearest DEA Registration Field Office at least 14 days before the date of the proposed transfer and provide the following information:

1. The name, address, and registration number of the registrant discontinuing business
2. The name, address, and registration number of the registrant acquiring the pharmacy
3. Whether the business activities will be continued at the location registered by the current business owner or moved to another location. If the latter, give the address of the new location.
4. The date on which the controlled substances will be transferred to the person acquiring the pharmacy

On the day the controlled substances are transferred, a complete controlled substances inventory must be taken and a copy of the inventory must be included in the records of both the person transferring the business and the person acquiring the business.[49]

If the registrant acquiring the pharmacy owns at least one other pharmacy licensed in the same state as the pharmacy being transferred, the registrant may apply for a new DEA registration before the date of transfer. The DEA will issue a registration that will authorize the registrant to obtain controlled substances at the time of transfer. However, the registrant may not dispense controlled substances until the pharmacy has been issued a valid state pharmacy license.[50]

A DEA registration application for transferring ownership of an existing pharmacy can be expedited if the applicant includes an affidavit verifying that the pharmacy has been registered by the state licensing agency. The affidavit verifying the existence of the state license should be attached to the initial application for registration.[51]

PRACTITIONERS

A practitioner as defined in the preceding may be issued a DEA registration number that authorizes that practitioner to prescribe controlled substances to patients. However, the issuance of a DEA number does not permit all practitioners to write prescriptions for any patient ailment. As discussed elsewhere, to be valid, a prescription for a controlled substance must be issued for a legitimate medical purpose by a practitioner acting in the usual course of sound professional practice. The practitioner is responsible for the proper prescribing and dispensing of controlled substances. However, a corresponding responsibility rests with the pharmacist who dispenses the prescription. An order for controlled substances that purports to be a valid prescription, but is not issued in the usual course of professional treatment, or for legitimate and authorized research, is not a valid prescription within the meaning and intent of the CSA. The individual who knowingly dispenses such a purported prescription, as well as the individual issuing it, is subject to criminal and/or civil penalties and administrative sanctions. A prescription may not be issued in order for an individual practitioner to obtain a supply of controlled substances for the purpose of general dispensing to his or her patients. Therefore, a prescription written for office stock or "medical bag" use is not valid.[52]

This means that a practitioner prescribes for a "legitimate medical purpose" (the use of the medication is for a medically acceptable course of treatment) and "acting in the usual course of sound professional practice" (the prescription is for an actual patient who has been diagnosed and has a medical record generated and is being treated for a medical condition that is within the usual treatment of the practitioner). Therefore, if the patient is being treated by a medical doctor who has studied all of the human organ systems, the practitioner's "scope of medical practice," and after "acting in the usual course of sound professional practice" (making the proper diagnosis), the physician practitioner may prescribe a controlled substance for any medical condition that the patient presents. In other words, medical doctors do not have a restricted scope of professional practice. This is not the case for other categories of practitioner. For example, veterinarians are restricted in their "usual course of sound professional practice" to the treatment of diseases found in animals. Dentists similarly are restricted to treating diseases of teeth, gums, and the oral cavity.

MID-LEVEL PRACTITIONERS

Mid-level practitioners (MLPs) are registered and authorized by the DEA and the state in which they practice to dispense, administer, and prescribe controlled substances in the course of professional practice. Examples of MLPs include, but are not limited to, healthcare providers such as nurse practitioners, nurse midwives, nurse anesthetists, clinical nurse specialists, physician assistants, optometrists, ambulance services, animal shelters, veterinarian euthanasia technicians, nursing homes, and homeopathic physicians.[53]

MLPs may receive individual DEA registration granting controlled substance privileges. However, such registration is contingent upon authority granted by the state in which they are licensed. The DEA registers MLPs whose states clearly authorize them to prescribe, dispense, and administer controlled substances in one or more schedules. The fact that an MLP has been issued a valid DEA registration number (beginning with the letter M) is evidence that he or she is authorized to prescribe, dispense, and/or administer at least some controlled substances.

However, it is still incumbent upon the pharmacist who fills the prescription to ensure that the MLP is prescribing within the parameters established by the state in which he or she practices. MLP authority to prescribe controlled substances varies greatly by state. Check with your state licensing or controlled substances authority to determine which MLP disciplines are authorized to prescribe controlled substances in your state.[54]

USE OF HOSPITAL DRUG ENFORCEMENT ADMINISTRATION REGISTRATION NUMBER

An individual practitioner (e.g., intern, resident, staff physician, mid-level practitioner) who is an agent or employee of a hospital or other institution may, when acting in the usual course of business or employment, administer, dispense, or prescribe controlled substances under the registration of the hospital or other institution in which he or she is employed, provided that:

1. The dispensing, administering, or prescribing is in the usual course of professional practice;
2. The practitioner is authorized to do so by the state in which he or she is practicing;
3. The hospital or institution has verified that the practitioner is permitted to dispense, administer, or prescribe controlled substances within the state;
4. The practitioner acts only within the scope of employment in the hospital or institution.

The hospital or institution authorizes the practitioner to dispense or prescribe under its registration and assigns a specific internal code number, in suffix, for each practitioner so authorized. For example, if Metropolitan Hospital's DEA registration number is BM1111119 and a visiting physician is granted practice privileges at that institution, the institution issues the physician an internal code that is required to appear on all prescriptions written. That code is included on the end of the DEA registration number for the hospital as a suffix (i.e., BM1111119-Q23).

A current list of internal codes and the corresponding individual practitioners is to be kept by the hospital or other institution. This list is to be available at all times to other registrants and law enforcement agencies upon request for the purpose of verifying the authority of the prescribing individual practitioner. Pharmacists should contact the hospital or other institution for verification if they have any doubts in dispensing such a prescription.

PRESCRIPTION BASICS

Federal law and regulation as well as those of many states require that prescriptions be complete with all requisite information. Prescriptions must be written in ink, typewritten, or in indelible pencil. Information may be entered onto a prescription by a designee, called an agent, of the prescriber or even by a pharmacist when a clarification is needed. The only information required to be in the prescriber's own handwriting is their personal signature. Federal law also allows prescriptions to be orally and routinely telephoned into pharmacies in Schedules III to V from prescribers or their agents, whereby pharmacists are required to record the name of that person onto that prescription.[55] These oral prescriptions then must be augmented by a written hard copy within 7 days of its issuance. This hard copy backup is the responsibility of the prescriber. Pharmacists who do not receive it are required to report this information to the DEA.

As alluded to previously, federal law categorizes prescription medications into schedules based on their abuse potential. As a result, they need to be handled by prescribers and pharmacists in some very specific ways. Schedule II controlled substances generally are used for moderate to severe pain and have the most restriction. Prescriptions written for medications listed in Schedule II are not refillable and require a written prescription only.[56]

Prescriptions for Schedule II controlled substances may be partially filled for quantities less than those prescribed because of the pharmacy being out-of-stock or a patient request for less provided that the pharmacy dispenses the remainder to the patient within 72 hours. If unable to do so, the prescription becomes void for further quantity and the prescriber is so informed. Pharmacists may dispense partial quantities of Schedule II medications to patients in long-term care facilities (LTCFs) or who are terminally ill for up to

60 days from the original date of the prescription's issuance. The dispensing pharmacist is required to record that the patient is in an LTCF or is terminally ill along with the date of dispensing, quantity dispensed and remaining, and dispensing pharmacist's signature on the back of the prescription.[57]

Schedule II medications also have restrictions on oral or telephone transmissions. The CSA allows for prescribers to call pharmacies and orally transmit prescriptions for Schedule II drugs only in an emergency situation. An emergency situation, under the Controlled Substance Act, means that immediate administration of the controlled substance is necessary for the proper treatment for the intended ultimate user; no appropriate alternative treatment is available, including administration of a drug that is not a controlled substance under Schedule II of the Act; and, it is not reasonably possible for the prescribing physician to provide a written prescription to be presented to the person dispensing the substance before dispensing.

In case of an emergency situation, a pharmacist may dispense a controlled substance in Schedule II upon receiving the orally transmitted authorization of a prescribing practitioner, provided that the quantity prescribed and dispensed is limited to the amount adequate to treat the patient during the emergency period. The prescribing practitioner then must provide a written prescription for the emergency quantity prescribed to be delivered or postmarked to the dispensing pharmacist within 7 days after authorizing an emergency oral prescription. In addition, the prescription shall have written on its face "Authorization for Emergency Dispensing." Upon receipt of the written prescription, the dispensing pharmacist must attach the prescription to the oral one. If the prescribing practitioner fails to deliver a written prescription within 7 days, the pharmacist shall notify the nearest office of the DEA.

The regulations for emergency situations can be cumbersome for home infusion pharmacies, hospices, and long-term care pharmacies. Frequent dosage modifications of parenteral or controlled-release narcotic substances for patients who require these services can place pharmacies and prescribers at a regulatory disadvantage in that the pharmacy would have to enforce the existing regulations. However, the DEA has provided an easier mechanism for handling prescriptions for CII pain medications. As of May 1994, the DEA has issued a rule that allows controlled substance prescription orders to be transmitted from a prescriber to a dispensing pharmacy by facsimile.[58] The rule covers all controlled substance prescriptions. Of interest to this discussion, the DEA allows pharmacies to receive facsimile prescriptions for intravenous pain therapy and retain them as the original prescription, thereby substantially reducing the need for oral emergency prescriptions in these settings. One must note that these rules do not apply to oral dosage forms.

Prescriptions written for Schedules III and IV have somewhat less stringent regulations attached to them. They are refillable up to five times if so authorized, or 6 months from their date of issue, whichever terminates first, and, when filled with a partial quantity, must have the quantity recorded on their back along with the date of refilling and initials of the dispensing pharmacist.[59] Prescriptions written for Schedules V are also refillable. However, the number of refills is not set by law and the authorized number of refills depends on good professional judgment by both the prescriber and pharmacist.[60]

Pharmacists and prescribers are also co-liable for prescriptions written in err or with obvious problems. This is called corresponding responsibility.[61] A prescription for a controlled substance must be issued in good faith and for a legitimate medical purpose by a practitioner in the usual course of his or her professional practice; likewise, pharmacists have the corresponding responsibility to ensure that the prescription is issued and dispensed in good faith for a legitimate medical purpose by a practitioner acting in the usual course of his practice. For example, if a pharmacist receives a prescription written by a radiologist for her child, what must the pharmacist do in order to protect herself from any corresponding responsibility? Radiologists are medical doctors with a specialty. However, this specialty does not preclude that person from prescribing medication outside that specialty provided that the prescription is written in good faith, for a legitimate medical purpose, and in the usual course of medical practice. If the radiologist conducted all of the medically required diagnosis and generated a patient record, thereby establishing a physician–patient relationship, the prescription would be fillable under federal law. Pharmacists question prescriptions such as this in order to protect themselves and their patients.

A prescription is considered complete when the following information is included on its face:

1. Date of issue
2. Name and address of practitioner
3. Controlled substance registration number
4. Name of patient
5. Address of patient
6. Name, strength, dose, and quantity of controlled substances
7. Directions for use and any cautionary statements required
8. Number of times to be refilled
9. Signature of prescriber

Prescriptions must be written in ink, indelible pencil, or typewritten. They may be prepared by a physician's secretary or agent, but must be manually signed by the physician who issues the order. In addition, prescriptions only may be issued by a physician, dentist, podiatrist, veterinarian, or other registered practitioner who is authorized to prescribe controlled substances by the jurisdiction in which he or she is licensed to practice.

ORAL PRESCRIPTIONS: A prescription may be transmitted both orally and routinely in Schedules III to V from any agent of the prescriber to the registered pharmacist. The pharmacist must place the name of the person who transmitted the prescription on the face of the oral prescription.

Prescriptions may be filled in a community pharmacy when written by interns, residents, and foreign physicians in a hospital who have been assigned a suffix to the institutional DEA number.

SCHEDULES III AND IV: Prescriptions written for Schedule III and IV are refillable up to five times or 6 months from the dater of issue, whichever terminates first if so authorized. The initials of the dispensing pharmacist and the quantity dispensed must appear on the back of the prescription when filling a partial quantity. All partial dispensing must be done within 6 months of the issuance of the original prescription.

SCHEDULE V: Prescriptions written for Schedule V drugs are refillable; however, the number of refills is not set by law and the authorized number of refills depends on good professional judgment by both the prescriber and pharmacist.

SCHEDULE V CONTROLLED SUBSTANCES SOLD OVER THE COUNTER

Regulations allow a pharmacist to sell Schedule V, non-narcotic, narcotic, and nonlegend preparations without a prescription with proper record keeping (as excepted compounds). Pharmacists may not sell more than 240 mL or 48 solid dosage units of opium containing substances, or 120 mL or 24 solid dosage units of non–opium containing controlled substances may be dispensed within a 48-hour period. The purchaser must be known to the pharmacist or provide identification to the pharmacist and must be at least 18 years of age at the time of sale. These preparations generally contain opium derivatives for the control of coughs or diarrhea.

The pharmacy must maintain a bound book to record the dispensing of Schedule V substances for a period of 2 years and include the following information:

1. Name and address of purchaser
2. Name and quantity of controlled substance
3. Date of sale
4. Initials or name of dispensing pharmacist

TRANSFERRING PRESCRIPTIONS

The transfer of existing, filled prescriptions are allowable under federal law for prescription drugs in Schedules III through V. The transfer may be conducted one time only. The transfer rule only applies in conjunction with state pharmacy law. Individual states may have more stringent requirements.

SCHEDULE II CONTROLLED SUBSTANCES

Prescriptions written for Schedule II controlled substances must be treated to a somewhat different standard than those in other schedules. The basic regulations are as follows:

1. CII prescriptions are not refillable.
2. They require a written prescription only
3. They are valid for 60 days from their date of issuance for patients in an LTCF or who are medically diagnosed to be terminally ill.
4. They must be secured in a locked and substantially constructed cabinet or dispersed throughout the stock of non-controlled substances in such a manner as to obstruct their theft or diversion.

ORAL EMERGENCY PRESCRIPTIONS FOR SCHEDULE II

Prescriptions may be called into a pharmacy by a prescriber in only certain, well-defined circumstances termed emergency situations. An emergency situation under the Controlled Substance Act means:

1. Immediate administration of the controlled substance is necessary for the proper treatment for the intended ultimate user.
2. No appropriate alternative treatment is available, including administration of a drug that is not a controlled substance under Schedule II of the Act.
3. It is not reasonably possible for the prescribing physician to provide a written prescription to be presented to the person dispensing the substance before dispensing.

In the case of an emergency situation a pharmacist may only dispense enough medication to carry the patient through the emergency or until the patient can access the prescriber. The pharmacist must copy the information in proper form onto a prescription blank and write the words EMERGENCY AUTHORIZATION on its face. A prescribing physician is required to mail or hand-deliver a written, hard copy prescription to the dispensing pharmacy to cover the oral emergency supply of medication within 7 days. Pharmacists are required to attach this hard copy to the oral copy on receipt. If the pharmacist does not receive the hard copy backup prescription from the physician within the 7-day period as prescribed by federal law and regulation, the pharmacist then is required to contact the DEA and report the missing prescription.

METHADONE

Prescriptions for methadone are valid provided that the drug is used as an analgesic. They are not valid through the typical retail pharmacy distribution channels for the purposes of detoxification or maintenance therapy for drug addiction. However, when written by a physician for an addicted patient, a single-day quantity for three consecutive days may be prescribed for the purposes of admitting that addicted person to an appropriately licensed treatment program.

PARTIAL FILLING

Prescriptions partially filled for Schedule II controlled substances require:

1. The quantity filled to be noted on the face of the prescription
2. The remainder to be filled within 72 hours
3. That beyond 72 hours the prescription becomes void for further quantity and the prescriber so informed
4. LTCF and terminally ill patients only

    A. The pharmacist must record that the patient is in an LTCF or is terminally ill.
    B. The pharmacist must record the date, quantity dispensed *and* remaining, and the initials or signature of the dispensing pharmacist on the back of the prescription.

ELECTRONICALLY TRANSMITTED AND FAXED PRESCRIPTIONS

Prescriptions or drug orders for controlled substances listed in Schedules III to V may be routinely transmitted by facsimile machine, computer modem, or other similar electronic device directly from an authorized prescribing practitioner or his or her expressly authorized agent to a pharmacy or pharmacy department of the patient's choice. The faxed copy may be retained as the hard copy original and is considered compliant with all federal regulations provided it contains all information as required under federal law and regulation. This electronically transmitted or faxed prescription may be filed with other prescriptions in the customary fashion.

SCHEDULE II FAXED PRESCRIPTIONS

Prescriptions faxed to pharmacies for medications listed in Schedule II must be treated somewhat differently based on where the patient resides. If the patient is "ambulatory" or resides at home, the original, signed prescription shall be presented to the dispensing pharmacist before the electronically transmitted filled prescription is released to the patient. However, federal law allows two exceptions to this rule:

1. Intravenous pain therapy, or home or hospice infusion: The original prescription need not be sent to the pharmacy either before or after the medication is de-

livered to a patient's home. The faxed copy is considered to be the original prescription and must be retained as such.
2. Long-term care facilities: Faxed prescriptions for patients in long-term care facilities are considered to be the original written prescription order.

UNITED STATES POSTAL REGULATIONS

United States postal regulations allow the mailing of any filled prescription containing a narcotic of any quantity or federal schedule to patients. When mailing controlled substances, two rules must be followed:

1. The inner container must be marked, sealed, and labeled with the name and address of the practitioner, or the name and address of the pharmacy or other person dispensing the prescription and the prescription number.
2. The outside wrapper or container must be plain with no markings of any kind that would indicate the contents contained within.

PRESCRIPTION LABELING

The prescription label must be affixed to a container and contain the following information:

1. Pharmacy name, address, and telephone number
2. Assigned serial number
3. Date of initial dispensing
4. Name of patient
5. Name of prescriber
6. Directions for use and any cautionary statements
7. Federal controlled substances warning label or "transfer label" for a Schedule II, III, and IV controlled substance

A controlled substance warning label, also known as the federal transfer label, must be affixed to prescription containers of any drug listed in Schedules II to IV. The label reads as follows:

CAUTION: Federal law prohibits the transfer of this drug to any person other than the patient for whom it was prescribed.

EXPIRATION OR BEYOND USE DATES

Expiration dates listed on a manufacturer's stock container are set based on appropriate stability data that would support some amount of shelf-life. However, many states require some form of expiration dating on prescription labels.

Most use the Standards as described by the United States Pharmacopoeia. USP XXI states:

> Unless otherwise specified in the individual monograph, such beyond-use date (expiration date) shall be not later than the expiration date on the manufacturer's container, or one year from the date from when the drug is dispensed, whichever is earlier.

In addition, the USP specifies that the expiration date for insulin products is 24 months from their date of manufacture. Expiration dates on OTC drug products are exempt from expiration dating if they are stabile for at least 3 years, have no dosing limitations, and are safe and suitable for frequent and prolonged use. Some examples of these products include toothpaste and medicated shampoo.

SAFETY CLOSURES AND CONTAINERS

In accordance with the Poison Prevention Packaging Act of 1970, child-resistant closures must be used on prescription containers unless the prescription is for an exempt drug (e.g., sublingual nitroglycerin, cholestyramine powder, unit dose or effervescent potassium supplements, erythromycin ethylsuccinate preparations, oral contraceptives packaged in mnemonic packages).

Patients may authorize conventional, easy-to-open packaging for good reason and even issue a "blanket waiver" for prescription containers. This authorization may be in writing or oral. A physician may *not* issue a "blanket waiver" for dispensing in conventional, easy-to-open packaging; the order must be on each prescription.

In addition, refills of prescriptions dispensed in plastic containers require new containers to assure that the locking mechanism does not become worn and ineffective through its constant use. Refills of prescriptions dispensed in glass containers require that only the caps be replaced.

PHARMACY REQUIREMENTS

Every pharmacy must be registered with the DEA and receive a certificate of registration to distribute or dispense controlled substances. Each pharmacy has its own DEA registration number. These certificates of registration must be renewed every 3 years. Every pharmacy registrant must keep and maintain an accurate record of each controlled substance received. Dated invoices for controlled substances in Schedules III, IV, and V constitute complete records for these drugs. Copy 3 of DEA Form 222 (discussed in the following) constitutes complete record for the receipt of Schedule II controlled substances. The DEA requires every registrant who changes his or her business address to notify them and receive their approval before moving. Registrants may keep records at a location other than

the registered location by notifying the nearest DEA office. Unless this request is denied, registrants may transfer records 14 days after notification.

RECORD KEEPING

One of the primary tasks of the pharmacy registrant is record keeping. The DEA as well as state agencies have specific requirements that all DEA registrants must follow. All records of receipt and distribution of controlled substances must be kept at the site for 2 years. For example, all DEA registrants must keep complete and accurate inventory of all federally controlled substances. The requirements are as follows.

INVENTORY REQUIREMENTS

An initial inventory must be taken as soon as controlled substance activities are engaged. If no controlled substances are on hand, a zero inventory should be recorded. The initial inventory must contain the name, address, and DEA number of the registrant; the date and time of the inventory; the signature of the person taking the inventory; as well as the name of the medication, dosage form, dosage, and quantity on hand. Then, once every 2 years, a *biennial inventory* must be taken of all federally controlled substances (CIIV) after the date on which the original inventory was taken. This biennial inventory may be taken on any date within the 2-year period. The DEA requires exact counting of medications listed in Schedule II. Medications listed in Schedules III, IV, and V may be estimated provided the original package size was less than 1000 solid, dosage units. IF the original package size is 1000 solid, dosage units or greater, an exact count must be made. Schedule II inventories must be kept separately from all other records of controlled substances. All controlled substance inventory records must be kept at the inventory location for a period of 2 years.

Federal regulation allows pharmacists to file filled prescriptions in one of three ways. Pharmacy practitioners should be cautioned that the laws and regulations of their home state may differ. The federal requirement is as follows:

1. Pharmacists may keep two files, one containing Schedule II drugs, and the other containing Schedule III, IV, V, and nonscheduled drugs. If this method is chosen, all federally controlled substances (i.e., III, IV, V) must be stamped with a large red C, no less than 1" high, in the lower right hand corner in order to make those prescriptions readily retrievable.
2. Pharmacists may also keep two files with all federally controlled substances in one, marking those prescriptions in Schedules III, IV, and V with a large red C, and the other containing noncontrolled substances.
3. The third method of filing prescriptions includes three separate files. One file is for Schedule II; one file for

Schedule III, IV, and V; and one file for noncontrolled substances.

COMPUTERIZED PRESCRIPTION PROCESSING SYSTEMS

Federal law and regulation permits its record keeping requirement to be accomplished via computerized prescription processing systems. A pharmacy may use such a system for the storage and retrieval of prescription information provided it can supply immediate retrieval of information by either cathode ray tube (CRT) display or hard copy printout for prescriptions currently being filled. The information necessary for retrieval must include, but not be limited to:

1. Date of issuance
2. Original prescription number
3. Name and address of patient
4. Physician's name and DEA number
5. Name, strength, dosage form, and quantity of controlled substance
6. Total number of refills authorized by the physician

The system must provide a refill history by CRT or hard copy for controlled substances that have been refilled during the past 6 months. Pharmacies who use a computerized prescription processing system must printout a hard copy or receive a hard copy from a central processor within 72 hours of dispensing. Pharmacists who dispense these prescriptions then must verify that the information on the hard copy is correct and then sign and date that printout. A hard copy printout or other documentation must be stored in a separate file for a period of 2 years.

DRUG ENFORCEMENT ADMINISTRATION FORMS

FORM 222: All Schedule I and II drugs ordered to stock a pharmacy or other registered location must be ordered using DEA Form 222. In addition, pharmacists wishing to borrow or transfer (from registrant to registrant) Schedule II controlled substances from other pharmacies may only do so by using a DEA Form 222. The form is in triplicate and may be signed by the registrant or any person who has written authorization to do so (e.g., power of attorney). Power of attorney refers to any individual or individuals authorized by the pharmacy to sign and obtain DEA 222 order forms on behalf of the pharmacy. These individuals do not necessarily need to be registered pharmacists.

Each form contains ten lines on which to write the CII medication to be ordered. One line on the order form should be used to describe one item ordered, if two lines are used for the same item, they count as only one line. These forms must be submitted to the supplier error free. Therefore, voiding a line on the order form because of an error is not permitted and the entire form should be voided. When complete, the person ordering the medication must separate the third copy of the form and retain it in the pharmacy. Upon receipt of the drugs, the person who has ordered them, or any other authorized person, must fill out the last two columns of the store's copy with quantity and date.

FORM 106: Loss of controlled substances (federally scheduled II to V) must be reported to the district DEA office on DEA Form 106. If the pharmacy is involved in a robbery or significant shortage of controlled substances is detected, after reporting to the local police department, a DEA Form 106 should be filled out in triplicate. Two copies must be sent to the regional DEA office as soon as possible, one copy must be kept on file by the pharmacy.

The information on DEA Form-106 should contain:

1. Name and address of the firm
2. DEA registration number
3. Date of theft
4. Local police department notified
5. Type of theft (robbery, break-in, etc.)
6. A listing of any symbols or cost codes used by the pharmacy, if any
7. A listing of any controlled substances that are missing

FORM 41: Used for the destruction of controlled substances. The DEA should be contacted for instructions when desiring to destroy outdated, damaged, or otherwise unusable controlled substances. The DEA has authorized private companies to administer controlled substances destruction. The agency should be contacted for further information.

MISCELLANEOUS

Patient package inserts (PPIs) are required by FDA regulation to be provided to the patient when dispensing certain drugs. Patient package inserts must be given to the patient on the initial dispensing and on refills if so requested.

All of the following are drugs that must be dispensed with a PPI:

1. Isoproterenol inhalation products
2. Oral contraceptives
3. Estrogen/progestogen-containing drug products
4. Intrauterine devices
5. Progestational drug products
6. Accutane R

A prescription for an approved drug may be filled for an unapproved use provided that the prescriber:

1. Is well-informed about the drug prescribed
2. Bases such use on firm scientific rationale or sound medical evidence
3. Maintains adequate records of drug use and effect

BIBLIOGRAPHY

1. Strauss S. Food and Drug Administration: An overview. In: *Strauss's Federal Drug Laws and Examination Review,* 5th edition. Lancaster, PA: Technomic Publishing Co., 1999:323.

2. FDCA, Sec.21(g)(1)

3. Strauss S. Food and Drug Administration: An overview. In: *Strauss's Federal Drug Laws and Examination Review,* 5th edition. Lancaster, PA: Technomic Publishing Co., 1999:176, 186.

4. Pinna K, Pines W. *The Drugs/Biologics Approval Process: A Practical Guide to Food and Drug Law and Regulation.* Washington, DC: FDLI, 1998:96.

5. 21CFR58

6. Pinna K, Pines W. *The Drugs/Biologics Approval Process: A Practical Guide to Food and Drug Law and Regulation.* Washington, DC: FDLI, 1998:98.

7. 21CFR56

8. Pinna K, Pines W. *The Drugs/Biologics Approval Process: A Practical Guide to Food and Drug Law and Regulation.* Washington, DC: FDLI, 1998:98.

9. 21CFR50

10. 21CFR314

11. Pinna K, Pines W. *The Drugs/Biologics Approval Process: A Practical Guide to Food and Drug Law and Regulation.* Washington, DC: FDLI, 1998:102,103.

12. Fed Reg, V.64(18), January 28, 1999

13. Pinna K, Pines W. *The Drugs/Biologics Approval Process: A Practical Guide to Food and Drug Law and Regulation.* Washington, DC: FDLI, 1998:103.

14. Strauss S. Food and Drug Administration: An overview. In: *Strauss's Federal Drug Laws and Examination Review,* 5th edition. Lancaster, PA: Technomic Publishing Co., 1999:280.

15. Food and Drug Administration Modernization Act of 1997, PL. 105, 1997

16. 42USC, Sec. 262

17. Form FDA 356h

18. The Orphan Drug Act of 1982, PL 97-414

19. The Orphan Drug Amendments of 1985, PL 99-91

20. Pinna K, Pines W. *The Drugs/Biologics Approval Process: A Practical Guide to Food and Drug Law and Regulation.* Washington, DC: FDLI, 1998:119.

21. USP/DI, Volume III, 13th Edition, Preface, v

22. USP/DI, p.I/7

23. USP/DI, p.I/9

24. USP/DI, p.I/10

25. USP/DI, p.I/12

26. Pinna K, Pines W. *The Drugs/Biologics Approval Process: A Practical Guide to Food and Drug Law and Regulation.* Washington, DC: FDLI, 1998:111.

27. Pinna K, Pines W. *The Drugs/Biologics Approval Process: A Practical Guide to Food and Drug Law and Regulation.* Washington, DC: FDLI, 1998:111.

28. Strauss S. Food and Drug Administration: An overview. In: *Strauss's Federal Drug Laws and Examination Review,* 5th edition. Lancaster, PA: Technomic Publishing Co., 1999:285.

29. Strauss S. Food and Drug Administration: An overview. In: *Strauss's Federal Drug Laws and Examination Review,* 5th edition. Lancaster, PA: Technomic Publishing Co., 1999:285.

30. 21USC301, et seq.

31. 21USC302, et seq.

32. 21USC304, et seq.

33. *Fundamentals of Regulatory Affairs.* Regulatory Affairs Professions Society, 1999:199.

34. *Fundamentals of Regulatory Affairs.* Regulatory Affairs Professions Society, 1999:200.

35. Fink JL, Marquardt KW, Simonsmeir LM. *Pharmacy Law Digest,* 26th edition. St. Louis, MO: Facts and Comparisons, 1995:CS-1.

36. Fink JL, Marquardt KW, Simonsmeir LM. *Pharmacy Law Digest,* 26th edition. St. Louis, MO: Facts and Comparisons, 1995:CS-2.

37. M.G.L., Ch.94c, Sec. 1, Definitions

38. Fink JL, Marquardt KW, Simonsmeir LM. *Pharmacy Law Digest,* 26th edition. St. Louis, MO: Facts and Comparisons, 1995:CS-2.

39. 21CFR1301.21

40. 21CFR1305 et seq

41. MGL, Ch.94c, Sec.23(b)

42. MGL, Ch.94c, Sec.23(b)(d)

43. Massachusetts law limits the filling of prescriptions for Schedule II drugs for up to a 30-day supply. However, dextroamphetamine and methylphenidate are the exception and fillable in Massachusetts for up to a 60-day supply on any single filling. M.G.L. Ch.94C, Sec. 23(d)

44. MGL, Ch.94c, Sec.2(a)

45. *DEA Pharmacists' Manual,* January 2001.

46. Strauss S. Food and Drug Administration: An overview. In: *Strauss's Federal Drug Laws and Examination Review,* 5th edition. Lancaster, PA: Technomic Publishing Co., 1999.

47. Strauss S. Food and Drug Administration: An overview. In: *Strauss's Federal Drug Laws and Examination Review,* 5th edition. Lancaster, PA: Technomic Publishing Co., 1999.

48. Strauss S. Food and Drug Administration: An overview. In: *Strauss's Federal Drug Laws and Examination Review,* 5th edition. Lancaster, PA: Technomic Publishing Co., 1999.

49. Strauss S. Food and Drug Administration: An overview. In: *Strauss's Federal Drug Laws and Examination Review,* 5th edition. Lancaster, PA: Technomic Publishing Co., 1999.

50. Strauss S. Food and Drug Administration: An overview. In: *Strauss's Federal Drug Laws and Examination Review,* 5th edition. Lancaster, PA: Technomic Publishing Co., 1999.

51. Strauss S. Food and Drug Administration: An overview. In: *Strauss's Federal Drug Laws and Examination Review,* 5th edition. Lancaster, PA: Technomic Publishing Co., 1999.

52. Strauss S. Food and Drug Administration: An overview. In: *Strauss's Federal Drug Laws and Examination Review,* 5th edition. Lancaster, PA: Technomic Publishing Co., 1999.

53. Strauss S. Food and Drug Administration: An overview. In: *Strauss's Federal Drug Laws and Examination Review,* 5th edition. Lancaster, PA: Technomic Publishing Co., 1999.

54. Strauss S. Food and Drug Administration: An overview. In: *Strauss's Federal Drug Laws and Examination Review,* 5th edition. Lancaster, PA: Technomic Publishing Co., 1999.

55. 21CFR1306.21

56. 21CFR1306.11

57. 21CFR1306.13

58. Federal Register, May 19, 1994

59. 21CFR1306.22

60. 21CFR1306.21

61. 21CFR1306.04

PATIENT PROFILE 1

FOOD AND DRUG ADMINISTRATION RECALLS

PRESENTATION

JJ is watching television one evening and sees a news brief describing a recall of the anticonvulsant medication he has used successfully for the last 20 years. The next morning he calls your pharmacy to ask whether you have also seen the news about this medication and what needs to be done about it. You explain there's nothing to worry about because the recall was only for newly open containers with recent lot numbers and resulted from off-coloring in the tablet that, although it poses no health risks, may cause confusion.

QUESTIONS

1. How would you characterize this incident?

   A. Class I, Consumer Level
   B. Class II, Consumer Level
   C. Class II, Retail Level
   D. Class III, Retail Level
   E. Class III, Consumer Level

2. If this product was shown to cause a decrease in efficacy which has resulted in patient death, what level of recall would one suppose would be called?

   A. Class I
   B. Class II
   C. Class IIb
   D. Class III
   E. Class IIIb

3. In the case study presented, could the pharmaceutical manufacturer refuse to recall the product citing economic reasons?

   A. Yes
   B. No

PATIENT PROFILE 2

CONTROLLED SUBSTANCES ACT

PRESENTATION

RD, a physician, calls you at your community pharmacy and asks you to fill a prescription for a controlled substance in Schedule II as an emergency supply for an elderly patron of your pharmacy. You ask about the nature of the emergency, and the prescriber indicates that the patient has fallen, has back pain, and doesn't feel quite like going out today.

The physician prescribes the following:

Oxycodone with acetaminophen tablets #30
Sig: Take 1 tablet every 6 hours as needed for pain.
No refills
DEA# AR1357938

You request that a hard-copy, written prescription be mailed to you. Instead, RD faxes the prescription to your pharmacy.

Before you have the opportunity to have the prescription delivered, the patient painfully walks into your pharmacy and requests the prescription. Your patient profile indicates that the patient is on Medicaid. You fill and dispense the prescription.

QUESTIONS

1. Which of the following factor(s) is/are true regarding the dispensing of an emergency supply of CIIs without a prescription?

   I.   The patient needs the drug immediately.
   II. The physician cannot get a written prescription to the patient or pharmacy.
   III. A Schedule III controlled substance will not alleviate the pain.
   IV. The physician has 72 hours to mail a hard copy to the patient.
   V.   The physician has 7 days to mail a hard copy to the pharmacist.

   A. I, II, III, and V
   B. I, II, and III
   C. I, II, III, and IV
   D. IV and V
   E. V

2. Which of the following DEA numbers is correct for RD?

   A. AR 1357938
   B. RD 1221390
   C. AD 1221388
   D. AD 3798611
   E. AR 1256734

3. If the prescriber in this case had telephoned an emergency prescription order for a CII into the pharmacy, how long would that prescriber have to send or mail a hard-copy prescription to the pharmacy to comply with the federal Controlled Substances Act?

   A. 72 hours
   B. 48 hours
   C. 7 days
   D. 5 days
   E. 6 months

4. Which of the following faxed prescriptions may not be kept as an original prescription (in place of a hand written hard copy) for CII drugs?

   A. Prescriptions for home infusion medications to patients in hospice care
   B. Prescriptions for solid, oral dosage forms for patients with terminal illnesses
   C. Prescriptions for solid, oral dosage forms for patients in long-term care facilities

   D. Prescriptions for solid, oral dosage forms for patients in hospice care
   E. Prescriptions for solid, oral dosage forms for ambulatory patients living at home who are chronically ill

5. With regard to the presented case and according to federal laws and regulations, the pharmacist filling this prescription

   I.   must use a child resistant closure.
   II. may use a non-child resistant closure if authorized by the patient.
   III. must affix a Federal Transfer label to the prescription vial.
   IV. must file CII hard-copy prescriptions separately.

   A. I and II
   B. II and III
   C. II and IV
   D. I and IV
   E. All of the above

6. Under federal Omnibus Budget Reconciliation Act of 1990 (OBRA 90) regulations, which of the following would be considered a legal offer to counsel?

   I.   Telephone communication with the patient
   II. An auxiliary label on a prescription vial
   III. A toll-free telephone number
   IV. A sign posted informing customers of their right to counseling
   V.   A cartoon illustration demonstrating how to take a medication for patients who do not speak English

   A. I, II, and III
   B. II, III, and IV
   C. III, IV, and V
   D. I, III, and IV
   E. II and IV

7. Federal OBRA 90 regulations require the offer to counsel be given to

   A. all patients on both new and refill prescriptions.
   B. Medicaid patients and only on new prescriptions.
   C. all patients on new prescriptions.
   D. Medicaid patients and on both new and refill prescriptions.
   E. none of the above.

8. A patient is injured after taking a medication in the wrong dosage. You, the pharmacist, had realized the error and informed the physician who wrote the prescription about the problem. The physician told you to "just fill the prescription," and you did. If the patient were to sue, the courts would take issue with the pharmacist because of a concept in the federal Controlled Substances Act called

A. professional accountability.
B. co-liability.
C. corresponding responsibility.
D. negligence.
E. tort suit.

9. If the following does not appear on a written prescription for phenobarbital, the prescription should not be filled by the pharmacist:

A. Federal legend
B. Expiration date
C. DEA number
D. Federal transfer label
E. NDC number

10. If the prescription in the case were written, "Give Bowser the Beagle (a dog) 1 tablet every 6 hours for pain," and called into the pharmacy by an assistant to Bowser's veterinarian, the pharmacist who received the prescription could legally fill and dispense it as in an emergency situation.

A. True. The federal CSA does not differentiate human and animal prescriptions for emergencies.
B. True. The federal CSA allows agents of prescribers to telephone prescription orders into pharmacies whether they are for humans, animals, emergencies, or otherwise.
C. False. The federal CSA does not permit pharmacists to dispense prescriptions for animals even in an emergency.
D. False. The federal CSA does not permit agents of prescribers to telephone prescription orders to pharmacies whether they are for humans, animals, emergencies, or otherwise.
E. A and B are true.

PATIENT PROFILE 3
ORPHAN DRUG APPROVAL

PRESENTATION

A good friend is diagnosed with an unfamiliar disease and has been prescribed a medication and treatment that you have not heard about in your practice as a pharmacy professional. After doing some research, you find that the disease is quite rare and the treatment is classified as an orphan drug. Because neither the disease nor its treatment is common, you begin to realize that you must familiarize yourself with all aspects of this problem so that you can best counsel your friend.

QUESTIONS

1. Orphan drugs may have more than one designation (as orphans or not) provided there are different indications for the same drug sponsored by the same or different companies.

A. True
B. False

2. Which of the following is *not* an incentive offered to the manufacturer of an orphan drug?

A. Seven years of market exclusivity
B. Open protocols
C. Tax credits
D. Use of compassionate or treatment investigational new drug (IND) applications
E. All of the above

3. Under the Orphan Drug Act, a company whose product has achieved orphan status may lose its market exclusivity if it cannot produce enough product.

A. True
B. False

PATIENT PROFILE 4
CONTROLLED SUBSTANCES ACT

PRESENTATION

A pharmacist takes over a pharmacy in June of a given year. That pharmacist applies for and is granted DEA registration for the pharmacy. Later the pharmacist realizes that she needs to take an inventory of all federally controlled substances. After taking this inventory, she finds that she is "short" a large quantity of several controlled substances. She reports the shortage to the DEA and takes appropriate measures to prevent this from happening again.

QUESTIONS

1. DEA Form-222 is used when

   A. pharmacists want to borrow CIIIs from other pharmacies.
   B. there is a theft or loss of controlled substances.
   C. pharmacists want to order more books of order forms.
   D. pharmacists want to destroy controlled substances.
   E. None of the above

2. Which of the following is true regarding the federal law on controlled substances inventories?

   A. Inventories for controlled substances in Schedule III and IV, regardless of original quantity in the stock bottle, must be counted exactly.
   B. Inventories for controlled substances must be taken at least once every 2 years of the initial inventory date.
   C. Inventories for controlled substances should be taken every other year (biennially) and may be changed after prior notification of the DEA.
   D. A and B
   E. A and C

3. Under federal law and regulation, if a pharmacist is granted power of attorney by a registrant, that pharmacist may

   A. sign all legal documents that concern the pharmacy.
   B. practice pharmacy law.
   C. open and manage other pharmacies.
   D. sign DEA Form-222 to order controlled substances in Schedule II.
   E. become the manager of the pharmacy.

4. DEA Form-106 is used when

   A. pharmacists want to borrow CIIIs from other pharmacies.
   B. there is a theft or loss of federally controlled substances.
   C. pharmacists want to order more books of order forms.
   D. pharmacists want to destroy controlled substances.
   E. None of the above

5. DEA Form-41 is used when

   A. pharmacists want to borrow CIIIs from other pharmacies.
   B. there is a theft or loss of federally controlled substances.
   C. pharmacists want to order more books of order forms.
   D. pharmacists want to destroy controlled substances.
   E. None of the above

PATIENT PROFILE 5

EXPIRATION DATING AND NATIONAL DRUG CODE

PRESENTATION

It's Tuesday morning in your busy hospital pharmacy, and your wholesaler delivers your prescription drug order. You ask a technician to put the order away and instruct him to be careful that all drugs are stocked in the correct place behind any open, existing bottles of the same medication. You also instruct him to check for product expiration dates. The technician replies that he is new to the job and is not sure he'll know which products are the same. He also asks how close to the printed expiration date he should use as a guide for removing the product from stock. You explain NDC numbers, how they are distinct, and how they identify products individually. You also tell him that it is the policy of the hospital pharmacy to remove from stock any product within 30 days of the printed expiration date.

QUESTIONS

1. Over-the-counter consumer products for human care, such as shampoo and toothpaste, are exempt from the FDA expiration dating regulations if

   A. they are stable for at least 5 years.
   B. the label bears dosage limitations.
   C. they are safe and effective.
   D. they are safe and suitable for frequent use and often prolonged use.
   E. None of the above

2. Which of the following is/are true regarding the use of the National Drug Code?

   A. It is requested by the FDA to be on all product labels for prescription drugs.

B. It consists of 12 digits.
C. The first set of digits identifies the product.
D. None of the above
E. All of the above

3. If an NDC number is used on a product label by a manufacturer, where must it appear?

A. On the top third of the principal display panel of all drug product labels from manufacturers
B. Anywhere on the manufacturer's product label
C. On the outer package only
D. On the prescription label
E. All of the above

P A T I E N T   P R O F I L E   6

PRACTITIONERS AND PRESCRIPTIVE AUTHORITY

PRESENTATION

On a busy afternoon in late September, Mrs. AD presents a prescription to you from an ophthalmologist for her first-grader who has been diagnosed with head lice. As awful as this may be, the presented prescription is written for a petroleum distillate product that is *not* indicated for ophthalmic use. You are unsure whether an ophthalmologist has the legal authority to write a prescription for a medication that is outside his scope of professional practice. You call the physician and he tells you that the nits (lice eggs) are in the patient's eyebrows and lashes and that he has instructed the mother on how to use the medication topically to rectify the problem.

QUESTIONS

1. Why can this practitioner write for this medication as described in the case?

A. He is permitted to treat any medical condition he encounters within his scope of medical specialty (the human eye).
B. He is permitted to treat any medical condition he encounters without regard to medical specialty.
C. He cannot treat any medical condition he encounters unless it is within his medical specialty

and is prescribing outside his scope of medical practice.
D. Answers A and B are true.
E. None of the above

2. Who is not considered to be a "practitioner" under federal law?

A. Physician
B. Chiropractor
C. Veterinarian
D. Dentist
E. Podiatrist

3. Which of the following are true in federal law about the prescribing by practitioners of methadone?

A. MDs can prescribe methadone to any patient whose medical condition merits methadone's pain control characteristics.
B. MDs cannot prescribe methadone to anyone for any reason.
C. MDs can prescribe methadone daily for up to 3 days to addicted individuals while clinic arrangements are being made.
D. A and B
E. A and C

P A T I E N T   P R O F I L E   7

MIDLEVEL PRACTITIONERS

PRESENTATIONS

A pharmacy intern is interested in honing her prescription-filling and patient-counseling skills. You tell her the only way she is going to learn is by doing. You tell her she's in charge. After about an hour and 20 or so prescriptions, she

has to stop. Here's a new one on her—a prescription written by a physician assistant for a controlled substance without a DEA registration number on it. "I know they can prescribe, but I'm not sure whether additional or different information has to be on the prescription," she says.

QUESTIONS

1. Which of the following DEA numbers is correct for Charles Frick, a PA who practices in your neighborhood?

   A. PA 1357938
   B. AF 1211399
   C. MF 1221388
   D. FA 3798611
   E. RF 1256734

2. If a state or other jurisdiction, such as a U.S. territory, does not permit a midlevel practitioner to act in the course of professional practice by granting prescriptive privilege, does federal law supersede state law in these cases?

   A. Yes, federal law takes precedence in all cases.
   B. No, states can refuse to permit any regulatory activity granted under the federal law.
   C. No, midlevel prescribes are subject to the more stringent regulation.
   D. B and C
   E. All of the above

3. Which of the following is/are true regarding midlevel practitioners and prescribing privileges?

   A. States require documentation regarding conditions of prescriptive privileges.
   B. Documentation should be kept readily available for inspection by the DEA.
   C. Practice agreements, practice guidelines, and protocols are examples of required documents.
   D. States are given authority by the DEA to set educational standards.
   E. All of the above

PATIENT PROFILE 8

FOOD, DRUG, AND COSMETIC ACT

PRESENTATION

Your pharmacy operation begins a new community outreach program. The basis of the program is to provide a pharmacist to community groups to speak about a disease, a particular medication, or a medical issue. A local business group comprising physicians, attorneys, and other professionals has invited you to speak about Medicaid. However, after several of the more typical questions about pricing and reimbursement have been asked, one of the local business owners begins to ask about how prescription medications "actually get on the market." This line of questioning consumes the next hour and thirty minutes of discussion.

QUESTIONS

1. Which of the following is/are false?

   I. The lot number of a prescription drug product is not required by federal law to be placed on manufacturers' stock bottles.
   II. All generic drug products are listed in the orange book.
   III. If a generic drug product were dispensed as the brand name, and the pharmacist put the brand name on the prescription label, this act would constitute misbranding.

   A. I only
   B. II only
   C. III only
   D. I and II only
   E. II and III only

2. Controlled substances such as morphine SO_4 are set into schedules on the basis of

   A. chemical classification.
   B. potential for abuse.
   C. criminal penalty.
   D. safe and effective dosage.
   E. None of the above

3. Which of the following is/are not listed in the orange book?

   A. Generic products not found to be therapeutically equivalent to those of another company
   B. B-rated drug products
   C. Drugs on patent for which there is no legal substitution product
   D. A and B
   E. A and C

4. A drug product given an A rating in the FDA "Approved Drugs with Therapeutic Equivalence Evaluations" would be characterized as

   A. pharmacotherapeutic.
   B. bioavailable.
   C. therapeutically equivalent.
   D. bioequivalent.
   E. pharmaceutically equivalent.

5. Which of the following is/are true regarding the use of the National Drug Code?

   A. It is not required by law to be on all product labels for prescription drugs.
   B. It consists of 12 digits, and the first set of digits identifies the product.
   C. If a product label has an NDC number on it, one can assume the product requires a prescription.
   D. A and B
   E. A and C

6. The _____ prohibit(s) pharmacies from storing, dispensing or purchasing prescription drug samples and requires state boards of pharmacy to license drug wholesalers.

   A. Poison Prevention Packaging Act
   B. Price Competition and Patent Restoration Act
   C. Prescription Drug Marketing Act
   D. Kefauver-Harris Amendments
   E. Food, Drug, and Cosmetic Act

7. The. _____ required the examination of all prescription medications manufactured between 1938 and 1962 to determine drug effectiveness.

   A. Poison Prevention Packaging Act
   B. Price Competition and Patent Restoration Act
   C. Prescription Drug Marketing Act
   D. Kefauver–Harris Amendments
   E. Food, Drug, and Cosmetic Act

8. _____ is the largest human testing phase in drug development. In this phase, data on safety and efficacy are gathered through a diverse test population.

   A. Phase I
   B. Phase II
   C. Phase III
   D. Phase IV
   E. Phase V

9. _____ is the phase during which long-term safety, efficacy, and monitoring are established after marketing approval is granted.

   A. Phase I
   B. Phase II
   C. Phase III
   D. Phase IV
   E. Phase V

10. Products contaminated after they are shipped to a retail outlet are considered _____ but not _____ .

    A. misdirected, inconsistent
    B. misbranded, adulterated
    C. adulterated, misbranded
    D. misbranded, USP
    E. USP, misbranded

11. Manufacturers who want to submit their generic products to the FDA for approval use a(n) _____ , which requires less documentation than a full drug review and approval.

    A. SNDA
    B. NDA
    C. INDA
    D. ANDA
    E. PANDA

12. The process used to describe the FDA panel review of ingredients for OTC products to determine safety and efficacy, labeling, indications, instructions, and warnings is _____ .

    A. Drug monograph
    B. Phase I
    C. Category I
    D. Phase II
    E. Category III

PATIENT PROFILE 9

CONTROLLED SUBSTANCES ACT

PRESENTATION

John the pharmacist receives a prescription from Mrs. AS. She lives in a warm southern state for the few months of the year when her home state is in a "deep freeze" during the winter. The prescription is for eye drops that she uses as therapy for glaucoma. She attaches a note to the prescription and asks whether you would be so kind as to mail her a few bottles of her filled prescription so that she'll have enough until she moves back home in the spring. You check her patient profile and realize that the dosage prescribed is different from that which she had been using. When you telephone, you find that the prescriber is a medical intern training in ophthalmology. The physician-intern states that AS's glaucoma has worsened, hence the change in the prescription. You fill the prescription and mail it in keeping with the patient's request.

QUESTIONS

1. According to U.S. postal regulations, which of the following filled prescriptions cannot be mailed to ultimate users?

   A. Derivatives of opium
   B. Cocaine
   C. Narcotics
   D. A and C
   E. A, B, and C

2. Soon after the prescription for the glaucoma medication is mailed to you, AS calls your pharmacy to request that you also send her whatever quantity is left on the remaining refills of her CV antidiarrheal medication. Again, you check her computer profile and find there are three refills remaining. However, the last time she refilled this prescription was 8 months ago. Under federal law, what should you do?

   A. Do not refill the prescription. Prescriptions for Schedule V drugs are valid for five refills or 6 months, whichever is earlier.
   B. Fill the prescription only for the quantity written on the face of the prescription, take it to the nearest U.S. post office, and mail it to the patient.
   C. Fill the prescription for the quantity of the remaining refills, take it to the nearest U.S. post office, and mail it to the patient.
   D. B and C
   E. A, B, and C are illegal under federal law.

3. Which of the following statements are true with regard to U.S. postal regulations?

   A. Pharmacists may not mail filled prescriptions for narcotics in Schedule II.
   B. Pharmacists must clearly label all outer packages containing filled prescriptions with the name and address of the pharmacy.
   C. Pharmacists need not label the inner container of a mailed package as long as that container has a child-resistant closure.
   D. Pharmacists can mail filled prescriptions in Schedule III to ultimate users.
   E. All of the above

4. AS's covering physician was a medical intern and so defined by federal law as a practitioner. Of the following, who would not be considered a practitioner?

   A. Allopathic physician
   B. Psychologist
   C. Psychiatrist
   D. Podiatrist
   E. Veterinarian

5. Pharmacists may lawfully fill prescriptions written by medical interns or foreign physicians when

   A. they are assigned a suffix to be used with the institutional (e.g., hospital) DEA registration number.
   B. they are assigned a prefix to be used with the institutional (e.g., hospital) DEA registration number.
   C. they write prescriptions which are then cosigned by the chief resident or other authorized practitioner within the institution.
   D. A and C
   E. B and C

6. A prescription for a controlled substance must be

   A. written in ink.
   B. written in indelible pencil.
   C. typewritten.
   D. signed by the prescriber in his or her own handwriting.
   E. all of the above.

7. The federal Controlled Substances Act limits prescription refills of up to five times within 6 months for

   A. emergency CII prescriptions only.
   B. telephoned CIII, CIV, and CV prescriptions only.
   C. any CII, CIII, and CIV prescriptions with authorized refills.
   D. any CIII and CIV prescriptions with authorized refills.
   E. all prescriptions.

PRESCRIPTION DRUG MARKETING ACT

PRESENTATION

One morning the telephone rings in your pharmacy. The caller is a local physician with whom you have a very cordial relationship. He asks if you're still on for golf on Sunday and tells you that he has a deal for you that you just can't refuse. It seems his office staff has been ordering prescription drug samples in fairly large quantities. He sheepishly tells you that he just signed the paperwork for these orders and never gave them much thought. Then yesterday he wanted a patient to have a few samples of a certain medication to get started and asked his nurse to get them. When she did, she brought several boxes. He asked, "How much of this stuff do we have?" Her answer was, "Enough to supply a small city!" He found thousands of dosage units of medication samples in his storage room. He knows that the cost price for all of these samples has to be more than ten thousand dollars. "Let's make a deal," he says. "Give me a thousand dollars, and you can have them all."

QUESTIONS

1. According to the Prescription Drug Marketing Act, which of the following is/are true?

    A. Pharmacists may purchase prescription drug samples provided they pay fair market price for them.
    B. Pharmacists may purchase prescription drug samples provided they add them to their inventory at the time of purchase.
    C. Pharmacists are prohibited by federal law from purchasing and redispensing prescription drug samples.

    D. Pharmacists may purchase prescription drug samples and designate them for resale to indigent patients at a reduced price.
    E. A, B, and D

2. Regarding hospital pharmacies and prescription drug samples, which of the following is/are permissible under the Prescription Drug Marketing Act?

    A. Hospital pharmacies may store prescription drug samples provided they are kept separate from other pharmacy stock.
    B. Hospital pharmacies must keep copies of prescribers' written requests to pharmaceutical companies for prescription drug samples.
    C. Hospital pharmacies may not offer prescription drug samples for sale to any individual.
    D. A and C
    E. All of the above

3. Regarding drug wholesalers, which of the following is/are true?

    A. The Prescription Drug Marketing Act requires drug wholesalers to become registered as such by the FDA.
    B. The Prescription Drug Marketing Act requires drug wholesalers to become registered as such by the state in which they operate.
    C. The Prescription Drug Marketing Act requirement for registration is voluntary for drug wholesalers who want to distribute prescription drug samples.
    D. The Prescription Drug Marketing Act does not include regulatory requirements for drug wholesalers.
    E. All of the above

STATUTORY AUTHORITY

PRESENTATION

One evening as you sit in front of your 51-inch plasma screen television, you see an advertisement for an arthritis headband that claims to be made from a space age material and has the ability to spontaneously relieve any musculoskeletal pain. The commercial states that this product is a "breakthrough" and is the most effective product of its kind in the world today. After thinking about it, you come to realize that many of your patients will be asking about it when you are in the pharmacy and you have concerns that the commercial is being misleading.

QUESTIONS

1. In the preceding case, which federal agency would be contacted about this type of product?

A. OSHA
B. FDA
C. FTC
D. DEA
E. NRA

2. Regarding the advertisement of prescription drugs, which of the following are true?

    A. The Food and Drug Administration (FDA) has the authority to determine the accuracy of prescription drug advertisements.
    B. The FDA has the authority to remove advertisements and commercials that it feels make false and misleading claims.

C. The FDA has no authority to remove advertisements and commercials that it feels make false and misleading claims.
D. A and B
E. A and C

3. In the case of any medical, food, or device product in which its labeling is considered incorrect but not in any way contaminated, the proper designation is _____ but not _____.

    A. Misdirected, inconsistent
    B. Misbranded, adulterated
    C. Adulterated, misbranded
    D. Misbranded, USP
    E. USP, misbranded

POISON PREVENTION PACKAGING ACT

PRESENTATION

RM, an elderly physician, has been in practice for many years. He likes the old way that medicine was practiced and spends a great deal of time with his few remaining patients. One of the things on which he insists on for all of his patients is that their prescriptions be dispensed without those "damn safety caps." "Too hard to get off by older folks," he states. "It gives them another reason not to take their medication!" Sometimes he authorizes non–child resistant closures on the prescriptions he writes, sometimes he does not.

QUESTIONS

1. According to the Poison Prevention Packaging Act, which of the following require complying containers?

    A. Prescription drugs for oral use
    B. Oral contraceptives in mnemonic packages
    C. Potassium supplements less than 50 mEq
    D. Powdered cholestyramine
    E. Topical creams and ointments

2. Which of the following comply with the requirements for packaging under the Poison Prevention Packaging Act?

A. Nitroglycerin sublingual tabs in non–child resistant containers
B. OTC ibuprofen tablets packaged in clearly marked, non–child resistant containers of 100 for elderly patients with arthritis
C. Children's aspirin in child resistant containers
D. Prescription medication packaged in non–child resistant containers with permission from the patient
E. All of the above require special packaging.

3. Which of the following is/are true under the PPPA?

    A. Plastic prescriptions containers must be discarded, and new containers must be provided when the refill is dispensed.
    B. Glass prescription containers must be discarded, and new containers must be provided when the refill is dispensed.
    C. Prescriptions can be dispensed in non–child resistant containers if a patient makes an oral request.
    D. A and C
    E. B and C

PATIENT PROFILE 13

FOOD, DRUG, AND COSMETIC ACT

PRESENTATION

Your pharmacy receives a letter from a pharmaceutical manufacturer that states it is conducting a recall of a certain product because of reports that the tablets are "breaking up" in the stock bottle during shipment, resulting in many unusable doses. The letter also states that the problem is not dangerous to patients in any way. You check your pharmacy shelves and find that you have two stock bottles on the shelf. One has been opened and has had tablets dispensed from it. The other bottle is unopened and has printed on its label the lot number of the product that has been recalled. You remove the recalled product and prepare to send it back to the manufacturer. However, you notice that the opened bottle appears to be within 3 months of its expiration date. You realize that you had opened it just the other day to make a few "bingo cards" or "blister packs" for a nursing home patient that you serve. These cards have not yet been delivered to the nursing home, and you wonder whether your technician has used the proper expiration date on the labels. You check the order and find that they have been labeled properly.

QUESTIONS

1. How would you characterize this incident?

    A. Class I, consumer level
    B. Class II, consumer level
    C. Class II, retail level
    D. Class III, retail level
    E. Class III, consumer level

2. Federal regulations regarding the expiration date on a manufacturer's stock bottle are based on the stability of product as packaged and as stored by the manufacturer. However, for products that are very stable, such as dry powders and capsules, what is the federal requirement for product expiration date?

    A. 5 years
    B. 7 years
    C. 10 years
    D. 2 years
    E. None of the above

3. What is the USP recommendation for the expiration date on a prescription label when a drug is dispensed from a community retail pharmacy?

    A. The date on the manufacturer's stock bottle
    B. 6 months from the date dispensed
    C. 1 year from the date dispensed
    D. A or B, whichever is earlier
    E. A or C, whichever is earlier

4. The proper expiration date used when hospital pharmacies repackage medications into unit-dose is

    A. 25% of the time remaining of the date on the manufacturers stock bottle.
    B. 6 months from the date repackaged.
    C. 1 year from the date repackaged.
    D. A or B, whichever is earlier.
    E. A or C, whichever is earlier.

5. The proper expiration date used on insulin products is

    A. any date the manufacturer proves the product to be stable.
    B. 6 months from the date manufactured.
    C. 1 year from the date manufactured.
    D. 2 years from the date manufactured.
    E. None of the above

PATIENT PROFILE 14

OVER-THE-COUNTER DRUGS

PRESENTATION

TM telephones the pharmacy to request a refill on his arthritis medicine. You tell him to hold on while you check his profile. You find there are no valid refills left. You tell TM that you'll contact his physician and deliver the prescription after you obtain authorization. He thanks you and hangs up. You call the physician and request the new prescription. The physician's nurse looks at the patient record and realizes that TM has not seen the physician for at least

18 months. She asks the physician about refilling the medication and he says, "No, tell him to see me." You call the patient and relay the news. The patient says the physician costs too much, that the drug he needs is OTC anyway, and that he'll just triple the dose to equal the prescription strength.

QUESTIONS

1. Which of the following is true regarding OTC medications?

   A. OTC product labels must by written in understandable language and provide information necessary for safe and effective use by consumers.
   B. OTC products must be appropriate for use by patients only for acute conditions consumers may identify after professional supervision.
   C. OTC products by design do not require consumers to read the label to use them appropriately.
   D. A and B
   E. A and C

2. The following can be generally said of the OTC drug review process:

   A. It allows a company to put new products on the market.
   B. It requires a company to use only ingredients and combinations described by the monograph for that product category.
   C. It permits scientific and public comment about OTC product categories and their ingredients and combinations.

   D. A and B
   E. All of the above

3. Regarding drugs considered for switch from prescription to OTC status, which of the following is false?

   A. In the change from prescription to OTC status, the entire review process does not have to be conducted on the product, such as submission of a new NDA, animal testing, and human testing.
   B. The monograph system can be used only when the product can be demonstrated as safe for use by consumers.
   C. A shortened NDA can be submitted to the FDA that contains information such as the desired indications, new labeling, and smaller dose if no OTC monograph exists.
   D. A petition may be filed by a product sponsor if that sponsor can prove a prescription is not necessary to protect public health.
   E. The monograph process can be used to facilitate a change from prescription to OTC status.

4. Which of the following criteria are used by the FDA to classify drugs as having prescription status?

   A. Habit-forming drugs are assigned prescription status.
   B. Homeopathic drugs diluted to IX are assigned to prescription status.
   C. Drugs that necessitate a physician's supervision are assigned to prescription status.
   D. A and B
   E. A and C

PATIENT PROFILE 15

CONTROLLED SUBSTANCES ACT

PRESENTATION

One quiet, rainy Friday morning, you are sitting in your pharmacy having a second cup of coffee and enjoying the slow pace thus far. A gentleman enters and walks up to the pharmacy counter. You greet him and ask, "May I help you?" He smiles and replies, "Yes, you may. I'm Agent Biggs from the U.S. Drug Enforcement Administration (DEA). I'm here on official business to conduct an audit." He shows you his badge and identification and your quiet, uneventful morning just became more interesting!

1. Which of the following would Agent Biggs wish to audit?

   A. Your posted DEA registration
   B. Your current biennial inventory

   C. Your 222 forms
   D. Your invoices and receipts for ordered CIII, CIV, and CV
   E. All of the above

2. The DEA agent will also look at prescriptions filled for federally controlled substances. Which of the following information is *not* required under federal law and regulation to be present on a presented prescription for a Schedule III?

   A. Name of practitioner
   B. Address of practitioner
   C. Name of patient
   D. Telephone number of prescriber
   E. Date of issue

3. Just before leaving the premises, Agent Biggs observes you filling a prescription for a Schedule IV antianxiety agent. He watches to see if you affix the proper federal transfer label to the container ("Caution: Federal law prohibits the transfer of this drug to any person other than the patient for whom it was prescribed"). On which containers must this required labeling appear?

A. Schedules II, III, and IV only
B. Schedules II, III, IV, and V only
C. Schedules II and III only
D. Schedule II only

PART III

ANSWERS WITH EXPLANATIONS
AND REFERENCES

OVER-THE-COUNTER PRODUCTS

ANSWERS

1. (C) β-Blockers and ACE inhibitors are appropriate initial therapy for patients who have undergone a myocardial infarction.

   Ref: The Joint National Committee on Prevention, Detection, Evaluation, and Treatment of High Blood Pressure. The Seventh Report of the Joint National Committee on Prevention, Detection, Evaluation, and Treatment of High Blood Pressure (JNC-7). *JAMA* 2003;289(19):2560–2572.

2. (A) Four grams is the maximum daily dosage for aspirin therapy.

   Ref: *Drug Facts and Comparisons,* 2003 ed. St. Louis: Facts and Comparisons, 2002.

3. (C) Nicotinic acid, not nicotinamide, is used in the treatment of hyperlipidemia.

   Ref: Talbert RL. Hyperlipidemia. In: DiPiro JT, Talbert RL, Yee GC, eds. *Pharmacotherapy: A Pathophysiologic Approach,* 5th ed. New York: McGraw-Hill, 2002:395–417.

4. (B) NSAIDs such as ibuprofen may reduce the effectiveness of ACE inhibitors.

   Ref: Jackson EK. Renin and angiotensin. In: Hardman JG, Limbird LE, Gilman A, eds. *Goodman & Gilman's The Pharmacological Basis of Therapeutics*, 10th ed. New York: McGraw Hill; 2001:829.

5. (E) All statements are true regarding aspirin administration in cardiac patients.

   Ref: Stringer KA, Lopez LM. Uncomplicated myocardial infarction. In: DiPiro JT, Talbert RL, Yee GC, eds. *Pharmacotherapy: A Pathophysiologic Approach,* 5th ed. New York: McGraw-Hill, 2002:262, 265.

6. (D) A nonproductive cough is a common side effect of ACE inhibitor therapy.

   Ref: *Drug Facts and Comparisons,* 2003 ed. St. Louis: Facts and Comparisons, 2002.

7. (B) Aspirin blocks thromboxane A_2 production, which inhibits platelet aggregation by permanently binding to the cyclooxygenase enzyme (the enzyme responsible for thromboxane A_2 production).

   Ref: Majerus PW, Tollefsen DM. Anticoagulant, thrombolytic, and antiplatelet drugs. In: Hardman JG, Limbird LE, Gilman A, eds. *Goodman & Gilman's The Pharmacological Basis of Therapeutics*, 10th ed. New York: McGraw Hill, 2001:1534.

8. (A) Aspirin overdose is associated with metabolic acidosis.

   Ref: *Drug Facts and Comparisons,* 2003 ed. St. Louis: Facts and Comparisons, 2002.

9. (C) Acetaminophen has analgesic and antipyretic properties. Acetaminophen has weak anti-inflammatory activity and does not inhibit platelet aggregation.

   Ref: Jackson Roberts L, Morrow JD. Analgesic-antipyretic and antinflammatory agents and drugs in the treatment of gout. In: Hardman JG, Limbird LE, Gilman AG, eds. *Goodman & Gilman's The Pharmacological Basis of Therapeutics*, 10th ed. New York: McGraw Hill; 2001:703.

10. (E) Pseudoephedrine, a vasoconstrictor, should be used with caution in patients with hypertension because it may elevate blood pressure and induce tachycardia.

    Ref: Hoffman BB. Catecholamines, sympathomimetic drugs, and adrenergic receptor antagonists. In: Hardman JG, Limbird LE, Gilman AG, eds. *Goodman & Gilman's The Pharmacological Basis of Therapeutics,* 10th ed. New York: McGraw Hill; 2001: 240.

CORONARY ARTERY DISEASE

ANSWERS

1. (E) Gout is not associated with the development of atherosclerosis.

   Ref: Talbert RL. Ischemic heart disease. In: DiPiro JT, Talbert RL, Yee GC, Matzke GR, Wells BG, Posey LM, eds. *Pharmacotherapy: A Pathophysiologic Approach.* 4th ed. Stamford, Conn: Appleton & Lange; 1999:182–210.

2. (D) Immediate administration of ASA has been proved to lower morbidity and mortality in unstable angina.

   Ref: Stringer KA, Lopez LM. Myocardial infarction. In: DiPiro JT, Talbert RL, Yee GC, Matzke GR, Wells BG, Posey LM, eds. *Pharmacotherapy: A Pathophysiologic Approach.* 4th ed. Stamford, Conn: Appleton & Lange; 1999:211–231.

3. (B) Immediate release nifedipine has been shown to worsen outcome when used in the treatment of patients with acute coronary syndromes.

   Ref: Stringer KA, Lopez LM. Myocardial infarction. In: DiPiro JT, Talbert RL, Yee GC, Matzke GR, Wells BG, Posey LM, eds. *Pharmacotherapy: A Pathophysiologic Approach.* 4th ed. Stamford, Conn: Appleton & Lange; 1999:211–231.

4. (B) This patient needs 40 mg lovastatin to attain the necessary LDL reduction.

   Ref: Talbert RL. Ischemic heart disease. In: DiPiro JT, Talbert RL, Yee GC, Matzke GR, Wells BG, Posey LM, eds. *Pharmacotherapy: A Pathophysiologic Approach.* 4th ed. Stamford, Conn: Appleton & Lange; 1999:182–210.

5. (C) To prevent moisture accumulation and degradation of the active drug, cotton should always be removed after a container is opened.

   Ref: Talbert RL. Ischemic heart disease. In: DiPiro JT, Talbert RL, Yee GC, Matzke GR, Wells BG, Posey LM, eds. *Pharmacotherapy: A Pathophysiologic Approach.* 4th ed. Stamford, Conn: Appleton & Lange; 1999:182–210.

   Ref: AHFS Drug Information, 1998.

PATIENT PROFILE 3

ATTENTION-DEFICIT/HYPERACTIVITY DISORDER (ADHD)

ANSWERS

1. (E) According to the *Diagnostic and Statistical Manual of Mental Disorders*, 4th edition, the diagnosis of ADHD can only be made in the presence of the following: six or more symptoms of hyperactivity/ impulsivity, inattention, or both; symptoms occurring prior to the age of 7 years; symptoms present in two or more settings; clear evidence of impairment in social and academic functioning; and symptoms determined to not be caused by an underlying mental disorder.

   Ref: American Psychiatric Association. *Diagnostic and Statistical Manual of Mental Disorders,* 4th ed. Washington: American Psychiatric Association, 2000.

2. (A) Behavior modification has been shown to be beneficial in the management of ADHD by teaching children to "stop and think" before acting. It is designed to facilitate self-control and enhance problem-solving skills. It is most useful in the presence of impulsivity and non-self-controlled behavior.

   Ref: Institute for Clinical Systems Improvement. *Diagnosis and Management of Attention Deficit Hyperactivity Disorder in Primary Care for School Age Children and Adolescents,* 5th ed. Bloomington, MN: Institute for Clinical Systems Improvement, 2003.

3. (C) The most commonly reported side effects associated with methylphenidate use include appetite suppression, insomnia, irritability, headaches, and nausea. Other side effects that occur less commonly include growth suppression, tachycardia, and changes in blood pressure (hypotension or hypertension), none of which have been considered to be dose-dependent effects. Only two case reports document the development of hematologic disorders (thrombocytopenia and eosinophilia) potentially owing to methylphenidate use. Routine complete blood counts (CBCs) are not necessary, but it may be prudent to obtain them periodically. Because of its central nervous system effects, methylphenidate can produce a withdrawal syndrome if discontinued abruptly. Doses should be reduced slowly to avoid withdrawal symptoms.

   Ref: Greenhill LL, et al. Stimulant medications. *J Am Acad Child Adolesc Psychiatry* 1999;38(5):502–512.

   Ref: Kuperman AA, et al. Methylphenidate as a possible cause of thrombocytopenia. *Ann Pharmacother* 2003;37:1146.

   Ref: Hayashi RJ, et al: The characteristics of eosinophilia in a series of intravenous methylphenidate abusers. *Drug Intell Clin Pharmacol* 1980;14:189–192.

4. (E) Tourette's syndrome may be precipitated or exacerbated in children treated with stimulant medications. It is often difficult to distinguish these symptoms from those associated with ADHD. Therefore, children who have Tourette's syndrome should not receive stimulant medications. If these symptoms develop during therapy, the medication should be discontinued. Anxiety or irritability is a common side effect of stimulant medications and may be exacerbated if used in children with such a history. Coadministration of MAO inhibitors and stimulant medications can lead to hypertensive crisis.

   Ref: Lowe TL, et al: Stimulant medications precipitate Tourette's syndrome. *JAMA* 1982;247:1168–1169.

   Ref: Product Information: Ritalin, methylphenidate, Novartis Pharmaceuticals.

   Ref: Hansten P, Horn J. *Drug Interactions Analysis and Management.* Vancouver, WA: Applied Therapeutics, 2000 (quarterly updates).

5. (B) A response to therapy should be seen within 2 weeks.

   Ref: Product Information: Ritalin, methylphenidate, Novartis Pharmaceuticals.

6. (A) The administration of methylphenidate close to bedtime can precipitate insomnia and irritability that could disrupt normal sleep patterns. Changing the administration

time of the second dose may alleviate these symptoms. All stimulant medications have been associated with the development of insomnia. The use of a hypnotic such as zolpidem is contraindicated in patients younger than 18 years of age. In addition, medication side effects should not be treated with another medication. Changing the time of administration, decreasing the dosage, or switching to a different medication should be sufficient to eliminate adverse effects.

Ref: Institute for Clinical Systems Improvement. *Diagnosis and Management of Attention Deficit Hyperactivity Disorder in Primary Care for School Age Children and Adolescents,* 5th ed. Bloomington, MN: Institute for Clinical Systems Improvement, 2003.

Ref: Product information: Ambien, zolpidem, Sanofi-Synthelabo.

7. (B) Strattera (atomoxetine) is not regulated as a controlled substance but does require a prescription. It has Food and Drug Administration (FDA) approval for use in both children and adults with ADHD. Strattera has a side-effect profile similar to the stimulant medications, and the same monitoring parameters should apply. Strattera is also contraindicated in patients taking MAO inhibitors owing to risk of the development of hypertensive crisis.

Ref: Product information: Strattera, atomoxetine, Lilly.

8. (D) Chewing Concerta tablets can break the formulation matrix and release all the medication at once, leading to a potential overdose. Inert substances from the tablet can pass through the stool, and patients should be told that this is normal and not harmful to them. Concerta can be given with or without food.

Ref: Product information: Concerta, extended-release methylphenidate, ALZA.

9. (B) Clonidine demonstrated an improvement in global impression scores of aggression in a small pilot study involving 17 children aged 5 to 15 years with various disruptive behavior disorders. The lack of evidence from large randomized, controlled trials limits its use in this setting. Clonidine has been studied more extensively as a second-line treatment for symptoms of ADHD refractory to stimulant medications. However, its side-effect profile limits its use as long-term therapy.

Ref: Kemph JP, et al. Treatment of aggressive children with clonidine: Results of an open pilot study. *J Am Acad Child Adolesc Psychiatry* 1993;32(3):577–581.

Ref: Hunt RD, et al. Clonidine benefits children with ADDH: Report of double-blind, placebo-crossover therapeutic trial. *J Am Acad Child Adolesc Psychiatry* 1985;24:617–629.

10. (D) From 1975 to 1999, 15 cases of acute liver failure that occurred as early as 6 months into pemoline therapy were reported to the FDA. Twelve cases resulted in either death or liver transplantation. Case reports of aplastic anemia also have been documented. Pemoline can cause nystagmus and other severe ocular side effects. For these reasons, pemoline should be avoided in the management of ADHD.

Ref: Product information: Cylert, pemoline, Abbott

PATIENT PROFILE 4
HYPERTENSION

ANSWERS

1. (E) The first appearance of sound is used to define systolic blood pressure. The disappearance of sound is used to define diastolic blood pressure.

Ref: Joint National Committee on Prevention, Detection, Evaluation, and Treatment of High Blood Pressure. The seventh report of the Joint National Committee of Prevention, Detection, Evaluation, and Treatment of High Blood Pressure. *Hypertension* 2003;42:1206–1252.

2. (E) Angiotensin-converting enzyme inhibitors such as enalapril are the preferred drug class in the care of patients with diabetes mellitus who are being treated for hypertension.

Ref: Joint National Committee on Prevention, Detection, Evaluation, and Treatment of High Blood Pressure. The seventh report of the Joint National Committee of Prevention, Detection, Evaluation, and Treatment of High Blood Pressure. *Hypertension* 2003;42:1206–1252.

3. (D) The goal blood pressure for patients with diabetes mellitus and hypertension is <130/80 mm Hg. The goal blood pressure among otherwise healthy patients is <140/90 mm Hg.

Ref: Joint National Committee on Prevention, Detection, Evaluation, and Treatment of High Blood Pressure. The seventh report of the Joint National Committee of Prevention, Detection, Evaluation, and Treatment of High Blood Pressure. *Hypertension* 2003;42:1206–1252.

4. (E) The risk factors for the development of cardiovascular disease are diabetes mellitus, smoking, sex (men and postmenopausal women), dyslipidemia, age older than 60 years, and a family history of cardiovascular disease (women older than 65 years and men younger than 55 years).

Ref: Joint National Committee on Prevention, Detection, Evaluation, and Treatment of High Blood Pressure. The seventh report of the Joint National Committee of Prevention, Detection, Evaluation, and Treatment of High Blood Pressure. *Hypertension* 2003;42:1206–1252.

DIABETES

ANSWERS

1. (C) KE was diagnosed with diabetes, and the goal blood pressure for a diabetic is less than 130/80 mm Hg.

   Ref: American Diabetes Association. Clinical practice guidelines. *Diabetes Care* 2004;27(1):S15–S35.

2. (C) He is a diabetic, and his goal should be an LDL level <100 mg/dL and an HDL level > 40 mg/dL.

   Ref: American Diabetes Association. Clinical practice guidelines. *Diabetes Care* 2004;27(1):S15–S35.

3. (A) KE should have an *eye* examination ASAP (since type 2 diabetics should have their first examination shortly after diagnosis) and yearly thereafter.

   Ref: American Diabetes Association. Clinical practice guidelines. *Diabetes Care* 2004;27(1):S15–S35.

4. (A) Current guidelines recommend annual influenza vaccination for diabetic patients.

   Ref: American Diabetes Association. Clinical practice guidelines. *Diabetes Care* 2004;27(1):S15–S35.

5. (C) Current guidelines recommend a full foot examination annually, and patients should visually inspect their feet daily. Health care professionals should examine the patient's feet at every routine visit.

   Ref: American Diabetes Association. Clinical practice guidelines. *Diabetes Care* 2004;27(1):S15–S35.

6. (D) Common side effects of metformin include nausea, vomiting, and gastrointestinal upset.

   Ref: Package Insert: Glucophage (metformin), Bristol-Myers Squibb Company, Princeton, NJ, 2004.

7. (C) The presence of other diabetes-related complications is a risk factor for a diabetic foot ulcer.

   Ref: American Diabetes Association. Clinical practice guidelines. *Diabetes Care* 2004;27(1):S15–S35.

8. (C) Patients with circulatory dysfunction (such as congestive heart failure) are at an increased risk for adverse reactions associated with metformin, especially lactic acidosis.

   Ref: Package Insert: Glucophage (metformin), Bristol-Myers Squibb Company, Princeton, NJ; 2004.

9. (C) KE's calculated BMI is 35.

   Ref: *NHLBI Clinical Guidelines on the Identification, Evaluation, and Treatment of Overweight and Obesity in Adults.* Washington: National Institutes of Health, National Heart, Lung, and Blood Institute, September 1998.

10. (A) KE meets the criteria for the metabolic syndrome.

    Ref: National Cholesterol Education Program. *Adult Treatment Panel III.* Washington: National Institutes of Health, National Heart, Lung, and Blood Institute, May 2001.

SEIZURE DISORDERS

ANSWERS

1. (C) Phenytoin is highly protein bound, particularly to albumin. A decrease in serum albumin can increase the concentration of free phenytoin, which is the pharmacologically active component. Patients with low albumin concentrations or impaired protein binding may have drug toxicity despite "normal" serum phenytoin concentrations.

   Ref: Phenytoin. In: *Basic Clinical Pharmacokinetics.* 3rd ed. Chapter 10.

2. (C) Hirsutism is a common side effect of phenytoin and is not correlated with serum phenytoin concentration. Ataxia and sedation are concentration-dependent side effects.

   Ref: Phenytoin. In: *Basic Clinical Pharmacokinetics.* 3rd ed. Chapter 10.

3. (D) Phenytoin is an enzyme inducer. It may increase the metabolism of oral contraceptives and reduce their efficacy. Patients should be advised to consider alternative methods of contraception to avoid unplanned pregnancy.

   Ref: Seizure disorders. In: Young LY, Koda-Kimble MA, eds. *Applied Therapeutics: The Clinical Use of Drugs.* 6th ed. Vancouver, Wash: Applied Therapeutics; 1995.

4. (D) Although folic acid may not reliably reduce the risk of birth defects in women receiving antiepileptic drugs, adequate folate supplementation is still recommended.

   Ref: Seizure disorders. In: Young LY, Koda-Kimble MA, eds. *Applied Therapeutics: The Clinical Use of Drugs.* 6th ed. Vancouver, Wash: Applied Therapeutics; 1995.

5. (D) Ethosuximide is considered the drug of choice for absence seizures, but it is of little value in the management of generalized seizures.

Ref: Seizure disorders. In: Young LY, Koda-Kimble MA, eds. *Applied Therapeutics: The Clinical Use of Drugs.* 6th ed. Vancouver, Wash: Applied Therapeutics; 1995.

PATIENT PROFILE 7

RESPIRATORY TRACT INFECTIONS

ANSWERS

1. (E) It is not uncommon to have a mixed infection between both typical and atypical organisms.

2. (C) PJ's lack of compliance suggests that once-daily therapy should be used if possible. His enrollment in an indigent care program will allow him to obtain free medication. The only medication listed that can be given once a day is azithromycin.

Ref: Mandell LA, Bartlett JG, Dowell SF, et al. Update of practice guidelines for the management of community-acquired pneumonia in immunocompetent adults. *Clin Infect Dis* 2003;37: 1405–1433.

3. (B) Azithromycin is the only choice listed that will cover both *S. pneumoniae* and *Legionella* organisms.

Ref: File TM Jr, Garau J, Blasi F, et al. Guidelines for empiric antimicrobial prescribing in community-acquired pneumonia. *Chest* 2004;125(5):1888–1901.

4. (E) A pneumococcal strain with an intermediate resistance pattern to penicillin still can be treated with penicillin. However, PJ also had the positive urine *Legionella* antigen. The fluoroquinolones are superb second-line agents for controlling infection. They also can be used as first-line agents as well; however, spectrum preservation should prevail. Because of PJ's situation, a once-daily drug with coverage against both pneumococci and *Legionella* organisms should be considered. Levofloxacin is the appropriate choice. Trovafloxacin also would work, but it has the broadest spectrum of activity of all the quinolones, and it should be reserved for patients who would benefit from therapy with such a broad-spectrum agent.

Ref: Gilbert DN, Moellering RC Jr, Eliopoulos GM, Sande MA, eds. *The Sanford Guide to Antimicrobial Therapy 2004,* 34th ed. Hyde Park, VT: Antimicrobial Therapy; 2004:55.

5. (B) Severe community-acquired pneumonia requires broad-spectrum coverage. Antibiotic coverage should include *S. pneumoniae, Haemophilus influenzae,* and atypical organisms such as *Legionella, Mycoplasma,* and *Chlamydia* species. Guidelines produced by both the American Thoracic Society and the Infectious Disease Society of America suggest use of a third-generation cephalosporin in combination with a macrolide to cover all possible pathogens in this setting. Both the third-generation cephalosporin and the macrolide will be useful in covering potentially penicillin-resistant strains of pneumococci. Doxycycline also may be useful, but it is not a first-line agent in this clinical situation.

Ref: Mandell LA, Bartlett JG, Dowell SF, et al. Update of practice guidelines for the management of community-acquired pneumonia in immunocompetent adults. *Clin Infect Dis* 2003;37:1405–1433.

PATIENT PROFILE 8

BUFFER SOLUTIONS

ANSWERS

1. (D) Maximum stability is determined as the minima of a graph of log k_{obs} versus pH. This is the point of minimum degradation but is independent of solubility.

Ref: Stocklosa M, Ansel H. *Physical Pharmacy.* 4th ed. Philadelphia: Lea & Febiger; 1993:301–310.

2. (D) pKa = –log (Ka)

Ref: Stocklosa M, Ansel H. *Pharmaceutical Calculations.* 10th ed. Baltimore: Williams & Wilkins; 1996:299.

3. (B) Solve the acid form of the Henderson-Hasselbalch equation for the ratio of salt to acid using a pH of 5.000 and a pKa of 4.757.

Ref: Stocklosa M, Ansel H. *Pharmaceutical Calculations.* 10th ed. Baltimore: Williams & Wilkins; 1996:301.

4. (C) Use the numbers for the salt (1.75) and acid (1) components from the molar ratio by total fraction of the total buffer concentration of 3.75×10^{-2} M to solve for the actual concentration.

Ref: Stocklosa M, Ansel H. *Pharmaceutical Calculations.* 10th ed. Baltimore: Williams & Wilkins; 1996:301–302.

5. (C) Grams of each ingredient are equal to concentration × volume × molecular weight.

Ref: Stocklosa M, Ansel H. *Pharmaceutical Calculations.* 10th ed. Baltimore: Williams & Wilkins; 1996:302.

END-STAGE RENAL DISEASE

ANSWERS

1. (A) Various equations are available to calculate creatinine clearance. However, using these equations is not appropriate for a patient on dialysis or with rapidly changing renal function. Because she is currently receiving hemodialysis, SG's estimated creatinine clearance is less than 10 mg/dL. The serum creatinine appears artificially low as a result of hemodialysis.

   Ref: Bakerman S. *ABC's of Interpretive Laboratory Data,* 4th ed. Scottsdale, AZ: Interpretive Laboratory Data, Inc., 2002:193–195.

2. (B) Hyperphosphatemia is a common problem in patients with end-stage renal disease, and dialysis does not correct it. These patients must restrict oral phosphorus intake (i.e., carbonated beverages) and may need drug treatment. Sevelamer is indicated when the serum calcium level is elevated, which is not the case with SG. Calcium acetate is the best choice at this time and should be prescribed with meals because it work by decreasing exogenous phosphorus absorption.

   Ref: Slatopolsky E. New developments in hyperphosphatemia management. *J Am Soc Nephrol* 2003;14(9 suppl 4):S297–299.

3. (B) Monitoring parameters required with the use of calcium acetate include serum calcium and phosphorus levels. Dialysis rather than hyperphosphatemia treatment will have an impact on potassium and renal function. Liver function should not be affected.

   Ref: Slatopolsky E. New developments in hyperphosphatemia management. *J Am Soc Nephrol* 2003;14(9 suppl 4):S297–299.

4. (E) All these medications have been associated with renal dysfunction and should be used only with careful monitoring of renal function.

   Ref: Gilbert DN, et al. *The Sanford Guide to Antimicrobial Therapy,* 34th ed. Hyde Park, NY: Antimicrobial Therapy, Inc, 2004:63–65.

5. (C) ACE inhibitors cause vasodilation of the efferent arteriole. This results in decreased glomerular pressure and has shown to be renoprotective in patients with documented proteinuria.

   Ref: Remuzzi G. Proteinuria predicting outcome in renal disease: Nondiabetic nephropathies (REIN). *Kidney Int* 2004; 92(suppl): S90–96.

6. (B) Typical adverse effects associated ACE inhibitor therapy include hyperkalemia, elevated serum creatinine, angioedema, and a dry, persistent cough. ACE inhibitors do not cause bradycardia, hyperphosphatemia, or erythrocytosis.

   Ref: Antiotensin-Converting Enzyme Inhibitors Drug Information, Micromedex, Thompson Healthcare, Inc., April 2001. Available at http://www.micromedex.com.

7. (D) Procrit (epoetin alfa) and Epogen (epoetin alfa) are both recombinant human erythropoietins that are identical to the endogenously produced hormone. Aranesp (darbepoetin alfa) is a hyperglycosylated analogue with a prolonged half-life.

   Ref: Procrit, Epogen, and Aranesp Drug Information, Micromedex, Thompson Healthcare, Inc., March 2004. Available at http://www.micromedex.com.

8. (D) Patients should respond to epoetin alfa within 2 to 4 weeks. If no response is noted by 4 to 8 weeks, the dose may be increased, and/or the etiology of anemia should be reassessed.

   Ref: Epogen Package Insert, Amgen, Inc., Thousand Oaks, CA, 2004.

9. (A) Epoetin alfa stimulates the bone marrow to expand the red cell mass, which increases the body's demand for iron. Patients with adequate iron stores on initiation of epoetin alfa do not necessarily require comcomitant iron-replacement therapy, but iron stores should be monitored routinely for the development of iron deficiency.

   Ref: Epogen Package Insert, Amgen, Inc., Thousand Oaks, CA, 2004.

10. (C) Oxacillin and nafcillin are the drugs of choice to treat methicillin-sensitive *S. aureus*.

    Ref: Gilbert DN, et al. *The Sanford Guide to Antimicrobial Therapy,* 34th ed. Hyde Park, NY: Antimicrobial Therapy, Inc., 2004:50.

PATIENT   PROFILE   10

BACTEREMIA AND SEPSIS

ANSWERS

1. (C) A suggests bacteremia. Bacteremia is not sepsis; however, there may be bacteria in the blood of patients with sepsis. B describes the systemic inflammatory response syndrome (SIRS). This syndrome may occur among patients with sepsis, but it is a response to sepsis rather than a definition. D and E focus specifically on blood pressure and end-organ damage. These responses can occur in sepsis but cannot serve as a definition of it. Thus C is a global definition of sepsis that encompasses all of the other selections.

   Ref: Bone RC, Balk RA, Cerra F, et al. American College of Chest Physicians/Society of Critical Care Medicine Consensus Conference: Definitions for sepsis and organ failure and guidelines for the use of innovative therapies in sepsis. *Crit Care Med* 1992;20:864–874.

2. (A) Gram-negative bacteremia can occur among patients who have been ill for some time or among patients who have an acute injury. The most common infectious source is the GI tract. Among patients with critical illnesses, bacteria may translocate across the membranes of the GI tract into the blood. In the presence of severe illness, acute injury, or impaired immune status, the result may be gram-negative bacteremia.

   Ref: Young LS. Gram-negative sepsis. In: Mandell GL, Douglas RG Jr, Bennett JE, eds. *Principles and Practice of Infectious Diseases.* New York: Churchill Livingstone, 1990;611–636.

3. (B) Norepinephrine is a pharmacologic vasopressor with adrenergic activity that stimulates primarily α_1 receptors with a small amount of β_1 activity. This yields the ability to squeeze the vessels while minimizing the chronotropic effect on the heart and minimizing cardiac arrhythmia. The doses of dopamine and phenylephrine listed are inadequate for maintaining blood pressure. Nitroprusside is a systemic vasodilator and is contraindicated in this scenario. Esmolol, a short-acting β-blocker that can be titrated, decreases heart rate and impairs systemic perfusion and oxygen delivery and also is contraindicated.

   Ref: Hardin TC, DiPiro JT. Sepsis and septic shock. In: DiPiro JT, Talbert RL, Yee GC, Matzke GR, Wells BG, Posey LM, eds. *Pharmacotherapy: A Pathophysiologic Approach.* 4th ed. Stamford, Conn: Appleton & Lange, 1999:1827–1838.

4. (E) The goal of empiric antibiotic selection is more or less a shotgun approach. A clear source of infection will naturally help you tailor your choices, but the infectious source is usually vague. With the knowledge that the GI tract possibly is the source, you direct therapy at covering organisms that reside in the GI tract. The regimen you choose also should possess the characteristics listed in answers A–D.

   Ref: Hardin TC, DiPiro JT. Sepsis and septic shock. In: DiPiro JT, Talbert RL, Yee GC, Matzke GR, Wells BG, Posey LM, eds. *Pharmacotherapy: A Pathophysiologic Approach.* 4th ed. Stamford, Conn: Appleton & Lange, 1999:1827–1838.

5. (B) Piperacillin-tazobactam with gentamicin is the only regimen that has activity against all of the organisms that may be present in an intraabdominal infection. Enterococci (group D streptococci), *Bacteroides fragilis* (gram-negative anaerobe), and enteric gram-negative rods are covered with this combination. All of the other regimens listed have holes in their coverage. A lacks gram-negative coverage, C lacks enteroccocal and anaerobic coverage, D lacks enterococcal and adequate gram-negative coverage (gram-negative organisms should be doubly covered).

   Ref: Hardin TC, DiPiro JT. Sepsis and septic shock. In: DiPiro JT, Talbert RL, Yee GC, Matzke GR, Wells BG, Posey LM, eds. *Pharmacotherapy: A Pathophysiologic Approach.* 4th ed. Stamford, Conn: Appleton & Lange, 1999:1827–1838.

PATIENT   PROFILE   11

DIABETES MELLITUS

ANSWERS

1. (B) Prednisone has been documented to cause hyperglycemia.

   Ref: Carlisle BA, Kroon LA, Koda-Kimble MA. Diabetes mellitus. In: Koda-Kimble MA, Young LY, Kradjan WA, Guglielmo BJ, eds. *Applied Therapeutics: The Clinical Use of Drugs,* 8th ed. Philadelphia: Lippincott Williams & Wilkins, 2005:50-1–50-80.

2. (E) Repaglinide, like glyburide, increases insulin secretion. Thus it would not be an effective strategy to improve blood sugar control. Glyburide and glipizide are in the same class, and the doses listed are equivalent, so switching would not improve blood sugar control. The maximum dose of glyburide is 10 mg twice daily. Metformin would be a possibility, but the dose is too high for initiation.

Ref: Carlisle BA, Kroon LA, Koda-Kimble MA. Diabetes mellitus. In: Koda-Kimble MA, Young LY, Kradjan WA, Guglielmo BJ, eds. *Applied Therapeutics: The Clinical Use of Drugs,* 8th ed. Philadelphia: Lippincott Williams & Wilkins, 2005:50-1–50-80.

3. (B) The LDL goal for someone with diabetes mellitus is less than 100 mg/dL. MB's triglycerides are at goal of less than 150 mg/dL, so adding gemfibrozil, which primarily lowers triglycerides, would not be appropriate. Atorvastatin is a more potent LDL-lowering agent than Niaspan. Niaspan at most decreases LDL by 25%. MB requires over a 40% reduction based on the baseline LDL of 180 mg/dL.

Ref: McKenney JM. Dyslipidemias, atherosclerosis and coronary heart disease. In: Koda-Kimble MA, Young LY, Kradjan WA, Guglielmo BJ, eds. *Applied Therapeutics: The Clinical Use of Drugs,* 8th ed. Philadelphia: Lippincott Williams & Wilkins, 2005:13-1-13-39.

4. (D) Glyburide is an insulin secretagogue and thus can cause hypoglycemia.

Ref: Carlisle BA, Kroon LA, Koda-Kimble MA. Diabetes mellitus. In: Koda-Kimble MA, Young LY, Kradjan WA, Guglielmo BJ, eds. *Applied Therapeutics: The Clinical Use of Drugs,* 8th ed. Philadelphia: Lippincott Williams & Wilkins, 2005:50-1–50-80.

5. (A) ACE inhibitors have been proven to decrease the progression of diabetic nephropathy in patients with microalbuminuria.

Ref: Carlisle BA, Kroon LA, Koda-Kimble MA. Diabetes mellitus. In: Koda-Kimble MA, Young LY, Kradjan WA, Guglielmo BJ, eds. *Applied Therapeutics: The Clinical Use of Drugs,* 8th ed. Philadelphia: Lippincott Williams & Wilkins, 2005:50-1–50-80.

6. (A) Thiazolidinediones rarely have been associated with liver damage. The manufacturers recommend liver function test monitoring at baseline, every 6 months for the first year, and then periodically.

Ref: Carlisle BA, Kroon LA, Koda-Kimble MA. Diabetes mellitus. In: Koda-Kimble MA, Young LY, Kradjan WA, Guglielmo BJ, eds. *Applied Therapeutics: The Clinical Use of Drugs,* 8th ed. Philadelphia: Lippincott Williams & Wilkins, 2005:50-1–50-80.

7. (A) Thiazolidinediones are associated with increasing the risk of heart failure exacerbation.

Ref: Carlisle BA, Kroon LA, Koda-Kimble MA. Diabetes mellitus. In: Koda-Kimble MA, Young LY, Kradjan WA, Guglielmo BJ, eds. *Applied Therapeutics: The Clinical Use of Drugs,* 8th ed. Philadelphia: Lippincott Williams & Wilkins, 2005:50-1–50-80.

8. (B) Primary side effects associated with acarbose are gastrointestinal in nature.

Ref: Carlisle BA, Kroon LA, Koda-Kimble MA. Diabetes mellitus. In: Koda-Kimble MA, Young LY, Kradjan WA, Guglielmo BJ, eds. *Applied Therapeutics: The Clinical Use of Drugs,* 8th ed. Philadelphia: Lippincott Williams & Wilkins, 2005:50-1–50-80.

9. (A) Acarbose should be taken with the first bite of each meal or with water immediately before a meal for maximum effectiveness.

Ref: Carlisle BA, Kroon LA, Koda-Kimble MA. Diabetes mellitus. In: Koda-Kimble MA, Young LY, Kradjan WA, Guglielmo BJ, eds. *Applied Therapeutics: The Clinical Use of Drugs,* 8th ed. Philadelphia: Lippincott Williams & Wilkins, 2005:50-1–50-80.

10. (B) Predinisone and other corticosteroids are associated with elevated blood pressures. This is a reversible dose-dependent side effect.

Ref: Carter BL, Saseen JJ. Hypertnsion. In: DiPiro JT, Talbert RL, Yee GC, et al, eds. *Pharmacotherapy: A Pathophysiologic Approach,* 5th ed. New York: McGraw-Hill, 2002:157–184.

PATIENT PROFILE 12

HIV, AIDS

ANSWERS

1. (A) Patients receiving zidovudine should be carefully monitored for hematologic toxicities, including anemia and granulocytopenia.

Ref: Hayden FG. Antiviral agents. In: Mandell GL, Douglas RG, Bennett JE. *Principles and Practice of Infectious Diseases.* 4th ed. New York: Churchill Livingstone; 1995:411–450.

2. (D) Adequate hydration is important for patients receiving indinavir because of a problem with nephrolithiasis. Monitoring for metabolic disturbances also is important. Disturbances have been reported among patients undergoing regimens that include protease inhibitor therapy.

Ref: Kaul DR, Ciniti SK, Carver PL, et al. HIV protease inhibitors: advances in therapy and adverse reactions, including metabolic complications. *Pharmacotherapy* 1999;19:281–298.

3. (E) Didanosine should be administered to adults as two tablets with each dosage on an empty stomach. Monitoring should include signs of peripheral neuropathy and pancreatitis.

Ref: Hayden FG. Antiviral agents. In: Mandell GL, Douglas RG, Bennett JE, eds. *Principles and Practice of Infectious Diseases.* 4th ed. New York: Churchill Livingstone; 1995:411–450.

4. (E) The frequency of rash can be decreased by use of a lead-in period when initiating therapy with nevirapine. Patients taking oral contraceptives should use an alternative form of birth control because of the induction effects of nevirapine.

    Ref: D'Aquila RT, Hughes MD, Johnson VA, et al. Nevirapine, zidovudine, and didanosine compared with zidovudine and didanosine in patients with HIV-1 infection. *Ann Intern Med* 1996;124: 1019–1029.

5. (E) Efavirenz, the first FDA-approved once a day antiretroviral agent, can cause adverse effects on the central nervous system. Barrier contraceptives are recommended for women of childbearing age who take this agent.

    Ref: SustivaTM [product information]. Wilmington, Del: DuPont Pharmaceuticals Company; 1999.

PATIENT PROFILE 13

HYPERLIPIDEMIA

ANSWERS

1. (C) Erythromycin and ketoconazole are medications that interact with lovastatin and would lead to inceased levels of lovastatin and increase the risk of myositis.

    Ref: McKenney JM. Dyslipidemias, atherosclerosis, and coronary heart disease. In: Young YL, Koda-Kimble MA, eds. *Applied Therapeutics: The Clinical Use of Drugs*. Vancouver, WA: Applied Therapeutics, 2005:13(1–39).

2. (E) Pravastatin is the only statin not metabolized through the cytochrome P450 system.

    Ref: McKenney JM. Dyslipidemias, atherosclerosis, and coronary heart disease. In: Young YL, Koda-Kimble MA, eds. *Applied Therapeutics: The Clinical Use of Drugs*. Vancouver, WA: Applied Therapeutics, 2005:13(1–39).

3. (A) This needs to occur within 24 hours of the event.

    Ref: Expert Panel on Detection, Evaluation, and Treatment of High Blood Cholesterol in Adults. Executive summary of the third report of the National Cholesterol Education Program (NCEP) on detection, evaluation, and treatment of high blood cholesterol in adults (Adult Treatment Panel III). *JAMA* 2001;285(19):2486–2497.

4. (B) Age, cigarette smoking, low HDL cholesterol are risk factors that modify the LDL cholesterol goals.

    Ref: Expert Panel on Detection, Evaluation, and Treatment of High Blood Cholesterol in Adults. Executive summary of the third report of the National Cholesterol Education Program (NCEP) on detection, evaluation, and treatment of high blood cholesterol in adults (Adult Treatment Panel III). *JAMA* 2001; 285(19):2486–2497.

5. (D) According to the ATP III guidelines, AM's LDL cholesterol goal would be less than 130 mg/dL.

    Ref: Expert Panel on Detection, Evaluation, and Treatment of High Blood Cholesterol in Adults. Executive summary of the third report of the National Cholesterol Education Program (NCEP) on detection, evaluation, and treatment of high blood cholesterol in adults (Adult Treatment Panel III). *JAMA* 2001;285(19):2486–2497.

6. (B) HMG-CoA reductase inhibitors exert their effects by competitively inhibiting the enzyme responsible for converting HMG-CoA to mevalonate in an early rate-limiting step in the pathway of cholesterol.

    Ref: McKenney JM. Dyslipidemias, atherosclerosis, and coronary heart disease. In: Young YL, Koda-Kimble MA, eds. *Applied Therapeutics: The Clinical Use of Drugs*. Vancouver, WA: Applied Therapeutics, 2005:13(1–39).

7. (C) Gemfibrozil interferes with the glucuronidation of statins, interfering with their renal clearance and resulting in a two- to fourfold increase in systemic statin levels.

    Ref: McKenney JM. Dyslipidemias, atherosclerosis, and coronary heart disease. In: Young YL, Koda-Kimble MA, eds. *Applied Therapeutics: The Clinical Use of Drugs*. Vancouver, WA: Applied Therapeutics, 2005:13(1–39).

8. (D) Weight management and limiting cholesterol intake to less than 200 mg/day are therapeutic lifestyle modifications.

    Ref: Expert Panel on Detection, Evaluation, and Treatment of High Blood Cholesterol in Adults. Executive summary of the third report of the National Cholesterol Education Program (NCEP) on detection, evaluation, and treatment of high blood cholesterol in adults (Adult Treatment Panel III). *JAMA* 2001;285(19):2486–2497.

9. (C) The flushing symptoms of niacin can be reduced by having patients take doses with food and by taking 325 mg aspirin 30 minutes before the morning dose of niacin.

    Ref: McKenney JM. Dyslipidemias, atherosclerosis, and coronary heart disease. In: Young YL, Koda-Kimble MA, eds. *Applied Therapeutics: The Clinical Use of Drugs*. Vancouver, WA: Applied Therapeutics, 2005:13(1–39).

10. (E) Lovastatin's side effects include rash, headache, abdominal pain, and muscle pain.

    Ref: McKenney JM. Dyslipidemias, atherosclerosis, and coronary heart disease. In: Young YL, Koda-Kimble MA, eds. *Applied Therapeutics: The Clinical Use of Drugs*. Vancouver, WA: Applied Therapeutics, 2005:13(1–39).

PATIENT   PROFILE   14

ONCOLOGY: BREAST CANCER

ANSWERS

1. (C) The most important risk factor for breast cancer is having a first-degree relative with the disease. Giving birth to a first child after 20 years of age is a lesser risk. Alcohol use and body weight may be associated with disease risk but are far less frequent risk factors.

   Ref: Lindley CM. Breast cancer. In: DiPiro JT, Talbert RL, Yee GC, Matzke GR, Wells BG, Posey LM, eds. *Pharmacotherapy: A Pathophysiologic Approach.* 4th ed. Stamford, Conn: Appleton & Lange; 1999:2013–2042.

2. (D) The dose-limiting toxicity of low-dose MTX and weekly 5-FU is bone marrow suppression.

   Ref: Valley AM, McManus C. Cancer treatment and chemotherapy. DiPiro JT, Talbert RL, Yee GC, Matzke GR, Wells BG, Posey LM, eds. *Pharmacotherapy: A Pathophysiologic Approach.* 4th ed. Stamford, Conn: Appleton & Lange; 1999:1957–2012.

   Ref: Herfindal ET, Gourley DR (eds). *Textbook of Therapeutics, Drug and Disease Management.* 6th ed. Baltimore: Williams & Wilkins; 1996.

3. (B) Systemic antineoplastic therapy is indicated to eradicate disease that has spread beyond the primary tumor site. The disease already has spread to the lymph nodes, and systemic treatment does not target a specific metastatic site (bone, CNS).

   Ref: Valley AM, McManus C. Cancer treatment and chemotherapy. DiPiro JT, Talbert RL, Yee GC, Matzke GR, Wells BG, Posey LM, eds. *Pharmacotherapy: A Pathophysiologic Approach.* 4th ed. Stamford, Conn: Appleton & Lange; 1999:1957–2012.

4. (A) The antiestrogen effects of tamoxifen have been shown to delay if not prevent recurrence of disease.

   Ref: Lindley CM. Breast cancer. In: DiPiro JT, Talbert RL, Yee GC, Matzke GR, Wells BG, Posey LM, eds. *Pharmacotherapy: A Pathophysiologic Approach.* 4th ed. Stamford, Conn: Appleton & Lange; 1999:2013–2042.

   Ref: Herfindal ET, Gourley DR (eds). *Textbook of Therapeutics, Drug and Disease Management.* 6th ed. Baltimore: Williams & Wilkins; 1996.

5. (A) Estrogen therapy is contraindicated in the care of patients who have or have had estrogen receptor-positive (ER+) breast cancer.

   Ref: Pugh MC, Mullins PM. Hormone replacement therapy. In: DiPiro JT, Talbert RL, Yee GC, Matzke GR, Wells BG, Posey LM, eds. *Pharmacotherapy: A Pathophysiologic Approach.* 4th ed. Stamford, Conn: Appleton & Lange; 1999: 1355–1365.

PATIENT   PROFILE   15

RESPIRATORY TRACT INFECTIONS

ANSWERS

1. (B) The potential pathogens that need attention include *S. pneumoniae* (pneumococcus), *Haemophilus influenzae*, and atypical organisms (*Legionella, Mycoplasma,* and *Chlamydia*). The lack of sputum and history of diarrhea suggest *Legionella*, but this organism is difficult to isolate. Empirical therapy for infection by the aforementioned organisms is warranted. Because the patient has been admitted to the hospital, IV administration of a third-generation cephalosporin and macrolide is warranted. The other selections lack the spectrum of coverage necessary to control pathogens that cause severe community-acquired pneumonia.

   Ref: Mandell LA, Bartlett JG, Dowell SF, et al. Update of practice guidelines for the management of community-acquired pneumonia in immunocompetent adults. *Clin Infect Dis* 2003;37: 1405–1433.

2. (A) Levofloxacin is a fluoroqquinolone with excellent gram-positive coverage that includes pneumococci. It also possesses an extended spectrum of coverage that includes atypical bacteria, such as *Legionella* species. Levofloxacin can be used as a primary agent in the care of these patients, but it is preferred as a second-line agent. This patient would benefit from a fluoroquinolone because of the rash caused by the primary antibiotic. The rash most likely is caused by the cephalosporin. With the substitution of a fluoroquinolone, the atypical bacteria are covered sufficiently. Because of this overlap in coverage, the macrolide antibiotic is discontinued, leaving the patient treated with only the fluoroquinolone for community-acquired pneumonia.

   Ref: Mandell LA, Bartlett JG, Dowell SF, et al. Update of practice guidelines for the management of community-acquired pneumonia in immunocompetent adults. *Clin Infect Dis* 2003;37: 1405–1433.

3. (D) It is difficult to isolate *Legionella* organisms. The *Legionella* urine antigen test has a high sensitivity but a low specificity. If the test result is positive, *Legionella* organisms are present, and the patient should be treated

accordingly. If the test result is negative, *Legionella* organisms still may be present. The test is not specific enough to allow a conclusion that the patient does not have infection. In this case the patient should be treated as though an infection is present.

Ref: Mandell LA, Bartlett JG, Dowell SF, et al. Update of practice guidelines for the management of community-acquired pneumonia in immunocompetent adults. *Clin Infect Dis* 2003;37:1405–1433.

4. (B) GI upset is the most frequent problem among patients who take erythromycin. This macrolide antibiotic stimulates motilin in the GI tract and causes GI discomfort. In addition to its antimicrobial properties, erythromycin has been used as a prokinetic agent in the care of patients who cannot tolerate metoclopramide or cisapride.

Ref: Gilbert DN, Moellering RC Jr, Eliopoulos GM, Sande MA, eds. *The Sanford Guide to Antimicrobial Therapy 2004,* 34th ed. Hyde Park, VT: Antimicrobial Therapy, 2004:69.

5. (E) Vancomycin is considered effective against almost all gram-positive organisms, including resistant pneumococci. The addition of rifampin to vancomycin provides synergistic killing of the organism. Changing antibiotic class from high-dose penicillin (effective against low- and intermediate-level resistance) to cephalosporins provides effective killing of resistant strains of pneumococci.

Ref: Gilbert DN, Moellering RC Jr, Eliopoulos GM, Sande MA, eds. *The Sanford Guide to Antimicrobial Therapy 2004,* 34th ed. Hyde Park, VT: Antimicrobial Therapy, 2004:55.

PATIENT PROFILE 16
MEDICINAL CHEMISTRY

ANSWER

1. (E) The patient is a truck driver and should not receive any medication that might cause drowsiness. Allegra® (fexofenadine) is the most suitable drug because it acts peripherally as an H_1 antagonist and has limited sedative effects. The polar hydroxyl groups and the amphoteric nature of the drug give it little chance to enter the CNS and exhibit sedative effects.

PATIENT PROFILE 17
SEIZURES

ANSWERS

1. (E) Phenytoin is bound to plasma albumin, which is low in RT. This increases the free concentration of phenytoin and can lead to toxicity even at normal total phenytoin levels in patients with hypoalbuminemia or renal failure. Formulas have been developed to normalize serum phenytoin concentrations for such patients.

Ref: Gidal BE, Garnett WR, Graves N. Epilepsy. In: Dipiro JT, Talbert RL, Yee GC, et al, eds. *Pharmacotherapy: A Pathophysiologic Approach.* New York: McGraw-Hill, 2002:1031–1059.

2. (E) All the side effects listed are associated with elevated serum phenytoin concentrations.

Ref: McAuley JW, Lott RS. Seizure disorders. In: Koda-Kimble MA, Young LY, Kradjian WA, Guglielmo BJ, eds. *Applied Therapeutics: The Clinical Use of Drugs.* Philadelphia: Lippincott Williams & Wilkins, 2004:54-1–54-42.

3. (B) Phenytoin, carbamazepine, and phenobarbital can induce the metabolism of oral contraceptives and reduce their efficacy. Valproate and gabapentin have not been shown to affect the metabolism of oral contraceptives.

Ref: McAuley JW, Lott RS. Seizure disorders. In: Koda-Kimble MA, Young LY, Kradjian WA, Guglielmo BJ, eds. *Applied Therapeutics: The Clinical Use of Drugs.* Philadelphia: Lippincott Williams & Wilkins, 2004:54-1–54-42.

4. (E) Folate supplementation can reduce the risk of congenital neural tube defects and is recommended for women with epilepsy.

Ref: McAuley JW, Lott RS. Seizure disorders. In: Koda-Kimble MA, Young LY, Kradjian WA, Guglielmo BJ, eds. *Applied Therapeutics: The Clinical Use of Drugs.* Philadelphia: Lippincott Williams & Wilkins, 2004:54-1–54-42.

5. (C) RT is experiencing classic signs of status epilepticus most likely caused by her discontinuing her medication.

Ref: McAuley JW, Lott RS. Seizure disorders. In: Koda-Kimble MA, Young LY, Kradjian WA, Guglielmo BJ, eds. *Applied Therapeutics: The Clinical Use of Drugs.* Philadelphia: Lippincott Williams & Wilkins, 2004:54-1–54-42.

6. (D) For rapid correction of her seizure, intravenous lorazepam is recommended.

Ref: McAuley JW, Lott RS. Seizure disorders. In: Koda-Kimble MA, Young LY, Kradjian WA, Guglielmo BJ, eds. *Applied Therapeutics: The Clinical Use of Drugs.* Philadelphia: Lippincott Williams & Wilkins, 2004:54-1–54-42.

7. (D) Intravenous phenytoin should be administered no faster than 50 mg/min to avoid cardiovascular toxicity.

Ref: McAuley JW, Lott RS. Seizure disorders. In: Koda-Kimble MA, Young LY, Kradjian WA, Guglielmo BJ, eds. *Applied Therapeutics: The Clinical Use of Drugs.* Philadelphia: Lippincott Williams & Wilkins, 2004:54-1–54-42.

8. (C) Fosphenytoin is a water-soluble prodrug that may be administered more rapidly than phenytoin.

Ref: McAuley JW, Lott RS. Seizure disorders. In: Koda-Kimble MA, Young LY, Kradjian WA, Guglielmo BJ, eds. *Applied Therapeutics: The Clinical Use of Drugs.* Philadelphia: Lippincott Williams & Wilkins, 2004:54-1–54-42.

9. (A) Ethosuximide is effective against absence seizures and is of little value for other types of seizures.

Ref: McAuley JW, Lott RS. Seizure disorders. In: Koda-Kimble MA, Young LY, Kradjian WA, Guglielmo BJ, eds. *Applied Therapeutics: The Clinical Use of Drugs.* Philadelphia: Lippincott Williams & Wilkins, 2004:54-1–54-42.

10. (E) Multiple-drug therapy is associated with increased cost, decreased compliance, and increased side effects and may not improve overall seizure control. For these reasons, monotherapy is preferred.

Ref: McAuley JW, Lott RS. Seizure disorders. In: Koda-Kimble MA, Young LY, Kradjian WA, Guglielmo BJ, eds. *Applied Therapeutics: The Clinical Use of Drugs.* Philadelphia: Lippincott Williams & Wilkins, 2004:54-1–54-42.

PATIENT PROFILE 18
PANIC DISORDER

ANSWERS

1. (D) The incidence of agoraphobia among patients with panic disorder is approximately 50%.

Ref: *Diagnostic and Statistical Manual of Mental Disorders.* 4th ed. Washington, DC: American Psychiatric Association; 1994.

2. (E) All can be the cause of anxiety and panic-type symptoms.

Ref: Roy-Byrne PR, Uhde TW. Exogenous factors in panic disorder: Clinical and research implications. *J Clin Psychiatry* 1988;49:56–61.

3. (E) All are considered effective for the management of panic disorder.

Ref: Otto MW, Pollack MH, Sachs GS, Reiter SR, Meltzer-Brody S, Rosenbaum JF. Discontinuation of benzodiazepine treatment:

Efficacy of cognitive/behavioral therapy for patients with panic disorder. *Am J Psychiatry* 1993;150:1485–1490.

4. (E) All are considered effective for the treatment of panic disorder.

Ref: den Boer JA. Pharmacotherapy of panic disorder: Differential efficacy from a clinical viewpoint. *J Clin Psychiatry* 1998;59(suppl 8):30–36.

5. (D) Because of the long half-life of fluoxetine and its nor-fluoxetine metabolite, the washout period is 5 weeks. If an MAO1 and fluoxetine are given together, there is a risk of development of the serotonin syndrome.

Ref: Ciraulo DA. *Drug Interactions in Psychiatry.* 2nd ed. Baltimore: Williams & Wilkins; 1995: chapter 2.

PATIENT PROFILE 19
BREAST CANCER

ANSWERS

1. (B)

Ref: Colvin OM. Antitumor alkylating agents. In: Devita VT, Hellman S, Rosenberg SA, eds. *Cancer: Principles and Practice of Oncology,* 6th ed. Philadelphia: Lippincott Williams & Wilkins, 2001:363.

2. (C)

Ref: Goodin S. Solid tumors. In: Koda-Kimbla MA, Young LY, Kradjan WA, et al, eds. *Applied Therapeutics: The Clinical Use of Drugs,* 8th ed. Philadelphia: Lippincott Williams & Wilkins, 2005:9-12.

3. (A)

Ref: Rowinsky EK, Tolcher AW. Antimicrotubule agents. In: Devita VT, Hellman S, Rosenberg SA, eds. *Cancer: Principles and Practice of Oncology,* 6th ed. Philadelphia: Lippincott Williams & Wilkins, 2001:440.

4. (B)

Ref: Lindley C. Adverse effects of chemotherapy. In: Koda-Kimbla MA, Young LY, Kradjan WA, et al, eds. *Applied Therapeutics: The Clinical Use of Drugs,* 8th ed. Philadelphia: Lippincott Williams & Wilkins, 2005:89-14.

5. (D)

Ref: Lindley CM. Breast cancer. In: Dipiro JT, Talbert RL, Yee GC, et al, eds. *Pharmacotherapy: A Pathophysiologic Approach,* 5th ed. New York: McGraw-Hill, 2002:2241.

6. (A)

Ref: Colvin OM. Antitumor alkylating agents. In: Devita VT, Hellman S, Rosenberg SA, eds. *Cancer: Principles and Practice of Oncology,* 6th ed. Philadelphia: Lippincott Williams & Wilkins, 2001:363.

7. (C)

Ref: Walther MM. Urologic emergencies. In: Devita VT, Hellman S, Rosenberg SA, eds. *Cancer: Principles and Practice of Oncology,* 6th ed. Philadelphia: Lippincott Williams & Wilkins, 2001:2646.

8. (A)

Ref: Lindley C. Adverse effects of chemotherapy. In: Koda-Kimbla MA, Young LY, Kradjan WA, et al, eds. *Applied Therapeutics: The Clinical Use of Drugs,* 8th ed. Philadelphia: Lippincott Williams & Wilkins, 2005:89-22.

9. (B)

Ref: Davis L, Lindley C. Neoplastic disorders and their treatment: general principles. In: Koda-Kimbla MA, Young LY, Kradjan WA, et al, eds. *Applied Therapeutics: The Clinical Use of Drugs,* 8th ed. Philadelphia: Lippincott Williams & Wilkins, 2005:88-7.

10. (D)

Ref: Gralla RJ, Osoba D, Kris MG, et al. Recommendations for the use of antiemetics: Evidence-based clinical practice guidelines. *J Clin Oncol* 1999;17:2971.

PATIENT PROFILE 20

RENAL TRANSPLANTATION

ANSWERS

1. (C) The microemulsion formulation of cyclosporine (Neoral®) is associated with less within-day variability in cyclosporine levels and increased cyclosporine absorption than is to Sandimmune®.

2. (B) Cyclosporine concentrations have to be monitored because cyclosporine is associated with a number of dose-related toxicities, such as nephrotoxicity.

3. (E) Two clinical signs associated with cyclosporine toxicity include tremors and hypertension.

4. (C) Monitoring of cyclosporine blood concentrations and measurements of renal function (BUN and SCr) are used to guide therapeutic decisions.

5. (E) Diltiazem inhibits the hepatic metabolism of cyclosporine and increases cyclosporine concentrations. It is used intentionally to decrease cyclosporine dosing requirements and drug costs.

Ref: Dupuis RE. Solid organ transplantation. In: Young LY, Koda-Kimble MA, eds. *Applied Therapeutics: The Clinical Use of Drugs.* 6th ed. Vancouver, Wash: Applied Therapeutics; 1995.

Ref: Tsunoda SM, Aweeka FT. Solid organ transplantation. In: Herfindal ET, Gourley DR, eds. *Textbook of Therapeutics, Drug and Disease Management.* Baltimore: Williams & Wilkins; 1996.

PATIENT PROFILE 21

DIABETES MELLITUS: COMPLICATIONS

ANSWERS

1. (D) Glycosylated hemoglobin measures the average blood glucose level over a period of 3 months in order to better determine compliance to therapy; daily finger-stick blood glucose readings provide point-in-time blood glucose readings.

Ref: American Diabetes Association. Clinical practice recommendations 2004. *Diabetes Care* 2004;27(1):S15–S35.

2. (C) Well-fitted shoes and daily visual foot inspections are some self-care techniques for caring for the diabetic foot.

Removal of calluses should be performed by an experienced health professional because it is most likely a case of a diabetes-related complication.

Ref: American Diabetes Association. Clinical practice recommendations 2004. *Diabetes Care* 2004;27(1):S63–S64.

3. (E) All are measured by a podiatrist during the annual visit. Skin integrity is evaluated owing to the chance of infection or dehydration. Vascular status is evaluated through assessment of posterior tibial and dorsalis pedis pulses. Protective sensation is assessed with a monofilament test.

Ref: American Diabetes Association. Clinical practice recommendations 2004. *Diabetes Care* 2004;27(1):S63–S64.

4. (D) Sexual dysfunction and retinopathy are both long-term microvascular complications of diabetes. Hypoglycemia is a short-term complication. Sexual dysfunction is an autonomic neuropathic complication; although sexual dysfunction is seen more commonly in males, females also experience the condition.

Ref: American Diabetes Association. Clinical practice recommendations 2004. *Diabetes Care* 2004;27(1):S15–S35.

5. (B) Blood pressure should be monitored at every diabetes visit to the primary care physician. Without risk factors or indications for the complication, a lipid panel, eye examinations, and microalbuminuria should be monitored annually. Cardiac stress test is only performed in patients with a history of occlusive disease, a sedentary lifestyle, and aged greater than 35 years.

Ref: American Diabetes Association. Clinical practice recommendations 2004. *Diabetes Care* 2004;27(1):S15–S35.

6. (D) Aspirin is used for primary and secondary therapy to prevent cardiovascular events. Atorvastatin use has demonstrated lower cardiovascular events. Ibuprofen does not have a role in cardiovascular protection.

Ref: American Diabetes Association. Clinical practice recommendations 2004. *Diabetes Care* 2004;27(1):S15–S35.

7. (E) Nondihydropyridine calcium channel blockers (i.e., verapamil, diltiazem), angiotensin-converting enzyme (ACE) inhibitors (e.g., lisinopril), and angiotension-receptor blockers (e.g., irbesartan) all may be used to prevent nephropathy. In a type 2 patient such as VB, ACE inhibitors and angiotensin-receptor blockers have been shown to delay the progression of macroalbuminuria. Dihydropyridine calcium channel blockers are not effective in prevention of nephropathy.

Ref: American Diabetes Association. Clinical practice recommendations 2004. *Diabetes Care* 2004;27(1):S15–S35.

8. (E) Low-dose tricyclic antidepressants (e.g., amitryptiline), anticonvulsants (e.g., gabapentin), and various pain medications (e.g., nonsteroidal anti-inflammatory drugs) typically are used for the off-label indication of neuropathic pain.

Ref: Oki JC, Isley WL. Diabetes mellitus. In: Dipiro JT, Talbert RL, Yee GC, et al, eds. *Pharmacotherapy: A Pathophysiologic Approach,* 5th ed. New York: McGraw-Hill, 2002:1335–1358.

9. (D) Metoclopramide is used often to promote gastric motility in patients suffering from gastroparesis.

Ref: Oki JC, Isley WL. Diabetes mellitus. In: Dipiro JT, Talbert RL, Yee GC, et al, eds. *Pharmacotherapy: A Pathophysiologic Approach,* 5th ed. New York: McGraw-Hill, 2002:1335–1358.

10. (B) The goal lipid panel for a male patient with diabetes is HDL >40 mg/dL, triglycerides <150 mg/dL, total cholesterol <200 mg/dL, and LDL <100mg/dL. An LDL level of less than 70 mg/dL is encouraged for only high-risk patients.

Ref: Grundy SM, Cleeman JI, Merz CNB, et al. Implications of recent clinical trials for the National Cholesterol Education Program Adult Treatment Panel III guidelines. *Circulation* 2004;110:227–239.

PATIENT PROFILE 22

ARRHYTHMIAS

ANSWERS

1. (D) The patient's hemodynamic condition is compromised, and immediate restoration of normal sinus rhythm is indicated.

Ref: Bauman JL, Schoen MD. Arrhythmias. In: DiPiro JT, Talbert RL, Yee GC, Matzke GR, Wells BG, Posey LM, eds. *Pharmacotherapy: A Pathophysiologic Approach.* 4th ed. Stamford, Conn: Appleton & Lange; 1999:232–264.

2. (B) The patient has asthma, and β-blockade is contraindicated.

Ref: Bauman JL, Schoen MD. Arrhythmias. In: DiPiro JT, Talbert RL, Yee GC, Matzke GR, Wells BG, Posey LM, eds. *Pharmacotherapy: A Pathophysiologic Approach.* 4th ed. Stamford, Conn: Appleton & Lange; 1999:232–264.

3. (A) Amiodarone is the best choice of treatment of patients with CHF.

Ref: Bauman JL, Schoen MD. Arrhythmias. In: DiPiro JT, Talbert RL, Yee GC, Matzke GR, Wells BG, Posey LM, eds. *Pharmacotherapy: A Pathophysiologic Approach.* 4th ed. Stamford, Conn: Appleton & Lange; 1999:232–264.

4. (D) Warfarin is the drug of choice for stroke prophylaxis for this patient with hypertension.

Ref: Bauman JL, Schoen MD. Arrhythmias. In: DiPiro JT, Talbert RL, Yee GC, Matzke GR, Wells BG, Posey LM, eds. *Pharmacotherapy: A Pathophysiologic Approach.* 4th ed. Stamford, Conn: Appleton & Lange; 1999:232–264.

5. (B) Amiodarone will increase serum digoxin concentration.

Ref: *Drug Interaction Facts.* St. Louis: Facts and Comparisons; 1999.

PATIENT PROFILE 23

RESPIRATORY TRACT INFECTIONS

ANSWERS

1. (C) Sputum color does not provide enough information to confirm a diagnosis of infection; however, there have been clinical reports of "rust-colored sputum" among patients with pneumococcal infection. A Gram stain of a sputum sample that yields gram-positive cocci in chains is highly suggestive of pneumococcal infection in a patient with clinical symptoms.

   Ref: Toltzis P, Witte MK, Reed MD. Lower respiratory tract infections. In: DiPiro JT, Talbert RL, Yee GC, et al, eds. *Pharmacotherapy: A Pathophysiolgoic Approach,* 5th ed. New York: McGraw-Hill, 2002:1856.

   Ref: Jaresko GS, Alexander DP. Respiratory tract infections. In: Koda-Kimble MA, Young LY, eds. *Applied Therapeutics: The Clinical Use of Drugs,* 7th ed. Baltimore: Lippincott Williams & Wilkins, 2001:58-1–58-27.

2. (A) Of the selections listed, ceftriaxone is the only one with adequate coverage against pneumococci.

   Ref: Toltzis P, Witte MK, Reed MD. Lower respiratory tract infections. In: DiPiro JT, Talbert RL, Yee GC, et al, eds. *Pharmacotherapy: A Pathophysiolgoic Approach,* 5th ed. New York: McGraw-Hill, 2002:1856.

   Ref: Jaresko GS, Alexander DP. Respiratory tract infections. In: Koda-Kimble MA, Young LY, eds. *Applied Therapeutics: The Clinical Use of Drugs,* 7th ed. Baltimore: Lippincott Williams & Wilkins, 2001:58-1–58-27.

3. (D) Clindamycin is the only agent listed that has both anaerobic and gram-positive coverage. It is useful for this reason in the treatment of patients with aspiration pneumonia. The patient should be monitored for signs and symptoms of *Clostridium difficile* colitis, a side effect of clindamycin therapy.

   Ref: Toltzis P, Witte MK, Reed MD. Lower respiratory tract infections. In: DiPiro JT, Talbert RL, Yee GC, et al, eds. *Pharmacother-*

apy: A Pathophysiolgoic Approach, 5th ed. New York: McGraw-Hill, 2002:1856.

   Ref: Jaresko GS, Alexander DP. Respiratory tract infections. In: Koda-Kimble MA, Young LY, eds. *Applied Therapeutics: The Clinical Use of Drugs,* 7th ed. Baltimore: Lippincott Williams & Wilkins, 2001:58-1–58-27.

4. (C) Underlying conditions predispose patients to increased risk of contracting gram-negaive infection from lactose-fermenting gram-negative bacilli. Underlying diseases may impair the immune system and other normal host defenses, making them more susceptible to those types of infections.

   Ref: Toltzis P, Witte MK, Reed MD. Lower respiratory tract infections. In: DiPiro JT, Talbert RL, Yee GC, et al, eds. *Pharmacotherapy: A Pathophysiolgoic Approach,* 5th ed. New York: McGraw-Hill, 2002:1856.

   Ref: Jaresko GS, Alexander DP. Respiratory tract infections. In: Koda-Kimble MA, Young LY, eds. *Applied Therapeutics: The Clinical Use of Drugs,* 7th ed. Baltimore: Lippincott Williams & Wilkins, 2001:58-1–58-27.

5. (D) "Beating" on one's chest loosens mucus in the lower respiratory tract. The patient is encouraged to cough deeply during and after the therapy in an effort to expectorate the secretions. Mobilization of the secretions helps to prevent organisms from being trapped deep in the lungs and helps prevent additional disease.

   Ref: Toltzis P, Witte MK, Reed MD. Lower respiratory tract infections. In: DiPiro JT, Talbert RL, Yee GC, et al, eds. *Pharmacotherapy: A Pathophysiolgoic Approach,* 5th ed. New York: McGraw-Hill, 2002:1856–1866.

   Ref: Jaresko GS, Alexander DP. Respiratory tract infections. In: Koda-Kimble MA, Young LY, eds. *Applied Therapeutics: The Clinical Use of Drugs,* 7th ed. Baltimore: Lippincott Williams & Wilkins, 2001:58-1–58-27.

PATIENT PROFILE 24

HYPERTENSION

ANSWERS

1. (B) β-Blockers and diuretics are first-line agents for the management of uncomplicated hypertension. They both have been shown to decrease morbidity and mortality.

   Ref: Joint National Committee on Prevention, Detection, Evaluation, and Treatment of High Blood Pressure. The seventh report of the Joint National Committee of Prevention, Detection, Evaluation,

and Treatment of High Blood Pressure. *Hypertension* 2003;42: 1206–1252.

2. (D) Atenolol may cause lightheadedness and bradycardia. α-Antagonists such as terazosin may cause first-dose syncope.

   Ref: Atenolol, terazosin hydrochloride. In: *American Hospital Formulary Service.* Bethesda, Md: American Society of Health-System Pharmacists; 1999:1390, 1634.

PATIENT   PROFILE   25

MENSTRUAL DISORDERS/VAGINAL INFECTION

ANSWERS

1. (A)

Ref: Parent-Stevens L, Sagraves R. Gynecologic and other disorders of women. In: Koda-Kimbla MA, Young LY, Kradjan WA, et al, eds. *Applied Therapeutics: The Clinical Use of Drugs,* 8th ed. Philadelphia: Lippincott Williams & Wilkins, 2005.

2. (C)

Ref: Parent-Stevens L, Sagraves R. Gynecologic and other disorders of women. In: Koda-Kimbla MA, Young LY, Kradjan WA, et al, eds. *Applied Therapeutics: The Clinical Use of Drugs,* 8th ed. Philadelphia: Lippincott Williams & Wilkins, 2005.

3. (B) Excedrin Migraine contains aspirin in combination with naproxen; may increase the risk of bleeding.

Ref: Micormedex healthcare series online, Micromedex, Inc., Greenwood Village, CO, 2004.

4. (A)

Ref: Grady-Welky T. Premenstrual dysphoric disorder. *N Engl J Med* 2003;348:433–438.

5. (A) Asthenia occurs in 9% to 21% of patients.

Ref: Micormedex healthcare series online, Micromedex, Inc., Greenwood Village, CO, 2004.

6. (C)

Ref: Micormedex healthcare series online, Micromedex, Inc., Greenwood Village, CO, 2004.

7. (C)

Ref: Sobel JD. Vaginitis. *N Engl J Med* 1997;337:1896–1903.

8. (C)

Ref: Micormedex healthcare series online, Micromedex, Inc., Greenwood Village, CO, 2004.

9. (D)

Ref: Sobel JD. Vaginitis. *N Engl J Med* 1997;337:1896–1903.

10. (C)

Ref: Krause U. Results of single-dose treatment of vaginal mycoses with 500-mg Canesten vaginal tablets. *Chemotherapy* 1982;28:99–105.

Ref: Mizuno S, Cho N. Clinical evaluation of three-day treatment of vaginal mycosis with clotrimazole vaginal tablets. *J Int Med Res* 1983;11:179–185.

PATIENT   PROFILE   26

SEIZURE DISORDER

ANSWERS

1. (D) During the first few weeks of therapy, carbamazepine may induce its own metabolism, resulting in lower serum drug concentrations. An increase in dose may be needed.

Ref: Seizure disorders. In: Young LY, Koda-Kimble MA, eds. *Applied Therapeutics: The Clinical Use of Drugs.* 6th ed. Vancouver, Wash: Applied Therapeutics; 1995: chapter 52.

2. (E) Leukopenia, visual disturbances, and syndrome of inappropriate antidiuretic hormone secretion (SIADH) all are side effects of carbamazepine therapy.

Ref: Seizure disorders. In: Young LY, Koda-Kimble MA, eds. *Applied Therapeutics: The Clinical Use of Drugs.* 6th ed. Vancouver, Wash: Applied Therapeutics; 1995: chapter 52.

3. (E) Unlike many agents, gabapentin to date has not been associated with serious drug interactions with other antiepileptic drugs.

Ref: Seizure disorders. In: Young LY, Koda-Kimble MA, eds. *Applied Therapeutics: The Clinical Use of Drugs.* 6th ed. Vancouver, Wash: Applied Therapeutics; 1995: chapter 52.

4. (A) One of the most serious side effects of valproate therapy is liver impairment. Baseline liver function tests should be performed before therapy is initiated.

Ref: Seizure disorders. In: Herfindal ET, Gourley DR, eds. *Textbook of Therapeutics, Drug and Disease Management.* 6th ed. Baltimore: Williams & Wilkins; 1996: chapter 50.

5. (E) Lamotrigene therapy is associated with a skin rash that is more common when doses are titrated too rapidly.

Ref: Seizure disorders. In: Herfindal ET, Gourley DR, eds. *Textbook of Therapeutics, Drug and Disease Management.* 6th ed. Baltimore: Williams & Wilkins; 1996: chapter 50.

PATIENT PROFILE 27
RENAL TRANSPLANTATION

ANSWERS

1. (C) The microemulsion formulation of cyclosporine (Neoral) is associated with less with-in day variability of serum cyclosporine concentrations owing to increased cyclosporine absorption compared with Sandimmune.

   Ref: Taber DJ, Dupuis RE. Solid organ transplantation. In: Koda-Kimble MA, et al, eds. *Applied Therapeutics: The Clinical Use of Drugs*, 8th ed. Philadelphia: Lippincott Williams & Wilkins, 2005:35(1–50).

2. (A) Phenytoin may decrease the serum concentration of CSA through cytochrome P450 3A/4 enzyme induction, a clinically significant drug interaction.

   Ref: Lake KD, Aaronson KD. Cardiac transplantation. In: DiPiro JT, Talbert RL, Yee GC, eds. *Pharmacotherapy: A Pathophysiologic Approach*, 5th ed. New York: McGraw-Hill, 2002:321–325

3. (E) OKT3, a therapeutic murine monoclonal antibody, is more expensive than methylprednisolone and is associated with potential toxicities requiring patient hospitalization during the 2-week course of treatment. Since the patient received one previous course of OKT3, preformed antibody titers >1:1000 may predispose the patient to severe hypersensitivity reactions and reduced efficacy.

   Ref: Taber DJ, Dupuis RE. Solid organ transplantation. In: Koda-Kimble MA, et al, eds. *Applied Therapeutics: The Clinical Use of Drugs*, 8th ed. Philadelphia: Lippincott Williams & Wilkins, 2005:35(1–50)

4. (E) CSA blood concentration monitoring and serum creatinine, BUN and blood pressure measurements are used to evaluate renal function and guide therapeutic decisions.

   Ref: Johnson HJ, Heim-Duthoy KL. Renal transplantation. In: DiPiro JT, Talbert RL, Yee GC, et al, eds. *Pharmacotherapy: A Pathophysiologic Approach*, 5th ed. New York: McGraw-Hill, 2002:843–866.

5. (D) Osteonecrosis, hyperglycemia, peptic ulcer disease, and hypertension are directly associated with either short- or long-term effects of prednisone therapy, and patients should be monitored carefully. Chronic rejection is usually associated with long-term use of CSA, not prednisone.

   Ref: Johnson HJ, Heim-Duthoy KL. Renal transplantation. In: DiPiro JT, Talbert RL, Yee GC, et al, eds. *Pharmacotherapy: A Pathophysiologic Approach*, 5th ed. New York: McGraw-Hill, 2002:843–866.

6. (A) Inhibition of cytochrome P450 metabolism of atorvastatin by CSA resulting in drug accumulation may lead to increased CK concentrations and rhabdomyolysis.

   Ref: Taber DJ, Dupuis RE. Solid organ transplantation. In: Koda-Kimble MA, et al, eds. *Applied Therapeutics: The Clinical Use of Drugs*, 8th ed. Philadelphia: Lippincott Williams & Wilkins, 2005:35(1–50).

7. (C) Ganciclovir is the antiviral agent of choice for the prevention of CMV infections associated with immunosuppressive therapy after renal transplantation.

   Ref: Johnson HJ, Heim-Duthoy KL. Renal transplantation. In: DiPiro JT, Talbert RL, Yee GC, et al, eds. *Pharmacotherapy: A Pathophysiologic Approach*, 5th ed. New York: McGraw-Hill, 2002:843–866.

8. (B) Previous acute allograft rejection episodes within the first year after renal transplantation and chronic use of CSA are known to predispose patients to an increased risk of chronic rejection or slow declining renal function leading to the loss of the allograft.

   Ref: Johnson HJ, Heim-Duthoy KL. Renal transplantation. In: DiPiro JT, Talbert RL, Yee GC, et al, eds. *Pharmacotherapy: A Pathophysiologic Approach*, 5th ed. New York: McGraw-Hill, 2002:843–866.

9. (C) Chronic rejection associated with long-term CSA use may be avoided by switching immunosuppressive therapy to tacrolimus.

   Ref: Taber DJ, Dupuis RE. Solid organ transplantation. In: Koda-Kimble MA, et al, eds. *Applied Therapeutics: The Clinical Use of Drugs*, 8th ed. Philadelphia: Lippincott Williams & Wilkins, 2005:35(1–50).

10. (E) Lymphomas have been reported in transplant patients receiving cyclosporine.

    Ref: Taber DJ, Dupuis RE. Solid organ transplantation. In: Koda-Kimble MA, et al, eds. *Applied Therapeutics: The Clinical Use of Drugs*, 8th ed. Philadelphia: Lippincott Williams & Wilkins, 2005:35(1–50).

PATIENT PROFILE 28
ANTIBIOTIC SUSPENSIONS

ANSWERS

1. (D) 1 tsp = 5 mL × 4 doses/day × 10 days = 200 mL

   Ref: Stocklosa M, Ansel H. *Pharmaceutical Calculations*. 10th ed. Baltimore: Williams & Wilkins; 1996:43.

2. (D) The nonconttstiluted product for a drug degraded by hydrolysis is more stable. When constituted, the product is anticipated to be stable for the expected time to completion of the dosage regimen.

   Ref: *Pharmaceutical Dosage Forms and Drug Delivery Systems*. 6th ed. Baltimore: Williams & Wilkins; 1995:253–254.

3. (D) Ampicillin is more stable in the dry state than in suspension or in solution. The nonconstituted product would then have a longer shelf life than the constituted product.

4. (C) For an ampicillin suspension, the particles to be suspended have a marked effect on the volume of the finished liquid preparation.

   Ref: Stocklosa M, Ansel H. *Pharmaceutical Calculations*. 10th ed. Baltimore: Williams & Wilkins; 1996:168–169.

5. (E) Increased temperature increases degradation. A suspension dosage form has an increased shelf life over a solution dosage form of the same drug because of pseudo-zero order kinetics.

   Ref: *Physical Pharmacy*. 4th ed. Philadelphia: Lea & Febiger; 1993:286–287, 295–296.

   Ref: *Pharmaceutical Dosage Forms and Drug Delivery Systems*. 6th ed. Baltimore: Williams & Wilkins; 1995:253–254.

PATIENT PROFILE 29
DIABETES

ANSWERS

1. (C) Blood sugar level above 120 mg/dL is considered high.

2. (B) The normal range is 80 to 100 mg\dL.

3. (B) Juvenile diabetes appears at earlier age; insulin-resistant diabetes does not appear all of a sudden.

4. (C) Osmotic diuretics such as sorbitol and mannitol are polyhydroxylated compounds; so is glucose.

5. (D) Both glucotrol and tolbutamide are sulfonylurea drugs for treating type 2 diabetes. Pioglitazone is not an antidiabetic agent by itself; it is used in cases of insulin-resistant diabetes to help regenerate insulin receptors on target cells.

6. (A) The chemical structures of the two agents show the sulfonylurea group.

7. (A) Since the sulfonylurea group is acidic in nature, rendering urine alkaline with antacids will increase the ionized species of the drug, leading to faster excretion of urine.

8. (B) Sulfonylurea drugs stimulate the release of insulin from the pancreatic beta cells. The mechanism is believed to be through partial blocking of the potassium channels.

9. (C) Insulin is secreted normally, but its receptors on target cell are defective owing to impaired protein synthesis.

10. (C) Nonresponsive type 2 diabetes to sulfonylurea drugs is indicative of insulin-resistant diabetes; pioglitazone will improve the efficacy of glucotrol.

PATIENT PROFILE 30
BACTEREMIA AND SEPSIS

ANSWERS

1. (C) The rationale is as follows: No cephalosporin has activity against enterococci. That rules out D and E.

Metronidazole is active against Bacteroides fragilis, an anaerobe, and is not useful in this situation because enterococci are gram-positive organisms. Vancomycin should be reserved for the control of enterococcal strains that are resistant to conventional therapy. When there are positive culture results, allow the results to guide therapy. Ampicillin and gentamicin in combination provide synergistic killing of the enterococci.

Ref: Moellering RC Jr. Enterococcus species, *Streptococcus bovis*, and *Leuconostoc* species. In: Mandell GL, Bennett JE, Dolin R, eds. *Principles and Practice of Infectious Diseases.* 4th ed. New York: Churchill Livingstone; 1995:1831.

2. (B) The drug of choice to control methicillin-resistant Staphylococcus aureus (MRSA) is vancomycin. The patient weighs 80 kg, which dictates that the vancomycin should be dosed 1 g IV q12h.

Ref: Rapp RP, Gorman SP, Adair CG. Nosocomial and device-related infections. In: DiPiro JT, Talbert RL, Yee GC, Matzke GR, Wells BG, Posey LM, eds. *Pharmacotherapy: A Pathophysiologic Approach.* 3rd ed. Stamford, Conn, Appleton & Lange; 1997:2390.

3. (D) Metronidazole is the drug of choice for initial management of *Clostridium difficile* colitis. Empiric treatment with metronidazole may allow for an adequate jump on treatment. If therapy with metronidazole fails, oral vancomycin at a dosage of 125–250 mg po q6h should be considered. No conclusive results have demonstrated the benefit of lactobacillus or yogurt.

Ref: Gilbert DN, Moellering RC Jr, Sande MA, eds. *The Sanford Guide to Antimicrobial Therapy* 1998. 28th ed. Vienna, Va: Antimicrobial Therapy; 1998:12.

4. (A) Vancomycin levels vary from publication to publication. A is safe. The other choices are inconsistent with the pharmacokinetics of vancomycin. Peak levels (if obtained at all) should be measured 1 hour after completion of the infusion. Vancomycin should be infused over 60–90 minutes to avoid "red man" syndrome. Vancomycin dose should be based on actual body weight. Vancomycin is not an aminoglycoside, and its clearance does not directly mimic serum creatinine level.

Ref: Rybak MJ, Aeschlimann JR. Laboratory tests to direct antimicrobial pharmacotherapy. In: DiPiro JT, Talbert RL, Yee GC, Matzke GR, Wells BG, Posey LM, eds. *Pharmaco-therapy: A Pathophysiologic Approach.* 4th ed. Stamford, Conn: Appleton & Lange; 1999:1597–1619.

5. (C) Vancomycin is not considered a nephrotoxic drug when used alone. However, in combination with other drugs that are nephrotoxic, such as aminoglycosides, amphotericin, and furosemide, vancomycin enhances the nephrotoxic potential of the other agents.

Ref: Gilbert DN, Moellering RC Jr, Sande MA, eds. *The Sanford Guide to Antimicrobial Therapy* 1998. 28th ed. Vienna, Va: Antimicrobial Therapy; 1998:68.

PATIENT PROFILE 31

ACUTE RENAL FAILURE

ANSWERS

1. (E) Metabolic acidosis, hyperkalemia, and oliguria are biochemical and hemodynamic manifestations commonly associated with acute renal failure.

Ref: Brophy D. Acute renal failure. In: Koda-Kimble MA, Young LY, Kradjan WA, et al, eds. *Applied Therapeutics: The Clinical Use of Drugs,* 8th ed. Philadelphia: Lippincott Williams & Wilkins, 2005:31(1–22).

2. (D) The calculated fractional excretion of sodium (FeNa) employing the patient's urinary chemistries for Na and Cr and urinalysis findings are used initially to differentiate prerenal from intrinsic renal failure. FeNa <1% and an unremarkable urinalysis may be associated prerenal azotemia. FeNa ≥ 1% and urinary sediment findings (RBC, WBC, casts, or protein) may be associated with intrinsic renal failure.

Ref: Brophy D. Acute renal failure. In: Koda-Kimble MA, Young LY, Kradjan WA, et al, eds. *Applied Therapeutics: The Clinical Use of Drugs,* 8th ed. Philadelphia: Lippincott Williams & Wilkins, 2005:31(1–22).

3. (C) Diuretics such as furosemide may cause false-positive FeNa values as a result of increased urinary Na from natriuresis.

Ref: Brophy D. Acute renal failure. In: Koda-Kimble MA, Young LY, Kradjan WA, et al, eds. *Applied Therapeutics: The Clinical Use of Drugs,* 8th ed. Philadelphia: Lippincott Williams & Wilkins, 2005:31(1–22).

4. (B) In patients at risk for developing prerenal azotemia, angiotensin-converting enzyme (ACE) inhibitors such as lisinopril lead to vasodilatation of the efferent arterioles and decrease intraglomerular pressure. Also, NSAIDs such as ibuprofen inhibit the vasodilatory effects of prostaglandins and may result in vasoconstriction of the afferent arterioles, reducing renal blood flow and intraglomerular pressure.

Ref: Mueller BA. Acute renal failure. In: DiPiro JT, Talbert RL, Yee GC, et al, eds. *Pharmacotherapy: A Pathophysiologic Approach,* 5th ed. New York: McGraw-Hill, 2002:771–795.

5. (E) Contributing factors leading to an increased risk of mortality associated with ARF include advanced age, oliguria, elevated serum creatinine, and septicemia, not hyperglycemia.

Ref: Mueller BA. Acute renal failure. In: DiPiro JT, Talbert RL, Yee GC, et al, eds. *Pharmacotherapy: A Pathophysiologic Approach,* 5th ed. New York: McGraw-Hill, 2002:771–795.

6. (A) Calcium gluconate directly antagonizes the effect of potassium in myocardial tissue and is indicated to reverse life-threatening ECG changes associated with hyperkalemia.

Ref: Brophy D. Acute renal failure. In: Koda-Kimble MA, Young LY, Kradjan WA, et al, eds. *Applied Therapeutics: The Clinical Use of Drugs,* 8th ed. Philadelphia: Lippincott Williams & Wilkins, 2005:31(1–22).

7. (D) Lisinopril may cause hyperkalemia in high-risk patients.

Ref: Hudson JQ, Johnson CA. Chronic kidney disease. In: Koda-Kimble MA, Young LY, Kradjan WA, et al, eds. *Applied Therapeutics: The Clinical Use of Drugs,* 8th ed. Philadelphia: Lippincott Williams & Wilkins, 2005:31(1–22), 32(1–36).

8. (D) NSAIDs should not be used in the presence of prerenal azotemia because they may worsen renal function.

Ref: Mueller BA. Acute renal failure. In: DiPiro JT, Talbert RL, Yee GC, et al, eds. *Pharmacotherapy: A Pathophysiologic Approach,* 5th ed. New York: McGraw-Hill, 2002:771–795.

9. (B) The loop diuretic furosemide is the drug of first choice in converting patients from oliguria to nonoliguria in ARF.

Ref: Mueller BA. Acute renal failure. In: DiPiro JT, Talbert RL, Yee GC, et al, eds. *Pharmacotherapy: A Pathophysiologic Approach,* 5th ed. New York: McGraw-Hill, 2002:771–795.

10. (D) Levofloxacin is renally dosed according to the patient-estimated creatinine clearance and the manufacturer's renal dosing guideline.

Ref: Guglielmo BJ. Principles of infectious diseases. In: Koda-Kimble MA, Young LY, Kradjan WA, et al, eds. *Applied Therapeutics: The Clinical Use of Drugs,* 8th ed. Philadelphia: Lippincott Williams & Wilkins, 2005:56(1–25).

PATIENT   PROFILE   32

OPPORTUNISTIC INFECTIONS: HIV, AIDS

ANSWERS

1. (A) Trimethoprim-sulfamethoxazole (TMP-SMZ, cotrimoxazole) is the preferred therapy for PCP. Early addition of adjunctive corticosteriod therapy to anti-PCP regimens has been shown to improve survival among patient with AIDS and moderate to severe PCP.

Ref: Kapusnik-Uner JE. Human immunodeficiency virus (HIV) infection and acquired immunodeficiency syndrome (AIDS). In: Herfindal ET, Gourley DR, eds. *Textbook of Therapeutics. Drug and Disease Management.* 6th ed. Baltimore: Williams & Wilkins; 1996:1405–1426.

2. (A) TMP-SMZ is the preferred agent for PCP prophylaxis (both primary and secondary) among adults, adolescents, and children.

Ref: Centers for Disease Control and Prevention. USPHS/IDSA guidelines for the prevention of opportunistic infections in persons infected with human immunodeficiency virus. *MMWR Morb Mortal Wkly Rep* 1997;46:1–46.

3. (B) Didanosine and zalcitabine have similar toxicity profiles and should be avoided in an antiretroviral regimen if it is possible to do so.

Ref: Carpenter CC, Fischl MA, Hammer SM. Antiretroviral therapy for HIV Infection in 1998: Updated recommendations of an international AIDS society USA Panel. *JAMA* 1998;280:78–86.

4. (E) Combivir® is a fixed-dose combination of lamivudine and zidovudine.

Ref: Combivir [product information]. Research Triangle Park, NC: GlaxoWellcome; 1999.

5. (D) First line choices for MAC prophylaxis are either azithromycin or clarithromycin.

Ref: Centers for Disease Control and Prevention. USPHS/IDSA guidelines for the prevention of opportunistic infections in persons infected with human immunodeficiency virus. *MMWR Morb Mortal Wkly Rep* 1997;46:1–46.

PATIENT   PROFILE   33

BACTEREMIA AND SEPSIS

ANSWERS

1. (C) A suggests bacteremia. Bacteremia is not sepsis; however, there may be bacteria in the blood of patients with sepsis. B describes the systemic inflammatory response syndrome (SIRS). This syndrome may occur among patients with sepsis, but the symptoms can result from a variety of inflammatory insults. D and E focus specifically

on blood pressure and end-organ damage. These responses can occur in sepsis but cannot serve as a definition of it. Thus C is a global definition of sepsis that encompasses all the other selections.

Ref: Jacobi J. Pathophysiology of sepsis. *Am J Health Syst Pharm* 2002;59:S3–S8.

2. (A) Gram-negative bacteremia can occur among patients who have been ill for some time or among patients who have an acute injury. The most common infectious source is the gastrointestinal (GI) tract. Among patients with critical illnesses, bacteria may translocate across the membranes of the GI tract into the blood. In the presence of severe illness, acute injury, or impaired immune status, the result may be gram-negative bacteremia.

Ref: Bochud PY, Glauser MP, Calandra T. Antibiotics in sepsis. *Intensive Care Med* 2001:27(suppl 1):S33–48.

3. (B) Norepinephrine is a pharmacologic vasopressor with adrenergic activity that stimulates primarily α_1 receptors with a small amount of β_1 activity. This yields the ability to squeeze the vessels while minimizing the chronotropic effect on the heart and minimizing cardiac arrhythmia. The doses of dopamine and phenylephrine listed are inadequate for maintaining blood pressure. Nitroprusside is a systemic vasodilator and is contraindicated in this scenario. Esmolol, a short-acting β-blocker that can be titrated, decreases heart rate and impairs systemic perfusion and oxygen delivery and also is contraindicated.

Ref: Kang-Birken SL, DiPiro JT. Sepsis and septic shock. In: DiPiro JT, Talbert RL, Yee GC, et al, eds. *Pharmacotherapy: A Pathophysiologic Approach,* 5th ed. New York: McGraw-Hill, 2002: 2038.

4. (E) The goal of empirical antibiotic selection is more or less a shotgun approach. A clear source of infection naturally will help you to tailor your choices, but the infectious source is usually vague. With the knowledge that the GI tract possibly is the source, you cover organisms that reside in the GI tract. The regiment you choose also should possess the characteristics listed in answers A–D.

Ref: Kang-Birken SL, DiPiro JT. Sepsis and septic shock. In: DiPiro JT, Talbert RL, Yee GC, et al, eds. *Pharmacotherapy: A Pathophysiologic Approach,* 5th ed. New York: McGraw-Hill, 2002: 2034.

5. (B) Piperacillin-tazobactam with gentamicin is the only regimen that has activity against all the organisms that may be present in an intraabdominal infection. Enterococci (group D streptococci), *B. fragilis* (gram-negative anaerobe), and enteric gram-negative rods are covered with this combination. All the other regimens listed have holes in their coverage. A lacks gram-negative coverage, C lacks enterococcal and anaerobic coverage, and D lacks enterococcal and adequate gram-negative coverage (gram-negative organisms should be doubly covered).

Ref: Kang-Birken SL, DiPiro JT. Sepsis and septic shock. In: DiPiro JT, Talbert RL, Yee GC, et al, eds. *Pharmacotherapy: A Pathophysiologic Approach,* 5th ed. New York: McGraw-Hill, 2002: 2035.

PATIENT PROFILE 34

ONCOLOGY: PROSTATE CANCER

ANSWERS

1. (B) Risk factors for prostate cancer are advanced age, genetic history, and previous vasectomy. Social history and the presence of BPH do not appear to be associated with increased risk of prostate cancer.

Ref: Kolesar JM, Goldspiel BR. Prostate cancer. In: DiPiro JT, Talbert RL, Yee GC, Matzke GR, Wells BG, Posey LM, eds. *Pharmacotherapy: A Pathophysiologic Approach.* 4th ed. Stamford, Conn: Appleton & Lange; 1999:2092–2109.

Ref: Herfindal ET, Gourley DR (eds). *Textbook of Therapeutics, Drug and Disease Management.* 6th ed. Baltimore: Williams & Wilkins; 1996: chapter 84.

2. (B) Current guidelines of the American Cancer Society are that a digital rectal examination be part of early detection methods for malignant disease. Yearly (not monthly) PSA measurement may replace this recommendation.

Ref: Valley AW, Balmer CM. Cancer treatment and chemotherapy. In: DiPiro JT, Talbert RL, Yee GC, Matzke GR, Wells BG, Posey LM, eds. *Pharmacotherapy: A Pathophysiologic Approach.* 4th ed. Stamford, Conn: Appleton & Lange; 1999:1957–2012.

Ref: Young LY, Koda-Kimble MA, eds. *Applied Therapeutics: The Clinical Use of Drugs.* 6th ed. Vancouver, Wash: Applied Therapeutics; 1995: chapter 90.

3. (D) Hormonal manipulation with LHRH agents and antiandrogens will ultimately decrease circulating testosterone, and the decrease stimulates tumor cell production.

Ref: Kolesar JM, Goldspiel BR. Prostate cancer. In: DiPiro JT, Talbert RL, Yee GC, Matzke GR, Wells BG, Posey LM, eds. *Pharmacotherapy: A Pathophysiologic Approach.* 4th ed. Stamford, Conn: Appleton & Lange; 1999:2092–2109.

Ref: Herfindal ET, Gourley DR (eds). *Textbook of Therapeutics, Drug and Disease Management.* 6th ed. Baltimore: Williams & Wilkins; 1996: chapter 84.

4. (C) It is likely that the introduction of this hormonal therapy will result in a disease flare until LH, FSH, and testosterone are suppressed.

Ref: Young LY, Koda-Kimble MA, eds. *Applied Therapeutics: The Clinical Use of Drugs.* 6th ed. Vancouver, Wash: Applied Therapeutics; 1995: chapter 93.

5. (A) Use of NSAIDs has been shown to be highly effective in the management of bone pain associated with metastatic disease.

Ref: Young LY, Koda-Kimble MA, eds. *Applied Therapeutics: The Clinical Use of Drugs.* 6th ed. Vancouver, Wash: Applied Therapeutics; 1995: chapter 7.

PATIENT PROFILE 35

PYELONEPHRITIS

ANSWERS

1. (D) Elevated WBC and differential are the most specific indicators of infection for LK. Her temperature may be influenced by the use of antipyretics such as acetaminophen and ibuprofen; her heart rate may be reflex tachycardia in the setting of hypotension (possibly induced by lisinopril use and dehydration).

Ref: Abate BJ, Barriere S. Antimicrobial regimen selection. In: Dipiro JT, Talbert RL, Yee GC, et al., eds. *Pharmacotherapy: A Pathophysiologic Approach,* 5th edition. New York: McGraw-Hill, 2002:1817–1829.

Ref: Gugliemo BJ. Principles of infectious diseases. In: Koda-Kimble MA, Young LY, Kradian WA, et al., eds. *Applied Therapeutics. The Clinical Use of Drugs,* 8th edition. Philadelphia: Lippincott Williams & Wilkins, 2004:56(1–25).

2. (B) The term "shift to the left" refers to the increased percentage of bands (immature neutrophils) in the differential. This is often seen in bacterial infections and indicates bone marrow response to an infectious process.

Ref: Gugliemo BJ. Principles of infectious diseases. In: Koda-Kimble MA, Young LY, Kradian WA, et al., eds. *Applied Therapeutics. The Clinical Use of Drugs,* 8th edition. Philadelphia: Lippincott Williams & Wilkins, 2004:56(1–25).

Ref: Rybak MJ, Aeschlimann JR. Laboratory tests to direct antimicrobial pharmacotherapy. In: Dipiro JT, Talbert RL, Yee GC, et al., eds. *Pharmacotherapy: A Pathophysiologic Approach,* 5th edition. New York: McGraw-Hill, 2002:1797–1815.

3. (C) Although *E. coli* is the primary pathogen in pyelonephritis (up to 50%), other gram-negative organisms (e.g., *Enterobacteriaceae* such as *Klebsiella pneumoniae, Proteus* spp., *Enterobacter* spp.) also may been seen. *Pseudomonas aeruginosa* and enterococci are possible pathogens in patients residing in nursing homes or with frequent or recent hospitalization.

Ref: Coyle EA, Prince RA. Urinary tract infections and prostatitis. In: Dipiro JT, Talbert RL, Yee GC, et al., eds. *Pharmacotherapy: A Pathophysiologic Approach,* 5th edition. New York: McGraw-Hill, 2002:1981–1996.

Fish DN. Urinary tract infections. In: Koda-Kimble MA, Young LY, Kradian WA, et al., eds. *Applied Therapeutics. The Clinical Use of Drugs,* 8th edition. Philadelphia: Lippincott Williams & Wilkins, 2004:64(1–22).

4. (A) IV therapy is indicated because of the patient's nausea and vomiting. Third-generation cephalosporins such as ceftriaxone IV are good choices because of their broad spectrum of activity against gram-negative organisms.

Ref: Coyle EA, Prince RA. Urinary tract infections and prostatitis. In: Dipiro JT, Talbert RL, Yee GC, et al., eds. *Pharmacotherapy: A Pathophysiologic Approach,* 5th edition. New York: McGraw-Hill, 2002:1981–1996.

Ref: Fish DN. Urinary Tract Infections. In: Koda-Kimble MA, Young LY, Kradian WA, et al., eds. *Applied Therapeutics. The Clinical Use of Drugs,* 8th edition. Philadelphia: Lippincott Williams & Wilkins, 2004:64(1–22).

5. (B) Considering her signs and symptoms (dry mucous membranes, nausea, and vomiting), and her low Na, Cl, and K levels, the patient appears to be dehydrated. IV fluids with the addition of KCl (initially 20 mEq) should be administered to rehydrate the patient and restore her electrolytes.

6. (E) The identified pathogen *Klebsiella pneumoniae* is sensitive to ciprofloxacin, and this drug is a reasonable choice for LK (400 mg IV q 12h). Oral cefazolin is not available; also, an oral regimen may not yet be suitable for the patient. Broad coverage with piperacillin/tazobactam or imipenem is not necessary.

Ref: Coyle EA, Prince RA. Urinary tract infections and prostatitis. In: Dipiro JT, Talbert RL, Yee GC, et al., eds. *Pharmacotherapy: A Pathophysiologic Approach,* 5th edition. New York: McGraw-Hill, 2002:1981–1996.

Ref: Fish DN. Urinary tract infections. In: Koda-Kimble MA, Young LY, Kradian WA, et al., eds. *Applied Therapeutics. The Clinical Use of Drugs,* 8th edition. Philadelphia: Lippincott Williams & Wilkins, 2004:64(1–22).

7. (D) Cefotaxime has no activity against *Pseudomonas aeruginosa.*

Ref: Abate BJ, Barriere S. Antimicrobial regimen selection. In: Dipiro JT, Talbert RL, Yee GC, et al., eds. *Pharmacotherapy: A Pathophysiologic Approach,* 5th edition. New York: McGraw-Hill, 2002:1817–1827.

Ref: Fish DN. Urinary tract infections. In: Koda-Kimble MA, Young LY, Kradian WA, et al., eds. *Applied Therapeutics. The Clinical Use of Drugs,* 8th edition. Philadelphia: Lippincott Williams & Wilkins, 2004:64(1–22).

8. (D) Patients who have symptomatically improved, are afebrile for 24 to 48 hours, and are able to take fluids should be switched to an oral antibiotic to complete a total antibiotic treatment course of 14 to 21 days for pyelonephritis. A good choice is ciprofloxacin 250 to 500 mg PO q 12H. To evaluate bacteriologic response, a urine C&S test should be done on the second day of therapy, 2 to 3 weeks after completion, and at 3 months.

    Ref: Coyle EA, Prince RA. Urinary tract infections and prostatitis. In: Dipiro JT, Talbert RL, Yee GC, et al., eds. *Pharmacotherapy: A Pathophysiologic Approach,* 5th edition. New York: McGraw-Hill, 2002:1981–1996.

    Ref: Fish DN. Urinary tract infections. In: Koda-Kimble MA, Young LY, Kradian WA, et al., eds. *Applied Therapeutics. The Clinical Use of Drugs,* 8th edition. Philadelphia: Lippincott Williams & Wilkins, 2004:64(1–22).

9. (D) Significantly decreased fluoroquinolone absorption (20% to 70%) occurs with the concurrent use of products containing divalent and trivalent cations (Al^{2+}, Mg^{2+}, Ca^{2+}, Zn^{2+}, Fe^{3+}). This may result in therapeutic failure. The patient should be instructed to best avoid intake of these products while taking fluoroquinolones, or to take them at least 2 hours before or 4 to 6 hours after the antibiotic dose.

    Ref: Fish DN. Urinary tract infections. In: Koda-Kimble MA, Young LY, Kradian WA, et al., eds. *Applied Therapeutics. The Clinical Use of Drugs,* 8th edition. Philadelphia: Lippincott Williams & Wilkins, 2004:64(1–22).

10. (E) All given options are suitable for this postmenopausal woman. Continuous antibiotic prophylaxis is a possibility for patients with two or more symptomatic UTIs during one 6-month period, or three or more UTIs over a 12-month period. Typically, low-dose antibiotics are taken at bedtime. Cranberry juice (200 to 750 mL/day) or cranberry tablets as well as topical estrogen cream have reduced symptomatic, recurrent infection.

    Ref: Coyle EA, Prince RA. Urinary tract infections and prostatitis. In: Dipiro JT, Talbert RL, Yee GC, et al., eds. *Pharmacotherapy: A Pathophysiologic Approach,* 5th edition. New York: McGraw-Hill, 2002:1981–1996.

    Ref: Finn SD. Acute uncomplicated urinary tract infection in women. *N Engl J Med* 2003;349(3):259–266.

PATIENT PROFILE 36

MEDICINAL CHEMISTRY

ANSWERS

1. (C) Because the patient is 80 years of age, her liver function may have declined. Sulindac and nabumetone are prodrugs that must be activated by the liver to be active as inhibitors of prostaglandin synthesis. Steroid therapy is not recommended for elderly patients for similar consideration of liver function. Naproxen is excreted mostly unchanged in the urine; only 30% is metabolized by the liver.

PATIENT PROFILE 37

HIV/AIDS

ANSWERS

1. (D) Zidovudine and lamivudine are both nucleoside reverse transcriptase inhibitors that target early stages of HIV-1 viral replication via inhibition of the reverse transcriptase enzyme of HIV-1.

    Ref: Department of Health and Human Services/Henry J Kaiser Family Foundation Panel on Clinical Practices for the Treatment of HIV Infection. Guidelines for the use of antiretroviral agents in HIV-infected adults and adolescents. Rockville, MD: HIV/AIDS Treatment Information Service, October 29, 2004 (available online at *http://AIDSinfo.nih.gov*).

2. (D) Zidovudine can be taken without regard to meals and RS should be counseled accordingly.

    Ref: Department of Health and Human Services/Henry J Kaiser Family Foundation Panel on Clinical Practices for the Treatment of HIV Infection. Guidelines for the use of antiretroviral agents in HIV-infected adults and adolescents. Rockville, MD: HIV/AIDS Treatment Information Service, October 29, 2004 (available online at *http://AIDSinfo.nih.gov*).

3. (D) Lamivudine can be taken without regard to meals and RS should be counseled accordingly.

    Ref: Department of Health and Human Services/Henry J Kaiser Family Foundation Panel on Clinical Practices for the Treatment of HIV Infection. Guidelines for the use of antiretroviral agents in HIV-infected adults and adolescents. Rockville, MD: HIV/AIDS Treatment Information Service, October 29, 2004 (available online at *http://AIDSinfo.nih.gov*).

4. (A) Ritonavir is the most potent inhibitor of cytochrome P450 within the protease inhibitor class.

    Ref: Piscitelli SC, Gallicano KD. Interactions among drugs for HIV and opportunistic infections. *N Engl J Med* 344(13):984–996, 2001.

5. (A) Ritonavir/lopinavir (Kaletra®) is a combination product that relies on the boosting effects of ritonavir to achieve adequate plasma concentrations of lopinavir.

    Ref: Department of Health and Human Services/Henry J Kaiser Family Foundation Panel on Clinical Practices for the Treatment of HIV Infection. Guidelines for the use of antiretroviral agents in HIV-infected adults and adolescents. Rockville, MD: HIV/AIDS Treatment Information Service, October 29, 2004 (available online at *http://AIDSinfo.nih.gov*).

6. (A) Patients receiving zidovudine should be monitored carefully for hematologic toxicities, including anemia and granulocytopenia.

    Ref: Kanmaz TJ, Lee NJ. Significant toxicities associated with anti-retroviral therapy. *J Pharm Pract* 13(6):457–474, 2000.

7. (C) Efavirenz can cause adverse effects of the central nervous system.

Ref: Kanmaz TJ, Lee NJ. Significant toxicities associated with anti-retroviral therapy. *J Pharm Pract* 13(6):457–474, 2000.

8. (D) In March 2003, the fusion inhibitor, enfuvirtide (T-20, Fuzeon), was the first inhibitor of HIV-1 entry to gain FDA approval.

    Ref: Lalezari JP, Henry K, O'Hearn M, et al. Enfuvirtide, an HIV-1 fusion inhibitor for drug-resistant HIV infection in North and South America. *N Engl J Med* 348:2186–2195, 2003.

9. (B) Enfuvirtide is a peptide that must be administered as a subcutaneous injection. The oral route of administration is not feasible given the peptide structure of the molecule and its degradation at gastric pH.

    Ref: Hardy H, Skolnik P. Enfuvirtide: A novel fusion inhibitor for therapy of HIV infection. *Pharmacotherapy* 2004;24(2): 198–211.

10. (A) Adequate hydration is important for patients taking indinavir in order to minimize the risk of nephrolithiasis. Patients taking indinavir should be advised to drink 48 ounces of liquids within 24 hours.

    Ref: Kanmaz TJ, Lee NJ. Significant toxicities associated with anti-retroviral therapy. *J Pharm Pract* 13(6):457–474, 2000.

PATIENT   PROFILE   38

GENERALIZED ANXIETY DISORDER

ANSWERS

1. (E) All the symptoms listed are characteristic of generalized anxiety disorder.

    Ref: American Psychiatric Association. *Diagnostic and Statistical Manual of Mental Disorders*. 4th ed. Washington, DC: American Psychiatric Association; 1994.

2. (D) Sexual dysfunction is one of the most common adverse effects of all SSRIs, although it is underreported.

    Ref: Herfindal ET, Gourley DR (eds). *Textbook of Therapeutics, Drug and Disease Management*. 6th ed. Baltimore: Williams & Wilkins; 1996: chapter 53.

3. (A) Cimetidine has been shown to significantly decrease diazepam metabolism through inhibition of CYP 3A4 and 2C19 in addition to possibly decreasing the volume

of distribution. Sertraline may decrease diazepam metabolism but not to any degree of clinical significance.

Ref: Young LY, Koda-Kimble MA, eds. *Applied Therapeutics: The Clinical Use of Drugs*. 6th ed. Vancouver, Wash: Applied Therapeutics; 1995: chapter 73.

4. (E) The principle route of elimination of lorazepam is glucuronidation. The inactive glucuronidate metabolite is renally excreted.

    Ref: *Goodman and Gilman's The Pharmacologic Basis of Therapeutics*. 9th ed. New York: McGraw-Hill; 1996: chapter 18.

5. (B) Buspirone has no hypnotic effect and is not likely to be abused.

    Ref: Herfindal ET, Gourley DR (eds). *Textbook of Therapeutics, Drug and Disease Management*. 6th ed. Baltimore: Williams & Wilkins; 1996: chapter 53.

RENAL TRANSPLANTATION

ANSWERS

1. (D) Intravenous administration of methylprednisolone in pulse doses (200–1000 mg qd for 3 days) then tapered rapidly is the primary therapy to manage acute episodes of allograft rejection.

2. (C) Administration of high-dose steroids such as methylprednisolone may lead to drug-induced psychosis.

3. (D) Patients with evidence of fluid overload on a chest radiograph (or >3% over their body weight) are at risk of pulmonary edema and respiratory distress caused by a cytokine-induced increase in capillary permeability associated with OKT3.

4. (B) OKT3 was introduced in the 1980s as the first monoclonal antibody approved for human use.

5. (A) A test dose of 1 mg OKT3 usually is administered before a therapeutic dose of 5 mg.

6. (E) The serum concentration of cytokine becomes acutely elevated within 1–4 hours after the first and second doses of OKT3. These high concentrations correlate with the onset of fever and cardiovascular symptoms such as hypertension and tachycardia.

Ref: Dupuis RE. Solid organ transplantation. In: *Applied Therapeutics: The Clinical Use of Drugs.* In: Young LY, Koda-Kimble MA, eds. *Applied Therapeutics: The Clinical Use of Drugs.* 6th ed. Vancouver, Wash: Applied Therapeutics; 1995: chapter 33.

Ref: Tsunoda SM, Aweeka FT. Solid organ transplantation. In: Herfindal ET, Gourley DR (eds). *Textbook of Therapeutics, Drug and Disease Management.* 6th ed. Baltimore: Williams & Wilkins; 1996: chapter 96.

ARRHYTHMIAS

ANSWERS

1. (C) The ventricular rate should be controlled before any attempt is made to restore normal sinus rhythm in the care of patients in stable hemodynamic condition.

Ref: Bauman JL, Schoen MD. Arrhythmias. In: DiPiro JT, Talbert RL, Yee GC, Matzke GR, Wells BG, Posey LM, eds. *Pharmacotherapy: A Pathophysiologic Approach.* 4th ed. Stamford, Conn: Appleton & Lange; 1999:232–264.

2. (A) The onset of atrial fibrillation was more than 48 hours ago. The patient needs 4 weeks of anticoagulation before cardioversion.

Ref: Bauman JL, Schoen MD. Arrhythmias. In: DiPiro JT, Talbert RL, Yee GC, Matzke GR, Wells BG, Posey LM, eds. *Pharmacotherapy: A Pathophysiologic Approach.* 4th ed. Stamford, Conn: Appleton & Lange; 1999:232–264.

3. (B) Mexiletine is not effective in the management of atrial arrhythmia.

Ref: Bauman JL, Schoen MD. Arrhythmias. In: DiPiro JT, Talbert RL, Yee GC, Matzke GR, Wells BG, Posey LM, eds. *Pharmacotherapy: A Pathophysiologic Approach.* 4th ed. Stamford, Conn: Appleton & Lange; 1999:232–264.

4. (C) Gemfibrizol has not been reported to interact with warfarin.

Ref: *Drug Interaction Facts.* St. Louis: Facts and Comparisons; 1999.

5. (D) The patient needs a drug that will lower total cholesterol and LDL cholesterol, not triglycerides.

Ref: Talbert RL. Ischemic heart disease. In: DiPiro JT, Talbert RL, Yee GC, Matzke GR, Wells BG, Posey LM, eds. *Pharmacotherapy: A Pathophysiologic Approach.* 4th ed. Stamford, Conn: Appleton & Lange; 1999:182–210.

Ref: Talbert RL. Hyperlipidemia. In: DiPiro JT, Talbert RL, Yee GC, Matzke GR, Wells BG, Posey LM, eds. *Pharmacotherapy: A Pathophysiologic Approach.* 4th ed. Stamford, Conn: Appleton & Lange; 1999:350–373.

PATIENT PROFILE 41

DIABETES

ANSWERS

1. (B) Impaired insulin secretion and tissue resistance to insulin are two of the three metabolic defects in type II diabetes. The third is insulin resistance.

    Ref: Oki JC, Isley WL. Diabetes mellitus. In: DiPiro JT, Talbert RL, Yee GC, et al., eds. *Pharmacotherapy: A Pathophysiologic Approach,* 5th edition. New York: McGraw-Hill, 2002:1335–1357.

2. (E) It is important not to miss a meal while on this medication because of the increased risk of hypoglycemia.

    Ref: Oki JC, Isley WL. Diabetes mellitus. In: DiPiro JT, Talbert RL, Yee GC, et al., eds. *Pharmacotherapy: A Pathophysiologic Approach,* 5th edition. New York: McGraw-Hill, 2002:1335–1357.

3. (D) Tachycardia is typically seen in a patient with hypoglycemia.

    Ref: Oki JC, Isley WL. Diabetes mellitus. In: DiPiro JT, Talbert RL, Yee GC, et al., eds. *Pharmacotherapy: A Pathophysiologic Approach,* 5th edition. New York: McGraw-Hill, 2002:1335–1357.

4. (D) The patient should take one to two glucose tablets to provide a short-term increase in blood sugar. The patient then should eat a meal to decrease the risk of recurrence.

    Ref: Oki JC, Isley WL. Diabetes mellitus. In: DiPiro JT, Talbert RL, Yee GC, et al., eds. *Pharmacotherapy: A Pathophysiologic Approach,* 5th edition. New York: McGraw-Hill, 2002:1335–1357.

5. (C) Glyburide stimulates insulin release from the pancreas via the pancreatic β cells.

6. (E) Allopurinol can decrease the urinary excretion of sulfonylureas.

    Ref: Oki JC, Isley WL. Diabetes mellitus. In: DiPiro JT, Talbert RL, Yee GC, et al., eds. *Pharmacotherapy: A Pathophysiologic Approach,* 5th edition. New York: McGraw-Hill, 2002:1335–1357.

7. (B) Actos is initiated at 15 to 30 mg a day with a max of 45 mg.

    Ref: Oki JC, Isley WL. Diabetes mellitus. In: DiPiro JT, Talbert RL, Yee GC, et al., eds. *Pharmacotherapy: A Pathophysiologic Approach,* 5th edition. New York: McGraw-Hill, 2002:1335– 1357.

8. (E) Use of contrast dye can result in an increased risk of lactic acidosis.

    Ref: Oki JC, Isley WL. Diabetes mellitus. In: DiPiro JT, Talbert RL, Yee GC, et al., eds. *Pharmacotherapy: A Pathophysiologic Approach,* 5th edition. New York: McGraw-Hill, 2002:1335–1357.

9. (B) Acarbose is an α-glucosidase inhibitor and flatulence is a common side effect that limits its use.

    Ref: Oki JC, Isley WL. Diabetes mellitus. In: DiPiro JT, Talbert RL, Yee GC, et al., eds. *Pharmacotherapy: A Pathophysiologic Approach,* 5th edition. New York: McGraw-Hill, 2002:1335–1357.

10. (D) Tolinase is a first-generation sulfonylurea.

    Ref: Oki JC, Isley WL. Diabetes mellitus. In: DiPiro JT, Talbert RL, Yee GC, et al., eds. *Pharmacotherapy: A Pathophysiologic Approach,* 5th edition. New York: McGraw-Hill, 2002:1335–1357.

PATIENT PROFILE 42

DIABETES MELLITUS

ANSWERS

1. (C) Insulin therapy should be initiated at 0.5–1.0 unit per kilogram per day.

    Ref: Koda-Kimble MA, Carlisle BA. Diabetes mellitus. In: Young LY, Koda-Kimble MA, eds. *Applied Therapeutics: The Clinical Use of Drugs.* 6th ed. Vancouver, Wash: Applied Therapeutics; 1995:48-1–48-62.

2. (B) This dosing schedule is one of several that mimics the activity of a functioning pancreas.

    Ref: Koda-Kimble MA, Carlisle BA. Diabetes mellitus. In: Young LY, Koda-Kimble MA, eds. *Applied Therapeutics: The Clinical Use of Drugs.* 6th ed. Vancouver, Wash: Applied Therapeutics; 1995:48-1–48-62.

3. (A) This sequence is the recommended way to mix regular insulin and NPH insulin to avoid contaminating the regular insulin vial with NPH insulin.

    Ref: Koda-Kimble MA, Carlisle BA. Diabetes mellitus. In: Young LY, Koda-Kimble MA, eds. *Applied Therapeutics: The Clinical Use of Drugs.* 6th ed. Vancouver, Wash: Applied Therapeutics; 1995:48-1–48-62.

4. (D) Massaging the area can disrupt absorption of the insulin and make absorption erratic and unpredictable.

    Ref: Koda-Kimble MA, Carlisle BA. Diabetes mellitus. In: Young LY, Koda-Kimble MA, eds. *Applied Therapeutics: The Clinical Use of Drugs.* 6th ed. Vancouver, Wash: Applied Therapeutics; 1995:48-1–48-62.

5. (E) Signs and symptoms of hyperglycemia include thirst, hunger, polyuria, nocturia, dry, itchy skin, sedation, and blurred vision.

Ref: Koda-Kimble MA, Carlisle BA. Diabetes mellitus. In: Young LY, Koda-Kimble MA, eds. *Applied Therapeutics: The Clinical Use of Drugs.* 6th ed. Vancouver, Wash: Applied Therapeutics; 1995:48-1–48-62.

P A T I E N T   P R O F I L E   4 3
SOLUTIONS (PHARMACEUTICALS)

ANSWERS

1. (B)

Ref: Zatz, J. *Pharmaceutical Calculations.* 3rd ed. New York: John Wiley & Sons; 1995:49–148.

2. (E)

Ref: Zatz, J. *Pharmaceutical Calculations.* 3rd ed. New York: John Wiley & Sons; 1995:49–148.

3. (D)

Ref: Zatz, J. *Pharmaceutical Calculations.* 3rd ed. New York: John Wiley & Sons; 1995:67–68.

4. (A)

Ref: Zatz, J. *Pharmaceutical Calculations.* 3rd ed. New York: John Wiley & Sons; 1995:149–182.

5. (E)

Ref: Zatz, J. *Pharmaceutical Calculations.* 3rd ed. New York: John Wiley & Sons; 1995:66–79.

6. (C)

Ref: Zatz, J. *Pharmaceutical Calculations.* 3rd ed. New York: John Wiley & Sons; 1995:255–268.

7. (D)

Ref: Zatz, J. *Pharmaceutical Calculations.* 3rd ed. New York: John Wiley & Sons; 1995:273.

8. (B)

Ref: Zatz, J. *Pharmaceutical Calculations.* 3rd ed. New York: John Wiley & Sons; 1995:247.

9. (E)

Ref: Zatz, J. *Pharmaceutical Calculations.* 3rd ed. New York: John Wiley & Sons; 1995:247.

10. (D)

Ref: Zatz, J. *Pharmaceutical Calculations.* 3rd ed. New York: John Wiley & Sons; 1995:247–252.

P A T I E N T   P R O F I L E   4 4
SEIZURE DISORDERS

ANSWERS

1. (C) This patient is experiencing status epilepticus, which is a medical emergency.

Ref: Seizure disorders. In: Young LY, Koda-Kimble MA, eds. *Applied Therapeutics: The Clinical Use of Drugs.* 6th ed. Vancouver, Wash: Applied Therapeutics; 1995: chapter 52.

2. (A) The agent of choice to manage convulsive status epilepticus is intravenous lorazepam because of the rapid onset of action.

Ref: Seizure disorders. In: Young LY, Koda-Kimble MA, eds. *Applied Therapeutics: The Clinical Use of Drugs.* 6th ed. Vancouver, Wash: Applied Therapeutics; 1995: chapter 52.

3. (D) To reduce the potential for cardiotoxicity, the maximum recommended administration rate for IV phenytoin is 50 mg/min.

Ref: Seizure disorders. In: Young LY, Koda-Kimble MA, eds. *Applied Therapeutics: The Clinical Use of Drugs.* 6th ed. Vancouver, Wash: Applied Therapeutics; 1995: chapter 52.

4. (E) Fosphenytoin is more water soluble than is phenytoin, is more rapidly absorbed after IM administration, and can be given at a rate that is three times faster than that of phenytoin.

Ref: Cerebyx [prescribing information]. Morris Plains, NJ: Parke-Davis; 1999.

5. (B) Compliance with antiepileptic drugs often is determined by the side effect profile. Weight gain caused by use of valproic acid may reduce compliance with the drug. The other side effects listed are more common with phenytoin therapy.

Ref: Seizure disorders. In: Herfindal ET, Gourley DR, eds. *Textbook of Therapeutics, Drug and Disease Management.* 6th ed. Baltimore: Williams & Wilkins; 1996: chapter 50.

PATIENT PROFILE 45

ALCOHOL WITHDRAWAL AND DEPENDENCE

ANSWERS

1. (B) Stage I occurs 6 to 8 hours after a decrease in blood ethanol levels. Clinical features involve moderate autonomic hyperactivity (e.g., anxiety, tremulousness, tachycardia, insomnia, nausea, vomiting, diaphoresis).

   Stage II occurs 24 hours after a decrease in blood ethanol levels. Clinical features involve autonomic hyperactivity with auditory and visual hallucinations.

   Stage III occurs in approximately 4% of untreated patients, 1 to 2 days after a decrease in blood ethanol levels. Clinical features involve grand mal seizures.

   Stage IV occurs in approximately 5% of untreated patients, 3 to 5 days after a decrease in blood ethanol levels. Clinical features involve delirium tremens (e.g., confusion, illusions, hallucinations, agitation, tachycardia, hyperthermia).

   There is no stage V.

   Ref: Jungnickel PW. Alcohol abuse. In: Koda-Kimble MA, Young LY, Kradjan WA, Guglielmo BJ, eds. *Applied Therapeutics: The Clinical Use of Drugs,* 8th edition. Baltimore: Lippincott Williams & Wilkins, 2005:84-6.

2. (E) Meta-analysis and evidence-based practice guidelines have established benzodiazepines as the drugs of choice for alcohol withdrawal symptoms because of proven efficacy in the management of agitation and seizures. Clinical experience is extensive with diazepam, lorazepam, and chlordiazepoxide, but all benzodiazepines appear to be equally effective when given in equivalent doses. Most patients can be managed with oral dosing, although parenteral therapy may be required in more acutely agitated and combative patients.

   Ref: Jungnickel PW. Alcohol abuse. In: Koda-Kimble MA, Young LY, Kradjan WA, Guglielmo BJ, eds. *Applied Therapeutics: The Clinical Use of Drugs,* 8th edition. Baltimore: Lippincott Williams & Wilkins, 2005:84-7.

3. (B) The Clinical Institute Withdrawal Assessment-Alcohol, Revised (CIWA-Ar) is a reliable and validated 10-item scale used to assess alcohol withdrawal symptoms and individualize therapy. The CAGE is used to assess the need for management of alcohol dependence. The Abnormal Involuntary Movement Scale (AIMS) is used to evaluate patients for movement disorders associated with the use of antipsychotic agents. The PANSS is the Positive and Negative Symptom Scale for Schizophrenia. The BPRS is the Brief Psychiatric Rating Scale, which is used to assess symptoms of schizophrenia.

   Ref: Jungnickel PW. Alcohol abuse. In: Koda-Kimble MA, Young LY, Kradjan WA, Guglielmo BJ, eds. *Applied Therapeutics: The*

   Clinical Use of Drugs, 8th edition. Baltimore: Lippincott Williams & Wilkins, 2005:84-7.

4. (C) Lorazepam has a shorter half-life (10 to 20 hours) than diazepam or chlordiazepoxide and is not oxidatively metabolized to active metabolites. Both diazepam and chlordiazepoxide have half-lives as long as 100 hours and are oxidatively metabolized to active metabolites. Lorazepam has predictable absorption after IM administration; both diazepam and chlordiazepoxide are erratically absorbed after IM administration.

   Ref: Jungnickel PW. Alcohol abuse. In: Koda-Kimble MA, Young LY, Kradjan WA, Guglielmo BJ, eds. *Applied Therapeutics: The Clinical Use of Drugs,* 8th edition. Baltimore: Lippincott Williams & Wilkins, 2005:84-7.

5. (D) β-Blockers can be used as ancillary therapy in the management of alcohol withdrawal by decreasing the adrenergic symptoms. The other statements are false.

   Ref: Jungnickel PW. Alcohol abuse. In: Koda-Kimble MA, Young LY, Kradjan WA, Guglielmo BJ, eds. *Applied Therapeutics: The Clinical Use of Drugs,* 8th edition. Baltimore: Lippincott Williams & Wilkins, 2005:84-7.

6. (C) ReVia (naltrexone) is a μ-opioid antagonist that appears to reduce ethanol cravings in patients who are abstinent and blocks the reinforcing effects of ethanol in patients who drink. The mechanism of its effects in managing alcoholism has not been established. Naloxone is also a μ-opioid agonist; the brand name is Narcan.

   Ref: Jungnickel PW. Alcohol abuse. In: Koda-Kimble MA, Young LY, Kradjan WA, Guglielmo BJ, eds. *Applied Therapeutics: The Clinical Use of Drugs,* 8th edition. Baltimore: Lippincott Williams & Wilkins, 2005:84-9.

7. (C) Acamprosate is an amino acid derivative that affects both GABA and glutamine (an excitatory amino acid) transmission; the precise mechanism of action is unknown. Disulfiram (Antabuse) blocks the enzyme aldehyde dehydrogenase causing unpleasant and potentially life-threatening effects when ethanol is coadministered (aversion therapy).

   Ref: Jungnickel PW. Alcohol abuse. In: Koda-Kimble MA, Young LY, Kradjan WA, Guglielmo BJ, eds. *Applied Therapeutics: The Clinical Use of Drugs,* 8th edition. Baltimore: Lippincott Williams & Wilkins, 2005:84-8,9.

8. (E) Medical complications of chronic alcoholism include gastrointestinal complications (e.g., diarrhea, gastritis, gastroesophageal reflux disease), pancreatitis, Wernicke-Korsakoff syndrome, cardiovascular complications

(e.g., cardiomyopathy, hypertension, arrhythmias), hypogonadism, myopathy, neuropathy, liver disease (e.g., hepatitis, cirrhosis), and hematologic complications (e.g., megaloblastic anemia, sideroblastic anemia, iron deficiency, thrombocytopenia).

Ref: Jungnickel PW. Alcohol abuse. In: Koda-Kimble MA, Young LY, Kradjan WA, Guglielmo BJ, eds. *Applied Therapeutics: The Clinical Use of Drugs,* 8th edition. Baltimore: Lippincott Williams & Wilkins, 2005:84-10,11.

9. (C) Disulfiram (Antabuse) blocks the enzyme aldehyde dehydrogenase, causing unpleasant and potentially life-threatening effects when ethanol is coadministered (aversion therapy).

Ref: Jungnickel PW. Alcohol abuse. In: Koda-Kimble MA, Young LY, Kradjan WA, Guglielmo BJ, eds. *Applied Therapeutics: The Clini-*

cal Use of Drugs, 8th edition. Baltimore: Lippincott Williams & Wilkins, 2005:84-8,9.

10. (C) Wernicke-Korsakoff syndrome is a neurologic disorder cause by thiamine deficiency. Wernicke's encephalopathy can be precipitated by a large glucose load and clinical features include central nervous system depression, ambulation problems, ocular problems, hypothermia, hypotension, and polyneuropathy. Korsakoff's psychosis manifests as retrograde amnesia, anterograde amnesia, and confabulation.

Ref: Jungnickel PW. Alcohol abuse. In: Koda-Kimble MA, Young LY, Kradjan WA, Guglielmo BJ, eds. *Applied Therapeutics: The Clinical Use of Drugs,* 8th edition. Baltimore: Lippincott Williams & Wilkins, 2005:84-11,14.

PATIENT PROFILE 46

BACTEREMIA AND SEPSIS

ANSWERS

1. (E) Patients treated in ICUs are colonized with gram-negative organisms within the first 24 hours of their stay. Patients in a ward other than an ICU are colonized with gram-negative bacilli within 4 days. Lactose-fermenting gram-negative bacilli include the following species: *Enterobacter, Citrobacter, Klebsiella, Listeria, E. coli, Serratia,* and *Proteus.*

Ref: Toltzis P, Glover ML, Reed MD. Lower respiratory tract infections. In: DiPiro JT, Talbert RL, Yee GC, Matzke GR, Wells BG, Posey LM, eds. *Pharmacotherapy: A Pathophysiologic Approach.* 4th ed. Stamford, Conn: Appleton & Lange; 1999:1651–1670.

2. (A) Of the choices provided, a third-generation cephalosporin such as ceftizoxime has the greatest spectrum of activity against lactose-fermenting gramnegative rods. Vancomycin and penicillin cover only gram-positive organisms. Ampicillin, like cefazolin, has limited gram-negative coverage, but ampicillin is the drug of choice in the treatment of patients with *Listeria* infection.

Ref: Gilbert DN, Moellering RC Jr, Sande MA, eds. *The Sanford Guide to Antimicrobial Therapy* 1998. 28th ed. Vienna, Va: Antimicrobial Therapy; 1998:52–54.

3. (A) The presence of non–lactose-fermenting gram-negative bacilli should lead one to believe that *Pseudomonas aeruginosa* is present. For adequate management of *P. aeruginosa* infection, two drug with activity against that

organism should be used. A is the only combination with that kind of activity. Other non–lactose-fermenting gram-negative bacilli, which are seen less frequently, are *Stenotrophomonas* and *Acinetobacter* species.

Ref: Toltzis P, Glover ML, Reed MD. Lower respiratory tract infections. In: DiPiro JT, Talbert RL, Yee GC, Matzke GR, Wells BG, Posey LM, eds. *Pharmacotherapy: A Pathophysiologic Approach.* 4th ed. Stamford, Conn: Appleton & Lange; 1999:1651–1670.

4. (C) Trimethoprim-sulfamethoxazole (Bactrim®) is the drug of choice to manage *Stenotrophomonas* infection. The double gram-negative therapy should be discontinued, and Bactrim® should be started.

Ref: Gilbert DN, Moellering RC Jr, Sande MA, eds. *The Sanford Guide to Antimicrobial Therapy* 1998. 28th ed. Vienna, Va: Antimicrobial Therapy; 1998:50.

5. (D) For treatment of patients with infection by resistant *Stenotrophomonas* organisms, piperacillin-tazobactam may be indicated. Resistant organisms clearly benefit from the use of two drugs with different mechanisms of action. In this case piperacillin-tazobactam works on the cell wall and ciprofloxacin works intracellularly. This combination should provide an additive killing effect.

Ref: Gilbert DN, Moellering RC Jr, Sande MA, eds. *The Sanford Guide to Antimicrobial Therapy* 1998. 28th ed. Vienna, Va: Antimicrobial Therapy; 1998:50.

PATIENT PROFILE 47

CONSTITUTION AND FLOW RATES

ANSWERS

1. (B) 1 g at 200 mg/mL is 5.0 mL final volume. Subtracting 4.6 mL solvent volume gives 0.4 mL powder volume.

   Ref: Stocklosa M, Ansel H. *Pharmaceutical Calculations*. 10th ed. Baltimore: Williams & Wilkins; 1996:171–173.

2. (C) 600 mg × (1 mL/200 mg) = 3.0 mL

   Ref: Stocklosa M, Ansel H. *Pharmaceutical Calculations*. 10th ed. Baltimore: Williams & Wilkins; 1996:172–173.

3. (A) 600 mg is dissolved in a total of 153 mL (IV solution + volume removed from vial). The 3 mL usually is ignored because it is less than 10% of the total volume. The concentration is found by use of these values in the standard concentration forms.

   Ref: Stocklosa M, Ansel H. *Pharmaceutical Calculations*. 10th ed. Baltimore: Williams & Wilkins; 1996:97–109.

4. (B) 60 drops/min × (30 min/150 mL) = 12 drops/mL.

   Ref: Stocklosa M, Ansel H. *Pharmaceutical Calculations*. 10th ed. Baltimore: Williams & Wilkins; 1996:180–182.

5. (C) 600 mg/(150 mL × 12 drops/mL) = 0.33 mg/drop.

   Ref: Stocklosa M, Ansel H. *Pharmaceutical Calculations*. 10th ed. Baltimore: Williams & Wilkins; 1996:180–182.

PATIENT PROFILE 48

HYPERCHOLESTEROLEMIA

ANSWERS

1. (D) Low-density lipoprotein is not directly measured. It is calculated using the formula: LDL = total cholesterol (TC) − high-density lipoprotein (HDL) + triglycerides (TG)/5, where TG has to be <400 mg/dL.

   Ref: *Third Report of the National Cholesterol Education Program (NCEP) Expert Panel on Detection, Evaluation, and Treatment of High Blood Cholesterol in Adults (Adult Treatment Panel III)*. Final report. *Circulation* 2002;106:3143–3421.

2. (B) Smoking and hypertension are the two CHD risk factors.

   Ref: *Third Report of the National Cholesterol Education Program (NCEP) Expert Panel on Detection, Evaluation, and Treatment of High Blood Cholesterol in Adults (Adult Treatment Panel III)*. Final report. *Circulation* 2002;106:3143–3421.

3. (A) Based on JW's number of risk factors and her 10-year risk factor, her goal LDL level is 130 mg/dL.

   Ref: *Third Report of the National Cholesterol Education Program (NCEP) Expert Panel on Detection, Evaluation, and Treatment of High Blood Cholesterol in Adults (Adult Treatment Panel III)*. Final report. *Circulation* 2002;106:3143–3421.

4. (B) HMG CoA reductase inhibitors (statins) have been shown to be the most efficient medications in lowering LDL and reducing mortality.

   Ref: *Third Report of the National Cholesterol Education Program (NCEP) Expert Panel on Detection, Evaluation, and Treatment of High Blood Cholesterol in Adults (Adult Treatment Panel III)*. Final report. *Circulation* 2002;106:3143–3421.

5. (E) Rosuvastatin has been shown to lower LDL levels more than any of the statins available.

   Ref: *Third Report of the National Cholesterol Education Program (NCEP) Expert Panel on Detection, Evaluation, and Treatment of High Blood Cholesterol in Adults (Adult Treatment Panel III)*. Final report. *Circulation* 2002;106:3143–3421.

6. (A) Elevated liver function tests (LFTs) are the most common adverse effects of statin therapy and thus need to be monitored periodically throughout therapy. A baseline LFT panel is required in all patients.

   Ref: *Third Report of the National Cholesterol Education Program (NCEP) Expert Panel on Detection, Evaluation, and Treatment of High Blood Cholesterol in Adults (Adult Treatment Panel III)*. Final report. *Circulation* 2002;106:3143–3421.

7. (C) The lowest initial dose for atorvastatin is 10 mg daily.

   Ref: *Third Report of the National Cholesterol Education Program (NCEP) Expert Panel on Detection, Evaluation, and Treatment of High Blood Cholesterol in Adults (Adult Treatment Panel III)*. Final report. *Circulation* 2002;106:3143–3421.

8. (D) Myopathy is one of the major adverse effects of statins that needs to be monitored throughout therapy.

   Ref: *Third Report of the National Cholesterol Education Program (NCEP) Expert Panel on Detection, Evaluation, and Treatment of High Blood Cholesterol in Adults (Adult Treatment Panel III)*. Final report. *Circulation* 2002;106:3143–3421.

9. (B) Active and chronic liver disease are absolute contraindications to statin therapy. They have been associated with elevating LFTs.

Ref: Third Report of the National Cholesterol Education Program (NCEP) Expert Panel on Detection, Evaluation, and Treatment of High Blood Cholesterol in Adults (Adult Treatment Panel III). Final report. *Circulation* 2002;106:3143–3421.

10. (A) Eighty milligrams daily is the maximum daily dose of lovastatin. It may be given in divided doses.

Ref: Third Report of the National Cholesterol Education Program (NCEP) Expert Panel on Detection, Evaluation, and Treatment of High Blood Cholesterol in Adults (Adult Treatment Panel III). Final report. *Circulation* 2002;106:3143–3421.

PATIENT PROFILE 49

SEXUALLY TRANSMITTED DISEASES

ANSWERS

1. (A) Coinfection with *Chlamydia trachomatis* often occurs among patients with gonococcal infection, and dual therapy is warranted. In the care of patients with a history of noncompliance, azithromycin is an appropriate option for chlamydial coverage, and ceftriaxone is an appropriate option for uncomplicated gonococcal infection.

   Ref: Centers for Disease Control and Prevention. 1998 guidelines for treatment of sexually transmitted diseases. *MMWR Morb Mortal Wkly Rep* 1998;47(RR-1):49-70.

2. (B) Quinolones and tetracyclines should be avoided in pregnancy. A regimen of ceftriaxone for gonococcal coverage and erythromycin base for chlamydial coverage is the most appropriate regimen during pregnancy.

   Ref: Centers for Disease Control and Prevention. 1998 guidelines for treatment of sexually transmitted diseases. *MMWR Morb Mortal Wkly Rep* 1998;47 (RR-1):49–70.

3. (B) Doxycycline is not adequate coverage for trichomoniasis or gonorrhea. Widespread resistance now prevents clinical use of this agent to manage gonorrhea.

   Ref: Centers for Disease Control and Prevention. 1998 guidelines for treatment of sexually transmitted diseases. *MMWR Morb Mortal Wkly Rep* 1998;47(RR-1):49–70.

4. (D) Ceftriaxone is approved for intramuscular administration and provides adequate coverage for gonorrhea but not for chlamydia or trichomoniasis.

   Ref: Centers for Disease Control and Prevention. 1998 guidelines for treatment of sexually transmitted diseases. *MMWR Morb Mortal Wkly Rep* 1998;47(RR-1):49–70.

5. (E) CD should be offered HIV counseling, HIV testing, and education on prevention strategies. Her sex partner(s) should be referred for evaluation.

   Ref: Centers for Disease Control and Prevention. 1998 guidelines for treatment of sexually transmitted diseases. *MMWR Morb Mortal Wkly Rep* 1998;47(RR-1):49–70.

PATIENT PROFILE 50

SOFT TISSUE INFECTIONS

ANSWERS

1. (B) Whenever an animal bite has occurred, one needs to consider the oropharyngeal pathogens of the animal. In general, animal bites are less severe than bites from humans, but infection by *P. multocida* with its delayed onset and high acuity should be considered.

   Ref: Danziger LH, Fish D, Pendlord SL. Skin and soft tissue infections. In: DiPiro JT, Talbert RL, Yee GC, et al, eds. *Pharmacotherapy: A Pathophysiolgoic Approach,* 5th ed. New York: McGraw-Hill, 2002:1894.

   Ref: McCormack JP, Brown G. Traumatic skin and soft tissue infections. In: Koda-Kimble MA, Young LY, eds. *Applied Therapeutics: The Clinical Use of Drugs,* 7th ed. Baltimore: Lippincott Williams & Wilkins, 2001:65-10–65-11.

   Ref: Gilbert DN, Moellering RC Jr, Eliopoulos GM, Sande MA, eds. *The Sanford Guide to Antimicrobial Therapy 2004,* 34th ed. Hyde Park, VT: Antimicrobial Therapy, 2004:35.

2. (D) Rabies and tetanus vaccinations should be considered after all animal bites, especially if the animal is not captured. If the animal is domestic, it usually is captured, and rabies vaccination becomes unnecessary. Hepatitis treatment is not indicated in the management of animal bites.

   Ref: Danziger LH, Fish D, Pendlord SL. Skin and soft tissue infections. In: DiPiro JT, Talbert RL, Yee GC, et al, eds. *Pharmacotherapy: A Pathophysiolgoic Approach,* 5th ed. New York: McGraw-Hill, 2002:1895.

   Ref: McCormack JP, Brown G. Traumatic skin and soft tissue infections. In: Koda-Kimble MA, Young LY, eds. *Applied Therapeutics: The Clinical Use of Drugs,* 7th ed. Baltimore: Lippincott Williams & Wilkins, 2001:65-10–65-11.

3. (C) A mild infection from a dog bite can be managed easily with amoxicillin-clavulanate (Augmentin). This agent covers most gram-positive organisms yet has a limited

gram-negative spectrum and good anaerobic coverage. This broad spectrum is needed to cover organisms that live on the skin and may have been introduced with the bite. It also covers organisms present in the dog's mouth and between its teeth that may have infectious potential.

Ref: Danziger LH, Fish D, Pendlord SL. Skin and soft tissue infections. In: DiPiro JT, Talbert RL, Yee GC, et al, eds. *Pharmacotherapy: A Pathophysiolgoic Approach,* 5th ed. New York: McGraw-Hill, 2002:1895.

Ref: McCormack JP, Brown G. Traumatic skin and soft tissue infections. In: Koda-Kimble MA, Young LY, eds. *Applied Therapeutics: The Clinical Use of Drugs,* 7th ed. Baltimore: Lippincott Williams & Wilkins, 2001:65-10–65-11.

Ref: Gilbert DN, Moellering RC Jr, Eliopoulos GM, Sande MA, eds. *The Sanford Guide to Antimicrobial Therapy 2004,* 34th ed. Hyde Park, VT: Antimicrobial Therapy, 2004:35.

4. (A) Patients who are unable to tolerate β-lactam therapy still need antimicrobial therapy similar to that provided by amoxicillin-clavulanate. Combining clindamycin and

levofloxacin provides a similar spectrum of coverage. Clindamycin covers gram-positive organisms and anaerobic organisms, including *B. fragilis.* Levofloxacin adds additional gram-positive coverage, but its focus is on the gram-negative spectrum. This regiment is not as convenient to take; the twice-daily Augmentin regiment may lead to adherence difficulties.

Ref: Gilbert DN, Moellering RC Jr, Eliopoulos GM, Sande MA, eds. *The Sanford Guide to Antimicrobial Therapy 2004,* 34th ed. Hyde Park, VT: Antimicrobial Therapy, 2004:35.

5. (E) The key is prophylaxis.

Ref: Danziger LH, Fish D, Pendlord SL. Skin and soft tissue infections. In: DiPiro JT, Talbert RL, Yee GC, et al, eds. *Pharmacotherapy: A Pathophysiolgoic Approach,* 5th ed. New York: McGraw-Hill, 2002:1895.

Ref: McCormack JP, Brown G. Traumatic skin and soft tissue infections. In: Koda-Kimble MA, Young LY, eds. *Applied Therapeutics: The Clinical Use of Drugs,* 7th ed. Baltimore: Lippincott Williams & Wilkins, 2001:65-10–65-11.

PATIENT PROFILE 51
ONCOLOGY: COLON CANCER

ANSWERS

1. (C) This regimen (5-FU with leucovorin) causes serious GI toxicity (stomatitis, diarrhea), which differs from the bone marrow suppression effects that occur with weekly low doses of 5-FU.

Ref: Herfindal ET, Gourley DR (eds). *Textbook of Therapeutics, Drug and Disease Management.* 6th ed. Baltimore: Williams & Wilkins; 1996: chapter 82.

2. (A) Optional therapy for colon cancer would still include 5-FU with levamisole substituted for leucovorin.

Ref: Davis LE, Horodysky MM. Colorectal cancer. In: DiPiro JT, Talbert RL, Yee GC, Matzke GR, Wells BG, Posey LM, eds. *Pharmacotherapy: A Pathophysiologic Approach.* 4th ed. Stamford, Conn: Appleton & Lange; 1999:2061–2091.

Ref: Herfindal ET, Gourley DR (eds). *Textbook of Therapeutics, Drug and Disease Management.* 6th ed. Baltimore: Williams & Wilkins; 1996: chapter 82.

3. (B) Tumor marker monitoring is not a good basis for diagnosis but is effective in assessing treatment efficacy.

Ref: Young LY, Koda-Kimble MA, eds. *Applied Therapeutics: The Clinical Use of Drugs.* 6th ed. Vancouver, Wash: Applied Therapeutics; 1995: chapter 93.

Ref: Ravel. Clinical Laboratory Medicine. 3rd ed.

4. (B) The use of megestrol acetate had been shown effective as an appetite stimulant. The use of sertraline would be indicated only if RR's lack of appetite is caused by depression.

Ref: AHFS, 1998 edition

Ref: Young LY, Koda-Kimble MA, eds. *Applied Therapeutics: The Clinical Use of Drugs.* 6th ed. Vancouver, Wash: Applied Therapeutics; 1995: chapter 93.

5. (B) The use of intraarterial infusion will direct the antineoplastic agent to the tumor site and provide the most benefit with the least systemic toxicity.

Ref: Davis LE, Horodysky MM. Colorectal cancer. In: DiPiro JT, Talbert RL, Yee GC, Matzke GR, Wells BG, Posey LM, eds. *Pharmacotherapy: A Pathophysiologic Approach.* 4th ed. Stamford, Conn: Appleton & Lange; 1999:2061–2091.

Ref: Young LY, Koda-Kimble MA, eds. *Applied Therapeutics: The Clinical Use of Drugs.* 6th ed. Vancouver, Wash: Applied Therapeutics; 1995: chapter 93.

PATIENT PROFILE 52

CHLAMYDIA AND EMERGENCY CONTRACEPTION

ANSWERS

1. (C) *C. trachomatis* is an intracellular parasite.

   Ref: Knodel LC. Sexually transmitted diseases. In: DiPiro JT, Talbert RL, Yee GC, et al, eds. *Pharmacotherapy: A Pathophysiologic Approach,* 5th edition. New York: McGraw-Hill, 2002:1997–2016.

2. (B) Azithromycin is the only single-dose therapy that is effective in treating *C. trachomatis*. Amoxicillin, doxycycline, erythromycin, and ofloxacin are all therapeutic choices but are dosed multiple times daily for 7 to 10 days.

   Ref: Knodel LC. Sexually transmitted diseases. In: DiPiro JT, Talbert RL, Yee GC, et al, eds. *Pharmacotherapy: A Pathophysiologic Approach,* 5th edition. New York: McGraw-Hill, 2002:1997–2016.

3. (E) All are accurate patient counseling information for azithromycin. Note the difference in administration recommendations in regard to taking with food for the two azithromycin dosage forms.

   Ref: Azithromycin (drug monograph). In: Klasco RK, ed. DRUGDEX® System. Thomson MICROMEDEX®. Greenwood Village, CO (Edition expires 9/2004).

4. (D) Permanent discoloration of the teeth during tooth development may occur with doxycycline. Arthropathy may occur with ciprofloxacin, disulfiram reaction with metronidazole and alcohol ingestion, kernicterus with sulfonamide administration in infants, and "red man" syndrome with rapid intravenous vancomycin administration.

   Ref: Doxycycline (drug monograph). In: Klasco RK, ed. DRUGDEX® System. Thomson MICROMEDEX®. Greenwood Village, CO (Edition expires 9/2004).

5. (E) All are accurate patient counseling information for doxycycline.

   Ref: Doxycycline (drug monograph). In: Klasco RK, ed. DRUGDEX® System. Thomson MICROMEDEX®. Greenwood Village, CO (Edition expires 9/2004).

6. (D) Treatment with oral therapy is recommended for sex partners to prevent reinfection.

   Ref: STD Facts: Chlamydia. Centers for Disease Control Web site. Available at: *http//www.cdc.gov/std/Chlamydia/STDFact-Chlamydia.htm.* Accessed October 17, 2004.

7. (E) Both Plan B® (product contains two white tablets, each containing 0.75 mg levonorgestrel; urine pregnancy test; and patient information booklet) and Preven® (contains four blue tablets, each containing 0.25 mg levonorgestrel/50 μg ethinyl estradiol) are FDA-approved products packaged for emergency contraception. Ovral® is an oral contraceptive that may be given for emergency contraception at a dose of two tablets followed by two tablets 12 hours after the first dose.

   Ref: Dickerson LM, Bucci KK. Contraception. In: DiPiro JT, Talbert RL, Yee GC, et al, eds. *Pharmacotherapy: A Pathophysiologic Approach,* 5th edition. New York: McGraw-Hill, 2002:1445–1461.

8. (A) The first dose of emergency contraception should be administered within 72 hours of unprotected intercourse. Beyond 72 hours, efficacy declines and is ineffective by 7 days after unprotected intercourse.

   Ref: Dickerson LM, Bucci KK. Contraception. In: DiPiro JT, Talbert RL, Yee GC, et al, eds. *Pharmacotherapy: A Pathophysiologic Approach,* 5th edition. New York: McGraw-Hill, 2002:1445–1461.

9. (B) All regimens for emergency contraception require a second dose administered 12 hours after the first.

   Ref: Dickerson LM, Bucci KK. Contraception. In: DiPiro JT, Talbert RL, Yee GC, et al, eds. *Pharmacotherapy: A Pathophysiologic Approach,* 5th edition. New York: McGraw-Hill, 2002:1445–1461.

10. (E) Emergency contraception may cause nausea, vomiting, and breast tenderness.

    Ref: Dickerson LM, Bucci KK. Contraception. In: DiPiro JT, Talbert RL, Yee GC, et al, eds. *Pharmacotherapy: A Pathophysiologic Approach,* 5th edition. New York: McGraw-Hill, 2002:1445–1461.

PATIENT PROFILE 53

MEDICINAL CHEMISTRY

ANSWER

1. (D) Valium is solubilized for injection with organic solvents (including 10% alcohol and 40% propylene glycol).

Valium injection should not be diluted with other aqueous vehicles to avoid changes in the percentages of organic solvents.

PATIENT PROFILE 54
SEIZURE DISORDERS

ANSWERS

1. (D) Many conditions can lead to seizure disorders such as head trauma, lack of sleep, and fever as well as electrolyte imbalances, hormonal changes, and emotional stress. All of these conditions can lead to seizures by causing fluctuation in the functioning of neurons.

Ref: Gidal BE, Garnett WR, Graves N. Epilepsy. In: DiPiro JT, Talbert RL, Yee GC, et al., eds. *Pharmacotherapy: A Pathophysiologic Approach,* 5th edition. New York: McGraw-Hill, 2002:1031–1060.

2. (C) The first-line drug therapy for tonic-clonic seizures includes valproic acid as well as phenytoin and carbamazepine. Lamotrigine is used as an adjunctive therapy. Phenobarbital is an alternative therapy, and ethosuximide is first line for absence seizures.

Ref: Gidal BE, Garnett WR, Graves N. Epilepsy. In: DiPiro JT, Talbert RL, Yee GC, et al., eds. *Pharmacotherapy: A Pathophysiologic Approach,* 5th edition. New York: McGraw-Hill, 2002:1031–1060.

3. (A) Gastrointestinal upset is a common side effect of valproic acid. Gingival hyperplasia, ataxia, and nystagmus are all adverse effects of phenytoin.

Ref: Gidal BE, Garnett WR, Graves N. Epilepsy. In: DiPiro JT, Talbert RL, Yee GC, et al., eds. *Pharmacotherapy: A Pathophysiologic Approach,* 5th edition. New York: McGraw-Hill, 2002:1031–1060.

4. (B) Salicylates interact with valproic acid by increasing the free concentration. Warfarin, isoniazid, and disulfiram all interact with phenytoin, causing an increase in its concentration.

Ref: Gidal BE, Garnett WR, Graves N. Epilepsy. In: DiPiro JT, Talbert RL, Yee GC, et al., eds. *Pharmacotherapy: A Pathophysiologic Approach,* 5th edition. New York: McGraw-Hill, 2002:1031–1060.

5. (B) The mechanism of action of valproic acid is postulated to be the inhibition of the breakdown of GABA or the stimulation of the synthesis of GABA. It also may increase the action of GABA.

Ref: Gidal BE, Garnett WR, Graves N. Epilepsy. In: DiPiro JT, Talbert RL, Yee GC, et al., eds. *Pharmacotherapy: A Pathophysiologic Approach,* 5th edition. New York: McGraw-Hill, 2002:1031–1060.

6. (C) Depakote® is an enteric coated tablet. This dosage form allows for slower dissolution of the tablet and a decrease in GI distress. Depakene® is available in an IV formulation and a sprinkle capsule. The dosing interval for both is the same.

Ref: Gidal BE, Garnett WR, Graves N. Epilepsy. In: DiPiro JT, Talbert RL, Yee GC, et al., eds. *Pharmacotherapy: A Pathophysiologic Approach,* 5th edition. New York: McGraw-Hill, 2002:1031–1060.

7. (D) The mechanism of action of lamotrigine is best described by its ability to impede sodium channels and calcium channels and prevent the release of glutamate as well as aspartate.

Ref: Gidal BE, Garnett WR, Graves N. Epilepsy. In: DiPiro JT, Talbert RL, Yee GC, et al., eds. *Pharmacotherapy: A Pathophysiologic Approach,* 5th edition. New York: McGraw-Hill, 2002:1031–1060.

8. (D) Diplopia (double vision) is an adverse effect of lamotrigine. Other adverse effects include drowsiness, ataxia, rash, and headache. Lamotrigine also can cause tremor when prescribed in combination with valproic acid.

Ref: Gidal BE, Garnett WR, Graves N. Epilepsy. In: DiPiro JT, Talbert RL, Yee GC, et al., eds. *Pharmacotherapy: A Pathophysiologic Approach,* 5th edition. New York: McGraw-Hill, 2002:1031–1060.

9. (B) When combined with valproic acid the dose of lamotrigine must be decreased because of enzyme inhibition by valproic acid, which affects the metabolism of lamotrigine.

Ref: Gidal BE, Garnett WR, Graves N. Epilepsy. In: DiPiro JT, Talbert RL, Yee GC, et al., eds. *Pharmacotherapy: A Pathophysiologic Approach,* 5th edition. New York: McGraw-Hill, 2002:1031–1060.

10. (C) Lorazepam is the preferred benzodiazepine for the treatment of status epilepticus, even though it is not Food and Drug Administration approved for this use. Lorazepam is less lipophilic than diazepam, allowing it to stay in the brain longer. Even though the time it takes for the seizures to stop is faster with diazepam there is less of a need for additional drug therapy with lorazepam.

Ref: Phelps SJ, Hovinga CA, Boucher BA. Status epilepticus. In: DiPiro JT, Talbert RL, Yee GC, et al., eds. *Pharmacotherapy: A Pathophysiologic Approach,* 5th edition. New York: McGraw-Hill, 2002:1061–1076.

MAJOR DEPRESSION

ANSWERS

1. (E) According to the *Diagnostic and Statistical Manual of Mental Disorders*, symptoms of depression include depressed mood, markedly diminished interest or pleasure, decrease or increase in appetite, insomnia or hypersomnia, psychomotor agitation or retardation, fatigue, feelings of worthlessness, decrease in ability to concentrate, and recurrent thoughts of death.

   Ref: American Psychiatric Association. *Diagnostic and Statistical Manual of Mental Disorders.* 4th ed. Washington, DC: American Psychiatric Association, 1994.

2. (D) Use of medications such as oral contraceptives and medical conditions such as hypothyroidism can cause depression.

   Ref: Young LY, Koda-Kimble MA, eds. *Applied Therapeutics: The Clinical Use of Drugs.* 6th ed. Vancouver, Wash: Applied Therapeutics; 1995: chapter 76.

3. (A) Fluoxetine would be the best choice for BC because of its lack of anti-cholinergic properties, which have a negative effect on the patients GERD.

   Ref: *Goodman and Gilman's The Pharmacologic Basis of Therapeutics.* 9th ed. New York: McGraw-Hill; 1996: chapter 19.

4. (E) Patients may have some symptomatic improvement in the first week, but full response is generally not recognized until 4 to 6 weeks later. Therefore all efficacy trials should continue for 6 weeks before it is concluded that treatment has failed.

   Ref: American Psychiatric Association. Practice guideline for major depressive disorder in adults. *Am J Psychiatry* 1993;150(suppl 4):1–26.

5. (B) Pharmacologic treatment should continue for 10–12 months after resolution of depressive symptoms.

   Ref: American Psychiatric Association. *Textbook of Psychopharmacology.* Washington, DC: American Psychiatric Press; 1995: chapter 28.

PEDIATRIC IMMUNIZATIONS

ANSWERS

1. (B) A family history of seizures or other central nervous system disorders are not contraindications to the vaccine.

   Ref: Luedtke S, Condren M, Haase M. Pediatric immunizations In: Koda-Kimble MA, Young LY, Kradjan WA, et al., eds. *Applied Therapeutics: The Clinical Use of Drugs,* 8th edition. Baltimore: Lippincott Williams & Wilkins, 2005:95-1–95-14.

2. (A) Some parents are concerned that the MMR vaccine may cause autism. Because of the rise in the incidence of autism as well as the development of autistic symptoms around the time of vaccination, it was suggested that MMR vaccination may cause autism. However, multiple epidemiologic studies have shown no correlation between vaccination and the development of autism.

   Ref: Luedtke S, Condren M, Haase M. Pediatric immunizations. In: Koda-Kimble MA, Young LY, Kradjan WA, et al., eds. *Applied Therapeutics: The Clinical Use of Drugs,* 8th edition. Baltimore: Lippincott Williams & Wilkins, 2005:95-1–95-14.

3. (D) Varicella vaccine contains live attenuated virus. The pneumococcal polysaccharide, meningococcal polysaccharide and DTaP vaccines all contain killed viruses.

   Ref: Bertino JS, Mayney MS. Vaccines, toxoids, and other immunobiologics. In: Dipiro JT, Talbert RL, Yee GC, et al., eds. *Pharmacotherapy: A Pathophysiologic Approach,* 5th edition. New York: McGraw-Hill, 2002:2123–2149.

4. (A) Contraindications to live attenuated vaccines include allergic reaction to previous exposure to vaccine components, immunosuppression (immunosuppressive therapy, immunodeficiency), recent administration of blood products, encephalopathy, and pregnancy. Premature infants should be vaccinated at the same chronologic age using the same schedule and precautions as full-term infants. Patients with chronic pulmonary, renal, hepatic, or metabolic disease who are not receiving immunosuppressants may receive both live attenuated and killed vaccines and toxoids. Aerosol steroids are not considered contraindications to immunization. Only patients receiving high-dose corticosteroids for greater than 2 weeks should wait 3 months before receiving immunization with a live attenuated virus.

   Ref: Luedtke S, Condren M, Haase M. Pediatric immunizations. In: Koda-Kimble MA, Young LY, Kradjan WA, et al., eds. *Applied Therapeutics: The Clinical Use of Drugs,* 8th edition. Baltimore: Lippincott Williams & Wilkins, 2005:95-1–95-14.

5. (B) OPV should only be used in cases of acute outbreaks of polio because it carries the risk of vaccine-associated paralytic polio (VAPP), especially after the first dose; in contrast, IPV has not been associated with VAPP. The first dose of MMR should not be given before the age of 12 months. HiB has led to a 95% reduction in the incidence of HiB disease in children younger than 5 years of age; therefore, it should be routinely given as part of childhood immunizations.

Ref: Luedtke S, Condren M, Haase M. Pediatric immunizations. In: Koda-Kimble MA, Young LY, Kradjan WA, et al., eds. *Applied Therapeutics: The Clinical Use of Drugs,* 8th edition. Baltimore: Lippincott Williams & Wilkins, 2005:95-1–95-14.

6. (C) Allergies to streptomycin, polymyxin B, and neomycin are contraindications to IPV use.

Ref: Bertino JS, Mayney MS. Vaccines, toxoids, and other immunobiologics. In: Dipiro JT, Talbert RL, Yee GC, et al., eds. *Pharmacotherapy: A Pathophysiologic Approach,* 5th edition. New York: McGraw-Hill, 2002:2123–2149.

7. (C) Measles, mumps, and rubella vaccine contains live virus; therefore, they should not be given to pregnant women or immunosuppressed patients, including patients with HIV. Although derived from chick embryo fibroblasts, the risk of measles vaccine administration to egg-allergic patients is exceedingly low; therefore, individuals in need of the vaccine should receive it, regardless of the history of egg allergy.

Ref: Bertino JS, Mayney MS. Vaccines, toxoids, and other immunobiologics. In: Dipiro JT, Talbert RL, Yee GC, et al., eds. *Pharmacotherapy: A Pathophysiologic Approach,* 5th edition. New York: McGraw-Hill, 2002:2123–2149.

8. (D) ProHIBiT is the *Haemophilus influenzae* type b diphtheria toxoid conjugate vaccine.

Ref: Bertino JS, Mayney MS. Vaccines, toxoids, and other immunobiologics. In: Dipiro JT, Talbert RL, Yee GC, et al., eds. *Pharmacotherapy: A Pathophysiologic Approach,* 5th edition. New York: McGraw-Hill, 2002:2123–2149.

9. (C) Live measles vaccine may suppress a positive tuberculin skin test for up to 6 weeks after administration.

Ref: Bertino JS, Mayney MS. Vaccines, toxoids, and other immunobiologics. In: Dipiro JT, Talbert RL, Yee GC, et al., eds. *Pharmacotherapy: A Pathophysiologic Approach,* 5th edition. New York: McGraw-Hill, 2002:2123–2149.

10. (B) Vaccines and toxoids containing inactivated bacteria often are combined with aluminum salts to increase their immunogenicity by prolonging antigen exposure. These adjuvants increase local tissue irritation where injected.

Ref: Bertino JS, Mayney MS. Vaccines, toxoids, and other immunobiologics. In: Dipiro JT, Talbert RL, Yee GC, et al., eds. *Pharmacotherapy: A Pathophysiologic Approach,* 5th edition. New York: McGraw-Hill, 2002:2123–2149.

PATIENT PROFILE 57
RENAL TRANSPLANTATION

ANSWERS

1. (D) Cyclosporine interacts with the HMG-CoA reductase inhibitors and may cause myopathy.

2. (B) Atorvastatin has the least potential effect on the cytochrome P450 enzyme in the liver and has the least potential for interaction with Neoral®.

3. (D) Immunosuppressive agents such as mycophenolate mofetil (CellCept®) must be taken long term on a daily basis to avoid allograft rejection. Gastrointestinal side effects commonly are associated with use of the drug and are managed by means of administering the daily dose tid rather than bid or by means of reducing the total daily dose under the direction of the prescribing physician.

4. (A) One of the most serious side effects of long-term use of steroids is hip necrosis.

Ref: Dupuis RE. Solid organ transplantation. In: Young LY, Koda-Kimble MA, eds. *Applied Therapeutics: The Clinical Use of Drugs.* 6th ed. Vancouver, Wash: Applied Therapeutics; 1995: chapter 33.

Ref: Tsunoda SM, Aweeka FT. Solid organ transplantation. In: Herfindal ET, Gourley DR (eds). *Textbook of Therapeutics, Drug and Disease Management.* 6th ed. Baltimore: Williams & Wilkins; 1996: chapter 96.

PATIENT PROFILE 58

ACNE

ANSWERS

1. (E) All three factors might exacerbate acne. Phenytoin is a known trigger that may exacerbate acne. Oil-based products are known to exacerbate acne by occluding the skin. DW's helmet may lead to acne by causing friction and obstruction of her forehead.

    Ref: Feldman S, Careccia RE, Barham KL, Hancox J. Diagnosis and treatment of acne. *Am Fam Physician* 2004;69:2123–2130.

2. (E) Mechanical irritation may occur while DW is playing the violin and the instrument is held next to her chin (the piano would not cause a problem). Chocolate has not been proved to cause acne. Gentle cleansing at least twice a day is recommended; vigorous scrubbing will not improve acne. Sexual activity does not exacerbate acne. Manipulating comedones may lead to scarring.

    Ref: Billow JA. Acne. In: Berardi RR, ed. *Handbook of Nonprescription Drugs,* 14th edition. Washington, DC: American Pharmacists Association, 2002:913–928.

3. (D) Ortho Tri-Cyclen® is approved by the Food and Drug Administration for the treatment of moderate acne. It contains ethinyl estradiol and norgestimate. Androgens play a role in the pathogenesis of acne; ethinyl estradiol has antiandrogenic effects and may improve acne. Norgestimate is a progestin with low androgenic activity. The other oral contraceptives listed have high androgenic activity and may exacerbate acne.

    Ref: Seaton TL. Acne. In: Koda-Kimble MA, Young LY, Kradjan WA, et al., eds. *Applied Therapeutics: The Clinical Use of Drugs,* 8th ed. Baltimore: Lippincott Williams & Wilkins, 2005:1–12.

4. (A) A closed comedone is formed when sebum is trapped under a blocked follicle. Engorged closed comedones form closed macrocomedones. Pustules are filled with pus and have a white tip. Papules are caused by an inflammatory reaction, these are solid and are red and raised in appearance. An open comedone is more commonly known as a blackhead.

    Ref: Gollnick H. Current concepts of the pathogenesis of acne. *Drugs* 2003;62:1579–1596.

5. (C) Several formulations of benzoyl peroxide are available without a prescription. Brand names for over-the-counter benzoyl peroxide include: Benoxyl 5 Lotion®, Clearasil Vanishing Acne Treatment Cream®, Dryoxy Gel®, and Oxy 10®. All other products listed require a prescription.

    Ref: Billow JA. Acne. In: Berardi RR, ed. *Handbook of Nonprescription Drugs,* 14th edition. Washington, DC: American Pharmacists Association, 2002:913–928.

6. (B) Most acne treatments may take 1 to 2 months to be effective. Therapy should not be altered for 1 to 2 months.

    Ref: Seaton TL. Acne. In: Koda-Kimble MA, Young LY, Kradjan WA, et al., eds. *Applied Therapeutics: The Clinical Use of Drugs,* 8th ed. Baltimore: Lippincott Williams & Wilkins, 2005:1–12.

7. (C) Isotretinoin is a known teratogen; use of this drug during pregnancy may cause birth defects. Cheilitis (chapped lips) is a common side effect of isotretinoin. Isotretinoin does not cause infertility.

    Ref: Accutane® (isotretinoin) capsules (product information). Nutley, NJ: Roche, August 2003.

    Ref: Seaton TL. Acne. In: Koda-Kimble MA, Young LY, Kradjan WA, et al., eds. *Applied Therapeutics: The Clinical Use of Drugs,* 8th ed. Baltimore: Lippincott Williams & Wilkins, 2005: 1–12.

8. (A) The brand name of isotretinoin capsules is Accutane®; it is manufactured and distributed by Roche Pharmaceuticals. Benzamycin® is a topical combination product containing benzoyl peroxide and erythromycin. Differin® is the brand name of topical adapalene. Minocin® is the brand name of minocycline capsules. Retin-A® is a topical retinoid, tretinoin.

    Ref: Seaton TL. Acne. In: Koda-Kimble MA, Young LY, Kradjan WA, et al., eds. *Applied Therapeutics: The Clinical Use of Drugs,* 8th ed. Baltimore: Lippincott Williams & Wilkins, 2005:1–12.

9. (E) All statements are true. Prescriptions for isotretinoin must comply with the *System to Manage Accutane Related Teratogenicity* (SMART). Other components of this system require the pharmacist to: ensure that each prescription has a yellow qualification sticker, dispense a maximum of 30 days supply, also, an Accutane Medication Guide® must accompany every prescription dispensed.

    Ref: Accutane® (isotretinoin) capsules (product information). Nutley, NJ: Roche, August 2003.

10. (C) Statements I and II are correct. Salicylic acid is effective as a keratolytic, but is less effective than benzoyl peroxide.

    Ref: Seaton TL. Acne. In: Koda-Kimble MA, Young LY, Kradjan WA, et al., eds. *Applied Therapeutics: The Clinical Use of Drugs,* 8th ed. Baltimore: Lippincott Williams & Wilkins, 2005:1–12.

PATIENT PROFILE 59

CORONARY ARTERY DISEASE

ANSWERS

1. (D) An increase in serum drug concentrations of theophylline after smoking cessation can stimulate the heart and increase myocardial oxygen demand.

   Ref: Talbert RL. Ischemic heart disease. In: DiPiro JT, Talbert RL, Yee GC, Matzke GR, Wells BG, Posey LM, eds. *Pharmacotherapy: A pathophysiologic approach.* 4th ed. Stamford, Conn: Appleton & Lange; 1999:182–210.

2. (C) β-Blockers are relatively contraindicated because of COPD, and longterm nitrate therapy should never be used as monotherapy for CAD.

   Ref: Talbert RL. Ischemic heart disease. In: DiPiro JT, Talbert RL, Yee GC, Matzke GR, Wells BG, Posey LM, eds. *Pharmacotherapy: A pathophysiologic approach.* 4th ed. Stamford, Conn: Appleton & Lange; 1999:182–210.

3. (A) HCTZ increases uric acid levels.

   Ref: AHFS Drug Information, 1998.

4. (C) Niacin may increase uric acid levels and precipitate an attack of gout.

   Ref: Talbert RL. Ischemic heart disease. In: DiPiro JT, Talbert RL, Yee GC, Matzke GR, Wells BG, Posey LM, eds. *Pharmacotherapy: A pathophysiologic approach.* 4th ed. Stamford, Conn: Appleton & Lange; 1999:182–210.

5. (C) Clopidogrel is an effective alternative to ASA in the prevention of AMI.

   Ref: Talbert RL. Ischemic heart disease. In: DiPiro JT, Talbert RL, Yee GC, Matzke GR, Wells BG, Posey LM, eds. *Pharmacotherapy: A pathophysiologic approach.* 4th ed. Stamford, Conn: Appleton & Lange; 1999:182–210.

PATIENT PROFILE 60

INHALATION ANTHRAX

ANSWERS

1. (A) Category A. According to CDC guidelines these pathogens are easy to disseminate and can be transmitted easily from person to person. They have a high mortality rate and have a major public health impact. Also, special action for public health preparedness is necessary. Anthrax fills all of these conditions.

   Ref: CDC update. Investigation of anthrax associated with intentional exposure and interim public health guidelines. *MMWR* 2001a;50(41):889–897.

   Ref: Sifton D. *PDR Guide to Biological and Chemical Warfare Response,* 1st edition. Montvale, NJ: Thompson, 2003.

   Ref: Weinstein R, Alibek K. *Biological and Chemical Terrorism: A Guide for Healthcare Providers and First Responders.* New York: Thieme, 2003.

2. (E) Diagnosis can be made with chest x-rays showing a widening of mediastinum, mediastinal adenopathy, with or without pleural effusions. You may or may not have infiltrates. Cultures grow gram-positive rods after 12 hours.

   Ref: Weinstein R, Alibek K. *Biological and Chemical Terrorism: A Guide for Healthcare Providers and First Responders.* New York: Thieme, 2003.

3. (C) *Bacillus anthracis,* which is an encapsulated gram-positive rod. *Bacillus anthracis* is a spore-forming bacterium that can survive for many years in the spore form.

Once the spore is in a host it changes to a vegetative form, quickly multiplying in the host.

   Ref: Sifton D. *PDR Guide to Biological and Chemical Warfare Response,* 1st edition. Montvale, NJ: Thompson, 2003.

   Ref: Weinstein R, Alibek K. *Biological and Chemical Terrorism: A Guide for Healthcare Providers and First Responders.* New York: Thieme, 2003.

4. (E) Doxycycline 100 mg IV q12 and rifampin 600 mg PO qd. Treatment guidelines per the CDC recommend several different options: ciprofloxacin 400 mg IV q12 hours *or* doxycycline 100 mg IV q12 hours *plus* rifampin 600 mg PO qd *or* clindamycin 900 mg IV q8 *or* vancomycin 1g IV q12 *or* imipenem 500 mg IM or IV q6 *or* ampicillin 500 mg IV q6 *or* clarithromycin 500 mg PO q12 along with fluid replacement and respiratory support.

   Ref: Sifton D. *PDR Guide to Biological and Chemical Warfare Response,* 1st edition. Montvale, NJ: Thompson, 2003.

   Ref: Weinstein R, Alibek K. *Biological and Chemical Terrorism: A Guide for Healthcare Providers and First Responders.* New York: Thieme, 2003.

5. (C) 60 days. CDC guidelines recommend treatment for 60 days. Once the patient is stable a switch from IV to PO medications can be made.

   Ref: CDC update. Investigation of anthrax associated with intentional exposure and interim public health guidelines. *MMWR* 2001a;50(41):889–897.

Ref: Sifton D. *PDR Guide to Biological and Chemical Warfare Response,* 1st edition. Montvale, NJ: Thompson, 2003.

Ref: Weinstein R, Alibek K. *Biological and Chemical Terrorism: A Guide for Healthcare Providers and First Responders.* New York: Thieme, 2003.

6. (A) 1 to 14 days. The typical incubation period for inhalation anthrax is 1 to 14 days, with occasional rare cases up to 60 days. The greater the number of bacterium exposed to the shorter the incubation period.

Ref: Centers for Disease Control and Prevention. Investigation of bioterrorism-related anthrax & interim guidelines for clinical evaluation of person with possible anthrax, *MMWR* 2001;50(43):941–948. *www.cdc.gov.* Accessed 10/25/2004.

Ref: Sifton D. *PDR Guide to Biological and Chemical Warfare Response,* 1st edition. Montvale, NJ: Thompson, 2003.

Ref: Weinstein R, Alibek K. *Biological and Chemical Terrorism: A Guide for Healthcare Providers and First Responders.* New York: Thieme, 2003.

7. (D) Both ciprofloxacin and doxycylcine are suitable options. Amoxicillin 500 mg PO q8 hours also is another acceptable option.

Ref: Centers for Disease Control and Prevention. Investigation of bioterrorism-related anthrax & interim guidelines for clinical evaluation of person with possible anthrax, *MMWR* 2001;50(43): 941–948. *www.cdc.gov.* Accessed 10/25/2004.

Ref: Sifton D. *PDR Guide to Biological and Chemical Warfare Response,* 1st edition. Montvale, NJ: Thompson, 2003.

Ref: Weinstein R, Alibek K. *Biological and Chemical Terrorism: A Guide for Healthcare Providers and First Responders.* New York: Thieme, 2003.

8. (D) 0, 2, and 4 weeks, and then 6, 12, and 18 months followed by yearly boosters for military personnel. The vaccine regimen consists of six 0.5-mL doses administered subcutaneously.

Ref: US Army. *USAMRIID'S Medical Management of Biological Casualties Handbook.* Fort Detrick, MD, 2001.

9. (C) I, II, and III are important counseling points for the postal employees. All employees need to complete the full course of therapy and should take the medication with a full glass of water. Use of antacids and iron products with ciprofloxacin and doxycycline should be avoided while taking these medications. If one is unable to avoid antacids or iron-containing products while on either medication, the dose of antibiotic should be separated by 2 hours *after* taking the antacid/iron product. Antacid/iron products should be avoided within 6 hours *before* taking ciprofloxacin and 2 hours with doxycycline. Although, ciprofoxacin has been shown to increase caffeine concentrations leading to increased central nervous system stimulation, it is not contraindicated. Excessive use of caffeine should be avoided.

Ref: Thomson MicroMedex. Micromedex® Healthcare Series Vol. 121. Expires 12/2004. *http://micromedex/ciprofloxacin/ overview.* Accessed 10/25/2004.

10. (C) Cutaneous anthrax is the most deadly form of anthrax. If untreated cutaneous anthrax has a 20% mortality rate. Inhalation anthrax has a 100% mortality rate if untreated. The CDC controls the anthrax vaccine. There are multiple forms of anthrax: inhalation, oropharnyngeal, gastrointestinal, and cutaneous.

Ref: Centers for Disease Control and Prevention. Investigation of bioterrorism-related anthrax & interim guidelines for clinical evaluation of person with possible anthrax, *MMWR* 2001;50(43): 941–948. *www.cdc.gov.* Accessed 10/25/2004.

Ref: Weinstein R, Alibek K. *Biological and Chemical Terrorism: A Guide for Healthcare Providers and First Responders.* New York: Thieme, 2003.

PATIENT PROFILE 61

DIABETES MELLITUS

ANSWERS

1. (B) A fasting plasma glucose level $\geq$126 mg/dL measured on subsequent days meets criteria for the diagnosis of diabetes mellitus. Fasting is defined as no caloric intake for at least 8 hours.

Ref: The Expert Committee on the Diagnosis and Classification of Diabetes Mellitus. Report of the Expert Committee on the Diagnosis and Classification of Diabetes Mellitus. *Diabetes Care* 1997;20: 1183–1194.

2. (D) Glipizide or glyburide may be used in the initial management of diabetes mellitus type II. Glucagon increases blood glucose concentrations by means of stimulating hepatic glucogenolysis.

Ref: American Hospital Formulary Service. Glipizide, glyburide, glucagon. Bethesda, Md: American Society of Health-System Pharmacists; 1999:2737, 2742, 2754.

3. (E) Palpitations, tachycardia, tremor, and confusion are blocked by the action propranolol, but sweating is not.

Ref: American Hospital Formulary Service. Propranolol. Bethesda, Md: American Society of Health-System Pharmacists; 1999:1499.

4. (E) The glucose from three glucose tablets, 1 cup of milk, ½ cup of juice or soda, or 1 tablespoon of sugar should help a patient with hypoglycemia.

Ref: Koda-Kimble MA, Carlisle BA. Diabetes mellitus. In: Young LY, Koda-Kimble MA, eds. *Applied Therapeutics: The Clinical Use of Drugs.* 6th ed. Vancouver, Wash: Applied Therapeutics; 1995:48-1–48-62.

PATIENT PROFILE 62

DEPRESSION

ANSWERS

1. (C) Venlafaxine. It has been shown that venlafaxine has a dose-dependent risk of increasing blood pressure; therefore, it is potentially less safe in a person with hypertension.

Ref: Schatzberg AF, Nemeroff CB, eds. *Essentials of Clinical Psychopharmacology.* Washington, DC: American Psychiatric Publishing, 2001.

2. (D) Amitriptyline. Amitriptyline is highly anticholinergic, which can worsen reflux. The other choices have minimal to no anticholinergic effects.

Ref: Schatzberg AF, Nemeroff CB, eds. *Essentials of Clinical Psychopharmacology.* Washington, DC: American Psychiatric Publishing, 2001.

3. (A) Mirtazapine is an alpha 2 antagonist while clonidine is an α_2 agonist.

Ref: Micromedex. Accessed 2004.

4. (B) Trazodone has potent antagonistic effects at the histamine 1 receptor that results in sedation.

Ref: Stahl S, ed. *Essential Psychopharmacology,* 2nd edition. New York: Cambridge University Press, 2000.

5. (A) Mirtazapine has been shown to increase total cholesterol.

Ref: Schatzberg AF, Nemeroff CB, eds. *Essentials of Clinical Psychopharmacology.* Washington, DC: American Psychiatric Publishing, 2001.

PATIENT PROFILE 63

SEIZURE DISORDERS

ANSWERS

1. (D) Febrile seizures are common in childhood. They may occur among as many as 5% of patients from 6 months to 6 years of age.

Ref: Seizure disorders. In: Young LY, Koda-Kimble MA, eds. *Applied Therapeutics: The Clinical Use of Drugs.* 6th ed. Vancouver, Wash: Applied Therapeutics; 1995: chapter 52.

2. (A) Because this child's condition is stable, no drug therapy is needed. However, fever reduction will help reduce the risk of further seizures.

Ref: Seizure disorders. In: Young LY, Koda-Kimble MA, eds. *Applied Therapeutics: The Clinical Use of Drugs.* 6th ed. Vancouver, Wash: Applied Therapeutics; 1995: chapter 52.

3. (C) Although a cause and effect relationship has not been clearly established, phenobarbital therapy has been reported to impair learning and intellectual quotient scores.

Ref: Graves NM, Garnett WR. Epilepsy. In: DiPiro JT, Talbert RL, Yee GC, Matzke GR, Wells BG, Posey LM, eds. *Pharmacotherapy: A Pathophysiologic Approach.* 4th ed. Stamford, Conn: Appleton & Lange; 1999:952–975.

4. (E) Diazepam is rapidly absorbed when administered rectally and is now commercially available in a rectal dosage form.

Ref: Seizure disorders. In: Young LY, Koda-Kimble MA, eds. *Applied Therapeutics: The Clinical Use of Drugs.* 6th ed. Vancouver, Wash: Applied Therapeutics; 1995: chapter 52.

5. (E) Soon after it became commercially available, there were reports of serious hepatotoxicity and aplastic anemia associated with felbamate. The drug remains on the market for patients refractory to other agents.

Ref: Seizure disorders. In: Herfindal ET, Gourley DR, eds. *Textbook of Therapeutics, Drug and Disease Management.* 6th ed. Baltimore: Williams & Wilkins; 1996: chapter 50.

PATIENT PROFILE 64

BACTEREMIA AND SEPSIS

ANSWERS

1. (A) Endocarditis can be caused by a variety of organisms. The most common are *Staphylococcus aureus* and *Streptococcus viridans*. Nafcillin with gentamicin is the only choice that provides adequate coverage against these organisms. Nafcillin, a cell-wall antibiotic, retains excellent activity against *S. aureus* and will cover most strains of *Streptococcus*. The synergistic combination with gentamicin in low doses is indicated for the initial treatment of patients with this life-threatening infection.

Ref: Berbari EF, Cockerill FR 3rd, Steckelberg JM. Infective endocarditis due to unusual or fastidious microorganisms. *Mayo Clin Proc* 1997;72:532–542.

2. (E) Rifampin has excellent activity against gram-positive organisms. Rifampin always should be used in combination with other antibiotics because it is susceptible to resistance fairly rapidly. When rifampin is used in combination with vancomycin, however, to treat patients with endocarditis, the synergistic benefits prevail.

Ref: Wilson WR, Karchmer AW, Dajani AS, et al. Antibiotic treatment of adults with infective endocarditis due to streptococci, enterococci, and HACEK microorganisms. American Heart Association. *JAMA* 1995;274:1706–1713.

3. (E) All of these effects should be monitored when a patient receives IV nafcillin.

Ref: Gilbert DN, Moellering RC Jr, Sande MA, eds. *The Sanford Guide to Antimicrobial Therapy* 1998. 28th ed. Vienna, Va: Antimicrobial Therapy; 1998:64.

4. (A) According to current guidelines for endocarditis prophylaxis before dental procedures, amoxicillin is the drug of choice because of its good bioavailability and low side effect profile.

Ref: Dajani AS, Taubert KA, Wilson W, et al. Prevention of bacterial endocarditis: recommendations by the American Heart Association. *JAMA* 1997;277:1794–1801.

5. (B) The presence of organisms that are resistant to penicillin does not preclude the use of penicillins provided that the resistance is low or of intermediate level. In this instance, however, the dose of penicillin should be increased to overcome the resistance.

Ref: Wilson WR, Karchmer AW, Dajani AS, et al. Antibiotic treatment of adults with infective endocarditis due to streptococci, enterococci, and HACEK microorganisms. American Heart Association. *JAMA* 1995;274:1706–1713.

PATIENT PROFILE 65

DIABETES

ANSWERS

1. (B) Combinations of antipsychotics and antidepressants can result in cardiotoxicity (QT-prolongation and torsades de pointes); thus, safer options can be explored first before using desipramine, amitriptyline, or fluphenazine that are appropriate first-line choices when patients do not have documented QT prolongation. Capsaicin cream or gel may be effective but is inconvenient because it requires three applications per day to adequately deplete substance P. Topiramate is a new option for the treatment of neuropathic pain that does not interact with JP's current medications and does not predispose her for risk of cardiotoxicity.

Ref: Chong MS, Libretto SE. The rationale and use of topiramate for treating neuropathic pain. *Clin J Pain* 2003;1:59–68.

Ref: Roden DM. Drug-induced prolongation of the QT interval. *N Engl J Med* 2004;350:1013–1022.

2. (C) Glimepiride is a major substrate of CYP 2C8/2C9. It is a newer sulfonylurea that stimulates insulin output from pancreatic ß-islet cells and may decrease hepatic glucose output from gluconeogenesis. It is only approved for type II diabetes because patients with type I diabetes have lost pancreatic ß-islet cell activity and the capability to produce endogenous insulin. Most importantly, sulfonylureas along with all oral medications for the treatment of diabetes require vigilant attention to diet and lifestyle to achieve and maintain control of HbA1c and prevent macrovascular and microvascular complications.

Ref: Glimepiride (Amaryl® [product information]. Aventis Pharmaceuticals.

3. (D) JP has limited exercise options because of fibromyalgia. Therefore, drug therapy must be maximized early to prevent early microvascular and ultimately macrovascular complications. Glimepiride monotherapy has been in place for 4 years and she continues to gain weight without real improvements in her blood glucose. Glimepiride alone will not help to bring her HbA1c to a desired target of ≤6.5. Dual therapy with metformin is the best option for JP because sulfonylurea and nonsulfonylurea secretagogues (nateglinide and repaglinide) do not produce reliable glucose control, and the combination is associated with frequent drug-induced hypoglycemia. Sulfonylureas and metformin reduce microvascular complications from diabetes, but only metformin reduces all-cause mortality in patients with diabetes.

Ref: Inzucchi SE. Oral antihyperglycemic therapy for type 2 diabetes. Scientific review. *JAMA* 2002;287:360–372.

4. **(B)** The Friedewald formula is commonly used to calculate LDL values when patients are in a fasting state (no food intake within 8 to 12 hours prior to the test). Patients who are not in a fasting state need a direct LDL measurement to correctly identify LDL levels. Patients with triglycerides >400 mg/dL also cannot have LDL accurately calculated with a Friedewald formula, nor does a direct LDL provide truly accurate results.

LDL-C = TC − HDL-C − (TG/5)
LDL-C = 250 − 50 − (300/5)
LDL-C = 140 mg/dL

Ref: McKenney JM. Dyslipidemias, atherosclerosis and coronary heart disease. In: Koda-Kimble MA, Young LY, Kradjan WA, Guglielmo BJ, eds. *Applied Therapeutics: The Clinical Use of Drugs,* 8th edition. Vancouver, WA: Applied Therapeutics, 2005:13–17.

5. **(A)** JP's risk factors, including uncontrolled diabetes, smoking, and metabolic syndrome, characterize her as being at a high risk for developing coronary disease in the future. New updates to the ATP III issued in 2004 summarize and provide new evidence that LDL-C levels ≤70 mg/dL are the ideal therapeutic target in patients with diabetes.

Ref: Grundy SM, Cleeman JI, Merz CNB, et al. Implications of recent clinical trials for the National Cholesterol Education Program Adult Treatment Panel III Guidelines. *Circulation* 2004;110: 227–239.

6. **(E)** The ATP III specifies that the primary target in a mixed hyperlipidemia is LDL-C. Gemfibrozil is reserved for patients who need a reduction in TG ≤150 mg/dL, often in addition to LDL-C reduction. Gemfibrozil can reduce LDL-C by 10%, reduce TG by 35%, and increase HDL by 10%. Niacin may reduce TG by 26% and decrease total cholesterol by 10%. Colestipol often is used as an adjunct because it may reduce LDL-C by 10% alone and is insufficient to reduce LDL-C to goal in the majority of patients. Simvastatin 40 mg was used in the Heart Protection Study (HPS) in patients with established coronary disease or a coronary heart disease (CHD) equivalent and was found to have an absolute risk reduction of any major cardiovascular event (nonfatal myocardial infarction, coronary death, nonfatal stroke, fatal stroke, coronary revascularization, and peripheral revascularization) of 5.4%. Treating 19 patients with simvastatin 40 mg daily for 5 years prevents one major cardiovascular event. JP has a CHD equivalent (diabetes) and may observe a LDL-C reduction of up to 70 mg/dL as observed in the HPS, bringing JP to her LDL-C target.

Ref: Heart Protection Study Collaborative Group. MRC/BHF Heart Protection Study of cholesterol lowering with simvastatin in 20,536 high-risk individuals; a randomized placebo-controlled trial. *Lancet* 2002;360:7–22.

7. **(A)** Smoking cessation is appropriate for all patients who continue to smoke; smoking cessation is the most cost-beneficial intervention for modifying CHD risk. Counseling about smoking cessation is appropriate at every visit for all patients who continue to actively smoke.

Ref: NCEP Expert Panel. Executive summary of the third report of the National Cholesterol Education Program (NCEP) expert panel on detection, evaluation, and treatment of high blood cholesterol in adults (adult treatment panel III). *JAMA* 2001;285:2486–2497.

8. **(A)** HMG-CoA reductase inhibitors (statins) that are currently available have excellent safety profiles and few serious adverse events arise from statin use unless a potential for drug interaction exists, patients have pre-existing liver dysfunction or muscle abnormalities. Most patients do not need routine evaluation of LFTs and muscle enzymes unless they have abnormal LFTs or muscle enzymes at baseline or receive other medications that are CYP 3A4 or CYP 2D6 inhibitors.

Ref: Snow V, Aronson MD, Hornbake ER, Mottur-Pilson C, Weiss KB. Clinical Efficacy Assessment Subcommittee of the American College of Physicians. Lipid control in the management of type 2 diabetes mellitus: a clinical practice guideline from the American College of Physicians. *Ann Intern Med* 2004;140(8):644–649.

9. **(D)** Clarithromycin is a potent inhibitor of CYP 3A4 and simvastatin is extensively metabolized by CYP 3A4. The combination of clarithromycin and simvastatin may place patients at serious risk of drug-induced rhabdomyolysis, resulting in acute renal failure and death.

Ref: Kahri AJ, Valkonen MM, Vuoristo MK, Pentikainen PJ. Rhabdomyolysis associated with concomitant use of simvastatin and clarithromycin. *Ann Pharmacother* 2004;38:719

Ref: Lee AJ, Maddix DS. Rhabdomyolysis secondary to a drug interaction between simvastatin and clarithromycin. *Ann Pharmacother* 2001;35:26–31.

10. **(C)** Discontinuing simvastatin permanently will be detrimental to JP in the future because she will need to be on simvastatin indefinitely to achieve her LDL-C goal. She can be treated for this new URI with clarithromycin as long as simvastatin is temporarily held while she receives clarithromycin. It is prudent to allow one additional day after the last dose of clarithromycin to allow it to be extensively metabolized and eliminated before reintroducing simvastatin. JP can resume simvastatin one additional day after finishing her clarithromycin. Options D and E introduce confusion, and both dirithromycin and azithromycin are minor substrates of CYP 3A4 that can still competitively displace simvastatin for metabolism.

Ref: Bauer LA. Clinical pharmacokinetics and pharmacodynamics. In: DiPiro JT, Talbert RL, Yee GC, et al., eds. *Pharmacotherapy: A Pathophysiologic Approach.* 4th edition. Stamford, CT: Appleton & Lange, 1999:21–43.

PATIENT PROFILE 66
RADIOPHARMACEUTICALS

ANSWERS

1. (C) 1 MBq = 2.7×10^{-2} mCi

   Ref: Stocklosa M, Ansel H. *Pharmaceutical Calculations.* 10th ed. Baltimore: Williams & Wilkins; 1996:217.

2. (D) The disintegration rate constant is found from 0.693/half-life.

   Ref: Stocklosa M, Ansel H. *Pharmaceutical Calculations.* 10th ed. Baltimore: Williams & Wilkins; 1996:218.

3. (E) The concentration later can be found from a first-order rate equation when the initial concentration and the disintegration rate constant are known.

Ref: Stocklosa M, Ansel H. *Pharmaceutical Calculations.* 10th ed. Baltimore: Williams & Wilkins; 1996:219–220.

4. (E) Dose/concentration = volume of dose

   Ref: Stocklosa M, Ansel H. *Pharmaceutical Calculations.* 10th ed. Baltimore: Williams & Wilkins; 1996:218–220.

5. (C) The parent molybdenum 99 compound degrades to give the daughter technetium 99m.

   Ref: Remington. *The Science and Practice of Pharmacy.* 19th ed. Easton, Pa: Mack Publishing; 1995:861.

PATIENT PROFILE 67
DOG BITE WOUND

ANSWERS

1. (D) The decision to initiate rabies and tetanus immunization after a bite wound depends on the immunization status of the patient, the type and degree of contamination of the wound, and the likelihood of rabies infection in the biting animal. In this case, the patient is current with his tetanus immunization. Although puncture wounds may be an indication for more aggressive tetanus immunization, a booster immunization would only be needed if one had not been administered during the last 5 years. The likelihood of rabies exposure is low given the nature of the attack and the immunization status of the animal. Rabies vaccination need not be initiated unless the dog begins to exhibit signs of rabid behavior.

   Ref: Goldstein EJ. Bites. In: Mandel GL, Bennett JE, Dolin R, eds. *Principles and Practice of Infectious Diseases,* 5th edition. Philadelphia: Churchill Livingstone, 2000:3202–3206.

2. (C) More than 80% of dog bite wounds harbor potential pathogens. When patients present early after a bite wound, it may not look infected because a clinical infection has not had time to be established. Although 15% to 20% of dog bite wounds become infected, for early-presenting patients (within 8 hours of the bite), it is difficult to predict which wounds will become infected. Therefore, a 3- to 5-day course of oral antibiotic therapy is recommended generally.

   Ref: Goldstein EJC. Bite wounds and infection. *Clin Infect Dis* 1992;14:633–638.

3. (D) The bacteriology of dog bite wounds is polymicrobial in nature. Therapy should be directed toward the typical cellulitis organisms (*S. aureus*) and organisms found in the dog's oral flora (anaerobes and *P. multocida*).

   Ref: Goldstein EJ. Bites. In: Mandel GL, Bennett JE, Dolin R, eds. *Principles and Practice of Infectious Diseases,* 5th edition. Philadelphia: Churchill Livingstone, 2000:3202–3206.

4. (D) Fluoroquinolones, tetracycline, and amoxicillin/clavulanate possess activity acceptable for infection prophylaxis against bite wound pathogens. The latter provides the most complete coverage for these organisms. Although erythromycin has activity against *S. aureus* and some oral anaerobes, it has poor activity against *P. multocida*. Because of concerns with arthropathy in animal fetal toxicity studies, fluoroquinolones typically are avoided in children unless other options are not available. Tetracycline can cause discoloration of teeth and affect normal bone growth in children.

   Ref: Goldstein EJ. Bites. In: Mandel GL, Bennett JE, Dolin R, eds. *Principles and Practice of Infectious Diseases,* 5th edition. Philadelphia: Churchill Livingstone, 2000:3202-3206.

5. (B) Clavulanic acid is a β-lactamase inhibitor that irreversibly binds to β-lactamase. This prevents these enzymes from splitting the amide bond on the β-lactam ring of other β-lactam antibiotics (i.e., amoxicillin). Clavulanic acid itself has poor intrinsic antimicrobial activity.

   Ref: Petri WA. Penicillins, cephalosporins, and other beta-lactam antibiotics. In: Hardman JG, Limbird LE, eds. *Goodman & Gilman's* the *Pharmacologic Basis of Therapeutics,* 10th edition. New York: McGraw-Hill, 2001:1189–1218.

6. (A) Ciprofloxacin is an inhibitor of cytochrome P450 1A2. Theophylline is a substrate of this hepatic enzyme.

Ref: Guay DRP. Implications of quinolone pharmacokinetic drug interactions. *Hosp Pharm* 1997;32:677–690.

7. (B) Ciprofloxacin is an inhibitor of cytochrome P450 1A2. The R-isomer of warfarin is a substrate of this hepatic enzyme.

Ref: Michalets EL. Update: clinically significant cytochrome P-450 drug interactions. *Pharmacotherapy* 1998;18:84–112.

8. (B) The absorption of oral fluoroquinolones is reduced when administered with foods or medications that contain large amounts of divalent cations (i.e., calcium, iron, aluminum, magnesium, zinc).

Ref: Guay DRP. Implications of quinolone pharmacokinetic drug interactions. *Hosp Pharm* 1997;32:677–690.

9. (A) Fluoroquinolones may cause QTc prolongation and torsades de pointes in patients at risk for this adverse effect. This is considered to be a class effect. Caution should be taken when administering these antibiotics to patients who are at risk for or are on medications that may prolong the QTc interval.

Ref: Owens RC, Ambrose PG. Torsades de pointes associated with fluoroquinolones. *Pharmacotherapy* 2002;22:663–668.

10. (B) The absorption of tetracycline is reduced when administered with foods or medications that containing large amounts of divalent cations (i.e., calcium, iron, aluminum, magnesium, zinc).

Ref: McEnvoy GK, ed. *AHFS Drug Information.* Bethesda, MD: American Society of Health-System Pharmacists, 2004.

PATIENT PROFILE 68
SEXUALLY TRANSMITTED DISEASE, HIV

ANSWERS

1. (C) Oral metronidazole is the therapy of choice for trichomoniasis among both men and women.

Ref: Centers for Disease Control and Prevention. 1998 guidelines for treatment of sexually transmitted diseases. *MMWR Morb Mortal Wkly Rep* 1998;47(RR-1):49–70.

2. (A) Parenteral penicillin G is the drug of choice for the management of all stages of syphilis.

Ref: Centers for Disease Control and Prevention. 1998 guidelines for treatment of sexually transmitted diseases. *MMWR Morb Mortal Wkly Rep* 1998;47(RR-1):49–70.

3. (E) The early diagnosis of HIV infection is important because the patient will benefit from counseling and the treatment regimens that are available. HIV disease also

affects the diagnosis, evaluation, management, and follow-up of many other diseases.

Ref: Centers for Disease Control and Prevention. 1998 guidelines for treatment of sexually transmitted diseases. *MMWR Morb Mortal Wkly Rep* 1998;47(RR-1):49–70.

4. (D) Nelfinavir may cause diarrhea and, like the other protease inhibitor, is metabolized by the CYP 3A4 isoenzyme.

Ref: Rana KZ, Dudley MN. Human immunodeficiency virus protease inhibitors. *Pharmacotherapy* 1999;19:35–59.

5. (D) The main dose-limiting toxicity of stavudine is peripheral neuropathy.

Ref: Hayden FG. Antiviral agents In: Mandell GL, Douglas RG, Bennett JE, eds. *Principles and Practice of Infectious Diseases.* 4th ed. New York: Churchill Livingstone; 1995.411–450.

PATIENT PROFILE 69
SOFT TISSUE INFECTIONS

ANSWERS

1. (C) The most common organisms found on the skin are gram-positive. Infections of the skin most commonly are caused by *Staphylococcus epidermidis, Staphylococcus aureus* (gram-positive cocci in clusters), or streptococci (gram-positive cocci in chains) infections.

Ref: Danziger LH, Fish D, Pendlord SL. Skin and soft tissue infections. In: DiPiro JT, Talbert RL, Yee GC, et al, eds. *Pharmacotherapy: A Pathophysiolgoic Approach,* 5th ed. New York: McGrwa-Hill, 2002:1886.

Ref: McCormack JP, Brown G. Traumatic skin and soft tissue infections. In: Koda-Kimble MA, Young LY, eds. *Applied Therapeutics: The Clinical Use of Drugs,* 7th ed. Baltimore: Lippincott Williams & Wilkins, 2001:65-1–65-12.

2. (A) Gram-positive organisms should be the focus in this type of infection. *S. aureus* is the only gram-positive organism listed.

Ref: Danziger LH, Fish D, Pendlord SL. Skin and soft tissue infections. In: DiPiro JT, Talbert RL, Yee GC, et al, eds. *Pharmacotherapy: A Pathophysiolgoic Approach,* 5th ed. New York: McGrwa-Hill, 2002:1887.

Ref: McCormack JP, Brown G. Traumatic skin and soft tissue infections. In: Koda-Kimble MA, Young LY, eds. *Applied Therapeutics: The Clinical Use of Drugs,* 7th ed. Baltimore: Lippincott Williams & Wilkins, 2001:65-1–65-12.

3. (D) When it is known that the organism is *S. aureus,* nafcillin is the most likely selection from the choices provided if the patient does not have a penicillin allergy. Nafcillin has the most specific coverage against staphylococci of all the antibiotics listed herein. Clindamycin and erythromycin also provide staphylococcal coverage, but these agents should be considered as second-line therapy in the care of patients with this type of infection.

Ref: Danziger LH, Fish D, Pendlord SL. Skin and soft tissue infections. In: DiPiro JT, Talbert RL, Yee GC, et al, eds. *Pharmacotherapy: A Pathophysiolgoic Approach,* 5th ed. New York: McGrwa-Hill, 2002:1888.

Ref: McCormack JP, Brown G. Traumatic skin and soft tissue infections. In: Koda-Kimble MA, Young LY, eds. *Applied Therapeutics: The Clinical Use of Drugs,* 7th ed. Baltimore: Lippincott Williams & Wilkins, 2001:65-1–65-12.

4. (B) Cefazolin, a first-generation cephalosporin, has excellent activity against gram-positive organisms. Patients who have a rash caused by penicillin may be given an appropriate cephalosporin. In this case, a first-generation cephalosporin (cefazolin) would be most appropriate because it is known that there is increased gram-positive activity with first-generation cephalosporins. Aztreonam, a monobactam, and cefazidime, a third-generation cephalosporin, are not effective against gram-positive infections. There is no clear reason to use imipenem in this instance. An organism has been identified, and until proved otherwise, it is susceptible to conventional therapy. Gentamicin covers gram-negative organisms and will not cover this type of infection. A first-generation cephalosporin will provide the best coverage (of the selections listed) in this type of infection.

Ref: Salkind AR, Cuddy PG, Foxworth JW. Is this patient allergic to penicillin? An evidence-based analysis of the likelihood of penicillin allergy. *JAMA* 2001;285(19):2498–2505.

5. (A) Vancomycin is a non-β-lactam antibiotic useful against almost all types of gram-positive infections. Anaphylaxis would exclude the use of any β-lactam antibiotic (penicillin). A single agent with superb gram-positive coverage is preferred. This excludes gentamicin and ciprofloxacin. Rifampin should not be used routinely as a single agent. Although rifampin has excellent gram-positive coverage, organisms become resistant rapidly when this drug is used alone.

Ref: Danziger LH, Fish D, Pendlord SL. Skin and soft tissue infections. In: DiPiro JT, Talbert RL, Yee GC, et al, eds. *Pharmacotherapy: A Pathophysiolgoic Approach,* 5th ed. New York: McGraw-Hill, 2002:1888.

Ref: McCormack JP, Brown G. Traumatic skin and soft tissue infections. In: Koda-Kimble MA, Young LY, eds. *Applied Therapeutics: The Clinical Use of Drugs,* 7th ed. Baltimore: Lippincott Williams & Wilkins, 2001:65-1–65-12.

PATIENT PROFILE 70

ONCOLOGY: LUNG CANCER

ANSWERS

1. (D) Smoking is a well-established cause of lung cancer. More than 70% of patients with lung cancer had smoked before the disease was diagnosed.

Ref: Felton SA, Finley RS. Lung cancer. In: DiPiro JT, Talbert RL, Yee GC, Matzke GR, Wells BG, Posey LM, eds. *Pharmacotherapy: A Pathophysiologic Approach.* 4th ed. Stamford, Conn: Appleton & Lange; 1999:2043–2060.

Ref: Herfindal ET, Gourley DR (eds). *Textbook of Therapeutics, Drug and Disease Management.* 6th ed. Baltimore: Williams & Wilkins; 1996: chapter 83.

2. (B) Nephrotoxicity is the dose-limiting toxicity. Neurotoxicity and bone marrow suppression also can occur.

Ref: Valley AW, Balmer CM. Cancer treatment and chemotherapy. In: DiPiro JT, Talbert RL, Yee GC, Matzke GR, Wells BG, Posey LM, eds. *Pharmacotherapy: A Pathophysiologic Approach.* 4th ed. Stamford, Conn: Appleton & Lange; 1999:1957–2012.

3. (C) The infusion rate is associated hypotension. Infusion should be slow (2 hours) to avoid this reaction.

Ref: Valley AW, Balmer CM. Cancer treatment and chemotherapy. In: DiPiro JT, Talbert RL, Yee GC, Matzke GR, Wells BG, Posey LM, eds. *Pharmacotherapy: A Pathophysiologic Approach.* 4th ed. Stamford, Conn: Appleton & Lange; 1999:1957–2012.

4. (A) The most commonly used agents for seizure prophylaxis among patients with brain metastases are phenytoin and dexamethasone. Use of other antiseizure medications has not been as thoroughly studied.

Ref: Felton SA, Finley RS. Lung cancer. In: DiPiro JT, Talbert RL, Yee GC, Matzke GR, Wells BG, Posey LM, eds. *Pharmacotherapy: A Pathophysiologic Approach.* 4th ed. Stamford, Conn: Appleton & Lange; 1999:2043–2060.

5. (D) Hypercalcemia is one of many paraneoplastic disorders. It is very common among patients with lung cancer.

Ref: Felton SA, Finley RS. Lung cancer. In: DiPiro JT, Talbert RL, Yee GC, Matzke GR, Wells BG, Posey LM, eds. *Pharmacotherapy: A Pathophysiologic Approach.* 4th ed. Stamford, Conn: Appleton & Lange; 1999:2043–2060.

PATIENT PROFILE 71

INSOMNIA

ANSWERS

1. (E) St. John's wort will have an additive effect with SSRIs and can cause serotonin syndrome. St. John's wort used with oral contraceptives can decrease steroid levels, resulting in breakthrough bleeding as well as pregnancy.

   Ref: St. John's Wort Detailed Information, Natural Medicines Comprehensive Database; accessed via Massachusetts College of Pharmacy and Health Sciences: *www.mcp.edu;* accessed August 9, 2004.

2. (E) St. John's wort is used most often to treat depression and anxiety because of its effects on neurotransmitters. It also has been associated with insomnia and restlessness.

   Ref: St. John's Wort Detailed Information, Natural Medicines Comprehensive Database; accessed via Massachusetts College of Pharmacy and Health Sciences: *www.mcp.edu;* accessed August 9, 2004.

3. (C) While there is evidence to support its use as an antianxiety treatment, kava has been reported to be a hepatotoxic agent.

   Ref: Kava Detailed Information, Natural Medicines Comprehensive Database; accessed via Massachusetts College of Pharmacy and Health Sciences: *www.mcp.edu;.*accessed August 9, 2004.

4. (D) The use of L-tryptophan is no longer recommended owing to its association with eosinophila-myalgia syndrome.

   Ref: Curtis JL, Jermaine DM. Sleep disorders. In: DiPiro JT, Talbert RL, Yee GC, eds. *Pharmacotherapy: A Pathophysiologic Approach,* 5th ed. New York: McGraw-Hill; 2002:1325.

5. (E) The safe use of valerian has only been established in regimens lasting less than 28 days.

   Ref: Valerian Detailed Information, Natural Medicines Comprehensive Database; accessed via Massachusetts College of Pharmacy and Health Sciences: *www.mcp.edu;* accessed August 9, 2004.

6. (D) Melatonin is synthesized endogenously in the pineal gland but is commonly taken for jet lag and is available parenterally.

   Ref: Melatonin Detailed Information, Natural Medicines Comprehensive Database; accessed via Massachusetts College of Pharmacy and Health Sciences: *www.mcp.edu;* accessed August 9, 2004.

7. (E) Drug-induced insomnia is seen with diuretic, steroid, SSRI, and anticonvulsant use but is not typically associated with HMG Co-A reductase inhibitors.

   Ref: Curtis JL, Jermaine DM. Sleep disorders. In: DiPiro JT, Talbert RL, Yee GC, eds. *Pharmacotherapy: A Pathophysiologic Approach,* 5th ed. New York: McGraw-Hill, 2002:1323–1333.

8. (D) Diphenhydramine blocks the histamine as well as the muscarinic receptors.

   Ref: Berardi RR, McDermott JH, et al. *Handbook of Nonprescription Drugs,* 14th ed. Washington: American Pharmacists Association. 2004:Chapter 48.

9. (C) Diphenhydramine should be used 1 to 2 h before bedtime to allow onset of action and should only be used for 3 nights before reevaluating sleep.

   Ref: Berardi RR, McDermott JH, et al. *Handbook of Nonprescription Drugs,* 14th ed. Washington: American Pharmacists Association. 2004:Chapter 48.

10. (A) Unisom Nighttime Sleep Aid contains doxylamine.

    Ref: Berardi RR, McDermott JH, et al. *Handbook of Nonprescription Drugs,* 14th ed. Washington: American Pharmacists Association, 2004:Chapter 48.

PATIENT PROFILE 72

MEDICINAL CHEMISTRY

ANSWER

1. (B) Both procaine and tetracaine can be metabolized into *p*-aminobenzoic acid. The latter antagonizes the action of sulfamethoxazole as an antibacterial agent. Sulfonamides act mechanistically by inhibiting the incorporation of *p*-aminobenzoic acid into bacterial folic acid synthesis. Because knee surggery may take a relatively long time, lidocaine, like procaine, is not a good choice because of its short duration of action.

PATIENT PROFILE 73

CHRONIC NONMALIGNANT PAIN

ANSWERS

1. (B) Because of the high incidence of constipation that occurs during opioid therapy, it is recommended that each patient be prescribed an appropriate prophylactic bowel regimen. This therapy must be individualized. CR should benefit from a stimulant laxative such as bisacodyl and a stool softener such as docusate. Additional counseling on increasing his intake of dietary fiber is also warranted. Patients should take no more than eight Vicodin tablets (40 mg hydrocodone and 4000 mg acetaminophen) per day. CR had been taking a total of 20 mg hydrocodone and 2000 mg acetaminophen daily, which is below the recommended maximum dose. Long-term use of Vicodin is limited by the toxicities associated with acetaminophen.

Ref: Reisner L, Koo JS. Pain and its management. In: Young YL, Koda-Kimble MA, eds. *Applied Therapeutics: The Clinical Use of Drugs.* Vancouver, WA: Applied Therapeutics, 2005: 9-1–9-40.

Ref: Product Information: Vicodin, hydrocodone and acetaminophen, Knoll Pharmaceuticals.

2. (E) A useful mnemonic in the management of chronic nonmalignant pain is the "4 A's." These parameters should be assessed, documented, and monitored continuously.

- Analgesia (pain relief, improved sleep and mood)
- Activities of daily living
- Adverse events (constipation, sedation, nausea, pruritus)
- Aberrant drug-taking behaviors (early refill requests, "lost" or "stolen" prescriptions, missed appointments)

Ref: Passik SD, Weinreb HJ. Managing chronic nonmalignant pain: Overcoming the obstacles to the use of opioids. *Adv Ther* 2000;17:70–83.

3. (A) Nonsteroidal anti-inflammatory drugs (NSAIDs) may be beneficial in the management of CR's chronic pain, particularly because there may be the presence of inflammation. Acetaminophen or acetaminophen-containing products (such as Percocet) would not be a good choice because of his daily use of Vicodin. Meperidine is not recommended for use in the management of chronic pain owing to its potential for the accumulation of toxic metabolites.

Ref: Reisner L, Koo JS. Pain and its management. In: Young YL, Koda-Kimble MA, eds. *Applied Therapeutics: The Clinical Use of Drugs.* Vancouver, WA: Applied Therapeutics, 2005: 9-1–9-40.

Ref: Portenoy RK, Kanner RM. Nonopioid and adjuvant analgesics. In: Portenoy RK, Kanner RM, eds. *Pain Management: Theory and Practice.* Philadelphia: FA Davis, 1996:219–247.

4. (A) Opioid tolerance is a physiologic state resulting from regular use of an opioid in which an increased dosage is needed to produce a specific effect or a reduced effect is observed with a constant dose over

time. CR has required a higher dose of Vicodin to sustain analgesia. Tolerance differs from addiction. Opioid addiction is a condition with genetic, psychosocial, and environmental factors influencing its development and manifestations. It is characterized by behaviors that include the following: impaired control over drug use, craving, compulsive use, and continued use despite harm. CR is not exhibiting signs commonly associated with opioid addiction.

Ref: Federation of State Medical Boards of the United States. Model guidelines for the use of controlled substances for the treatment of pain; available at *http://www.fsmb.org.*

5. (B) CR is currently taking a total of 30 mg hydrocodone per day. The equivalent daily morphine dose is 30 mg. The appropriate dosing regimen for CR would be extended-release morphine 15 mg PO BID for a total daily morphine dose of 30 mg.

Ref: American Pain Society. *Principles of Analgesic Use in the Treatment of Acute Pain and Cancer Pain,* 5th ed. Glenview, IL: American Pain Society, 2003:14–17.

6. (B) The occurrence of breakthrough pain is not uncommon in patients treated with long-acting opioids. The pain that breaks through the analgesia should be managed with an immediate-release, short-acting opioid. CR is not exhibiting signs and symptoms of addiction. It is difficult to determine if CR is experiencing tolerance to his morphine regimen. Initiation and assessment of a short-acting opioid for breakthrough pain may help to provide further information about tolerance to his current morphine dose. If CR was experiencing tolerance, a morphine dosage increase would be appropriate. Morphine lacks a "ceiling dose" and therefore does not have a recommended maximum daily dose.

Ref: Portenoy RK. Opioid analgesics. In: Portenoy RK, Kanner RM, eds. *Pain Management: Theory and Practice.* Philadelphia: FA Davis, 1996:248–276.

Ref: Portenoy RK, Hagen NA. Breakthrough pain: Definition, prevalence and characteristics. *Pain* 1990;41:273–281.

7. (D) Side effects that generally subside after the initiation of opioid therapy include nausea and sedation. Constipation, insomnia, sexual dysfunction, and diaphoresis are considered side effects that may persist but to varying degrees among patients treated.

Ref: Fishman SM, Mao J. Opioid therapy in chronic nonmalignant pain. In: Ballantyne J, Fishman SM, Abdi. S, Fields HL, eds. *Massachusetts General Hospital Handbook of Pain,* 2d ed. Philadelphia: Lippincott Williams & Wilkins, 2002:428–436.

8. (D) Signs of addiction also include self-escalation of dosage, drug intolerances described as "allergies," and focusing visits mainly around opioid therapy.

Ref: Wilsey BL, Fishman SM. Chronic opioid therapy, drug abuse and addiction. In: Ballantyne J, Fishman SM, Abdi, S, Fields HL, eds. *Massachusetts General Hospital Handbook of Pain*, 2d ed. Philadelphia: Lippincott Williams & Wilkins, 2002:495–505.

9. (C) Several anticonvulsants have been found to be beneficial in the management of neuropathic pain–related syndromes. Gabapentin has been well tolerated in patients with chronic pain because of its minimal side-effect profile. Doses greater than 2200 mg are required in this population to obtain a clinical benefit.

Ref: Markman JD, Oaklander AL. Neuropathic pain syndromes. In: Ballantyne J, Fishman SM, Abdi. S, Fields HL, eds. *Massachusetts General Hospital Handbook of Pain*, 2d ed. Philadelphia: Lippincott Williams & Wilkins, 2002:341–359.

10. (E) Various organizations, such as the American Pain Society, the American Academy of Pain Medicine, and the Federation of State Medical Boards in the United States, have created consensus statements and "model" guidelines for the use of opioids in chronic nonmalignant pain. The lack of current standardized guidelines is due largely to physician fear of regulatory scrutiny, patient and physician fears of addiction, and the presence of social stigmas regarding the use of opioids.

Ref: Federation of State Medical Boards of the United States. Model guidelines for the use of controlled substances for the treatment of pain; available at *http://www.fsmb.org*.

Ref: Purvis JM. Pain management. In: Ballantyne J, Fishman SM, Abdi S, Fields HL, eds. *Massachusetts General Hospital Handbook of Pain*, 2d ed. Philadelphia: Lippincott Williams & Wilkins, 2002:685–691.

Ref: American Pain Society and American Academy of Pain Medicine. Consensus statement on the use of opioids in chronic pain; available at *http://www.ampainsoc.org*.

P A T I E N T   P R O F I L E   7 4

MAJOR DEPRESSION

ANSWERS

1. (D) All tricyclic antidepressants have proarrhythmic effects and should be avoided in the treatment of patients with preexisting arrhythmias.

Ref: Seizure disorders. In: Young LY, Koda-Kimble MA, eds. *Applied Therapeutics: The Clinical Use of Drugs*. 6th ed. Vancouver, Wash: Applied Therapeutics; 1995: chapter 76.

2. (B) Clonidine has been shown to cause depression. Depression is a relative contraindication to use of this agent.

Ref: Seizure disorders. In: Young LY, Koda-Kimble MA, eds. *Applied Therapeutics: The Clinical Use of Drugs*. 6th ed. Vancouver, Wash: Applied Therapeutics; 1995: chapter 76.

3. (C) Sertraline has the least amount of enzymatic inhibition on the CYP450 system.

Ref: *Goodman and Gilman's The Pharmacologic Basis of Therapeutics*. 9th ed. New York: McGraw-Hill; 1996: chapter 19.

4. (B) Sertraline has a minimal effect on the ability of warfarin to produce anti-coagulation. Dosage adjustment of warfarin usually is not necessary.

Ref: Mitchell PB. Drug interactions of clinical significance with selective serotonin reuptake inhibitors. *Drug Saf* 1997;17: 390–406.

5. (A) Fatigue, nausea, dizziness and light-headedness, tremors, chills, insomnia, anxiety and diaphoresis are the most common effects of abrupt discontinuation of SSRIs. Fluoxetine, because of its long half-life and active metabolite, is the least likely agent to cause these symptoms.

Ref: Zajecka J, Tracey KA, Mitchell S. Discontinuation symptoms after treatment with serotonin reuptake inhibitors: a literature review. *J Clin Psychiatry* 1997;58:291–297.

P A T I E N T   P R O F I L E   7 5

DIABETES AND PERIPHERAL NEUROPATHY

ANSWERS

1. (C) DR is diabetic, and his goal blood pressure should be less than 130/80 mm Hg.

Ref: American Diabetes Association. Clinical practice guidelines. *Diabetes Care* 2004;27(S1):S15–S35.

2. (B) Hypertension is not considered a direct risk factor for a foot ulcer in DR. The other factors listed are established risk factors applicable to DR.

Ref: American Diabetes Association. Clinical practice guidelines. *Diabetes Care* 2004;27(S1):S15–S35.

3. (C) Circulatory dysfunction (like congestive heart failure) and an increased serum creatinine above 1.5 mg/dL in males are both contraindications to metformin therapy. These factors put patients at an increased risk of lactic acidosis.

   Ref: Package Insert: Glucophage (metformin), Bristol-Myers Squibb Company, Princeton, NJ; 2004.

4. (D) DR is a diabetic, and his LDL goal should be less than 100 mg/dL.

   Ref: American Diabetes Association. Clinical practice guidelines. *Diabetes Care* 2004;27(S1):S15–S35.

5. (D) These are all symptoms of hypoglycemia.

   Ref: Carlisle BA, Kroon AL, Koda-Kimble MA. Diabetes mellitus. In: Koda-Kimble MA, Young LY, Kradjan WA, et al, eds. *Applied Therapeutics: The Clinical Use of Drugs,* 8th ed. Philadelphia: Lippincott Williams & Wilkins, 2005:50(41).

6. (B) The UKPDS demonstrated a decrease in the microvascular complications of diabetes mellitus in patients in the intensive blood glucose control group.

   Ref: American Diabetes Association. Clinical practice guidelines. *Diabetes Care* 2004;27(S1):S15–S35.

7. (D) Hypoglycemia is strictly defined as a blood glucose level of less than 50 mg/dL, although some patients will feel symptoms at blood glucose levels higher than this.

   Ref: American Diabetes Association. Clinical practice guidelines. *Diabetes Care* 2004;27(S1):S15–S35.

8. (C) Gabapentin is approved to treat neuropathic pain.

   Ref: Package Insert: Neurontin (gabapentin), Pfizer, New York, 2004.

9. (B) This is an appropriate titration for gabapentin. Gabapentin is approved to treat neuropathic pain.

   Ref: Package Insert: Neurontin (gabapentin), Pfizer, New York, 2004.

10. (B) Gabapentin is well tolerated, although it may cause drowsiness, especially at higher doses. Gabapentin is approved to treat neuropathic pain.

    Ref: Package Insert: Neurontin (gabapentin), Pfizer, New York, 2004.

PATIENT PROFILE 76
URINARY TRACT INFECTION

ANSWERS

1. (D) *Escherichia coli* accounts for 80%–90% of community-acquired and uncomplicated UTIs.

2. (D) Empiric drug treatment of a lower UTI often is started before culture and sensitivity results are known because the likely pathogen can be predicted and is sensitive to antibiotics. A single antibiotic dose of Bactrim® DS (trimethoprim-sulfamethoxazole) is reasonably effective in the management of acute lower UTI among young women who are allergic to penicillin.

3. (D) Single-dose Bactrim® (trimethoprim-sulfamethoxazole) therapy is contraindicated among patients with diabetes mellitus because of the high incidence of relapse.

4. (A) Bactrim® (trimethoprim-sulfamethoxazole) is not heat labile and does not have to be stored in the refrigerator.

   Ref: Sahai J. Urinary tract infections. In: Young LY, Koda-Kimble MA, eds. *Applied Therapeutics: The Clinical Use of Drugs.* Vancouver, Wash: Applied Therapeutics; 1995: chapter 63.

5. (E) Fluoroquinolones such as ciprofloxacin have excellent activity against most gram-negative organisms and good activity against many gram-positive organisms. These agents are considered as effective as Bactrim® (trimethoprim-sulfamethoxazole) in the management of uncomplicated UTI. Ciprofloxacin would be appropriate in the treatment of a patient who is highly allergic to both trimethoprim-sulfamethoxazole and penicillin.

   Ref: Romac DR. Urinary tract infections. In: Herfindal ET, Gourley DR, eds. *Textbook of Therapeutics, Drug and Disease Management.* Baltimore: Williams & Wilkins; 1996: chapter 65.

PATIENT PROFILE 77

KIDNEY TRANSPLANTATION

ANSWERS

1. (A) Concomitant use of calcineurin inhibitors (cyclosporine) and statins (atorvastatin) results in elevated statin levels. Clinically, this translates to an increased risk of myopathy or rhabdomyolysis, and periodic monitoring of CK is necessary.

   Ref: Pasternak RC, et al. ACA/AHA/NHLBI clinical advisory on use and safety of statins. *J Am Coll Cardiol* 2002;40(3):567–572.

2. (E) Increasing the metoprolol dose or initiating labetalol is not appropriate owing to KT's borderline bradycardia. Verapamil has a significant drug interaction with cyclosporine, and concomitant use should be avoided. Lisinopril and amlodipine are both reasonable options, but initiating amlodipine is the best choice at this time. Calcium channel blockers historically have been considered the treatment of choice for hypertension in transplant recipients. Lisinopril is a reasonable option and has renoprotective effects but can cause a rise in the serum creatinine. In the first few months, renal transplant recipients are at the highest risk for rejection, and introducing outside factors that can complicate the clinical presentation of rejection should be avoided.

   Ref: Baroletti SA, et al. Calcium channel blockers as the treatment of choice for hypertension in renal transplant recipients: Fact or fiction. *Pharmacotherapy* 2003;23(6):788–801.

3. (A) Hypophosphatemia is common after renal transplantation and may result in osteopenia if left untreated. All oral phosphorus preparations also contain potassium, which may be a problem in this patient. K-Phos Neutral, Neutra-Phos, and Neutra-Phos-K each contain 250 mg phosphorus and 1.1, 7.1, and 14.2 mEq potassium, respectively. Because of its low potassium content and KT's high-normal potassium level, K-Phos Neutral is the best option.

   Ref: K-Phos Neutral, Neutra-Phos, and Neutra-Phos-K Drug Information, Micromedex, Thompson Healthcare, Inc., September 2003. Available at http://www.micromedex.com.

4. (B) All three of these are risk factors for developing CMV disease after transplantation. This patient did not receive induction immunosuppression with a polyclonal antibody—basiliximab is a monoclonal antibody. This patient was CMV seronegative prior to transplant, so reactivation of virus is not possible. KT's risk factor for CMV disease is receiving a graft from a seropositive donor.

   Ref: Schnitzler MA. Costs and consequences of cytomegalovirus disease. *Am J Health Syst Pharm* 2003;60(suppl 1):S5–8.

5. (A) Cyclosporine is a calcineurin inhibitor (not inducer) whose ultimate action is preventing the production of interleukin 2 (IL-2), among other immunomodulatory factors. IL-2 is a major player in T-cell activation.

   Ref: Neoral Package Insert, Novartis Pharmaceuticals Corp., East Hanover, NJ, 2002.

6. (D) Cyclosporine has numerous adverse effects. Some of the major and/or most common effects include renal dysfunction, hypertension, hyperglycemia, headache, tremor, hypomagnesemia, hyperkalemia, gingival hyperplasia, and hirsutism. It has not been associated with rhabdomyolysis, hair loss, leukocytosis, nor hyperphosphatemia.

   Ref: Neoral Package Insert, Novartis Pharmaceuticals Corp., East Hanover, NJ, 2002.

7. (B) IL-2 receptor antagonists (basiliximab and daclizumab) are indicated for induction immunosuppression in solid-organ transplantation. Using these agents for long-term immunosuppression is not appropriate owing to their cost and the questionable need for this degree of long-term immunosuppression. They are not useful in treating rejection.

   Ref: Berard JL, et al. A review of interleukin-2 receptor antagonists in solid organ transplantation. *Pharmacotherapy* 1999;19:1127–1137.

8. (C) Sulfamethoxazole-trimethoprim is the preferred agent for PCP prophylaxis. Other options include dapsone, pentamadine, and atovaquone. Doxycycline does not have activity against this pathogen and would not be an appropriate choice.

   Ref: Gilbert DN, et al. *The Sanford Guide to Antimicrobial Therapy,* 34th ed. Hyde Park, NY: Antimicrobial Therapy, Inc., 2004:96.

9. (B) A drug interaction between fluconazole and cyclosporine is present. Fluconazole significantly increases cyclosporine concentrations, which may result in increased serum creatinine levels and cyclosporine toxicity. Careful drug level monitoring and dose titration are necessary when these two medications are used concomitantly.

   Ref: Anaizi N. Drug interactions involving immunosuppressive agents. *Graft* 2001;4(4):232–247.

10. (D) Two formulations of cyclosporine are currently available. Cyclosporine, nonmodified, is the generic equivalent of Sandimmune. This was the first cyclosporine product available and is also the formulation of the intravenous

preparation. Cyclosporine, modified release, is equivalent to Neoral and Gengraf. This is a newer cyclosporine formulation with better bioavailability compared with the original product. Generic substitution can be done within formulations in the absence of an "NDPS," but nonmodified products may not be substituted for modified-release products. Of note, many practitioners prefer "no substitution" in order to minimize interproduct variation even within equivalent formulations.

Ref: Dunn CJ, et al. Cyclosporine: An updated review of the pharmacokinetic properties, clinical efficacy and tolerability of a microemulsion-based formulation (neural) in organ transplantation. *Drugs* 2001;61(13):1957–2016.

PATIENT PROFILE 78
CORONARY ARTERY DISEASE

ANSWERS

1. (B) β-Blockers are contraindicated in the treatment of patients with asthma.

   Ref: Talbert RL. Ischemic heart disease. In: DiPiro JT, Talbert RL, Yee GC, Matzke GR, Wells BG, Posey LM, eds. *Pharmacotherapy: A pathophysiologic approach.* 4th ed. Stamford, Conn: Appleton & Lange; 1999:182–210.

2. (A) NSAIDs may blunt the effect of antihypertensive agents.

   Ref: Hawkins DW, Bussey HI, Prisant LM. Hypertension. In: DiPiro JT, Talbert RL, Yee GC, Matzke GR, Wells BG, Posey LM, eds. *Pharmacotherapy: A Pathophysiologic Approach.* 4th ed. Stamford, Conn: Appleton & Lange; 1999:131–152.

3. (D) Nitroglycerin SL administered before exertion may prevent the onset of chest pain.

   Ref: Talbert RL. Ischemic heart disease. In: DiPiro JT, Talbert RL, Yee GC, Matzke GR, Wells BG, Posey LM, eds. *Pharmacotherapy: A pathophysiologic approach.* 4th ed. Stamford, Conn: Appleton & Lange; 1999:182–210.

4. (C) Aspirin would be an appropriate intervention.

   Ref: Talbert RL. Ischemic heart disease. In: DiPiro JT, Talbert RL, Yee GC, Matzke GR, Wells BG, Posey LM, eds. *Pharmacotherapy: A pathophysiologic approach.* 4th ed. Stamford, Conn: Appleton & Lange; 1999:182–210.

PATIENT PROFILE 79
SOFT TISSUE INFECTIONS

ANSWERS

1. (C) Diabetic foot infections typically are mixed infections. Many organisms may be present. Impairment of host defenses, poor blood circulation, and neuropathy caused by diabetes mellitus make it difficult for patients to ward off infection. Foot infections can have many organisms present. Daily events such as showering can carry many organisms from other parts of the body and deposit them in an open wound in the foot. Adding host impairment makes severe infection possible. Fastidious foot care is essential for persons with diabetes.

   Ref: Danziger LH, Fish D, Pendlord SL. Skin and soft tissue infections. In: DiPiro JT, Talbert RL, Yee GC, et al, eds. *Pharmacotherapy: A Pathophysiolgoic Approach,* 5th ed. New York: McGraw-Hill, 2002:1891.

   Ref: Gilbert DN, Moellering RC Jr, Eliopoulos GM, Sande MA, eds. *The Sanford Guide to Antimicrobial Therapy 2004,* 34th ed. Hyde Park, VT: Antimicrobial Therapy, 2004:10.

2. (A) Broad-spectrum antibiotics, including fluoroquinolones, allow adequate management of infections from osteomyelitis. These infections are severe and may necessitate hospitalization.

   Ref: Danziger LH, Fish D, Pendlord SL. Skin and soft tissue infections. In: DiPiro JT, Talbert RL, Yee GC, et al, eds. *Pharmacotherapy: A Pathophysiolgoic Approach,* 5th ed. New York: McGraw-Hill, 2002:1891.

   Ref: McCormack JP, Brown G. Traumatic skin and soft tissue infections. In: Koda-Kimble MA, Young LY, eds. *Applied Therapeutics: The Clinical Use of Drugs,* 7th ed. Baltimore: Lippincott Williams & Wilkins, 2001:65-6–65-8.

3. (D) Of the selections listed, piperacillin-tazobactam has the broadest spectrum of coverage. Diabetic foot infections often are polymicrobial. Until a definitive organism is cultured with proper technique, a broad-spectrum antibiotic directed at gram-positive organisms, including enterococci and gram-negative organisms, and at anaerobic

organisms, including *B. fragilis*, should be considered. Ampicillin-sulbactam is another antibiotic frequently selected for its spectrum of this type of infection.

Ref: Lipsky BA, Berendt AR, Deery HG, et al. ISDA guidelines: Diagnosis and treatment of diabetic foot infections. *Clin Infect Dis* 2004;39:885–904.

Ref: Danziger LH, Fish D, Pendlord SL. Skin and soft tissue infections. In: DiPiro JT, Talbert RL, Yee GC, et al, eds. *Pharmacotherapy: A Pathophysiolgoic Approach,* 5th ed. New York: McGrwa-Hill, 2002:1888.

Ref: McCormack JP, Brown G. Traumatic skin and soft tissue infections. In: Koda-Kimble MA, Young LY, eds. *Applied Therapeutics: The Clinical Use of Drugs,* 7th ed. Baltimore: Lippincott Williams & Wilkins, 2001:65-6–65-8.

Ref: Gilbert DN, Moellering RC Jr, Eliopoulos GM, Sande MA, eds. *The Sanford Guide to Antimicrobial Therapy 2004,* 34th ed. Hyde Park, VT: Antimicrobial Therapy, 2004:10.

4. (C) Although piperacillin-tazobactam has activity against *P. aeruginosa*, single agents should be avoided when treating patients with this type of infection. Adding a second agent such as an aminoglycoside or a fluoroquinolone with activity against *P. aeruginosa* would be useful to this patient. *P. aeruginosa* is the only deficiency in antibiotic coverage in this patient.

Ref: Danziger LH, Fish D, Pendlord SL. Skin and soft tissue infections. In: DiPiro JT, Talbert RL, Yee GC, et al, eds. *Pharmacotherapy: A Pathophysiolgoic Approach,* 5th ed. New York: McGraw-Hill, 2002:1892.

5. (E) Proper foot care is paramount in preventing diabetic foot infections. Avoidance truly is the best treatment in this case. Once an infection is present, poor circulation, impaired nerve responses, and maintenance of foot care become difficult and often necessitate hospitalization.

Ref: Lipsky BA, Berendt AR, Deery HG, et al. ISDA guidelines: Diagnosis and treatment of diabetic foot infections. *Clin Infect Dis* 2004;39:885–904.

Ref: Danziger LH, Fish D, Pendlord SL. Skin and soft tissue infections. In: DiPiro JT, Talbert RL, Yee GC, et al, eds. *Pharmacotherapy: A Pathophysiolgoic Approach,* 5th ed. New York: McGraw-Hill, 2002:1888.

Ref: McCormack JP, Brown G. Traumatic skin and soft tissue infections. In: Koda-Kimble MA, Young LY, eds. *Applied Therapeutics: The Clinical Use of Drugs,* 7th ed. Baltimore: Lippincott Williams & Wilkins, 2001:65–8.

PATIENT PROFILE 80

DIABETES MELLITUS

ANSWERS

1. (D) The contraindications to metformin therapy include renal disease or dysfunction suggested by a serum creatinine level of 1.5 mg/dL or more for men and a serum creatinine of 1.4 mg/dL or more for women, congestive heart failure that necessitates pharmacologic management, and acute or metabolic acidosis.

Ref: Glucophage [package insert]. Princeton, NJ: Bristol-Myers Squibb; 1998.

2. (B) Diarrhea occurs among approximately 30% of patients who take metformin. Lactic acidosis occurs in approximately 0.03 cases per 1000 patient years.

Ref: Glucophage [package insert]. Princeton, NJ; Bristol-Myers Squibb; 1998.

3. (D) To decrease the incidence of diarrhea caused by metformin therapy, doses should be gradually titrated.

Ref: Glucophage [package insert]. Princeton, NJ: Bristol-Myers Squibb; 1998.

4. (C) The IV contrast agents used in some radiographic procedures may decrease creatinine clearance and cause accumulation of metformin. This increases the risk of lactic acidosis. To avoid lactic acidosis, metformin should be held for 48 hours after the use of IV contrast agents and restarted after renal function is assessed and determined to be normal.

Ref: Glucophage [package insert]. Princeton, NJ: Bristol-Myers Squibb; 1998.

PATIENT PROFILE 81

DIABETES MELLITUS

ANSWERS

1. (C) RL has neuropathic pain. Amitriptyline is the only choice that is a first-line treatment for neuropathic pain.

Ref: Baumann RJ. Pain management. In: DiPiro JT, Talbert RL, Yee GC, et al, eds. *Pharmacotherapy: A Pathophysiologic Approach,* 5th ed. New York: McGraw-Hill, 2002:1103–1118.

2. (C) To minimize side effects, gabapentin should be titrated. The minimum effective dose for neuropathy is 300 mg tid. Maximum effect takes 6 to 8 weeks.

Ref: Baumann RJ. Pain management. In: DiPiro JT, Talbert RL, Yee GC, et al, eds. *Pharmacotherapy: A Pathophysiologic Approach,* 5th ed. New York: McGraw-Hill, 2002:1103–1118.

3. (A) Drowsiness is a common side effect associated with gabapentin use.

Ref: Baumann RJ. Pain management. In: DiPiro JT, Talbert RL, Yee GC, et al, eds. *Pharmacotherapy: A Pathophysiologic Approach,* 5th ed. New York: McGraw-Hill, 2002:1103–1118.

4. (B) Tramadol should be titrated to minimize the occurrence of side effects and maximize tolerability.

Ref: Baumann RJ. Pain management. In: DiPiro JT, Talbert RL, Yee GC, et al, eds. *Pharmacotherapy: A Pathophysiologic Approach,* 5th ed. New York: McGraw-Hill, 2002:1103–1118.

5. (E) Tramadol is known to reduce the seizure threshold.

Ref: Baumann RJ. Pain management. In: DiPiro JT, Talbert RL, Yee GC, et al, eds. *Pharmacotherapy: A Pathophysiologic Approach,* 5th ed. New York: McGraw-Hill, 2002:1103–1118.

6. (E) RL has white coat hypertension, which means that her blood pressures are elevated only when she is in healthcare settings. Her home blood pressures are at goal, so no treatment for blood pressure is necessary.

Ref: Carter BL, Saseen JJ. In: DiPiro JT, Talbert RL, Yee GC, et al, eds. *Pharmacotherapy: A Pathophysiologic Approach,* 5th ed. New York: McGraw-Hill, 2002:157–184.

7. (E) RL has type 1 diabetes and requires insulin therapy. Oral agents are only effective in the presence of insulin.

Ref: Carlisle BA, Kroon LA, Koda-Kimble MA. Diabetes mellitus. In: Koda-Kimble MA, Young LY, Kradjan WA, Guglielmo BJ, eds. *Applied Therapeutics: The Clinical Use of Drugs,* 8th ed. Philadelphia: Lippincott Williams & Wilkins, 2005:50-1–50-80.

8. (C) Patients with type 1 diabetes mellitus typically do not have insulin resistance. Thus a physiologic dose of insulin (0.5 units/kg/day) is an appropriate dose.

Ref: Carlisle BA, Kroon LA, Koda-Kimble MA. Diabetes mellitus. In: Koda-Kimble MA, Young LY, Kradjan WA, Guglielmo BJ, eds. *Applied Therapeutics: The Clinical Use of Drugs,* 8th ed. Philadelphia: Lippincott Williams & Wilkins, 2005:50-1–50-80.

9. (A) RL's morning blood sugars may be elevated secondary to the Somogyi effect (rebound hyperglycemia secondary to hypoglycemia). A 2 AM blood sugar should be checked before any changes are made to her insulin regimen.

Ref: Carlisle BA, Kroon LA, Koda-Kimble MA. Diabetes mellitus. In: Koda-Kimble MA, Young LY, Kradjan WA, Guglielmo BJ, eds. *Applied Therapeutics: The Clinical Use of Drugs,* 8th ed. Philadelphia: Lippincott Williams & Wilkins, 2005:50-1–50-80.

10. (C) Salicylic acid should not be used in patients with diabetes mellitus, especially those with neuropathy because they may not be able to feel if the salicylic acid is causing damage. A pumice stone also could result in damage in someone with decreased sensation.

Ref: United States National Library of Medicine; available at *http://www.nlm.nih.gov/medline plus/druginfo/uspdi/202516. html;* accessed September 2004.

PATIENT PROFILE 82
ASTHMA CASE

ANSWERS

1. (C) Because inflammation is important in the pathogenesis of asthma, NHLBI guidelines recommend daily antiinflammatory medication for patients with persistent forms of asthma. Inhaled corticosteroids are recommended for mildly and moderately persistent asthma because of a more favorable side effect profile than that of oral steroids.

Ref: National Asthma Education Panel Prevention Program. Expert Panel Report II. Guidelines for the Diagnosis and Management of Asthma. www.nhlbi.nih.gov/nhlbi/nhlbi.htm

2. (B) Peak expiratory flow rate (PEFR) correlates most closely with forced expiratory volume in the first second (FEV_1), which is used to assess the degree of small airway obstruction.

Ref: Asthma. In: Young LY, Koda-Kimble MA, eds. *Applied Therapeutics: The Clinical Use of Drugs.* 6th ed. Vancouver, Wash: Applied Therapeutics; 1995: chapter 19.

3. (E) A PEFR of 80% or greater of a patient's personal best is indicative of good asthma control.

Ref: Asthma. In: Young LY, Koda-Kimble MA, eds. *Applied Therapeutics: The Clinical Use of Drugs.* 6th ed. Vancouver, Wash: Applied Therapeutics; 1995: chapter 19.

4. (E) Patients with asthma classify their PEFR recordings in terms of traffic signals. Green is good control. Yellow means caution or suboptimal control, perhaps necessitating a change in medication regimen. A PEFR in the red zone signals that the patient is in danger of acute bronchospasm and that immediate action is needed.

Ref: Asthma. In: Young LY, Koda-Kimble MA, eds. *Applied Therapeutics: The Clinical Use of Drugs.* 6th ed. Vancouver, Wash: Applied Therapeutics; 1995: chapter 19.

5. (A) Because PEFR is important objective assessment of a patient's control of asthma, measurements should be obtained daily.

Ref: Asthma. In: Young LY, Koda-Kimble MA, eds. *Applied Therapeutics: The Clinical Use of Drugs.* 6th ed. Vancouver, Wash: Applied Therapeutics; 1995: chapter 19.

P A T I E N T   P R O F I L E   8 3

HYPERLIPIDEMIA

ANSWERS

1. (A) According to the ATP III, diabetes is considered a risk equivalent.

Ref: Expert Panel on Detection, Evaluation, and Treatment of High Blood Cholesterol in Adults. Executive summary of the third report of the National Cholesterol Education Program (NCEP) on detection, evaluation, and treatment of high blood cholesterol in adults (Adult Treatment Panel III). *JAMA* 2001;285(19):2486–2497.

2. (E) Less than 100 mg/dL is the current LDL cholesterol goal for patients with existing cardiovascular disease or a coronary heart disease risk equivalent.

Ref: Expert Panel on Detection, Evaluation, and Treatment of High Blood Cholesterol in Adults. Executive summary of the third report of the National Cholesterol Education Program (NCEP) on detection, evaluation, and treatment of high blood cholesterol in adults (Adult Treatment Panel III). *JAMA* 2001;285(19): 2486–2497.

3. (B) Liver function tests should be monitored before and after initiating HMG-CoA reductase inhibitor therapy.

Ref: McKenney JM. Dyslipidemias, atherosclerosis, and coronary heart disease. In: Young YL, Koda-Kimble MA, eds. *Applied Therapeutics: The Clinical Use of Drugs.* Vancouver, WA: Applied Therapeutics, 2005:13(1–39).

4. (A) Hypertension, low HDL cholesterol, and age are JF's positive risk factors for heart disease based on the National Cholesterol Education Program's Adult Treatment Panel III.

Ref: Expert Panel on Detection, Evaluation, and Treatment of High Blood Cholesterol in Adults. Executive summary of the third report of the National Cholesterol Education Program (NCEP) on detection, evaluation, and treatment of high blood cholesterol in adults (Adult Treatment Panel III). *JAMA* 2001;285(19): 2486–2497.

5. (D) Disagree; her LDL cholesterol goal is less than 100 mg/dL, and follow-up should be in 6 weeks.

Ref: Expert Panel on Detection, Evaluation, and Treatment of High Blood Cholesterol in Adults. Executive summary of the third report of the National Cholesterol Education Program (NCEP) on detection,

evaluation, and treatment of high blood cholesterol in adults (Adult Treatment Panel III). *JAMA* 2001;285(19):2486– 2497.

6. (C) Myositis is myalgia and an increase in serum creatine phosphokinase (CPK) of greater than 10 times the upper limit of normal. We should monitor CPK levels when there are unexplained symptoms of muscle aches.

Ref: McKenney JM. Dyslipidemias, atherosclerosis, and coronary heart disease. In: Young YL, Koda-Kimble MA, eds. *Applied Therapeutics: The Clinical Use of Drugs.* Vancouver, WA: Applied Therapeutics, 2005:13(1–39).

7. (D) Revisit and emphasize lifestyle modifications and smoking cessation but also add ezetimibe 10 mg PO qd.

Ref: Expert Panel on Detection, Evaluation, and Treatment of High Blood Cholesterol in Adults. Executive summary of the third report of the National Cholesterol Education Program (NCEP) on detection, evaluation, and treatment of high blood cholesterol in adults (Adult Treatment Panel III). *JAMA* 2001;285(19):2486–2497.

8. (A) Hydrochlorothiazide increases total cholesterol on a transient basis.

Ref: McKenney JM. Dyslipidemias, atherosclerosis, and coronary heart disease. In: Young YL, Koda-Kimble MA, eds. *Applied Therapeutics: The Clinical Use of Drugs.* Vancouver, WA: Applied Therapeutics, 2005:13(1–39).

9. (B) Ezetimibe has been shown to cause fatigue but not flatulence and flushing.

Ref: McKenney JM. Dyslipidemias, atherosclerosis, and coronary heart disease. In: Young YL, Koda-Kimble MA, eds. *Applied Therapeutics: The Clinical Use of Drugs.* Vancouver, WA: Applied Therapeutics, 2005:13(1–39).

10. (D) A therapeutic lifestyle change (TLC) diet is comprised of a limit of saturated fat to less than 7% of calories, increased viscous (soluble) fiber (10–25 g/ day), and increased plant stanols/sterols (2 g/day).

Ref: Expert Panel on Detection, Evaluation, and Treatment of High Blood Cholesterol in Adults. Executive summary of the third report of the National Cholesterol Education Program (NCEP) on detection, evaluation, and treatment of high blood cholesterol in adults (Adult Treatment Panel III). *JAMA* 2001;285(19):2486–2497.

PATIENT PROFILE 8 4
ANTACID SUSPENSIONS

ANSWERS

1. (E) The molecular weight would be the sum of the atomic frequencies multiplied by atomic weight.

   Ref: Stocklosa M, Ansel H. *Pharmaceutical Calculations*. 10th ed. Baltimore: Williams & Wilkins; 1996:305–306.

2. (E) Reduction in particle size, levigation with a nonsolvent, and thickening the vehicle all are steps that slow the rate of settling and produce a better suspension.

   Ref: Ansel H, Popavitch N, Allen L. *Pharmaceutical Dosage Forms and Drug Delivery Systems*. 6th ed. Baltimore: Williams & Wilkins; 1995:262–264.

3. (D) This is a simple sedimentation ratio based on Stokes'law of settling.

Ref: Martin A. *Physical Pharmacy*. 4th ed. Philadelphia: Lea & Febiger; 1993:479–480.

4. (E) According to the molecular formula, there would be 14 total positive charges, or 14 mEq/mmol. Multiplying this value by the millimoles of magaldrate found in 1 g would give the number of milliequivalents of magaldrate.

   Ref: Stocklosa M, Ansel H. *Pharmaceutical Calculations*. 10th ed. Baltimore: Williams & Wilkins; 1996:156–162.

5. (D) There is no scientific reason for the packaging. It has nothing to do with stability. The appearance of settled suspensions is not elegant.

   Ref: Ansel H, Popavitch N, Allen L. *Pharmaceutical Dosage Forms and Drug Delivery Systems*. 6th ed. Baltimore: Williams & Wilkins; 1995:253–262.

PATIENT PROFILE 8 5
ASTHMA

ANSWERS

1. (D) Asthma is a chronic inflammatory disorder that results in air obstruction.

   Ref: Self TH. Asthma. In: Koda-Kimble MA, Young LY, Kradjian WA, Guglielmo BJ, eds. *Applied Therapeutics: The Clinical Use of Drugs*. Philadelphia: Lippincott Williams & Wilkins, 2004:23-1–23-43.

2. (C) National Asthma Education Program Expert Panel Guidelines recommend short acting β-agonists for quick relief of symptoms.

   Ref: National Asthma Education Program Expert Panel Report: Guidelines for the Diagnosis and Management of Asthma: Update on Selected Topics 2002; available at *http://www.nhlbi. nih.gov/guidelines/asthma*.

3. (D) The recommended route of administration in this age group is by nebulizer.

   Ref: National Asthma Education Program Expert Panel Report: Guidelines for the Diagnosis and Management of Asthma: Update on Selected Topics 2002; available at *http://www.nhlbi.nih.gov/ guidelines/asthma*.

4. (B) Of these agents, isoproterenol is considered a nonselective β-agonist.

   Ref: Kelly HW, Sorkness CA. Asthma. In: Diporo JT, Talbert RL, Yee GC, et al, eds. *Pharmacotherapy: A Pathophysiologic Approach*. New York: McGraw Hill, 2002:475–510.

5. (B) β_2-Selectivity is less likely to be associated with cardiac effects.

   Ref: Self TH. Asthma. In: Koda-Kimble MA, Young LY, Kradjian WA, Guglielmo BJ, eds. *Applied Therapeutics: The Clinical Use of Drugs*. Philadelphia: Lippincott Williams & Wilkins, 2004:23-1–23-43.

6. (B) Because asthma is an inflammatory disorder, for patients with mild disease, low-dose inhaled corticosteroids are recommended as a maintenance medication.

   Ref: National Asthma Education Program Expert Panel Report: Guidelines for the Diagnosis and Management of Asthma: Update on Selected Topics 2002; available at *http://www.nhlbi. nih.gov/guidelines/asthma*.

7. (B) An Aerochamber is an example of a spacer device.

   Ref: Self TH. Asthma. In: Koda-Kimble MA, Young LY, Kradjian WA, Guglielmo BJ, eds. *Applied Therapeutics: The Clinical Use of Drugs*. Philadelphia: Lippincott Williams & Wilkins, 2004:23-1–23-43.

8. (D) An ultrasonic nebulizer uses sound waves rather than a propellant or airflow to generate an aerosol.

   Ref: Self TH. Asthma. In: Koda-Kimble MA, Young LY, Kradjian WA, Guglielmo BJ, eds. *Applied Therapeutics: The Clinical Use of Drugs*. Philadelphia: Lippincott Williams & Wilkins, 2004:23-1–23-43.

9. (A) Necrodomil and cromolyn are anti-inflammatory agents that work by stabilizing mast cells, thus preventing the release of mediators of inflammation. They are not

effective in treating acute bronchospasm. They are both administered by inhalation and are relatively free of side effects. They are considered alternatives to inhaled corticosteroids for mild persistent disease.

Ref: Self TH. Asthma. In: Koda-Kimble MA, Young LY, Kradjian WA, Guglielmo BJ, eds. *Applied Therapeutics: The Clinical Use of Drugs.* Philadelphia: Lippincott Williams & Wilkins, 2004:23-1–23-43.

10. (D) Oral corticosteroid therapy may be associated with growth retardation in children.

Ref: Self TH. Asthma. In: Koda-Kimble MA, Young LY, Kradjian WA, Guglielmo BJ, eds. *Applied Therapeutics: The Clinical Use of Drugs.* Philadelphia: Lippincott Williams & Wilkins, 2004:23-1–23-43.

PATIENT PROFILE 86

METASTATIC BREAST CANCER

ANSWERS

1. (D)

Ref: Hillner BE, Ingle JN, Chlebowski RT, et al. American Society of Clinical Oncology 2003 update on the role of bisphosphonates and bone health issues in women with breast cancer. *J Clin Oncol* 2003;21:4042–4057.

2. (C)

Ref: Lau AH. Fluid and electrolyte disorders. In: Koda-Kimbla MA, Young LY, Kradjan WA, et al, eds. *Applied Therapeutics: The Clinical Use of Drugs,* 8th ed. Philadelphia: Lippincott Williams & Wilkins, 2005:12(20).

3. (D)

Ref: Hillner BE, Ingle JN, Chlebowski RT, et al. American Society of Clinical Oncology 2003 update on the role of bisphosphonates and bone health issues in women with breast cancer. *J Clin Oncol* 2003;21:4042–4057.

4. (A)

Ref: Anderson CM. Drug profiles. In: Pine JW, ed. *Companion Handbook to the Chemotherapy Sourcebook.* Philadelphia: Lippincott Williams & Wilkins, 1999:115.

5. (C)

Ref: Reisner L, Koo PJS. Pain and its management. In: Koda-Kimbla MA, Young LY, Kradjan WA, et al, eds. *Applied Therapeutics: The Clinical Use of Drugs,* 8th ed. Philadelphia: Lippincott Williams & Wilkins, 2005:9(16).

6. (C) The patient is receiving 200 mg/day of OxyContin. The equianalgesic dose of MS Contin is approximately 300 mg. Since we are changing to a new agent and cross-tolerance between the opiates is not 100%, the dose of the new agent can be 75% of the equianalgesic dose, which equals 225 mg. MS Contin is available as 100-mg tablets, so the dose will be 100 mg PO q12h.

Ref: Reisner L, Koo PJS. Pain and its management. In: Koda-Kimbla MA, Young LY, Kradjan WA, et al, eds. *Applied Therapeutics: The Clinical Use of Drugs,* 8th ed. Philadelphia: Lippincott Williams & Wilkins, 2005:9(12–16).

7. (C)

Ref: Reisner L, Koo PJS. Pain and its management. In: Koda-Kimbla MA, Young LY, Kradjan WA, et al, eds. *Applied Therapeutics: The Clinical Use of Drugs,* 8th ed. Philadelphia: Lippincott Williams & Wilkins, 2005:9(12–16).

8. (B)

Ref: Rowinsky EK, Tolcher AW. Antimicrotubule agents. In: Devita VT, Hellman S, Rosenberg SA, eds. *Cancer: Principles and Practice of Oncology,* 6th ed. Philadelphia: Lippincott Williams & Wilkins, 2001:432.

9. (C)

Ref: Rowinsky EK, Tolcher AW. Antimicrotubule agents. In: Devita VT, Hellman S, Rosenberg SA, eds. *Cancer: Principles and Practice of Oncology,* 6th ed. Philadelphia: Lippincott Williams & Wilkins, 2001:436.

10. (D)

Ref: Rowinsky EK, Tolcher AW. Antimicrotubule agents. In: Devita VT, Hellman S, Rosenberg SA, eds. *Cancer: Principles and Practice of Oncology,* 6th ed. Philadelphia: Lippincott Williams & Wilkins, 2001:433.

PATIENT PROFILE 87

RESPIRATORY TRACT INFECTION

ANSWERS

1. (A) The most likely pathogen is *Streptococcus pneumoniae*. A culture frequently is performed, and there is no growth. It is difficult to grow pathogens from the lung. *Legionella* species, which are atypical organisms, also cause community-acquired pneumonia, although less commonly than *S. pneumoniae*. It is unlikely that community-acquired pneumonia would be caused by *Pseudomonas aeruginosa* (a gram-negative non–lactose fermenting bacillus commonly found in institutional settings that can cause nosocomial pneumonia), *Bacteroides fragilis* (an anaerobe typically found in the GI tract), or *Peptostreptococcus,* an oral anaerobe. Anaerobic bacteria may be present in persons with aspiration pneumonia.

   Ref: Bartlett JG, Breiman RF, Mandell LA, et al. Community-acquired pneumonia in adults: guidelines for management. *Clin Infect Dis* 1998;26.811–838.

2. (C) PJ's lack of compliance suggests that once-daily therapy be used if possible. His enrollment in an indigent care program will allow him to obtain free medication. The only medication listed that can be given as once a day is azithromycin.

   Ref: Bartlett JG, Breiman RF, Mandell LA, et al. Community-acquired pneumonia in adults: guidelines for management. *Clin Infect Dis* 1998;26:811–838.

3. (B) Azithromycin is the only choice listed that will cover both *Streptococcus pneumoniae* and *Legionella* organisms.

   Ref: Bartlett JG, Breiman RF, Mandell LA, et al. Community-acquired pneumonia in adults: guidelines for management. *Clin Infect Dis* 1998;26:811–838.

4. (E) A pneumococcal strain with an intermediate resistance pattern to penicillin can still be treated with penicillin. However, PJ also had the positive urine *Legionella* antigen. The fluoroquinolones are superb second-line agents for controlling infection. They also can be used as first-line agents as well; however, spectrum preservation should prevail. Because of PJ's situation, a once-daily drug with coverage against both pneumococci and *Legionella* organisms should be considered. Levofloxacin is the appropriate choice. Trovafloxacin also would work, but it has the broadest spectrum of activity of all the quinolones, and it should be reserved for patients who would benefit from therapy with such a broad-spectrum agent.

   Ref: Bartlett JG, Breiman RF, Mandell LA, et al. Community-acquired pneumonia in adults: guidelines for management. *Clin Infect Dis* 1998;26:811–838.

5. (B) Severe community-acquired pneumonia requires broad-spectrum coverage. Antibiotic coverage should include *Streptococcus pneumoniae, Haemophilus influenzae,* and atypical organisms such as *Legionella, Mycoplasma,* and *Chlamydia* species. Guidelines produced by both the American Thoracic Society and the Infectious Disease Society of America suggest use of a third-generation cephalosporin in combination with a macrolide to cover all possible pathogens in this setting. Both the third-generation cephalosporin and the macrolide will be useful in covering potentially penicillin-resistant strains of pneumococci. Doxycycline also may be useful, but it is not a firstline agent in this clinical situation.

   Ref: Bartlett JG, Breiman RF, Mandell LA, et al. Community-acquired pneumonia in adults: guidelines for management. *Clin Infect Dis* 1998;26:811–838.

PATIENT PROFILE 88

DIABETES MELLITUS: COMPLICATIONS

ANSWERS

1. (B) A fasting plasma glucose concentration of 126 mg/dL or greater is a diagnostic criterion for diabetes mellitus. A 2-hour postload glucose concentration of 200 mg/dL or greater during an oral glucose tolerance test or a casual blood glucose concentration of 200 mg/dL or greater plus symptoms of diabetes (e.g., polydipsia, polyuria, and unexplained weight loss) is diagnostic for diabetes mellitus.

   Ref: American Diabetes Association. Clinical practice recommendations 2004. *Diabetes Care* 2004;27(1):S9.

2. (B) Common symptoms indicating hyperglycemia include polyuria, polydipsia, weight loss, and occasionally, polyphagia and blurred vision. The patient complains of thirst.

   Ref: American Diabetes Association. Clinical practice recommendations 2004. *Diabetes Care* 2004;27(1):S5.

3. (D) Glyburide (a sulfonylurea) and regular insulin both work by increasing insulin production—which may lead to a hypoglycemic event owing to increased effects of insulin. On the other hand, metformin works by increasing

insulin sensitivity. Atenolol blocks the counterregulatory response of the body to a hypoglycemic event and has no effect on causing a hypoglycemic response.

Ref: Oki JC, Isley WL. Diabetes mellitus. In: Dipiro JT, Talbert RL, Yee GC, et al, eds. *Pharmacotherapy: A Pathophysiologic Approach,* 5th ed. New York: McGraw-Hill, 2002:1335–1358.

4. (C) Approximately 15 to 20 g oral glucose is adequate to treat a hypoglycemia event. Thus 4 to 6 oz fruit juice fulfills the criterion. Other options include 8 to 10 Life Savers, 3 to 6 glucose tablets, and a tube of glucose gel. Chocolate candies usually are not recommended owing to unreliable carbohydrate absorption.

Ref: Oki JC, Isley WL. Diabetes mellitus. In: Dipiro JT, Talbert RL, Yee GC, et al, eds. *Pharmacotherapy: A Pathophysiologic Approach,* 5th ed. New York: McGraw-Hill, 2002:1335–1358.

5. (C) Sweating most likely will appear as WV's first symptom of hypoglycemia. Since WV is taking a β-blocker, sympathetic symptoms of hypoglycemia will be blunted (i.e., palpitations, tachycardia). The other listed neuroglycopenic symptoms (i.e., seizure, confusion) will occur later when the hypoglycemic event had worsened.

Ref: Oki JC, Isley WL. Diabetes mellitus. In: Dipiro JT, Talbert RL, Yee GC, et al, eds. *Pharmacotherapy: A Pathophysiologic Approach,* 5th ed. New York: McGraw-Hill, 2002:1335–1358.

6. (A) Patients like WV, diagnosed with type 2 diabetes, always should be screened for complications immediately on diagnosis. Patients with type 1 diabetes often are screened for certain complications at 5 years after diagnosis.

Ref: American Diabetes Association. Clinical practice recommendations 2004. *Diabetes Care* 2004;27(1):S21–35.

7. (D) Patients like WV, with type 2 diabetes, are more likely to experience hyperglycemia as HHNS rather than DKA; DKA is associated with type 1 diabetes. Retinopathy,

neuropathy, and cardiovascular complications may be present when WV was diagnosed with diabetes.

Ref: American Diabetes Association. Clinical practice recommendations 2004. *Diabetes Care* 2004;27(1):S94–102.

8. (C) WV is diagnosed with autonomic neuropathy, which includes erectile dysfunction. Other autonomic neuropathies include inactive bladder and decreased intestinal and gastric peristalsis. Peripheral neuropathy may include loss of sensation in the feet or a foot ulcer.

Ref: American Diabetes Association. Clinical practice recommendations 2004. *Diabetes Care* 2004;27(1):S15–35.

9. (B) The prevention of cardiovascular complications in a patient with diabetes involves control of blood pressure and lipids, use of antiplatelets, smoking cessation, and coronary heart disease screening and treatment. The goal blood pressure for a patient with diabetes is 130/80 mm Hg. Other goal values include preprandial glucose concentration od between 90 and 130 mg/dL, postprandial glucose concentration of less than 180 mg/dL, LDL of less than 100 mg/dL, HDL of greater than 40 mg/dL, and triglycerides of less than 150 mg/dL.

Ref: American Diabetes Association. Clinical practice recommendations 2004. *Diabetes Care* 2004;27(1):S15–35.

10. (B) According to the patient case, WV's blood pressure of 132/90 mm Hg falls as a risk factor for the metabolic syndrome. According to ATP III guidelines, risk factors for the metabolic syndrome for a male patient are defined as triglycerides of 150 mg/dL or greater, blood pressure of 130/85 mm Hg or greater, HDL of less than 40 mg/dL, fasting glucose concentration of greater than 110 mg/dL, and waist circumference of greater than 40 in.

Ref: Grundy SM, Cleeman JI, Merz CN, et al. Implications of recent clinical trials for the National Cholesterol

Ref: Education Program Adult Treatment Panel III guidelines. *Circulation* 2004;110:227–239.

PATIENT PROFILE 89

MEDICINAL CHEMISTRY

ANSWERS

1. (D) Cholestyramine is a nonabsorbable polymeric material that lowers plasma cholesterol levels through complexing with bile acids in the GI tract that normally

are reabsorbed to be reused for cholesterol biosynthesis. The polymer similarly binds to the steroidal compound ethinyl estradiol. Lovastatin works through a systemic mechanism, so no potential interaction is expected.

TUBERCULOSIS

ANSWERS

1. (D) The Mantoux tuberculin skin test is an intradermal injection of 5 tuberculin units of PPD of killed tubercle bacilli. The test usually is administered on the inner forearm. The area tested is examined induration and the result interpreted by a trained health care provider 48 to 72 hours after injection.

   Ref: Zeind CS, Gourley GA, Corbett CE. Tuberculosis. In: Herfindal ET, Gourley DR, eds. *Textbook of Therapeutics, Drug and Disease Management.* 6th ed. Baltimore: Williams & Wilkins; 1996:1283–1306.

2. (A) Pyridoxine (vitamin B$_6$) should be given with isoniazid to persons who have conditions in which neuropathy is common. It also should be given to pregnant patients and persons with a history of seizure disorders.

   Ref: Zeind CS, Gourley GA, Corbett CE. Tuberculosis, In: Herfindal ET, Gourley DR, eds. *Textbook of Therapeutics. Drug and Disease Management.* 6th ed. Baltimore: Williams & Wilkins; 1996:1283–1306.

3. (D) Optic neuritis is most toxic effect of ethambutol.

   Ref: Zeind CS, Gourley GA, Corbett CE. Tuberculosis. In: Herfindal ET, Gourley DR, eds. *Textbook of Therapeutics. Drug and Disease Management.* 6th ed. Baltimore: Williams & Wilkins; 1996:1283–1306.

4. (B) The addition of rifampin, which is a potent inducer of CYP450, may decrease phenytoin serum concentrations.

   Ref: Zeind CS, Gourley GA, Corbett CE. Tuberculosis. In: Herfindal ET and Gourley DR, eds. *Textbook of Therapeutics, Drug and Disease Management.* 6th ed. Baltimore: Williams & Wilkins; 1996:1283–1306.

5. (A) Hepatoxicity is the most toxic effect of pyrazinamide.

   Ref: Zeind CS, Gourley GA, Corbett CE. Tuberculosis. In: Herfindal ET and Gourley DR, eds. *Textbook of Therapeutics, Drug and Disease Management.* 6th ed. Baltimore: Williams & Wilkins; 1996:1283–1306.

OSTEOPOROSIS

ANSWERS

1. (B)

   Ref: Osteoporosis Prevention, Diagnosis, and Therapy, NIH Consensus Statement Online, March 27–29; 2000 (November 4, 2004);17(1):1–36; *http://consensus.nih.gov/cons/111/111_statement .htm.*

2. (D)

   Ref: Osteoporosis Prevention, Diagnosis, and Therapy, NIH Consensus Statement Online, March 27–29; 2000 (November 4, 2004);17(1):1–36; *http://consensus.nih.gov/cons/111/111_statement .htm.*

3. (D)

   Ref: Osteoporosis Prevention, Diagnosis, and Therapy, NIH Consensus Statement Online, March 27–29; 2000 (November 4, 2004);17(1):1–36; *http://consensus.nih.gov/cons/111/111_statement .htm.*

4. (C)

   Ref: Egsmose C, Hegedus L, Lund B, et al. Bone minerals and levothyroxine (letter). *Lancet* 1992;340:345–346.

   Ref: Ross DS. Monitoring L-thyroxine therapy: Lessons from the effects of L-thyroxine on bone mineral density. *Am J Med* 1991;91:1–4.

5. (B)

   Ref: Package insert: Fosamax (alendronate), Merck and Co., Inc., Whitehouse Station, NJ; 2004.

6. (B)

   Ref: Osteoporosis Prevention, Diagnosis, and Therapy, NIH Consensus Statement Online, March 27–29; 2000 (November 4, 2004);17(1):1–36; *http://consensus.nih.gov/cons/111/111_ statement .htm.*

7. (C)

   Ref: Package insert: Fosamax (alendronate), Merck and Co., Inc., Whitehouse Station, NJ, 2004.

8. (D)

   Ref: Package insert: Fosamax (alendronate), Merck and Co., Inc., Whitehouse Station, NJ, 2004.

9. (A)

   Ref: Package insert: Forteo (teriparatide), Eli Lilly and Co., Indianapolis, IN, 2002.

10. (C)

    Ref: Micromedex Healthcare series online, Micromedex, Inc., Greenwood Village, CO, 2004.

PATIENT PROFILE 92
URINARY TRACT INFECTION

ANSWERS

1. (E) Although *E. coli* is the predominant urinary tract pathogen, other gram-negative bacteria such as *Proteus* and *Pseudomonas* organisms are common with hospital-acquired UTI. The sensitivity of hospital-acquired bacteria to antibiotics has been shown to differ from that of community-acquired bacteria and is associated with a higher incidence of antibiotic resistance.

2. (B) Regardless of renal function, the first dose or loading dose of gentamicin is administered in the usual 1.5–2.0 mg/kg range for all patients. It is imperative that subsequent maintenance doses of the aminoglycoside are dose adjusted to renal function to avoid toxicity.

3. (A) Trough concentrations of gentamicin must be monitored and maintained at less than 2 mg/L to avoid dose-related nephro- and ototoxicity.

4. (A) Gentamicin is excreted unchanged in the urine. Declining renal function may elevate drug concentrations.

5. (E) Cefotaxime is a third-generation cephalosporin that has activity against gram-positive and gram-negative organisms, including *Pseudomonas* organisms.

6. (D) The criteria for conversion from intravenous to oral antibiotics are based on clinical presentation, response to the initial IV treatment, and whether the gastrointestinal tract is functioning. Age is not considered a criteria for conversion.

Ref: Sahai J. Urinary tract infections. In: Young LY, Koda-Kimble MA, eds. *Applied Therapeutics: The Clinical Use of Drugs.* 6th ed. Vancouver, Wash: Applied Therapeutics; 1995: chapter 63.

Ref: Romac DR. Urinary tract infections. In: Herfindal ET, Gourley DR, eds. *Textbook of Therapeutics, Drug and Disease Management.* Baltimore: Williams & Wilkins; 1996: chapter 65.

PATIENT PROFILE 93
ONCOLOGY: OVARIAN CANCER

ANSWERS

1. (E) CA-125 is not specific enough or sensitive enough for use as the sole diagnostic criterion. The level may be elevated in patients with benign ovarian disease.

Ref: Zamboni W, Goldspiel BR. Ovarian cancer. In: DiPiro JT, Talbert RL, Yee GC, Matzke GR, Wells BG, Posey LM, eds. *Pharmacotherapy: A Pathophysiologic Approach.* 4th ed. Stamford, Conn: Appleton & Lange; 1999:2136–2148.

Ref: Young LY, Koda-Kimble MA, eds. *Applied Therapeutics: The Clinical Use of Drugs.* 6th ed. Vancouver, Wash: Applied Therapeutics; 1995: chapter 90.

2. (D) JP has CHF, and the cardiotoxicity associated with doxorubicin therapy is severe enough to warrant a change to mitoxantrone, a synthetic anthracycline with less cardiotoxicity.

Ref: Valley AW, Balmer CM. Cancer treatment and chemotherapy. In: DiPiro JT, Talbert RL, Yee GC, Matzke GR, Wells BG, Posey LM, eds. *Pharmacotherapy: A Pathophysiologic Approach.* 4th ed. Stamford, Conn: Appleton & Lange; 1999:1957–2012.

3. (C) Pretreatment recommendations for patients receiving paclitaxel include both H_1 and H_2 blockers and a steroid.

Ref: Herfindal ET, Gourley DR (eds). *Textbook of Therapeutics, Drug and Disease Management.* 6th ed. Baltimore: Williams & Wilkins; 1996: chapter 86.

4. (B) All the adverse effects listed are associated with the use of paclitaxel, but the dose-limiting toxicity is bone marrow suppression.

Ref: Valley AW, Balmer CM. Cancer treatment and chemotherapy. In: DiPiro JT, Talbert RL, Yee GC, Matzke GR, Wells BG, Posey LM, eds. *Pharmacotherapy: A Pathophysiologic Approach.* 4th ed. Stamford, Conn: Appleton & Lange; 1999:1957–2012.

5. (D) Intraperitoneal administration of antineoplastic agents has been studied for use by patients with ovarian cancer. The goal is to maximize tumor exposure and minimize systemic effects.

Ref: Zamboni W, Goldspiel BR. Ovarian cancer. In: DiPiro JT, Talbert RL, Yee GC, Matzke GR, Wells BG, Posey LM, eds. *Pharmacotherapy: A Pathophysiologic Approach.* 4th ed. Stamford, Conn: Appleton & Lange; 1999:2136–2148.

Ref: Young LY, Koda-Kimble MA, eds. *Applied Therapeutics: The Clinical Use of Drugs.* 6th ed. Vancouver, Wash: Applied Therapeutics; 1995: chapter 93.

P A T I E N T   P R O F I L E   9 4

ASTHMA

ANSWERS

1. (E) All three drugs relieve asthma through different mechanisms.

2. (C) Cromolyn sodium inhibits mast cells degradation and release of histamine, a predisposing agent for asthmatic attacks.

3. (E) Ipratropium bromide is an anticholinergic agent that antagonizes acetylcholine effects on the bronchial smooth muscles.

4. (C)

5. (D) I, II, and IV are β_2-selective agonists; metoprolol is a β_1-selective antagonist.

6. (E) The ester groups in bitolterol increase lipophilicity; hence better absorption. Esterification of the catechol groups of colterol also increases volatlity, and delays deactivation by the enzyme COMT.

7. (C) Ipratropium is an anticholinergic agent. Carbachol is a cholinomimetic antiglaucoma drug. Administration of an anticholinergic agent such as ipratropium will decrease the effectiveness of carbachol.

8. (B) Propranolol is a nonselective β-blocker. Blocking of β_2 receptors by propranolol exacerbates asthma.

9. (A) Isoproterenol is a nonselective β agonist; the β_1 agonists cause blood vessels to constrict, leading to worsening of hypertension.

10. (C) Corticosteroids represent a major class of anti-inflammatory agents, and inflammation is one of the predisposing factors for asthmatic attacks.

P A T I E N T   P R O F I L E   9 5

BIPOLAR DISORDER

ANSWERS

1. (D) The *Diagnostic and Statistical Manual of Mental Disorders*, 4th edition, states that symptoms of mania include abnormally elevated mood, grandiosity, decreased need for sleep, talkativeness, flight of ideas, distractibility, psychomotor agitation, and excessive involvement in pleasurable activities that have a high potential for painful consequences.

Ref: American Psychiatric Association. *Diagnostic and Statistical Manual of Mental Disorders*. 4th ed. Washington, DC: American Psychiatric Association; 1994.

2. (B) Increased use of caffeinated beverages is the most likely option that would lead to a manic state. A and D would lead to lithium toxicity, and C would most likely lead to hypothyroidism and depressive symptoms (although hypothyroidism is thought to have induced mania in a few cases).

Ref: Young LY, Koda-Kimble MA, eds. *Applied Therapeutics: The Clinical Use of Drugs*. 6th ed. Vancouver, Wash: Applied Therapeutics; 1995: chapter 77.

3. (B) The patient is not effectively treated with lithium. Because she cycles rapidly, she is a good candidate for treatment with valproic acid.

Ref: Suppes T, Rush AJ, Kraemer HC, et al. Treatment algorithm use to optimize management of symptomatic patients with a history of mania. *J Clin Psychiatry* 1998;59:89–96.

4. (D) ACE inhibitors and thiazide diuretics both have been shown to markedly increase serum lithium levels.

Ref: Finley PR, Warner MD, Peabody CA. Clinical relevance of drug interactions with lithium. *Clin Pharmacokinet* 1995;29: 172–191.

5. (D) The therapeutic range for lithium is 0.6–1.0 mEq/L, although this range may vary slightly among institutions.

Ref: Young LY, Koda-Kimble MA, eds. *Applied Therapeutics: The Clinical Use of Drugs*. 6th ed. Vancouver, Wash: Applied Therapeutics; 1995: chapter 77.

PATIENT PROFILE 96

ACUTE OR CHRONIC RENAL FAILURE

ANSWERS

1. (B) Oliguria as compared with nonoliguria is associated with an increased risk of morbidity and mortality in ARF patients.

    Ref: Brophy D. Acute renal failure. In: Koda-Kimble MA, Young LY, Kradjan WA, et al, eds. *Applied Therapeutics: The Clinical Use of Drugs,* 8th ed. Philadelphia: Lippincott Williams & Wilkins, 2005:31(1–22).

2. (D) Baseline serum creatinine and BUN are necessary to establish the patient's preadmission renal function and classify the degree of renal failure. EF would help classify her CHF. ABGs and blood pH are used to assess metabolic acidosis.

    Ref: Hudson JQ, Johnson CA. Chronic kidney disease. In: Koda-Kimble MA, Young LY, Kradjan WA, et al, eds. *Applied Therapeutics: The Clinical Use of Drugs,* 8th ed. Philadelphia: Lippincott Williams & Wilkins, 2005:32(1–36).

3. (A) Nonoliguria is associated with improved patient outcomes in ARF.

    Ref: Brophy D. Acute renal failure. In: Koda-Kimble MA, Young LY, Kradjan WA, et al, eds. *Applied Therapeutics: The Clinical Use of Drugs,* 8th ed. Philadelphia: Lippincott Williams & Wilkins, 2005:31(1–22).

4. (A) Renal laboratory values such as serum creatinine and BUN and serum potassium are significantly elevated, indicating a sudden deterioration in renal function.

    Ref: Brophy D. Acute renal failure. In: Koda-Kimble MA, Young LY, Kradjan WA, et al, eds. *Applied Therapeutics: The Clinical Use of Drugs,* 8th ed. Philadelphia: Lippincott Williams & Wilkins, 2005:31(1–22).

5. (C) FeNa <1% is indicative of prerenal azotemia.

    Ref: Mueller BA. Acute renal failure. In: DiPiro JT, Talbert RL, Yee GC, et al, eds. *Pharmacotherapy: A Pathophysiologic Approach,* 5th ed. New York: McGraw-Hill, 2002:771–795.

6. (A) Sodium polysterene sulfonate removes potassium from the body and may be used to reduce serum potassium in patients with persistent hyperkalemia.

    Ref: Lau AH. Fluid and electrolyte disorders. In: Koda-Kimble MA, Young LY, Kradjan WA, et al, eds. *Applied Therapeutics: The Clinical Use of Drugs,* 8th ed. Philadelphia: Lippincott Williams & Wilkins, 2005:12(1–33).

7. (B) Furosemide is the loop diuretic of choice in converting patients from oliguria to nonoliguria in the presence of ARF.

    Ref: Brophy D. Acute renal failure. In: Koda-Kimble MA, Young LY, Kradjan WA, et al, eds. *Applied Therapeutics: The Clinical Use of Drugs,* 8th ed. Philadelphia: Lippincott Williams & Wilkins, 2005:31(1–22).

8. (e) Nifedipine may precipitate reflex tachycardia and should be used with caution in patients with an elevated heart rate.

    Ref: Trujillo TC, Nolan PE. Ischemic heart disease: Anginal syndromes. In: Koda-Kimble MA, Young LY, Kradjan WA, et al, eds. *Applied Therapeutics: The Clinical Use of Drugs,* 8th ed. Philadelphia: Lippincott Williams & Wilkins, 2005:17(1–33).

9. (E) In the presence of worsening renal or cardiac function, volume overload, and hypoalbuminemia, higher than usual loop diuretic doses may be necessary.

    Ref: Brophy D. Acute renal failure. In: Koda-Kimble MA, Young LY, Kradjan WA, et al, eds. *Applied Therapeutics: The Clinical Use of Drugs,* 8th ed. Philadelphia: Lippincott Williams & Wilkins, 2005:31(1–22).

10. (b) Diuretic resistance may occur in patients with advanced kidney disease, hypoalbuminemia, and sodium and fluid retention.

    Ref: Hudson JQ, Johnson CA. Chronic kidney disease. In: Koda-Kimble MA, Young LY, Kradjan WA, et al, eds. *Applied Therapeutics: The Clinical Use of Drugs,* 8th ed. Philadelphia: Lippincott Williams & Wilkins, 2005:32(1–36).

PATIENT PROFILE 97

CORONARY ARTERY DISEASE

ANSWERS

1. (D) The use of clopidogrel in the setting of acute MI has not been shown to improve outcome.

    Ref: Stringer KA, Lopez LM. Myocardial infarction. In: DiPiro JT, Talbert RL, Yee GC, Matzke GR, Wells BG, Posey LM, eds. *Pharmacotherapy: A Pathophysiologic Approach.* 4th ed. Stamford, Conn: Appleton & Lange; 1999:211–231.

2. (B) Verapamil is a negative inotrope and can worsen left ventricular failure.

Ref: Johnson JA, Parker RB, Geraci SA. Heart failure. In: DiPiro JT, Talbert RL, Yee GC, Matzke GR, Wells BG, Posey LM, eds. *Pharmacotherapy: A Pathophysiologic Approach.* 4th ed. Stamford, Conn: Appleton & Lange; 1999:153–181.

3. (D) Diltiazem has not been demonstrated to improve outcome after AMI.

Ref: Stringer KA, Lopez LM. Myocardial infarction. In: DiPiro JT, Talbert RL, Yee GC, Matzke GR, Wells BG, Posey LM, eds. *Pharmacotherapy: A Pathophysiologic Approach.* 4th ed. Stamford, Conn: Appleton & Lange; 1999:211–231.

4. (A) Use of ACE inhibitors after MI have been shown to prevent remodeling and the onset of CHF after MI.

Ref: Stringer KA, Lopez LM. Myocardial infarction. In: DiPiro JT, Talbert RL, Yee GC, Matzke GR, Wells BG, Posey LM, eds. *Pharmacotherapy: A Pathophysiologic Approach.* 4th ed. Stamford, Conn: Appleton & Lange; 1999:211–231.

5. (D) Nitrates have not been shown to decrease mortality during or after AMI despite their hemodynamic and analgesic benefits.

Ref: Stringer KA, Lopez LM. Myocardial infarction. In: DiPiro JT, Talbert RL, Yee GC, Matzke GR, Wells BG, Posey LM, eds. *Pharmacotherapy: A Pathophysiologic Approach.* 4th ed. Stamford, Conn: Appleton & Lange; 1999:211–231.

PATIENT PROFILE 98
BACTEREMIA AND SEPSIS

ANSWERS

1. (C) The rationale is as follows: No cephalosporin has activity against enterococi. That rules out D and E. Metronidazole is active against *B. fragilis*, an anaerobe, and is not useful in this situation because enterococci are gram-positive organisms. Vancomycin should be reserved for the control of enterococcal strains that are resistant to conventional therapy. When there are positive culture results, allow the results to guide therapy. Ampicillin and gentamicin in combination provide synergistic killing of the enterococci.

Ref: Moellering RC Jr. Enterococcus species, *Streptococcus bovis*, and *Leuconostoc* species. In: Mandell GL, Bennett JE, Dolin R, eds. *Principles and Practice of Infectious Diseases*, 5th ed. New York: Churchill Livingstone, 2000:2147–2152.

2. (B) The drug of choice to control MRSA is vancomycin. The patient weighs 80 kg, which dictates that the vancomycin should be dosed 1 g IV q12h.

Ref: Gilbert DN, Moellering RC Jr, Eliopoulos GM, Sande MA, eds. *The Sanford Guide to Antimicrobial Therapy 2004,* 34th ed. Hyde Park, VT: Antimicrobial Therapy, 2004:55.

3. (D) Metronidazole is the drug of choice for initial management of *C. difficile* colitis. Empirical treatment with metronidazole may allow for an adequate jump on treatment. If therapy with metronidazole fails, oral vancomycin at a dosage of 125 to 250 mg PO q6h should be considered. No conclusive results have demonstrated the benefit of *Lactobacillus* or yogurt.

Ref: Gilbert DN, Moellering RC Jr, Eliopoulos GM, Sande MA, eds. *The Sanford Guide to Antimicrobial Therapy 2004,* 34th ed. Hyde Park, VT: Antimicrobial Therapy, 2004:11.

4. (A) Vancomycin levels vary from publication to publication. A is safe. The other choices are inconsistent with the pharmacokinetics of vancomycin. Peak levels (if obtained at all) should be measured 1 hour after completion of the infusion. Vancomycin should be infused over 60 to 90 minutes to avoid "red man" syndrome. Vancomycin doses should be based on actual body weigh. Vancomycin is not an aminoglycoside, and its clearance does not directly mimic serum creatinine level.

Ref: Rybak MJ, Aeschlimann JR. Laboratory tests to direct antimicrobial pharmacotherapy. In: DiPiro JT, Talbert RL, Yee GC, et al, eds. *Pharmacotherapy: A Pathophysiolgoic Approach,* 5th ed. New York: McGraw-Hill, 2002:1812.

5. (C) Vancomycin is not considered a nephrotoxic drug when used alone. However, in combination with other drugs that are nephrhotoxic, such as aminoglycosides, amphotericin, and furosemide, vancomyin enhances the nephrotoxic potential of the other agents.

Ref: Gilbert DN, Moellering RC Jr, Eliopoulos GM, Sande MA, eds. *The Sanford Guide to Antimicrobial Therapy 2004,* 34th ed. Hyde Park, VT: Antimicrobial Therapy, 2004:65.

PATIENT PROFILE 99
ASTHMA

ANSWERS

1. (D) Inhaled albuterol and cromolyn are both appropriate for prevention of exercise-induced asthma. An optimal response to inhaled corticosteroids may take a few weeks; therefore these agents must be taken on a regular basis to be effective.

   Ref: Asthma. In: Young LY, Koda-Kimble MA, eds. *Applied Therapeutics: The Clinical Use of Drugs.* 6th ed. Vancouver, Wash: Applied Therapeutics; 1995: chapter 19.

2. (A) Because of its rapid onset of action, albuterol is classified as a quick-relief medication and would be the agent of choice for relief of acute bronchospasm. Cromolyn and fluticasone are considered maintenance therapies and are not used for immediate treatment.

3. (C) Salmeterol is a long-acting β-agonist with a delayed onset of action. It should be inhaled within 60 minutes before exercise for maximum benefit.

   Ref: AHFS Drug Information 98, Salmeterol Monograph.

4. (D) Tremors are a common side effect of therapy with β_2 agonists. Weight gain, growth suppression, oral thrush, and gastric ulceration are complications of corticosteroid therapy.

   Ref: Asthma. In: Young LY, Koda-Kimble MA, eds. *Applied Therapeutics: The Clinical Use of Drugs.* 6th ed. Vancouver, Wash: Applied Therapeutics; 1995: chapter 19.

5. (B) Isoproterenol is a nonselective β-agonist. It affects β-receptors in both the lung and heart. Compared with more selective β_2 agents, it may be associated with an increase in cardiovascular side effects such as hypertension and arrhythmias.

   Ref: Asthma. In: Herfindal ET, Gourley DR (eds). *Textbook of Therapeutics, Drug and Disease Management.* 6th ed. Baltimore: Williams & Wilkins; 1996: chapter 35.

PATIENT PROFILE 100
SKIN AND SOFT TISSUE INFECTIONS AND OSTEOMYELITIS

ANSWERS

1. (C) *Staphylococcus aureus* and group A streptococci (*S. pyogenes*) are the most common etiologic agents in cellulitis.

   Ref: Danziger LH, Fish DN, Pendland SL. Skin and soft tissue infections. In Koda-Kimble MA, Young LY, Kradian WA, et al., eds. *Applied Therapeutics. The Clinical Use of Drugs,* 8th edition. Philadelphia: Lippincott Williams & Wilkins, 2004: 1885–1898.

   Ref: McCormack JP, Brown G. Traumatic skin and soft tissue infections. In: Dipiro JT, Talbert RL, Yee GC, et al., eds. *Pharmacotherapy: A Pathophysiologic Approach,* 5th edition. New York: McGraw-Hill, 2002:67(1–11).

2. (D) Dicloxacillin has excellent coverage against gram-positive cocci and is the appropriate oral treatment for mild to moderate infection (PO 250 to 500 mg PO Q6H for 7 to 10 days). Local care includes elevation and immobilization of her leg and cool saline dressings to decrease the pain.

   Ref: Danziger LH, Fish DN, Pendland SL. Skin and soft tissue infections. In Koda-Kimble MA, Young LY, Kradian WA, et al., eds. *Applied Therapeutics. The Clinical Use of Drugs,* 8th edition. Philadelphia: Lippincott Williams & Wilkins, 2004: 1885–1898.

   Ref: McCormack JP, Brown G. Traumatic skin and soft tissue infections. In: Dipiro JT, Talbert RL, Yee GC, et al., eds. *Pharmacotherapy: A Pathophysiologic Approach,* 5th edition. New York: McGraw-Hill, 2002:67(1–11).

3. (E) Intravenous therapy is indicated in patients who are moderately to severely ill, who show systemic responses (e.g., chills and fever with temperatures of more than 37.8°C), or whose cellulitis is rapidly spreading. All drugs are reasonable treatment options except aztreonam, which does not cover gram-positive organisms.

   Ref: Danziger LH, Fish DN, Pendland SL. Skin and soft tissue infections. In Koda-Kimble MA, Young LY, Kradian WA, et al., eds. *Applied Therapeutics. The Clinical Use of Drugs,* 8th edition. Philadelphia: Lippincott Williams & Wilkins, 2004:1885–1898.

   Ref: McCormack JP, Brown G. Traumatic skin and soft tissue infections. In: Dipiro JT, Talbert RL, Yee GC, et al., eds. *Pharmacotherapy: A Pathophysiologic Approach,* 5th edition. New York: McGraw-Hill, 2002:67(1–11).

   Ref: Swartz MN. Cellulitis. *NEJM* 2004;305(9):904–912.

4. (E) Imipenem has no activity against MRSA.

Ref: Gugliemo BJ. Principles of infectious diseases. In Koda-Kimble MA, Young LY, Kradian WA, et al., eds. *Applied Therapeutics. The Clinical Use of Drugs,* 8th edition. Philadelphia: Lippincott Williams & Wilkins, 2004:56(1–25).

5. (B) Red man syndrome is a pseudoallergic reaction associated with vancomycin infusion. It is characterized by facial flushing, tachycardia, hypotension, and pruritus and occurs when large doses of the drug are administered rapidly. Infusion of vancomycin over longer time periods (2 hours) or preadministration of antihistamines is effective ways to prevent the reaction. Ototoxicity (associated with high doses) and phlebitis are other ADRs.

Ref: Middleton RK, Beringer PM. Anaphylaxis and drug allergies. In Koda-Kimble MA, Young LY, Kradian WA, et al., eds. *Applied Therapeutics. The Clinical Use of Drugs,* 8th edition. Philadelphia: Lippincott Williams & Wilkins, 2004:4(1–25).

6. (A) Linezolid has been associated with hematologic toxicities and MAO inhibition.

Ref: Gugliemo BJ. Principles of infectious diseases. In Koda-Kimble MA, Young LY, Kradian WA, et al., eds. *Applied Therapeutics. The Clinical Use of Drugs,* 8th edition. Philadelphia: Lippincott Williams & Wilkins, 2004:56(1–25).

7. (C) Imipenem can cause seizures, especially if given in large doses and if doses are not adjusted for renal function. Allergic reactions may occur, and there is cross-sensitivity with penicillin.

Ref: Abate BJ, Barriere SL. Antimicrobial selection. In Dipiro JT, Talbert RL, Yee GC, et al., eds. *Pharmacotherapy: A Pathophysiologic Approach,* 5th edition. New York: McGraw-Hill 2002:1817–1829.

8. (D) Either metronidazole or clindamycin could be added to the MRSA treatment because both drugs have excellent anaerobic coverage.

Ref: Danziger LH, Fish DN, Pendland SL. Skin and soft tissue infections. In Koda-Kimble MA, Young LY, Kradian WA, et al., eds. *Applied Therapeutics. The Clinical Use of Drugs,* 8th edition. Philadelphia: Lippincott Williams & Wilkins, 2004:1885–1898.

Ref: McCormack JP, Brown G. Traumatic skin and soft tissue infections. In: Dipiro JT, Talbert RL, Yee GC, et al., eds. *Pharmacotherapy: A Pathophysiologic Approach,* 5th edition. New York: McGraw-Hill, 2002:67(1–11).

9. (E) Osteomyelitis secondary to contiguous spread (spread of an infection to the bone from adjacent tissue) may involve multiple organisms including gram-positive pathogens (*S. aureus, S. epidermidis,* streptococci), gram-negative pathogens (e.g., *Pseudomonas aeruginosa, Proteus* sp., *E. coli*), and anaerobes. Parenteral antibiotic regimens in high doses for 4 to 6 weeks usually are necessary to achieve adequate bone levels. In patients with recent disease onset, oral quinolones may be used effectively with an identified pathogen and compliance.

Ref: Armstrong EP. Bone and joint infections. In: Dipiro JT, Talbert RL, Yee GC, et al., eds. *Pharmacotherapy: A Pathophysiologic Approach,* 5th edition. New York: McGraw-Hill, 2002:2017–2027.

Ref: Raasch RH. Osteomyelitis and septic arthritis. In: Koda-Kimble MA, Young LY, Kradian WA, et al., eds. *Applied Therapeutics. The Clinical Use of Drugs,* 8th edition. Philadelphia: Lippincott Williams & Wilkins, 2004:66(1–13).

10. (A) Gentamicin plus ceftazidime is a synergistic and effective combination against *Pseudomonas aeruginosa.*

Ref: Armstrong EP. Bone and joint infections. In: Dipiro JT, Talbert RL, Yee GC, et al., eds. *Pharmacotherapy: A Pathophysiologic Approach,* 5th edition. New York: McGraw-Hill, 2002:2017–2027.

Ref: Raasch RH. Osteomyelitis and septic arthritis. In: Koda-Kimble MA, Young LY, Kradian WA, et al., eds. *Applied Therapeutics. The Clinical Use of Drugs,* 8th edition. Philadelphia: Lippincott Williams & Wilkins, 2004:66(1–13).

PATIENT PROFILE 101

OINTMENTS

ANSWERS

1. (B) The concentration of drug in ointment is converted to total grams.

Ref: Stocklosa M, Ansel H. *Pharmaceutical Calculations.* 10th ed. Baltimore: Williams & Wilkins; 1996:101–103.

2. (D) Medicated ointment is diluted to a lower concentration through the addition of ointment base (diluent).

Ref: Stocklosa M, Ansel H. *Pharmaceutical Calculations.* 10th ed. Baltimore: Williams & Wilkins; 1996:117–120.

3. (B) The alternative alligation technique is used with the pure drug powder (100%) as the high concentration value.

Ref: Stocklosa M, Ansel H. *Pharmaceutical Calculations.* 10th ed. Baltimore: Williams & Wilkins; 1996:130–135.

4. (D) The percentage strength concentration is converted to grams (and then milligrams) of drug per gram of ointment.

Ref: Stocklosa M, Ansel H. *Pharmaceutical Calculations.* 10th ed. Baltimore: Williams & Wilkins; 1996:107–108.

5. (E) The addition of powder makes a stiffer ointment (more like a paste), but incorporation can be eased with the use of a levigating agent.

Ref: Stocklosa M, Ansel H. *Pharmaceutical Dosage Forms and Drug Delivery Systems.* 6th ed. Baltimore: Williams & Wilkins; 1995:375–380.

PATIENT   PROFILE   1 0 2
OPPORTUNISTIC INFECTIONS

ANSWERS

1. (A) Trimethoprim-sulfamethoxazole (TMP-SMZ, co-trimoxazole) is the preferred therapy for PCP. Early addition of adjunctive corticosteroid therapy to anti-PCP regimens has been shown to improve survival among patient with AIDS and moderate to severe PCP.

   Ref: Centers for Disease Control and Prevention. *USPHS/IDSA Guidelines for the Prevention of Opportunistic Infections in Persons with Human Immunodeficiency Virus, 2001.*

2. (A) TMP-SMZ is the preferred agent for PCP prophylaxis (both primary and secondary) among adults, adolescents, and children.

   Ref: Centers for Disease Control and Prevention. *USPHS/IDSA Guidelines for the Prevention of Opportunistic Infections in Persons with Human Immunodeficiency Virus, 2001.*

3. (B) Didanosine and zalcitabine have similar toxicity profiles and should be avoided in an antiretroviral regimen if possible.

   Ref: Department of Health and Human Services/Henry J Kaiser Family Foundation Panel on Clinical Practices for the Treatment of HIV Infection. Guidelines for the use of antiretroviral agents in HIV-infected adults and adolescents. Rockville, MD: HIV/AIDS Treatment Information Service, October 29, 2004 (available online at *http://AIDSinfo.nih.gov).*

4. (A) Stavudine (Zerit®); nucleoside reverse transcriptase inhibitor; peripheral neuropathy.

   Ref: Department of Health and Human Services/Henry J Kaiser Family Foundation Panel on Clinical Practices for the Treatment of HIV Infection. Guidelines for the use of antiretroviral agents in HIV-infected adults and adolescents. Rockville, MD: HIV/AIDS Treatment Information Service, October 29, 2004 (available online at *http://AIDSinfo.nih.gov).*

5. (D) First-line choices for MAC prophylaxis are either azithromycin or clarithromycin.

   Ref: Centers for Disease Control and Prevention. *USPHS/IDSA Guidelines for the Prevention of Opportunistic Infections in Persons with Human Immunodeficiency Virus, 2001.*

6. (B) Amphotericin B, an antifungal agent plus flucytosine, is appropriate therapy of choice for treatment of acute cryptococcal meningitis in patients with AIDS.

   Ref: Centers for Disease Control and Prevention. *USPHS/IDSA Guidelines for the Prevention of Opportunistic Infections in Persons with Human Immunodeficiency Virus, 2001.*

7. (B) Neutropenia is the dose-limiting toxicity of ganciclovir.

   Ref: Centers for Disease Control and Prevention. *USPHS/IDSA Guidelines for the Prevention of Opportunistic Infections in Persons with Human Immunodeficiency Virus, 2001.*

8. (B) Cidofovir's intracellular half-life is long, enabling the drug to be administered less frequently.

   Ref: Centers for Disease Control and Prevention. *USPHS/IDSA Guidelines for the Prevention of Opportunistic Infections in Persons with Human Immunodeficiency Virus, 2001.*

9. (A) Sulfadiazine is a para-aminobenzoic acid (PABA) analogue that competitively inhibits dihydropteroate synthase and prevents synthesis of folic acid in bacteria.

   Ref: Centers for Disease Control and Prevention. *USPHS/IDSA Guidelines for the Prevention of Opportunistic Infections in Persons with Human Immunodeficiency Virus, 2001.*

10. (C) Nephrotoxicity.

    Ref: Centers for Disease Control and Prevention. *USPHS/IDSA Guidelines for the Prevention of Opportunistic Infections in Persons with Human Immunodeficiency Virus, 2001.*

PATIENT   PROFILE   1 0 3
RESPIRATORY TRACT INFECTION

ANSWERS

1. (B) The potential pathogens that need attention include *Streptococcus pneumoniae* (pneumococcus), Haemophilus influenzae, and atypical organisms (*Legionella, Mycoplasma,* and *Chlamydia*). The lack of sputum and history of diarrhea suggest *Legionella,* but this organism is difficult to isolate. Empiric therapy for infection by the aforementioned organisms is warranted.

Because the patient has been admitted to the hospital, IV administration of a third-generation cephalosporin and macrolide is warranted. The other selections lack the spectrum of coverage necessary to control pathogens that cause severe community-acquired pneumonia.

Ref: Bartlett JG, Breiman RF, Mandell LA, et al. Community-acquired pneumonia in adults: guidelines for management. *Clin Infect Dis* 1998;26:811–838.

2. (A) Levofloxacin is a fluoroquinolone with excellent gram-positive coverage that includes pneumococci. It also possesses an extended spectrum of coverage that includes atypical bacteria, such as *Legionella* species. Levofloxacin can be used as a primary agent in the care of these patients, but it is preferred as a second-line agent. This patient needs a fluoroquinolone because of the rash caused by the primary antibiotic. The rash is most likely caused by the cephalosporin. With addition of the fluoroquinolone, the atypical bacteria are doubly covered. Because of this overlap in coverage, the macrolide antibiotic is discontinued, leaving the patient treated with only the fluoroquinolone for community-acquired pneumonia.

    Ref: Bartlett JG, Breiman RF, Mandell LA, et al. Community-acquired pneumonia in adults: guidelines for management. *Clin Infect Dis* 1998;26:811–838.

3. (D) It is difficult to isolate *Legionella* organisms. The *Legionella* urine antigen test has a high sensitivity but a low specificity. If the test result is positive, *Legionella* organisms are present, and the patient should be treated accordingly. If the test result is negative, *Legionella* organisms still may be present. The test is not specific enough to allow a conclusion that the patient does not have

infection. In this case the patient should be treated as though an infection is present.

    Ref: Bartlett JG, Breiman RF, Mandell LA, et al. Community-acquired pneumonia in adults: guidelines for management. *Clin Infect Dis* 1998;26:811–838.

4. (B) GI upset is the most frequent problem among patients who take erythromycin. This macrolide antibiotic stimulates motilin in the GI tract and causes GI discomfort. In addition to its antimicrobial properties, erythromycin has been used as a prokinetic agent in the care of patients who cannot tolerate metoclopramide or cisapride.

    Ref: Gilbert DN, Moellering RC Jr, Sande MA, eds. *The Sanford Guide to Antimicrobial Therapy 1998*. 28th ed. Vienna, Va: Antimicrobial Therapy; 1998:68.

5. (E) Vancomycin is considered effective against almost all gram-positive organisms, including resistant pneumococci. The addition of rifampin to vancomycin provides synergistic killing of the organism. Changing antibiotic class from high-dose penicillin (effective against low and intermediate-level resistance) to cephalosporins provides effective killing of resistant strains of pneumococci.

    Ref: Gold HS, Moellering RC Jr. Antimicrobial-drug resistance. *N Engl J Med* 1996;335:1445–1453.

PATIENT PROFILE 104

ASTHMA

ANSWERS

1. (C) Step 2: Mild persistent asthma caused by having daily symptoms three times per week.

    Ref: Kelly HW, Sorkness CA. Asthma. In: DiPiro JT, Talbert RL, Yee GC, et al., eds. *Pharmacotherapy: A Pathophysiologic Approach,* 5th edition. New York: McGraw-Hill, 2002:475–510.

2. (C) Receive the influenza vaccine because of its ability to decrease morbidity and mortality in asthmatic patients.

    Ref: Kelly HW, Sorkness CA. Asthma. In: DiPiro JT, Talbert RL, Yee GC, et al., eds. *Pharmacotherapy: A Pathophysiologic Approach,* 5th edition. New York: McGraw-Hill, 2002:475–510.

3. (D) Ibuprofen 200 mg as needed for occasional aches and pains. Nonsteroidal anti-inflammatory drugs have been shown to exacerbate asthma attacks in some asthmatic patients.

    Ref: National Asthma Education and Prevention Program, Expert Panel Report 2. *Guidelines for the Diagnosis and Management of Asthma.* NIH Publication No. 97-4051. Bethesda, MD: US Department of Health and Human Services, 1997.

4. (E) Albuterol as needed and fluticasone 44-µg inhaler one puff by mouth two times a day. Albuterol will be the

"rescue" inhaler, and an inhaled corticosteroid is the first-line agent in the treatment of chronic asthma.

    Ref: Kelly HW, Sorkness CA. Asthma. In: DiPiro JT, Talbert RL, Yee GC, et al., eds. *Pharmacotherapy: A Pathophysiologic Approach,* 5th edition. New York: McGraw-Hill, 2002:475–510.

5. (E) The dose of the medication can tail off toward the end of the canister.

    Ref: Kelly HW, Sorkness CA. Asthma. In: DiPiro JT, Talbert RL, Yee GC, et al., eds. *Pharmacotherapy: A Pathophysiologic Approach,* 5th edition. New York: McGraw-Hill, 2002:475–510.

6. (B) Tremor caused by the β_2 effect on skeletal muscle.

    Ref: Kelly HW, Sorkness CA. Asthma. In: DiPiro JT, Talbert RL, Yee GC, et al., eds. *Pharmacotherapy: A Pathophysiologic Approach,* 5th edition. New York: McGraw-Hill, 2002:475–510.

7. (E) Less patient technique dependent because of dry powder inhaler (DPI) only requiring the patient to breath in forcefully.

    Ref: Kelly HW, Sorkness CA. Asthma. In: DiPiro JT, Talbert RL, Yee GC, et al., eds. *Pharmacotherapy: A Pathophysiologic Approach,* 5th edition. New York: McGraw-Hill, 2002:475–510.

8. (C) Montelukast is the best option because of its safety profile compared to theophylline.

Ref: National Asthma Education and Prevention Program, Expert Panel Report 2. *Guidelines for the Diagnosis and Management of Asthma.* NIH Publication No. 97-4051. Bethesda, MD: US Department of Health and Human Services, 1997.

9. (D) Initiate Serevent Diskus® inhale one puff by mouth twice a day because of the product's proven efficacy in treating nocturnal symptoms.

Ref: National Asthma Education and Prevention Program, Expert Panel Report 2. *Guidelines for the Diagnosis and Management of Asthma.* NIH Publication No. 97-4051. Bethesda, MD: US Department of Health and Human Services, 1997.

10. (B) Three to six months would be an appropriate time frame for a patient to be reassessed after an addition to their therapy.

Ref: National Asthma Education and Prevention Program, Expert Panel Report 2. *Guidelines for the Diagnosis and Management of Asthma.* NIH Publication No. 97-4051. Bethesda, MD: US Department of Health and Human Services, 1997.

PATIENT PROFILE 105

TUBERCULOSIS

ANSWERS

1. (B) Tuberculosis is acquired through inhalation of infectious airborne particles, called *droplet nuclei.*

Ref: Zeind CS, Gourley GA, Corbett CE. Tuberculosis. In: Herfindal ET, Gourley DR, eds. *Textbook of Therapeutics. Drug and Disease Management.* 6th ed. Baltimore: Williams & Wilkins; 1996:1283–1306.

2. (B) Although rare, progressive liver dysfunction, jaundice, bilirubinuria, and severe and sometimes fatal hepatitis have been associated with the use of isoniazid.

Ref: Zeind CS, Gourley GA, Corbett CE. Tuberculosis. In: Herfindal ET, Gourley DR, eds. *Textbook of Therapeutics. Drug and Disease Management.* 6th ed. Baltimore: Williams & Wilkins; 1996:1283–1306.

3. (A) Persons who have conditions in which neuropathy is common, such as diabetes, should be given pyridoxine (vitamin B_6) with isoniazid. Isoniazid is not an inducer of cytochrome P450 and does not frequently cause hyperuricemia.

Ref: Zeind CS, Gourley GA, Corbett CE. Tuberculosis. In: Herfindal ET, Gourley DR, eds. *Textbook of Therapeutics. Drug and Disease Management.* 6th ed. Baltimore: Williams & Wilkins; 1996: 1283–1306.

4. (D) The main toxicities associated with streptomycin, an aminoglycoside, are nephrotoxicity and ototoxicity.

Ref: Zeind CS, Gourley GA, Corbett CE. Tuberculosis. In: Herfindal ET, Gourley DR, eds. *Textbook of Therapeutics. Drug and Disease Management.* 6th ed. Baltimore: Williams & Wilkins; 1996:1283–1306.

5. (D) Rifampin, a potent inducer of hepatic microsomal enzymes, may decrease the efficacy of oral contraceptives. This agent may impart an orange discoloration to the urine, feces, sputum, tears, and sweat and may permanently discolor soft contact lenses.

Ref: Zeind CS, Gourley GA, Corbett CE. Tuberculosis. In: Herfindal ET, Gourley DR, eds. *Textbook of Therapeutics. Drug and Disease Management.* 6th ed. Baltimore: Williams & Wilkins; 1996: 1283–1306.

PATIENT PROFILE 106

^{32}P CONSIDERATIONS

ANSWERS

1. D

Ref: Saha, GP. *Fundamentals of Nuclear Pharmacy.* 4th ed. New York: Springer-Verlag; 1997:29.

2. C

Ref: Saha, GP. *Fundamentals of Nuclear Pharmacy.* 4th ed. New York: Springer-Verlag; 1997:29.

3. B

Ref: Wang CH, Willis DL, Loveland WD. *Radiotracer Methodology in the Biological, Environmental, and Physical Sciences.* New Jersey: Prentice Hall; 1975:350.

4. A

Ref: Wang CH, Willis DL, Loveland WD. *Radiotracer Methodology in the Biological, Environmental, and Physical Sciences.* New Jersey: Prentice Hall; 1975:155.

5. E

Ref: Saha, GP. *Fundamentals of Nuclear Pharmacy*. 4th ed. New York: Springer-Verlag; 1997:20–21.

6. A

Ref: Saha, GP. *Fundamentals of Nuclear Pharmacy*. 4th ed. New York: Springer-Verlag; 1997:20–21.

7. D

Ref: Wang CH, Willis DL, Loveland WD. *Radiotracer Methodology in the Biological, Environmental, and Physical Sciences.* New Jersey: Prentice Hall; 1975:155.

8. B

Ref: Stoklosa MJ, Ansel HC. *Pharmaceutical Calculations*. 10th ed. Baltimore: Williams & Wilkins; 1996:221.

9. D

Ref: Shargel L, Mutnick AH, Souney PF, et al. *Comprehensive Pharmacy Review.* 4th ed. Philadelphia: Lippincott Williams & Wilkins; 2001:386.

10. B

Ref: Saha, GP. *Fundamentals of Nuclear Pharmacy*. 4th ed. New York: Springer-Verlag; 1997:326.

PATIENT PROFILE 107
ONCOLOGY: HODGKIN'S LYMPHOMA

ANSWERS

1. (B) Pulmonary toxicity is a known adverse effect of bleomycin. The cumulative dose of doxorubicin should not be high enough after only three cycles (alternating courses) to cause the cardiomyopathy that may manifest as shortness of breath.

Ref: Valley AW, Balmer CM. Cancer treatment and chemotherapy. In: DiPiro JT, Talbert RL, Yee GC, Matzke GR, Wells BG, Posey LM, eds. *Pharmacotherapy: A Pathophysiologic Approach.* 4th ed. Stamford, Conn: Appleton & Lange; 1999:1957–2012.

2. (C) These two agents are least likely to affect the bone marrow.

Ref: Valley AW, Balmer CM. Cancer treatment and chemotherapy. In: DiPiro JT, Talbert RL, Yee GC, Matzke GR, Wells BG, Posey LM, eds. *Pharmacotherapy: A Pathophysiologic Approach.* 4th ed. Stamford, Conn: Appleton & Lange; 1999:1957–2012.

3. (B) The combination of doxorubicin and chest irradiation increases the risk of cardiotoxicity.

Ref: Adams VR, Morris AK. Malignant lymphomas. In: DiPiro JT, Talbert RL, Yee GC, Matzke GR, Wells BG, Posey LM, eds. *Pharmacotherapy: A Pathophysiologic Approach.* 4th ed. Stamford, Conn: Appleton & Lange; 1999:2110–2135.

Ref: Herfindal ET, Gourley DR (eds). *Textbook of Therapeutics, Drug and Disease Management.* 6th ed. Baltimore: Williams & Wilkins; 1996: chapter 79.

4. (D) Because of the high emetogenicity of the antineoplastic regimen, the literature supports the use of a 5-HT3 antagonist and a steroid. The other options, although containing agents used for control of nausea and vomiting, are not administered in a regimen that would be effective.

Ref: Taylor AT. Nausea and vomiting. In: DiPiro JT, Talbert RL, Yee GC, Matzke GR, Wells BG, Posey LM, eds. *Pharmacotherapy: A Pathophysiologic Approach.* 4th ed. Stamford, Conn: Appleton & Lange; 1999:586–598.

Ref: Herfindal ET, Gourley DR (eds). *Textbook of Therapeutics, Drug and Disease Management.* 6th ed. Baltimore: Williams & Wilkins; 1996: chapter 25.

5. (A) The risk of a secondary malignant tumor among patients aggressively treated for lymphoma is well documented.

Ref: Adams VR, Morris AK. Malignant lymphomas. In: DiPiro JT, Talbert RL, Yee GC, Matzke GR, Wells BG, Posey LM, eds. *Pharmacotherapy: A Pathophysiologic Approach.* 4th ed. Stamford, Conn: Appleton & Lange; 1999:2110–2135.

PATIENT PROFILE 108
OBSESSIVE COMPULSIVE DISORDER

ANSWERS

1. (E) All of the statements about OCD are true and are based on the DSM-IV diagnostic criteria for OCD.

Ref: Augustin SG. Anxiety disorders. In: Koda-Kimble MA, Young LY, Kradjan WA, Guglielmo BJ, eds. *Applied Therapeutics: The Clinical Use of Drugs,* 8th edition. Baltimore: Lippincott Williams & Wilkins, 2005:1–47.

2. (C) A compulsion is defined as a behavior or ritual that is performed in a repetitive way in order to reduce anxiety associated with obsessions or to prevent some future event or situation.

   Ref: Augustin SG. Anxiety disorders. In: Koda-Kimble MA, Young LY, Kradjan WA, Guglielmo BJ, eds. *Applied Therapeutics: The Clinical Use of Drugs,* 8th edition. Baltimore: Lippincott Williams & Wilkins, 2005:1–47.

3. (B) One leading hypothesis for the etiology of OCD is that of serotonergic dysfunction. This hypothesis is supported by the fact that the only effective medication treatments for OCD primarily influence serotonergic transmission. However, the exact role of serotonin in OCD has not been determined.

   Ref: Augustin SG. Anxiety disorders. In: Koda-Kimble MA, Young LY, Kradjan WA, Guglielmo BJ, eds. *Applied Therapeutics: The Clinical Use of Drugs,* 8th edition. Baltimore: Lippincott Williams & Wilkins, 2005:1–47.

4. (E) Clomipramine is a potent inhibitor of serotonin reuptake, and is the only TCA that is FDA approved for the treatment of OCD.

   Ref: Augustin SG. Anxiety disorders. In: Koda-Kimble MA, Young LY, Kradjan WA, Guglielmo BJ, eds. *Applied Therapeutics: The Clinical Use of Drugs,* 8th edition. Baltimore: Lippincott Williams & Wilkins, 2005:1–47.

5. (A) SSRIs (e.g., fluvoxamine, fluoxetine, paroxetine, sertraline, citalopram) are the only first-line medication treatments for OCD. Clomipramine is currently reserved as a second-line treatment. There is no evidence that venlafaxine is useful in the treatment of OCD.

   Ref: Augustin SG. Anxiety disorders. In: Koda-Kimble MA, Young LY, Kradjan WA, Guglielmo BJ, eds. *Applied Therapeutics: The Clinical Use of Drugs,* 8th edition. Baltimore: Lippincott Williams & Wilkins, 2005:1–47.

6. (E) Benzodiazepines generally are not beneficial in treating OCD. Clonazepam appears to have serotonergic activity and may be helpful with anxiety symptoms; it can also interfere with the effectiveness of cognitive behavioral therapy and should not be used concurrently.

Fluvoxamine and fluoxetine can significantly reduce serum levels of clonazepam.

Ref: Augustin SG. Anxiety disorders. In: Koda-Kimble MA, Young LY, Kradjan WA, Guglielmo BJ, eds. *Applied Therapeutics: The Clinical Use of Drugs,* 8th edition. Baltimore: Lippincott Williams & Wilkins, 2005:1–47.

7. (D) Response to medication treatment in OCD is gradual and often delayed. Initial improvements begin to appear within the first month, but 5 to 6 months may be necessary for maximal response. Nonetheless, complete elimination of symptoms is rare with currently available treatments. Patients may only experience a 25% to 35% reduction on their symptoms and be considered responders.

Ref: Augustin SG. Anxiety disorders. In: Koda-Kimble MA, Young LY, Kradjan WA, Guglielmo BJ, eds. *Applied Therapeutics: The Clinical Use of Drugs,* 8th edition. Baltimore: Lippincott Williams & Wilkins, 2005:1–47.

8. (B) The initial recommended dosage for fluvoxamine in adults is 50 mg per day (25 mg in children). It is best taken in the evening because of its sedating effects. The dosage can be increased by 50-mg increments every 3 to 4 days, based on patient tolerability, to an initial targeted effective dose of 150 to 200 mg per day.

Ref: Augustin SG. Anxiety disorders. In: Koda-Kimble MA, Young LY, Kradjan WA, Guglielmo BJ, eds. *Applied Therapeutics: The Clinical Use of Drugs,* 8th edition. Baltimore: Lippincott Williams & Wilkins, 2005:1–47.

9. (C) Fluvoxamine is an SSRI.

Ref: Augustin SG. Anxiety disorders. In: Koda-Kimble MA, Young LY, Kradjan WA, Guglielmo BJ, eds. *Applied Therapeutics: The Clinical Use of Drugs,* 8th edition. Baltimore: Lippincott Williams & Wilkins, 2005:1–47.

10. (C) Most clinical trials in OCD define clinical response as a 25% to 35% reduction in Y-BCOS scores.

Ref: Augustin SG. Anxiety disorders. In: Koda-Kimble MA, Young LY, Kradjan WA, Guglielmo BJ, eds. *Applied Therapeutics: The Clinical Use of Drugs,* 8th edition. Baltimore: Lippincott Williams & Wilkins, 2005:1–47.

PATIENT PROFILE 109

MEDICINAL CHEMISTRY

ANSWER

1. (D) Oxazepam is a short-acting hypnosedative drug. Its polar hydroxyl group makes it susceptible to direct phase II metabolism into inactive products. Butabarbital, a long-acting barbiturate, is not recommended for daily sleep induction because of the risk of habit formation. Neither B nor C is correct because the Valium® (diazepam) molecule does not contain an acidic or basic functional group to make excretion of the drug dependent on urinary pH. E is not appropriate; TJ is already suffering from sleep deprivation, and caffeine will worsen it.

MIXED DYSLIPIDEMIA

ANSWERS

1. (D) SS exhibits four independent risk factors for CHD other than elevated LDL: (a) being a man more than 45 years old, (b) having a first-degree relative with CHD less than 55 years old, (c) smoking, and (d) hypertension.

   Ref: Third Report of the National Cholesterol Education Program Expert Panel on Detection, Evaluation, and Treatment of High Blood Cholesterol in Adults (Adult Treatment Panel III). Final report. *Circulation* 2002;106:3143–3421.

2. (A) SS has both elevated triglycerides (TGs) and LDL in combination with an elevated glucose. Both fibrates and niacin can decrease elevated TGs, but niacin can worsen a patient's elevated glucose.

   Ref: Third Report of the National Cholesterol Education Program Expert Panel on Detection, Evaluation, and Treatment of High Blood Cholesterol in Adults (Adult Treatment Panel III). Final report. *Circulation* 2002;106:3143–3421.

3. (C) Ciprofibrate is not available in the United States.

   Ref: Third Report of the National Cholesterol Education Program Expert Panel on Detection, Evaluation, and Treatment of High Blood Cholesterol in Adults (Adult Treatment Panel III). Final report. *Circulation* 2002;106:3143–3421.

4. (D) The daily dose of fenofibrate is 200 mg daily.

   Ref: Third Report of the National Cholesterol Education Program Expert Panel on Detection, Evaluation, and Treatment of High Blood Cholesterol in Adults (Adult Treatment Panel III). Final report. *Circulation* 2002;106:3143–3421.

5. (E) Renal insufficiency is not a major adverse reaction of fenofibrate.

   Ref: Third Report of the National Cholesterol Education Program Expert Panel on Detection, Evaluation, and Treatment of High Blood Cholesterol in Adults (Adult Treatment Panel III). Final report. *Circulation* 2002;106:3143–3421.

6. (C) Severe hepatic insufficiency is an absolute contraindication of fibrates.

   Ref: Third Report of the National Cholesterol Education Program Expert Panel on Detection, Evaluation, and Treatment of High Blood Cholesterol in Adults (Adult Treatment Panel III). Final report. *Circulation* 2002;106:3143–3421.

7. (B) Both fibrates and statins have been associated with causing myopathy. When used together they are associated with potentially increasing the risk of myopathy.

   Ref: Third Report of the National Cholesterol Education Program Expert Panel on Detection, Evaluation, and Treatment of High Blood Cholesterol in Adults (Adult Treatment Panel III). Final report. *Circulation* 2002;106:3143–3421.

8. (E) The use of niacin may cause hyperglycemia.

   Ref: Third Report of the National Cholesterol Education Program Expert Panel on Detection, Evaluation, and Treatment of High Blood Cholesterol in Adults (Adult Treatment Panel III). Final report. *Circulation* 2002;106:3143–3421.

9. (B) The usual daily dose of regular release crystalline niacin that is effective in lowering LDL levels is 1.5 to 3.0 g/day.

   Ref: Third Report of the National Cholesterol Education Program Expert Panel on Detection, Evaluation, and Treatment of High Blood Cholesterol in Adults (Adult Treatment Panel III). Final report. *Circulation* 2002;106:3143–3421.

10. (A) Flushing caused by niacin can be blunted from the use of an anti-inflammatory dose of aspirin (650 mg) taken about 30 to 45 minutes before ingestion of niacin.

    Ref: Third Report of the National Cholesterol Education Program Expert Panel on Detection, Evaluation, and Treatment of High Blood Cholesterol in Adults (Adult Treatment Panel III). Final report. *Circulation* 2002;106:3143–3421.

BIPOLAR DISORDER

ANSWERS

1. (E) The *Diagnostic and Statistical Manual of Mental Disorders*, 4th edition, states that the symptoms of a manic episode are abnormally and persistently elevated, expansive or irritable mood, grandiosity, decreased need for sleep, talkativeness, flight of ideas, distractibility, psychomotor agitation, and involvement in pleasurable activities that have a high potential for painful consequences.

Ref: American Psychiatric Association. *Diagnostic and Statistical Manual for Mental Disorders.* 4th ed. Washington, DC: American Psychiatric Association; 1994.

2. (A) Valproic acid appears to have better efficacy than lithium, clonazepam, or chlorpromazine in the management of bipolar disorder when the patient has the subtype of rapid cycling.

Ref: Keck PE, McElroy SL, Strakowski SM. Anticonvulsants and antipsychotics in the treatment of bipolar disorder. *J Clin Psychiatry* 1998;59(suppl 6):74–81.

3. (E) Use of valproic acid requires that the patient have a complete blood cell count initially and then periodically because of the risk of thrombocytopenia. Liver function must be monitored because the drug may cause fatal hepatotoxicity. Serum valproate levels are monitored because levels between 50 and 120 μg/mL correlate with efficacy.

Ref: Young LY, Koda-Kimble MA, eds. *Applied Therapeutics: The Clinical Use of Drugs.* 6th ed. Vancouver, Wash: Applied Therapeutics; 1995: chapter 77.

4. (D) Lithium levels of 0.6–1.0 mEq/L correlate with efficacy. Higher levels cause toxicity. Lithium use also can cause hypothyroidism, so thyroid function tests are recommended every 6 months.

Ref: *Textbook of Psychopharmacology.* Washington DC: American Psychiatric Press; 1995: chapter 29.

5. (A) Therapeutic doses of aspirin have caused valproic acid toxicity, probably because of displacement of valproic acid from proteins.

Ref: Ciraulo DA. *Drug Interactions in Psychiatry.* 2nd ed. Baltimore: Williams & Wilkins; 1995: chapter 6.

PATIENT PROFILE 112

CONTRACEPTION

ANSWERS

1. (A) To ensure effectiveness, Depo-Provera® must be given during the first 5 days of a normal menstrual cycle. Day 1 is considered the day of menses onset.

Ref: Medroxyprogesterone acetate (drug monograph). In: Klasco RK, ed. DRUGDEX® System. Greenwood Village, CO: Thomson MICROMEDEX®. (edition expires 9/2004).

2. (C) Depo-Provera® should be administered every 12 weeks or 3 months. If the patient is more than 1 week late for a repeat injection, it is recommended to first exclude pregnancy.

Ref: Dickerson LM, Bucci KK. Contraception. In: DiPiro JT, Talbert RL, Yee GC, et al., eds. *Pharmacotherapy: A Pathophysiologic Approach,* 5th edition. New York: McGraw-Hill, 2002:1445–1461.

3. (A) Intramuscular injection is the route of administration for Depo-Provera®.

Ref: Dickerson LM, Bucci KK. Contraception. In: DiPiro JT, Talbert RL, Yee GC, et al., eds. *Pharmacotherapy: A Pathophysiologic Approach,* 5th edition. New York: McGraw-Hill, 2002:1445–1461.

4. (E) Depo-Provera® may cause adverse effects, including but not limited to breast tenderness, depression, dizziness, headache, insomnia, menstrual abnormalities, and weight gain.

Ref: Dickerson LM, Bucci KK. Contraception. In: DiPiro JT, Talbert RL, Yee GC, et al., eds. *Pharmacotherapy: A Pathophysiologic Approach,* 5th edition. New York: McGraw-Hill, 2002:1445–1461.

5. (A) Deep vein thrombosis is one contraindication to combined oral contraceptives. Other contraindications include breast cancer, diabetes with vascular disease, heart disease, hypertension, liver disease, and pregnancy.

Ref: Dickerson LM, Bucci KK. Contraception. In: DiPiro JT, Yee GC, et al., eds. *Pharmacotherapy: A Pathophysiologic Approach,* 5th edition. New York: McGraw-Hill, 2002: 1445–1461.

6. (D) To ensure efficacy, it is recommended to start oral contraceptive therapy either on the first day of menses or the first Sunday after the onset of menses. In many patients, the Sunday-start allows for menses during the week without any bleeding during the weekend.

Ref: Dickerson LM, Bucci KK. Contraception. In: DiPiro JT, Talbert RL, Yee GC, et al., eds. *Pharmacotherapy: A Pathophysiologic Approach,* 5th edition. New York: McGraw-Hill, 2002:1445–1461.

7. (B) Tetracycline use, as well as griseofulvin and rifampin therapy, require the use of a back-up method of contraception because of the decreased contraceptive effect.

Ref: Dickerson LM, Bucci KK. Contraception. In: DiPiro JT, Talbert RL, Yee GC, et al., eds. *Pharmacotherapy: A Pathophysiologic Approach,* 5th edition. New York: McGraw-Hill, 2002: 1445–1461.

8. (E) The onset of menses occurs during the placebo week or within 1 to 3 days after the last active pill.

Ref: Dickerson LM, Bucci KK. Contraception. In: DiPiro JT, Talbert RL, Yee GC, et al., eds. *Pharmacotherapy: A Pathophysiologic Approach,* 5th edition. New York: McGraw-Hill, 2002:1445–1461.

9. (E) Blurred vision, calf pain, and severe headache should be reported by an individual taking an oral contraceptive. The pneumonic ACHES (abdominal pain, chest pain, headaches, eye problems, severe leg pain) can be used to recall symptoms that may indicate a serious problem. Patients should be educated to report any of these symptoms to their provider.

Ref: Dickerson LM, Bucci KK. Contraception. In: DiPiro JT, Talbert RL, Yee GC, et al., eds. *Pharmacotherapy: A Pathophysiologic Approach,* 5th edition. New York: McGraw-Hill, 2002: 1445–1461.

10. (D) Seasonale® is the first Food and Drug Administration–approved product marketed as an extended-cycle oral contraceptive. It is a 91-day regimen with 84 active pills (levonorgestrel 0.15 mg/ethinyl estradiol 30 μg) and seven placebo pills.

Ref: Medroxyprogesterone acetate (drug monograph). In: Klasco RK, ed. DRUGDEX® System. Greenwood Village, CO: Thomson MICROMEDEX®. (edition expires 9/2004).

PATIENT PROFILE 113
URINARY TRACT INFECTIONS

ANSWERS

1. (E) Although the patient has no symptoms, she should receive antibiotic treatment because acute symptoms of pyelonephritis may develop in pregnant women with untreated bacteriuria. Maternal UTI during pregnancy has been implicated in preterm delivery and low birth weight.

2. (C) Trimethoprim (TMP) is a folic acid antagonist and should be avoided during the first trimester of pregnancy.

3. (A) Ampicillin is relatively safe to administer during pregnancy. Sulfonamides can cause kernicterus if given to mothers during the third trimester of pregnancy and in breast milk can cause hemolytic anemia in infants with G6PD deficiency.

4. (B) Cure rates with single-dose oral antibiotic therapy are lower than those with 7–10 day regimens in the management of UTI during pregnancy.

Ref: Sahai J. Urinary tract infections. In: Young LY, Koda-Kimble MA, eds. *Applied Therapeutics: The Clinical Use of Drugs.* Vancouver, Wash: Applied Therapeutics; 1995: chapter 63.

Romac DR. Urinary tract infections. In: Herfindal ET, Gourley DR, eds. *Textbook of Therapeutics, Drug and Disease Management.* Baltimore: Williams & Wilkins; 1996: chapter 65.

PATIENT PROFILE 114
PARKINSON'S DISEASE

ANSWERS

1. (A) Parkinson's disease is characterized by a decrease in dopamine. As the disease progresses, the decrease in dopamine becomes even more significant because of the destruction of dopaminergic neurons causing symptoms to increase in intensity.

Ref: Nelson MV, Berchou, RC, LeWitt PA. Parkinson's disease. In: DiPiro JT, Talbert RL, Yee GC, et al., eds. *Pharmacotherapy: A Pathophysiologic Approach,* 5th edition. New York: McGraw-Hill, 2002:1089–1102.

2. (D) The hallmark symptoms of Parkinson's disease include tremor at rest, bradykinesia, postural instability, and muscle rigidity. JB's diagnosis includes tremor at rest, which is typically unilateral initially.

Ref: Nelson MV, Berchou, RC, LeWitt PA. Parkinson's disease. In: DiPiro JT, Talbert RL, Yee GC, et al., eds. *Pharmacotherapy: A Pathophysiologic Approach,* 5th edition. New York: McGraw-Hill, 2002:1089–1102.

3. (C) Amantadine has been shown to be effective in treating tremor, making it a good choice for JB's initial therapy.

Ref: Nelson MV, Berchou, RC, LeWitt PA. Parkinson's disease. In: DiPiro JT, Talbert RL, Yee GC, et al., eds. *Pharmacotherapy: A Pathophysiologic Approach,* 5th edition. New York: McGraw-Hill, 2002:1089–1102.

4. (C) Livedo reticularis is a common side effect of amantadine but is reversible on discontinuation. It is characterized by mottling of the skin. Other common side effects include dry mouth, sedation, and vivid dreams.

Ref: Nelson MV, Berchou, RC, LeWitt PA. Parkinson's disease. In: DiPiro JT, Talbert RL, Yee GC, et al., eds. *Pharmacotherapy: A Pathophysiologic Approach,* 5th edition. New York: McGraw-Hill, 2002:1089–1102.

5. (B) Benztropine, an anticholinergic agent, has been shown to be useful in treating tremor associated with Parkinson's disease. It is not useful against bradykinesia,

postural instability, and muscle rigidity. It is typically used in younger rather than elderly patients because of its adverse effect profile, which is particularly bothersome in elderly patients.

Ref: Nelson MV, Berchou, RC, LeWitt PA. Parkinson's disease. In: DiPiro JT, Talbert RL, Yee GC, et al., eds. *Pharmacotherapy: A Pathophysiologic Approach,* 5th edition. New York: McGraw-Hill, 2002:1089–1102.

6. (D) The side effects of benztropine include the typical anticholinergic effects, such as dry mouth, constipation, and blurred vision. Other side effects include urinary retention, confusion, depression, and anxiety.

Ref: Nelson MV, Berchou, RC, LeWitt PA. Parkinson's disease. In: DiPiro JT, Talbert RL, Yee GC, et al., eds. *Pharmacotherapy: A Pathophysiologic Approach,* 5th edition. New York: McGraw-Hill, 2002:1089–1102.

7. (C) Benadryl® has anticholinergic properties and can be used to treat Parkinson-induced tremor. It is an over-the-counter drug, but should not be used without the advice of a physician.

Ref: Nelson MV, Berchou, RC, LeWitt PA. Parkinson's disease. In: DiPiro JT, Talbert RL, Yee GC, et al., eds. *Pharmacotherapy: A Pathophysiologic Approach,* 5th edition. New York: McGraw-Hill, 2002:1089–1102.

8. (A) JB should discontinue his use of Benadryl® because it may have additive anticholinergic side effects with benztropine.

Ref: Nelson MV, Berchou, RC, LeWitt PA. Parkinson's disease. In: DiPiro JT, Talbert RL, Yee GC, et al., eds. *Pharmacotherapy: A Pathophysiologic Approach,* 5th edition. New York: McGraw-Hill, 2002:1089–1102.

9. (C) JB is in the very early stages of Parkinson's disease and can continue to function as a lawyer. His job does not require fine motor skills and his resting hand tremor should not interfere with his performance.

Ref: Ernst M, Gottwald MD, Gidal BE. Parkinson's disease. In: Koda-Kimble MA, Young LY, Kradjan, WA, et al., eds. *Applied Therapeutics: The Clinical Use of Drugs,* 8th edition. Philadelphia: Lippincott Williams & Wilkins, 2005:1–30.

10. (B) The Hoehn and Yahr staging is a good monitoring tool for JB. JB is in stage I, with tremor only on one side of the body and the ability to function independently.

Ref: Ernst M, Gottwald MD, Gidal BE. Parkinson's disease. In: Koda-Kimble MA, Young LY, Kradjan, WA, et al., eds. *Applied Therapeutics: The Clinical Use of Drugs,* 8th edition. Philadelphia: Lippincott Williams & Wilkins, 2005:1–30.

PATIENT PROFILE 115
CORONARY ARTERY DISEASE

ANSWERS

1. (C) The patient has a low cardiac index.

Ref: Stringer KA, Lopez LM. Myocardial infarction. In: DiPiro JT, Talben RL, Yee GC, Matzke GR, Wells BG, Posey LM, eds. *Pharmacotherapy: A Pathophysiologic Approach.* 4th ed. Stamford, Conn: Appleton & Lange; 1999:211–231.

Ref: Erstad BL. Hypovolemic shock. In: DiPiro JT, Talbert RL, Yee GC, Matzke GR, Wells BG, Posey LM, eds. *Pharmacotherapy: A Pathophysiologic Approach.* 4th ed. Stamford, Conn: Appleton & Lange; 1999:408–421.

2. (D) A positive inotrope is most appropriate for a patient who has left ventricular dysfunction.

Ref: Stringer KA, Lopez LM. Myocardial infarction. In: DiPiro JT, Talbert RL, Yee GC, Matzke GR, Wells BG, Posey LM, eds. *Pharmacotherapy: A Pathophysiologic Approach.* 4th ed. Stamford, Conn: Appleton & Lange; 1999:211–231.

Ref: Erstad BL. Hypovolemic shock. In: DiPiro JT, Talbert RL, Yee GC, Matzke GR, Wells BG, Posey LM, eds. *Pharmacotherapy: A Pathophysiologic Approach.* 4th ed. Stamford, Conn: Appleton & Lange; 1999:408–421.

3. (E) Lidocaine is the drug of choice in the acute treatment of ventricular arrhythmias in the setting of an acute MI.

Ref: Stringer KA, Lopez LM. Myocardial infarction. In: DiPiro JT, Talbert RL, Yee GC, Matzke GR, Wells BG, Posey LM, eds. *Pharmacotherapy: A Pathophysiologic Approach.* 4th ed. Stamford, Conn: Appleton & Lange; 1999:211–231.

Ref: Bauman JL, Schoen MD. Arrhythmias. In: DiPiro JT, Talbert RL, Yee GC, Matzke GR, Wells BG, Posey LM, eds. *Pharmacotherapy: A Pathophysiologic Approach.* 4th ed. Stamford, Conn: Appleton & Lange; 1999:232–264.

Ref: Erstad BL. Hypovolemic shock. In: DiPiro JT, Talbert RL, Yee GC, Matzke GR, Wells BG, Posey LM, eds. *Pharmacotherapy: A Pathophysiologic Approach.* 4th ed. Stamford, Conn: Appleton & Lange; 1999:408–421.

4. (D) Amiodarone will increase serum drug concentration.

Ref: *Drug Interaction Facts.* St. Louis: Facts and Comparisons; 1999.

5. (A) β-Blocker therapy will improve mortality after MI and for CHF.

Ref: Talbert RL. Ischemic heart disease. In: DiPiro JT, Talbert RL, Yee GC, Matzke GR, Wells BG, Posey LM, eds. *Pharmacotherapy: A Pathophysiologic Approach.* 4th ed. Stamford, Conn: Appleton & Lange; 1999:182–210.

PATIENT PROFILE 116

ADULT IMMUNIZATIONS

ANSWERS

1. (C) Annual influenza vaccination is strongly recommended for individuals over the age of 6 months with chronic medical conditions that make them at increased risk for the complications of influenza.

   Ref: Bertino JS, Mayney MS. Vaccines, toxoids, and other immunobiologics. In: Dipiro JT, Talbert RL, Yee GC, et al., eds. *Pharmacotherapy: A Pathophysiologic Approach,* 5th edition. New York: McGraw-Hill, 2002:2123–2149.

2. (C) The optimal time period for influenza vaccination is October through mid-November. However, the vaccine can be administered to unvaccinated individuals throughout the influenza season, which typically lasts until April.

   Ref: Bertino JS, Mayney MS. Vaccines, toxoids, and other immunobiologics. In: Dipiro JT, Talbert RL, Yee GC, et al., eds. *Pharmacotherapy: A Pathophysiologic Approach,* 5th edition. New York: McGraw-Hill, 2002:2123–2149.

3. (A) Administration of the influenza vaccination is contraindicated in persons with a known anaphylactic reaction to eggs or other components of the vaccine; however, the vaccine does not contain neomycin. The influenza vaccine is indicated for women who will be in their second or third trimester of pregnancy during flu season.

   Ref: Bertino JS, Mayney MS. Vaccines, toxoids, and other immunobiologics. In: Dipiro JT, Talbert RL, Yee GC, et al., eds. *Pharmacotherapy: A Pathophysiologic Approach,* 5th edition. New York: McGraw-Hill, 2002:2123–2149.

4. (A) Amantadine is highly effective in preventing influenza A infection.

   Ref: Bertino JS, Mayney MS. Vaccines, toxoids, and other immunobiologics. In: Dipiro JT, Talbert RL, Yee GC, et al., eds. *Pharmacotherapy: A Pathophysiologic Approach,* 5th edition. New York: McGraw-Hill, 2002:2123–2149.

5. (E) In the pre-exposure setting, the hepatitis B vaccine has been recommended for persons with occupational risk (healthcare workers, public safety workers), persons in training for healthcare fields, clients and staff of institutions for developmentally disabled, hemodialysis patients, recipients of clotting factor concentrate, household contacts and sexual partners of hepatitis B carriers, adoptees from countries where hepatitis B is endemic, international travelers (those spending more than 6 months in areas with high rates of hepatitis B infection or high-risk, short-term travelers), injecting drug users, sexually active homosexual or bisexual men, sexually active heterosexual men and women, and inmates of long-term correctional facilities. In addition, the American Academy of Pediatrics recommends universal immunization of all newborns.

6. (D) College freshman, particularly those living in dormitories or residence halls, are at modestly increased risk of invasive meningococcal disease compared to the rest of the population in this age group. The ACIP recommends that healthcare workers inform college students and parents about the increased risk and that a safe effective vaccine is available. The meningococcal polysaccharide vaccine should be made easily available for those college freshmen wishing to decrease their risk for meningococcal disease.

   Ref: Bertino JS, Mayney MS. Vaccines, toxoids, and other immunobiologics. In: Dipiro JT, Talbert RL, Yee GC, et al., eds. *Pharmacotherapy: A Pathophysiologic Approach,* 5th edition. New York: McGraw-Hill, 2002:2123–2149.

7. (C) Pneumococcal vaccination is recommended in for the following: immunocompromised patients, persons 65 years of age or older, persons aged 2 to 64 with a chronic illness, persons aged 2 to 64 with functional or anatomic splenectomy, persons aged 2 to 64 living in environments where the risk of invasive pneumococcal disease or its complications are increased. Children younger than 2 years of age do not respond adequately to this vaccine; therefore, the pneumococcal conjugate vaccine is recommended in them.

   Ref: Bertino JS, Mayney MS. Vaccines, toxoids, and other immunobiologics. In: Dipiro JT, Talbert RL, Yee GC, et al., eds. *Pharmacotherapy: A Pathophysiologic Approach,* 5th edition. New York: McGraw-Hill, 2002:2123–2149.

8. (B) The BCG vaccine protects against tuberculosis.

   Ref: Bertino JS, Mayney MS. Vaccines, toxoids, and other immunobiologics. In: Dipiro JT, Talbert RL, Yee GC, et al., eds. *Pharmacotherapy: A Pathophysiologic Approach,* 5th edition. New York: McGraw-Hill, 2002:2123–2149.

9. (B) A slight increase in the risk of Guillain-Barré syndrome may follow in the weeks after influenza vaccination. The risk is estimated to be one case per million doses of vaccine administered.

   Ref: Bertino JS, Mayney MS. Vaccines, toxoids, and other immunobiologics. In: Dipiro JT, Talbert RL, Yee GC, et al., eds. *Pharmacotherapy: A Pathophysiologic Approach,* 5th edition. New York: McGraw-Hill, 2002:2123–2149.

10. (D) All adults should receive booster doses of Td every 10 years.

    Ref: Bertino JS, Mayney MS. Vaccines, toxoids, and other immunobiologics. In: Dipiro JT, Talbert RL, Yee GC, et al., eds. *Pharmacotherapy: A Pathophysiologic Approach,* 5th edition. New York: McGraw-Hill, 2002:2123–2149.

HYPERCHOLESTEROLEMIA

ANSWERS

1. (D) The risk factors for coronary heart disease are age (men 45 years and older, women 55 years and older or with premature menopause without estrogen replacement therapy), family history of premature coronary heart disease (definite myocardial infarction or sudden death before 55 years of father or other first-degree male relative or before 65 years of mother or other first-degree female relative), current cigarette smoking, hypertension (blood pressure $\geq140/90$ mm Hg or taking antihypertensive medication), low HDL cholesterol (<35 mg/dL), and diabetes mellitus. The negative risk factor is high HDL cholesterol (≥60 mg/dL).

   Ref: Expert Panel on Detection, Evaluation, and Treatment of High Blood Cholesterol in Adults. Summary of the second report of the National Cholesterol Education Program (NCEP) Expert Panel on Detection, Evaluation, and Treatment of High Blood Cholesterol in Adults (Adult Treatment Panel II). *JAMA* 1993;269:3015–3023.

2. (A) A total cholesterol level <200 mg/dL is considered within the desirable level. Total cholesterol and HDL should be rechecked in 5 years.

   Ref: Expert Panel on Detection, Evaluation, and Treatment of High Blood Cholesterol in Adults. Summary of the second report of the National Cholesterol Education Program (NCEP) Expert Panel on Detection, Evaluation, and Treatment of High Blood Cholesterol in Adults (Adult Treatment Panel II). *JAMA* 1993;269:3015–3023.

3. (B) The goal LDL level for a patient with two or more risk factors and using on dietary therapy is <130 mg/dL.

   Ref: Expert Panel on Detection, Evaluation, and Treatment of High Blood Cholesterol in Adults. Summary of the second report of the National Cholesterol Education Program (NCEP) Expert Panel on Detection, Evaluation, and Treatment of High Blood Cholesterol in Adults (Adult Treatment Panel II). *JAMA* 1993;269:3015–3023.

4. (E) Drug therapy should be recommended as secondary prevention for a patient with a history of coronary heart disease. Diet and exercise should be used as adjunctive nonpharmacologic therapy.

   Ref: Expert Panel on Detection, Evaluation, and Treatment of High Blood Cholesterol in Adults. Summary of the second report of the National Cholesterol Education Program (NCEP) Expert Panel on Detection, Evaluation, and Treatment of High Blood Cholesterol in Adults (Adult Treatment Panel II). *JAMA* 1993;269:3015–3023.

5. (C) The goal LDL level for a patient with coronary heart disease is <100 mg/dL.

   Ref: Expert Panel on Detection, Evaluation, and Treatment of High Blood Cholesterol in Adults. Summary of the second report of the National Cholesterol Education Program (NCEP) Expert Panel on Detection, Evaluation, and Treatment of High Blood Cholesterol in Adults (Adult Treatment Panel II). *JAMA* 1993;269:3015–3023.

ACNE

ANSWERS

1. (A) Prednisone has been associated with triggering or exacerbating acne. Methylphenidate and salmeterol have not been associated with acne.

   Ref: Feldman S, Careccia RE, Barham KL, Hancox J. Diagnosis and treatment of acne. *Am Fam Physician* 2004;69:2123–2130.

2. (E) Mild acne should be treated with a topical product. Initial treatment with tretinoin should begin with a weaker formulation applied every other day or once daily. Azelaic acid is available in a 20% cream, not 2%. Clindamycin solution should only be applied twice a day. Erythromycin gel should be applied twice a day. Tazarotene is available in a 0.1% gel and cream.

   Ref: Patel NM, Elias SS, Cheigh NH. Acne and psoriasis In: DiPiro JT, Talbert RL, Yee GC, et al., eds. *Pharmacotherapy: A Pathophysiologic Approach,* 5th edition. New York: McGraw-Hill, 2002:1689–1702.

3. (D) Klaron® is a brand name for sulfacetamide lotion, a sulfonamide derivative. Given his severe reaction to SMZ-TMP, any sulfa drug is contraindicated for AA. Azelex® (Azelaic acid), A/T/S® (erythromycin gel), Benzamycin® (erythromycin and benzoyl peroxide), and Vibramycin® (doxycycline) is not contraindicated with a sulfa allergy.

   Ref: Feldman S, Careccia RE, Barham KL, Hancox J. Diagnosis and treatment of acne. *Am Fam Physician* 2004;69:2123–2130.

4. (D) Patients should be made aware that benzoyl peroxide may bleach colored fabric clothing, washcloths because of its oxidizing effects. Common side effects of benzoyl peroxide include stinging, burning, moderate erythema, and pruritus; the gel formulation is associated with increase incidence of irritation and dryness. Skin should be clean and dry when benzoyl peroxide is applied; moist skin is more sensitive to side effects.

Ref: Patel NM, Elias SS, Cheigh NH. Acne and psoriasis In: DiPiro JT, Talbert RL, Yee GC, et al., eds. *Pharmacotherapy: A Pathophysiologic Approach,* 5th edition. New York: McGraw-Hill, 2002:1689–1702.

5. (A) Azelaic acid (Azelex®) is a topical agent with moderate antibacterial and keratolytic properties; it also exhibits weak anti-inflammatory effects. Differin® (adapalene), Tazorac® (tazarotene), and Retin-A® (tretinoin) are all topical retinoids.

Ref: Gollnick H. Current concepts of the pathogenesis of acne. *Drugs* 2003;62:1579–1596.

6. (D) Adapalene is a third-generation topical retinoid; tretinoin belongs to the first generation. The onset of adapalene is slightly quicker than tretinoin. Both agents are equally effective in antimicrobial activity and in treating acne, but adapalene is better tolerated because it is less irritating.

Ref: Gollnick H. Current concepts of the pathogenesis of acne. *Drugs* 2003;62:1579–1596.

7. (B) Doxycycline 50 to 100 mg bid is the appropriate regimen for acne. Ciprofloxacin is not indicated for acne. The proper dosage of erythromycin stearate for acne is 250 to 500 mg bid. Tetracycline should be administered qid and minocycline should be given bid.

Ref: Feldman S, Careccia RE, Barham KL, Hancox J. Diagnosis and treatment of acne. *Am Fam Physician* 2004;69:2123–2130.

8. (D) Oral antibiotics, such as Minocin® (minocycline), have moderate anti-inflammatory properties. Benzoyl peroxide has no anti-inflammatory activity. Topical antibiotics, such as Cleocin® have are weakly anti-inflammatory. BenzaClin® is a combination of clindamycin and benzoyl peroxide formulated as a topical gel. Tazarotene has no anti-inflammatory properties.

Ref: Gollnick H. Current concepts of the pathogenesis of acne. *Drugs* 2003;62:1579–1596.

9. (C) Isotretinoin is only indicated for severe recalcitrant nodular acne. Closed comedones (white heads), macrocomedones (enlarged closed comedones), and open comedones (black heads) are associated with mild to moderate acne. Papules, although inflammatory in nature, are not severe enough to warrant therapy with isotretinoin.

Ref: Accutane® (isotretinoin) capsules (product information). Nutley, NJ: Roche, August 2003.

Ref: Gollnick H. Current concepts of the pathogenesis of acne. *Drugs* 2003;62:1579–1596.

10. (E) Isotretinoin does induce photosensitivity; it has been associated with psychosis, suicidal ideation, and depression. Also, isotretinoin can increase serum triglycerides elevations exceeding 800 mg/dL have been reported, this is reversible on discontinuation of the drug.

Ref: Accutane® (isotretinoin) capsules (product information). Nutley, NJ: Roche, August 2003.

PATIENT PROFILE 119

ASTHMA

ANSWERS

1. (B) Because beclomethasone is not a bronchodilator, patients do not experience the immediate relief they do after inhaling a β-agonist and often believe the drug is of no value. Patients need to understand that asthma is an inflammatory disease and that antiinflammatory agents are needed for optimal control of the disease.

Ref: National Asthma Education Panel Prevention Program. Expert Panel Report II. Guidelines for the Diagnosis and Management of Asthma. www.nhlbi.nih.gov/nhlbi/nhlbi.htm

2. (D) Because maximum benefit may not be realized for several weeks, inhaled corticosteroids are used for long-term control of asthma and not for quick relief of symptoms. Administration of albuterol first will aid optimal disposition of steroid into airways. Rinsing the mouth after the use of a steroid inhaler will help minimize the risk of oral candidiasis.

Ref: Asthma. In: Young LY, Koda-Kimble MA, eds. *Applied Therapeutics: The Clinical Use of Drugs.* 6th ed. Vancouver, Wash: Applied Therapeutics; 1995: chapter 19.

3. (C) Because it is a long acting β-agonist that provides relief for 12 hours, salmeterol may be used for management of nocturnal symptoms.

Ref: Asthma. In: Young LY, Koda-Kimble MA, eds. *Applied Therapeutics: The Clinical Use of Drugs.* 6th ed. Vancouver, Wash: Applied Therapeutics; 1995: chapter 19.

4. (D) Zafirlukast, a leukotriene receptor antagonist, is one of a new class of agents called leukotriene modifiers. Leukotrienes are major mediators of inflammation in the pathogenesis of asthma, and these drugs are selectively designed to reduce the effects of leukotrienes.

Ref: National Asthma Education Panel Prevention Program. Expert Panel Report II. Guidelines for the Diagnosis and Management of Asthma. www.nhlbi.nih.gov/nhlbi/nhlbi.htm

5. (E) When inhaling more than one puff from a metered-dose inhaler, patients should wait at least 30 seconds between puffs to achieve maximum benefit from the second puff.

Ref: Asthma. In: Young LY, Koda-Kimble MA, eds. *Applied Therapeutics: The Clinical Use of Drugs.* 6th ed. Vancouver, Wash: Applied Therapeutics; 1995: chapter 19.

CUTANEOUS ANTHRAX

ANSWERS

1. (C) If untreated has almost 100% fatality. Without proper treatment approximately 20% of patients develop a fatal systemic form of anthrax. The bacteria can enter through a scratch or abrasion on the skin and is only transmitted by direct contact. Cattle farmers working with infected animals may develop cutaneous anthrax.

   Ref: Weinstein R, Alibek K. *Biological and Chemical Terrorism: A Guide for Healthcare Providers and First Responders.* New York: Thieme, 2003.

2. (D) Flavivirus is the causative organism of Dengue fever, castor bean extract causes ricin and *Coxiella burnetii* is the causative organism of Q-fever.

   Ref: Weinstein R, Alibek K. *Biological and Chemical Terrorism: A Guide for Healthcare Providers and First Responders.* New York: Thieme, 2003.

3. (B) Once exposed to the bacteria and the time the initial sore appears can range from 1 to 12 days.

   Ref: Weinstein R, Alibek K. *Biological and Chemical Terrorism: A Guide for Healthcare Providers and First Responders.* New York: Thieme, 2003.

4. (A) Ciprofloxacin 500 mg po q12 hours or doxycycline 100 mg po q12 hours are both in the Centers for Disease Control (CDC) guidelines, but DM is allergic to minocycline; therefore, ciprofloxacin is the drug of choice for this patient.

   Ref: Weinstein R, Alibek K. *Biological and Chemical Terrorism: A Guide for Healthcare Providers and First Responders.* New York: Thieme, 2003.

5. (D)

   Ref: Thomson MICROMEDEX® Healthcare Series Vol. 121. Expires 12/2004. *http://micromedex/ciprofloxacin/overview.* Accessed 10/25/2004.

6. (C) The CDC recommends the treatment for 60 days because of the possibility of inhaled spores, especially in a possible biological attack. Zoonotic cutaneous anthrax is treated for 7 to 10 days.

   Ref: Bell D, Kozarsky P, Stephens D. Clinical issues in the prophylaxis, diagnosis, and treatment of anthrax. *Emerg Infect Dis* 2002;8(2):222–225.

7. (B) Ciprofloxacin has been shown to cause arthropathy in immature animals. Some say use the drug with caution in adolescents if skeletal growth is incomplete. The American Academy of Pediatrics states that the use of a quinolone in children under 18 may be justified under certain conditions and used only after careful assessment of risks versus benefits.

   Ref: AHFS DI Bioterrorism Resource Manual. Bethesda, MD: *American Society of Health-System Pharmacists,* 2002.

8. (C) The CDC guidelines recommend at least 60 days of prophylaxis therapy. Some suggest 100 days of antibiotics or 100 days of antibiotics plus anthrax vaccine (three doses over a 4-week period).

   Ref: Bell D, Kozarsky P, Stephens D. Clinical issues in the prophylaxis, diagnosis, and treatment of anthrax. *Emerg Infect Dis* 2002;8(2):222–225.

   Ref: Weinstein R, Alibek K. *Biological and Chemical Terrorism: A Guide for Healthcare Providers and First Responders.* New York: Thieme, 2003.

9. (A) To prevent "burning" of the esophagus, the patient needs to drink a full (8-oz) glass of water and remain upright after ingesting the medication.

   Ref: Thomson MICROMEDEX® Healthcare Series Vol. 121. Expires 12/2004. *http://micromedex/ciprofloxacin/overview.* Accessed 10/25/2004.

10. (E) Successful mass prophylaxis after a biological attack requires a great of collaboration and planning between public health officials and healthcare workers. Policies must be in place before an attack to identify who is eligible fro prophylaxis treatment; public health officials must have a local spokesperson as a liaison between the public and healthcare facilities. Distribution centers must have sites picked out beforehand. Each site must consider management of traffic control, security, supplies, and personnel to man the distribution centers 24 hours a day. Providing drug information sheets and having multilingual staff and follow-up assessments are necessary. Follow-up assessments monitor illnesses, adverse drug reactions, and adherence problems.

    Ref: Bell D, Kozarsky P, Stephens D. Clinical issues in the prophylaxis, diagnosis, and treatment of anthrax. *Emerg Infect Dis* 2002;8(2):222–225.

PATIENT PROFILE 121

ELIXIRS

ANSWERS

1. (C) The common-system dry and liquid measures need to be converted to the metric system. Those amounts are converted to a percentage strength.

   Ref: Stocklosa M, Ansel H. *Pharmaceutical Calculations*. 10th ed. Baltimore: Williams & Wilkins; 1996:52,98–99.

2. (E) Alcohol, USP, is used in formulations for its cosolvent and preservation properties.

   Ref: Ansel H, Popavitch N, Allen L. *Pharmaceutical Dosage Forms and Drug Delivery Systems*. 6th ed. Baltimore: Williams & Wilkins; 1995:247.

3. (D) The amount of alcohol, USP, to be used can be found from simple dilution techniques. Because of the contrac-

tion that occurs when alcohol, USP, and water are mixed, we cannot determine the exact amount of water needed.

   Ref: Stocklosa M, Ansel H. *Pharmaceutical Calculations*. 10th ed. Baltimore: Williams & Wilkins; 1996:125–126.

4. (B) The simple method is % v/v × SG = % w/v. A more complicated solution is found in the reference.

   Ref: Stocklosa M, Ansel H. *Pharmaceutical Calculations*. 10th ed. Baltimore: Williams & Wilkins; 1996:101.

5. (B) Use simple enlargement after the conversion to metric-system quantity.

   Ref: Stocklosa M, Ansel H. *Pharmaceutical Calculations*. 10th ed. Baltimore: Williams & Wilkins; 1996:79–83.

PATIENT PROFILE 122

DEPRESSION

ANSWERS

1. (A) Desipramine is fatal in overdose with the dose being as little as 1 week's worth of medication.

   Ref: Goldfrank L, Nelson R, Hoffman M, et al., eds. *Goldfrank's Toxicologic Emergencies,* 7th ed. New York: McGraw-Hill, 2002.

2. (C) Terazosin is a potent α_1 receptor blocker. Nortriptyline also has potent α_1 receptor blocking effects.

   Ref: MICROMEDEX.® Accessed 2004.

   Ref: Schatzberg AF, Nemeroff CB, eds. *Essentials of Clinical Psychopharmacology*. Washington, DC: American Psychiatric Publishing, 2001.

3. (B) Lorazepam has been shown to induce depression in patients not treated with antidepressants.

   Ref: Schatzberg AF, Nemeroff CB, eds. *Essentials of Clinical Psychopharmacology*. Washington, DC: American Psychiatric Publishing, 2001.

4. (A) Nefazodone is a potent inhibitor of cytochrome P450 3A4. Amlodipine is metabolized via 3A4. Amlodipine serum levels could dramatically increase and become fatal if nefazodone were added.

   Ref: MICROMEDEX.® Accessed 2004.

5. (D) Acetaminophen overdose results in prolonged increases of AST and ALT.

   Ref: POISONDEX.® Accessed 2004.

PATIENT PROFILE 123

RESPIRATORY TRACT INFECTION

ANSWERS

1. (C) Sputum color does not provide enough information to confirm a diagnosis of infection; however, there have been clinical reports of "rust-colored sputum" among

patients with pneumococcal infection. A Gram stain of a sputum sample that yields gram-positive cocci in chains is highly suggestive of pneumococcal infection in a patient with clinical symptoms.

Ref: Toltzis P, Witte MK, Reed MD. Lower respiratory tract infections. In: DiPiro JT, Talbert RL, Yee GC, Matzke GR, Wells BG, Posey LM, eds. *Pharmacotherapy: A Pathophysiologic Approach.* 4th ed. Stamford, Conn: Appleton & Lange; 1999:1651–1670.

Ref: Jaresko GS, Alexander DP. Respiratory tract infections. In: Young LY, Koda-Kimble MA, eds. *Applied Therapeutics: The Clinical Use of Drugs.* 6th ed. Vancouver, Wash: Applied Therapeutics; 1995:58-1–58-16.

2. (A) Of the selections listed, ceftriaxone is the only one with adequate coverage against pneumococci.

Ref: Toltzis P, Witte MK, Reed MD. Lower respiratory tract infections. In: DiPiro JT, Talbert RL, Yee GC, Matzke GR, Wells BG, Posey LM, eds. *Pharmacotherapy: A Pathophysiologic Approach.* 4th ed. Stamford, Conn: Appleton & Lange; 1999:1651–1670.

Ref: Jaresko GS, Alexander DP. Respiratory tract infections. In: Young LY, Koda-Kimble MA, eds. *Applied Therapeutics: The Clinical Use of Drugs.* 6th ed. Vancouver, Wash: Applied Therapeutics; 1995:58-1–58-16.

3. (D) Clindamycin is the only agent listed that has both anaerobic and grampositive coverage. It is useful for this reason in the treatment of patients with aspiration pneumonia. The patient should be monitored for signs and symptoms of *Clostridium difficile* colitis, a side effect of clindamycin therapy.

Ref: Toltzis P, Witte MK, Reed MD. Lower respiratory tract infections. In: DiPiro JT, Talbert RL, Yee GC, Matzke GR, Wells BG, Posey LM, eds. *Pharmacotherapy: A Pathophysiologic Approach.* 4th ed. Stamford, Conn: Appleton & Lange; 1999:1651–1670.

Ref: Jaresko GS, Alexander DP. Respiratory tract infections. In: Young LY, Koda-Kimble MA, eds. *Applied Therapeutics: The Clin-*

ical Use of Drugs. 6th ed. Vancouver, Wash: Applied Therapeutics; 1995:58-1–58-16.

4. (C) Underlying conditions predispose patients to increased risk of contracting gram-negative infection from lactose-fermenting gram-negative bacilli. Underlying diseases may impair the immune system and other normal host defenses, making them more susceptible to those types of infections.

Ref: Toltzis P, Witte MK, Reed MD. Lower respiratory tract infections. In: DiPiro JT, Talbert RL, Yee GC, Matzke GR, Wells BG, Posey LM, eds. *Pharmacotherapy: A Pathophysiologic Approach.* 4th ed. Stamford, Conn: Appleton & Lange; 1999:1651–1670.

Ref: Jaresko GS, Alexander DP. Respiratory tract infections. In: Young LY, Koda-Kimble MA, eds. *Applied Therapeutics: The Clinical Use of Drugs.* 6th ed. Vancouver, Wash: Applied Therapeutics; 1995:58-1–58-16.

5. (D) "Beating" on one's chest loosens mucus in the lower respiratory tract. The patient is encouraged to cough deeply during and after the therapy in an effort to expectorate the secretions. Mobilization of the secretions helps prevent organisms from being trapped deep in the lungs and helps prevent additional disease.

Ref: Toltzis P, Witte MK, Reed MD. Lower respiratory tract infections. In: DiPiro JT, Talbert RL, Yee GC, Matzke GR, Wells BG, Posey LM, eds. *Pharmacotherapy: A Pathophysiologic Approach.* 4th ed. Stamford, Conn: Appleton & Lange; 1999:1651–1670.

Ref: Jaresko GS, Alexander DP. Respiratory tract infections. In: Young LY, Koda-Kimble MA, eds. *Applied Therapeutics: The Clinical Use of Drugs.* 6th ed. Vancouver, Wash: Applied Therapeutics; 1995:58-1–58-16.

PATIENT PROFILE 124

DIABETES

ANSWERS

1. (C) Intensive physiologic strategies using multiple insulins often result in improved control of HbA1c at the risk of frequent hypoglycemia. Stacking occurs when regular insulin and NPH insulin are administered too close together in time. This results in excessive insulin concentrations and can lead to marked hypoglycemia. This occurs commonly in conventional physiologic insulin regimens using the "split-mix" rule when dosing regular and NPH insulins. NPH insulin lasts from 10 to 16 hours and has a distinct peak that limits NPH from being considered a basal insulin. Answers A and B alone do not completely describe the clinical presentation. Lipodystrophy would delay the absorption but otherwise would not change the peaking effect. Degradation of NPH insulin protein structure would reduce its effect rather than delaying absorption.

Ref: DeWitt DE, Dugdale DC. Using new insulin strategies in the outpatient treatment of diabetes: clinical applications. *JAMA* 2003;289:2265–2269.

2. (A) Spacing out evening doses of regular and NPH insulin apart by 3 to 4 hours allows regular insulin to wear off before NPH begins to peak. This strategy helps to reduce the stacking effect but does not completely protect against nocturnal hypoglycemia, especially if patients skip an evening meal. Reducing the NPH dose by 10% still results in stacking and nocturnal hypoglycemia because evening doses of regular insulin and NPH are given together. Reducing regular insulin by 30% is inappropriate because it results in several hours of impaired glucose disposal postprandial hyperglycemia at bedtime and through the evening. Eating snacks at bedtime is associated with significant weight gain and worsening insulin resistance over time, resulting in increase insulin requirements

and lack of metabolic control. Discontinuing NPH is inappropriate as SP would have no long-acting insulin to work on glucose disposal overnight.

Ref: DeWitt DE, Dugdale DC. Using new insulin strategies in the outpatient treatment of diabetes: clinical applications. *JAMA* 2003;289:2265–2269.

3. (D) SP's previous physiologic insulin strategy was resulting in nocturnal hypoglycemia forcing her to snack and progressively gain weight. This weight gain leads to long-term worsened insulin resistance and metabolic syndrome, requires increased insulin doses and increases the risk of cardiovascular events. A new strategy is necessary to prevent nocturnal hypoglycemia that necessitates in frequent snacking. Combination therapy using insulin glargine and insulin lispro reduces nocturnal hypoglycemia and HbA1c, preventing further weight gain, worsening insulin resistance and improves glucose control. This combination also allows more flexibility than NPH based regimens because it can allow patients to skip meals or change mealtimes. Regimens using Ultralente insulin are inappropriate with SP because of the stacking phenomenon, resulting in worsened hypoglycemia in the day and night. An NPH/lispro regimen may work but remains difficult to adjust because NPH can be either prandial or basal in relation to its timing. An insulin glargine/regular combination also may work as well but the benefit of this combination is not well documented.

Ref: Kelly JL, Trence DL, Hirsch IB. Rapid decrease in clinically significant hypoglycemia with insulin glargine. *Diabetes* 2002;51: A123.

Ref: Porcellati F, Rossetti P, Fanelli CG, et al. Glargine vs NPH as basal insulin in intensive treatment of t1dm given lispro at meals. *Diabetes* 2002;51(suppl 2):A53.

4. (E) Insulin lispro cannot be mixed with insulin glargine. Insulin glargine must always be administered separately in a separate syringe.

Ref: Insulin glargine (Lantus® [product information]. Aventis Pharmaceuticals Inc.

5. (B) Insulin glargine has a pharmacodynamic profile that is closest to basal physiologic insulin release. Insulin glargine must be administered separately and causes hypoglycemia less often than insulin NPH and Ultralente.

Ref: Insulin glargine (Lantus® [product information]. Aventis Pharmaceuticals Inc.

6. (A) To convert to a basal-prandial regimen with a combination of insulin glargine and insulin lispro provide 50% of the total daily insulin requirement as insulin glargine and 50% insulin lispro initially and adjust basal and prandial requirements based on the glucose log. SP has been receiving a form of basal insulin NPH for years and is accustomed to managing her glucose so she will be the best judge of success. Calculate SP's total daily insulin requirement (NPH = 100 Units, Regular 75 units = 175 Units total daily insulin requirement) When beginning this regimen in patients who

have never received insulin, it's prudent to lower this 50% basal requirement by 20% to reduce the risk of hypoglycemia while patients are adjusting to insulin supplementation. Once patients who are new to exogenous insulin become comfortable then basal requirements can be increased to 50%. Using this strategy, 33% of patients will be receiving the correct dose, 33% will require more basal insulin and 33% will require less basal insulin. Thus SP may receive 88 Units of insulin glargine once daily and the other 87 units can be divided equally among 3 meals at 29 units of lispro at each meal. It's important to provide flexibility for carbohydrate intake so allow SP to experiment with the insulin lispro by using 19–29 units of lispro at each meal based on carbohydrate intake.

Ref: DeWitt DE, Dugdale DC. Using new insulin strategies in the outpatient treatment of diabetes: clinical applications. *JAMA* 2003;289:2265–2269.

Ref: Kelly JL, Trence DL, Hirsch IB. Rapid decrease in clinically significant hypoglycemia with insulin glargine. *Diabetes* 2002;51: A123.

7. (C) Each milliliter of insulin glargine contains 100 units. SP requires 88 units of insulin glargine per day or 0.88 mL. One vial contains 10 mL or 1000 units of insulin glargine. SP will use a full vial every 11 days. Thus, to fill a 28 day prescription, 2.5 full vials of insulin lispro are required. Since vials of insulin glargine cannot be partially dispensed you will need to provide 3 full vials for 28 days while SP receives a 50/50 basal prandial regimen requiring 88 units of insulin glargine daily.

Ref: Insulin glargine (Lantus® [product information]. Aventis Pharmaceuticals Inc.

8. (C) Each milliliter of insulin lispro contains 100 units. SP requires 87 units of insulin lispro per day or 0.88 mL. This is further divided as 29 units or approximately 0.3 mL prior to each meal. One vial contains 10 mL or 1000 units insulin lispro. SP will use a full vial every 11 days. Thus, to fill a 28 day prescription, 2.5 full vials of insulin lispro are required. Vials of insulin lispro cannot be partially dispensed, so you will need to provide 3 full vials for 28 days while SP receives a 50/50 basal prandial regimen requiring 87 units of insulin lispro daily.

Ref: Isulin lispro (Humalog® [product information]. Eli Lilly and Co.

9. (E) The carbohydrate content of a snack or meal has the greatest influence on capillary blood glucose. SP can use 1 unit of insulin lispro for every 10–15 grams of extra carbohydrate in a meal or snack. The advantage of this regimen is that SP will feel empowered to control her glucose and is more likely to implement control of her glucose while enjoying life. Most patients with type 1 diabetes prefer qualitative strategies with multiple options for controlling blood glucose rather than rigid fixed doses and lack of self-guided glucose control. The disadvantage of this strategy is weight gain. If SP gains weight, insulin resistance often worsens and she may need more insulin to cover each 10–15 grams of extra carbohydrate.

Ref: DeWitt DE, Dugdale DC. Using new insulin strategies in the outpatient treatment of diabetes: clinical applications. *JAMA* 2003;289:2265–2269.

Ref: DeWitt DE, Hirsch IB. Outpatient insulin therapy in type 1 and type 2 diabetes mellitus: scientific review. *JAMA* 2003;289:2254–2264.

10. (B) Helping patients to adjust pre-meal glucose engenders patient empowerment and encourages tight glucose control in patients with type 1 or patients with type 2 diabetes who require insulin. Patients with a glucose ≥150 mg/dL can begin experimenting with 1 unit of insulin lispro to reduce blood glucose 50 mg/dL. Thus, a patient with a premeal glucose of 300 mg/dL would require 3 units of insulin lispro plus 1 unit of additional insulin lispro for every 10–15 grams of extra carbohydrate. The drawback with this strategy is weight gain and worsening insulin resistance when patients decide to eat increasing amounts of calorically dense carbohydrate rich foods without discretion.

Ref: DeWitt DE, Dugdale DC. Using new insulin strategies in the outpatient treatment of diabetes: clinical applications. *JAMA* 2003;289:2265–2269.

Ref: DeWitt DE, Hirsch IB. Outpatient insulin therapy in type 1 and type 2 diabetes mellitus: scientific review. *JAMA* 2003;289:2254–2264.

PATIENT PROFILE 125
DERMATOLOGY

ANSWERS

1. (E) At initiation of benzoyl peroxide therapy, application once daily (apply sparingly and avoid the periorbital, perinasal, and perioral skin) minimizes irritation If the medication is applied at bedtime, erythema should be minimal by the next morning;

   Ref: Menon M, Ghorbani A, Sloan L, et al. Common skin disorders. In: Herfindal ET, Gourley DR, eds. *Textbook of Therapeutics. Drug and Disease Management.* 6th ed. Baltimore: Williams & Wilkins; 1996:889–921.

2. (E) Tolerance to adverse effects occurs as therapy continues. The full therapeutic benefit may not be experienced for 4 to 8 weeks. Benzoyl peroxide can bleach hair and clothes.

   Ref: Menon M, Ghorbani A, Sloan L, et al. Common skin disorders. In: Herfindal ET, Gourley DR, eds. *Textbook of Therapeutics. Drug and Disease Management.* 6th ed. Baltimore: Williams & Wilkins; 1996:889–921.

3. (E) Minocycline may cause vestibular toxicity and esophagitis from reflux, so it should not be taken just before retiring. Minocycline and other tetracyclines should be avoided in pregnancy.

   Ref: Menon M, Ghorbani A, Sloan L, et al. Common skin disorders. In: Herfindal ET, Gourley DR, eds. *Textbook of Therapeutics. Drug and Disease Management.* 6th ed. Baltimore: Williams & Wilkins; 1996:889–921.

4. (B) The combination of erythromycin and astemizole should be avoided because of an interaction that can cause cardiac effects such as prolongation of the QRS or QT interval.

   Ref: Astemizole (Hismanal®) [product information]. Janssen.

5. (E) Photosensitivity can occur with use of tetracyclines, as can vaginal yeast infections. Patients should separate administration of tetracyclines with that of diary products, antacids, iron products, and bismuth salts.

   Ref: Menon M, Ghorbani A, Sloan L, et al. Common skin disorders. In: Herfindal ET, Gourley DR, eds. *Textbook of Therapeutics. Drug and Disease Management.* 6th ed. Baltimore: Williams & Wilkins; 1996:889–921.

PATIENT PROFILE 126
HUMAN IMMUNODEFICIENCY VIRUS

ANSWERS

1. (C) Patients infected with *N. gonorrhoeae* are often coinfected with *C. trachomatis*. If the physician is considering treatment, it should be directed at both organisms.

   Ref: Centers for Disease Control and Prevention. Sexually transmitted diseases. Treatment guidelines 2002. *MMWR Morbd Mortal Wkly Rep* 2002;51(RR-6):1–84.

2. (A) Ceftriaxone 125 mg IM is one of the recommended therapies for *N. gonorrhoeae* urethritis. It is considered safe in pregnancy. Erythromycin is one of the recommended therapies for *C. trachomatis* in pregnant patients. (Do not use the estolate salt because of concerns for hepatic toxicity in pregnant patients.) Doxycycline has a pregnancy category rating of D because of its

effects on the fetus. Although ciprofloxacin has a category C rating, its use is typically avoided in pregnancy because of arthropathy observed in animal fetal toxicity studies. Although a 1-g dose of azithromycin is considered an option for *C. trachomatis* infection, it is not considered sufficient for *N. gonorrhoeae*.

Ref: Centers for Disease Control and Prevention. Sexually transmitted diseases. Treatment guidelines 2002. *MMWR Morbd Mortal Wkly Rep* 2002;51(RR-6):1–84.

3. (C) The AIDS surveillance case definition traditionally has been based on the acquisition of one of several AIDS-associated opportunistic infections. The most recent guidelines also included a CD4 cell count threshold of 200 cell/mm^3 in its definition of AIDS. Although this patient has had several sexually transmitted diseases, they are not unique to HIV/AIDS patients and are not considered opportunistic. The AIDS case definition does not address viral load or overall white blood cell counts in its definition.

Ref: Centers for Disease Control and Prevention. Sexually transmitted diseases. Treatment guidelines 2002. *MMWR Morbd Mortal Wkly Rep* 2002;51(RR-6):1–84.

4. (A) Although d4T has a pregnancy category rating of C and ddI a rating of B, the Food and Drug Administration and the drug's manufacturers have issued a warning about the increased risk of fatal lactic acidosis in pregnant women prescribed a regimen that includes the concomitant administration of these two antiretrovirals. Amprenavir oral solution contains propylene glycol as an excipient that may accumulate in pregnant women and children. Amprenavir oral capsules do not contain this excipient. Although efavirenz has a category C rating, its use should be avoided during the first trimester of pregnancy because of its potential teratogenic effects.

Ref: US Department of Health and Human Services. Safety and toxicity of individual antiretroviral agents in pregnancy. 2004 Jun 23 [cited 2004 Oct 12]:1–22. Available from: *http://aidsinfo. nih.gov/guidelines/perinatal/ST_062304.pdf*

5. (B) Triple-nucleoside antiretroviral regimens should only be considered when nonnucleoside-based or protease-inhibitor–based regimens cannot be administered. These regimens are less virologically potent than nonnucleoside-based or protease-inhibitor–based regimens.

Ref: US Department of Health and Human Services. Safety and toxicity of individual antiretroviral agents in pregnancy. 2004 Jun 23 [cited 2004 Oct 12]:1–22. Available from: *http://aidsinfo. nih.gov/guidelines/perinatal/ST_062304.pdf*

6. (D) The AZT protocol for preventing mother-to-child transmission includes three components: AZT administration to the mother during the pregnancy to protect the child *in utero*, AZT administration to the mother during delivery to protect the child during delivery, and AZT administration to the child after delivery.

Ref: US Department of Health and Human Services. Recommendations for the use of antiretroviral drugs in pregnant HIV-1–infected women for maternal health and interventions to reduce perinatal HIV-1 transmission in the United States. 2004 June 23 [cited 2004 Oct 12]:1–52. Available from: *http://aidsinfo. nih.gov/guidelines/perinatal/PER_062304.pdf*

7. (A) Ritonavir is both an inhibitor and inducer of the cytochrome P450 enzyme 3A4. It also may be an inducer of CYP 2C9. Methadone is a substrate of these enzymes. The net effect of coadministration is induction of methadone metabolism, decreased methadone concentrations, and possible appearance of opiate withdrawal symptoms. Nelfinavir also may cause decreases in methadone concentrations.

Ref: Geletko SM, Erickson AD. Decreased methadone effect after ritonavir initiation. *Pharmacotherapy* 2000; 20:93–94.

8. (C) Protease inhibitors and nonnucleoside reverse transcriptase inhibitors undergo hepatic metabolism. They make required dose reduction in patients with hepatic failure and may cause hepatic toxicity.

Ref: US Department of Health and Human Services. Recommendations for the use of antiretroviral drugs in pregnant HIV-1–infected women for maternal health and interventions to reduce perinatal HIV-1 transmission in the United States. 2004 June 23 [cited 2004 Oct 12]:1–52. Available from: *http://aidsinfo. nih.gov/guidelines/perinatal/PER_062304.pdf*

9. (A) Lipodystrophy is a syndrome associated with lipoatrophy in the face, extremities, and buttocks and excessive fat deposition in the abdomen, neck, and breasts. Although it can be observed with all antiretrovirals, it is most commonly associated with protease inhibitors.

Ref: US Department of Health and Human Services. Recommendations for the use of antiretroviral drugs in pregnant HIV-1–infected women for maternal health and interventions to reduce perinatal HIV-1 transmission in the United States. 2004 June 23 [cited 2004 Oct 12]:1–52. Available from: *http://aidsinfo. nih.gov/guidelines/perinatal/PER_062304.pdf*

10. (B) Lactic acidosis is a manifestation of mitochondrial toxicity caused by nucleoside reverse transcriptase inhibitors. Symptoms are vague and nonspecific: feeling unwell, abdominal pain, nausea, vomiting, diarrhea, weakness, myalgias, and tachypnea.

Ref: US Department of Health and Human Services. Recommendations for the use of antiretroviral drugs in pregnant HIV-1–infected women for maternal health and interventions to reduce perinatal HIV-1 transmission in the United States. 2004 June 23 [cited 2004 Oct 12]:1–52. Available from: *http://aidsinfo.nih. gov/guidelines/perinatal/PER_062304.pdf*

PATIENT PROFILE 127

ONCOLOGY: PEDIATRIC ACUTE LYMPHOCYTIC LEUKEMIA

ANSWERS

1. (C) The large number of malignant cells and destruction of the cells by the antineoplastic agents release uric acid. To avoid elevated uric acid serum concentrations, patients are routinely pretreated with allopurinol.

   Ref: Young LY, Koda-Kimble MA, eds. *Applied Therapeutics: The Clinical Use of Drugs.* 6th ed. Vancouver, Wash: Applied Therapeutics; 1995: chapter 92.

2. (B) The neuropathy associated with vincristine use commonly affects the intestine and causes constipation.

   Ref: Young LY, Koda-Kimble MA, eds. *Applied Therapeutics: The Clinical Use of Drugs.* 6th ed. Vancouver, Wash: Applied Therapeutics; 1995: chapter 92.

3. (A) Prevention of disease recurrence is the primary objective of maintenance therapy. CNS prophylaxis with intrathecal methotrexate is a therapeutic option in addition to maintenance.

   Ref: In: Herfindal ET, Gourley DR, eds. *Textbook of Therapeutics. Drug and Disease Management.* 6th ed. Baltimore: Williams & Wilkins; 1996: chapter 78.

   Ref: Smith SP, Beltz SE. Acute leukemias. In: DiPirc JT, Talbert RL, Yee GC, Matzke GR, Wells BG, Posey LM, eds. *Pharmacotherapy: A Pathopysiologic Approach.* 4th ed. Stamford, Conn: Appleton & Lange; 1999:2149–2168.

   Ref: Young LY, Koda-Kimble MA, eds. *Applied Therapeutics: The Clinical Use of Drugs.* 6th ed. Vancouver, Wash: Applied Therapeutics; 1995: chapter 92.

4. (D) Combination therapy administered by the intrathecal route has decreased the incidence of CNS spread.

   Ref: In: Herfindal ET, Gourley DR, eds. *Textbook of Therapeutics. Drug and Disease Management.* 6th ed. Baltimore: Williams & Wilkins; 1996: chapter 78.

   Ref: Smith SP, Beltz SE. Acute leukemias. In: DiPiro JT, Talbert RL, Yee GC, Matzke GR, Wells BG, Posey LM, eds. *Pharmacotherapy: A Pathophysiologic Approach.* 4th ed. Stamford, Conn: Appleton & Lange; 1999:2149–2168.

   Ref: Young LY, Koda-Kimble MA, eds. *Applied Therapeutics: The Clinical Use of Drugs.* 6th ed. Vancouver, Wash: Applied Therapeutics; 1995: chapter 92.

5. (D) This adverse effect, especially among children, has resulted in decreased use of this modality for CNS prophylaxis.

   Ref: In: Herfindal ET, Gourley DR, eds. *Textbook of Therapeutics. Drug and Disease Management.* 6th ed. Baltimore: Williams & Wilkins; 1996: chapter 78.

   Ref: Smith SP, Beltz SE. Acute leukemias. In: DiPiro JT, Talbert RL, Yee GC, Matzke GR, Wells BG, Posey LM, eds. *Pharmacotherapy: A Pathophysiologic Approach.* 4th ed. Stamford, Conn: Appleton & Lange; 1999:2149–2168.

   Ref: Young LY, Koda-Kimble MA, eds. *Applied Therapeutics: The Clinical Use of Drugs.* 6th ed. Vancouver, Wash: Applied Therapeutics; 1995: chapter 92.

PATIENT PROFILE 128

OVER-THE-COUNTER PRODUCTS

ANSWERS

1. (D) Nicotinic acid (niacin) is considered the first-line treatment for hypertriglyceridemia.

   Ref: Talbert RL. Hyperlipidemia. In: DiPiro JT, Talbert RL, Yee GC, eds. *Pharmacotherapy: A Pathophysiologic Approach,* 5th ed. New York: McGraw-Hill, 2002:408.

2. (B) Maalox contains aluminum and magnesium, which can bind to fluoroquinolones and decrease the absorption of the antibiotic, possibly resulting in treatment failure.

   Ref: Henderson RP. Acid-peptic disorders and intestinal gas. In: *Handbook of Nonprescription Drugs,* 13th ed. Washington: RR Donnelley and Sons, 2002:268–303.

3. (A) Diphenydramine is a histamine H_1-receptor antagonist that has anticholinergic effects. JA is currently on tolteridine for urinary incontinence, which is an anticholinergic agent. Antihistamines should be used with caution in patients on anticholinergic therapy.

   Ref: May JR. Allergic rhinitis. In: DiPiro JT, Talbert RL, Yee GC, eds. *Pharmacotherapy: A Pathophysiologic Approach,* 5th ed. New York: McGraw-Hill, 2002:1683.

4. (D) Acetaminophen is the oral analgesic of choice in the treatment of osteoarthritis.

Ref: Boh LE, Elliott ME. Osteoarthritis. In: DiPiro JT, Talbert RL, Yee GC, eds. *Pharmacotherapy: A Pathophysiologic Approach,* 5th ed. New York: McGraw-Hill, 2002:1647.

5. (C) Vitamin C is given with iron to improve iron absorption.

Ref: Huckleberry Y, Rollins CJ. Prevention of nutritional deficiencies. In: *Handbook of Nonprescription Drugs,* 13th ed. Washington: RR Donnelley and Sons, 2002:451–492.

6. (C) Choices I and III are correct; choice II would be correct if it read, "Absorption of fat-soluble vitamins is altered by the administration of mineral oil."

Ref: Curry CE Jr, Butler DM. Constipation. In: *Handbook of Nonprescription Drugs.* 13th ed. Washington: RR Donnelley and Sons, 2002:6–334.

7. (B) High doses of calcium supplementation decrease iron absorption.

Ref: Huckleberry Y, Rollins CJ. Prevention of nutritional deficiencies. In: *Handbook of Nonprescription Drugs,* 13th ed. Washington: RR Donnelley and Sons, 2002:451–492.

8. (A) Ferrous sulfate should be administered separately from levothyroxine because iron can interfere with the absorption of levothyroxine.

Ref: Talbert RL. Thyroid disorders. In: DiPiro JT, Talbert RL, Yee GC, ed. *Pharmacotherapy: A Pathophysiologic Approach,* 5th ed. New York: McGraw-Hill, 2002.1372.

9. (D) Iron supplementation commonly causes constipation, nausea, abdominal pain/diarrhea, and black and tarry stools.

Ref: Huckleberry Y, Rollins CJ. Prevention of nutritional deficiencies. In: *Handbook of Nonprescription Drugs,* 13th ed. Washington: RR Donnelley and Sons, 2002:451–492.

10. (C) Vitamin C may increase estrogen serum levels.

Ref: Huckleberry Y, Rollins CJ. Prevention of nutritional deficiencies. In: *Handbook of Nonprescription Drugs,* 13th ed. Washington: RR Donnelley and Sons, 2002:451–492.

PATIENT PROFILE 129

MEDICINAL CHEMISTRY

ANSWER

1. (E) The duration of action of first-generation sulfonylureas is directly related to the rate of metabolism (through oxidation) at the *para* position of the aromatic ring into inactive metabolites. The chlorine atom cannot be oxidized, so the metabolism of chlorpropamide at this site is greatly reduced. B is incorrect both because the butyl is more lipophilic than the propyl group and because lipophilicity is not the determinant of sulfonylurea activity. C is incorrect because first-generation sulfonylureas, unlike the second generation, do not go through the enterohepatic circulation. D is incorrect because all sulfonylureas are characterized by having very strong plasma protein binding with no substantial difference among them.

PATIENT PROFILE 130

IRRITABLE BOWEL SYNDROME

ANSWERS

1. (E) Irritable bowel syndrome can be exacerbated by changes in diet, exercise, and stress level. Further assessment is warranted to determine the cause of FP's exacerbation.

Ref: Wall GC. Lower gastrointestinal disorders. In: Young YL, Koda-Kimble MA, eds. *Applied Therapeutics: The Clinical Use of Drugs.* Vancouver, WA: Applied Therapeutics, 2005:28-17–28-24.

2. (C) Gastrointestinal bleeding may be indicative of a more severe complication. Additional "alarm" symptoms include weight loss, anemia, fever, and frequent nocturnal symptoms. FP does not currently exhibit any alarm signs.

Ref: Fass R, et al. Evidence and consensus-based practice guidelines for the diagnosis of irritable bowel syndrome. *Arch Intern Med* 2001;161:2081.

3. (C) Hydrochlorothiazide, a thiazide diuretic, facilitates fluid and electrolyte loss. Therefore, patients with gastrointestinal losses secondary to a disease process may be at higher risk of developing dehydration and electrolyte abnormalities.

Ref: Product Information: Hydrodiuril, hydrochlorothiazide, Merck & Co, Inc.

4. (B) Although a theoretical interaction, the slowing of intestinal transit time could progress to the increased absorption of concomitant medications.

Ref: Wall GC. Lower gastrointestinal disorders. In: Young YL, Koda-Kimble MA, eds. *Applied Therapeutics: The Clinical Use of Drugs*. Vancouver, WA: Applied Therapeutics, 2005:28-17–28-24.

5. (C) The manufacturer recommended maximum daily dose is 16 mg or eight 2-mg capsules.

Ref: Product information: Imodium, loperamide, McNeil.

6. (A) The anticholinergic properties of atropine could place FP at risk for falls. Most medications with anticholinergic properties should be avoided in the elderly. Diphenoxylate/atropine does not interact with selective serotonin reuptake inhibitors (SSRIs). It has been implicated in the development of hypertensive crisis when used in combination with monoamine oxidase (MAO) inhibitors. Diphenoxylate/atropine is not contraindicated in patients with hypertension.

Ref: Wall GC. Lower gastrointestinal disorders. In: Young YL, Koda-Kimble MA, eds. *Applied Therapeutics: The Clinical Use of Drugs*. Vancouver, WA: Applied Therapeutics, 2005: 28-17–28-24.

Ref: Product Information: Lomotil, diphenoxylate/atropine, G.D. Searle & Co.

7. (D) Cholestyramine has been shown to be an effective, inexpensive alternative to standard antidiarrheal therapy, particularly in patients with bile acid malabsorption. This

is not suspected in FP. Regardless, palatability and risk of drug-drug interactions are reasons to avoid its use in FP.

Ref: Wall GC. Lower gastrointestinal disorders. In: Young YL, Koda-Kimble MA, eds. *Applied Therapeutics: The Clinical Use of Drugs*. Vancouver, WA: Applied Therapeutics, 2005:28-17–28-24.

8. (D) Zelnorm (tegaserod) is a partial 5-HT$_4$ agonist approved for the treatment of constipation-predominant IBS. It has been associated with the development of severe diarrhea requiring hospitalization for rehydration therapy. It is only approved for use in women.

Ref: Product information: Zelnorm, tegaserod, Novartis.

9. (D) Prior to the initiation of alosetron, patients should be well informed of the risks associated with its use. They should be monitored closely for the signs and symptoms associated with severe constipation and ischemic colitis. Treatment should be discontinued after 1 month if there is no clinical response.

Ref: Wall GC. Lower gastrointestinal disorders. In: Young YL, Koda-Kimble MA, eds. *Applied Therapeutics: The Clinical Use of Drugs*. Vancouver, WA: Applied Therapeutics, 2005:28-17–28-24.

Ref: Product information: Lotronex, alosetron, GlaxoSmithKline.

10. (D) Although headache occurs frequently during alosetron therapy, it is not considered a reason to discontinue therapy. Rectal bleeding may indicate ischemic colitis or a more severe gastrointestinal complication.

Ref: Wall GC. Lower gastrointestinal disorders. In: Young YL, Koda-Kimble MA, eds. *Applied Therapeutics: The Clinical Use of Drugs*. Vancouver, WA: Applied Therapeutics, 2005:28-17–28-24.

Ref: Product information: Lotronex, alosetron, GlaxoSmithKline.

PATIENT PROFILE 131

SCHIZOPHRENIA

ANSWERS

1. (C) The efficacy of traditional antipsychotic agents in the treatment of patients with hallucinations is related to their ability to block dopamine-2 receptors.

Ref: *Textbook of Psychopharmacology*. Washington, DC: American Psychiatric Press; 1995: chapter 30.

2. (C) Extrapyramidal symptoms are caused by excessive blockade of dopamine receptors in the nigrostriatal region of the brain.

Ref: *Textbook of Psychopharmacology*. Washington, DC: American Psychiatric Press; 1995: chapter 30.

3. (A) The anticholinergic agent benztropine mesylate is very effective at relieving extrapyramidal symptoms.

Ref: Young LY, Koda-Kimble MA, eds. *Applied Therapeutics: The Clinical Use of Drugs*. 6th ed. Vancouver, Wash: Applied Therapeutics; 1995: chapter 75.

4. (D) Blocking the α_1 receptor prevents vasoconstriction and hinders the body from maintaining blood pressure when the person stands.

Ref: *Textbook of Psychopharmacology*. Washington, DC: American Psychiatric Press; 1995: chapter 13.

5. (C) Use of clozapine is associated with a dose-dependent and rapid titration seizure risk that is higher than that with the other antipsychotics. The risk with clozapine is approximately 6% among patients taking 600 mg/d or more.

Ref: Young LY, Koda-Kimble MA, eds. *Applied Therapeutics: The Clinical Use of Drugs*. 6th ed. Vancouver, Wash: Applied Therapeutics; 1995: chapter 75.

PATIENT PROFILE 132
DIABETES AND NEPHROPATHY

ANSWERS

1. (C) GP is a diabetic, so his blood pressure goal is less than 130/80 mm Hg.

    Ref: American Diabetes Association. Clinical practice guidelines. *Diabetes Care* 2004;27(S1):S15–S35.

2. (C) Dihydropyridine calcium channel blockers have not been shown to prevent the progression of nephropathy in diabetics.

    Ref: American Diabetes Association. Clinical practice guidelines. *Diabetes Care* 2004;27(S1):S15–S35.

3. (C) GP's calculated creatinine clearance is 33 mL/min.

    Ref: Brophy DF. Acute renal failure. In: Koda-Kimble MA, Young LY, Kradjan WA, et al, eds. *Applied Therapeutics: The Clinical Use of Drugs,* 8th ed. Philadelphia: Lippincott Williams & Wilkins, 2005:31(5).

4. (A) Quinapril must be adjusted based on the creatinine clearance. The dose should be reduced to 5 mg PO qd.

    Ref: Package Insert: Accupril (quinapril), Pfizer, New York, 2003.

5. (B) Metformin is contraindicated in this patient because of her serum creatinine.

    Ref: Package Insert: Glucophage (metformin), Bristol-Myers Squibb, Princeton, NJ, 2004.

6. (D) GP's HDL goal is greater than 50 mg/dL. Females tend to have higher HDL levels, so female patients often have HDL goals roughly 10 points higher than males.

    Ref: National Cholesterol Education Program Adult Treatment Panel III. Washington: National Institutes of Health, National Heart, Lung, and Blood Institute, May 2001.

7. (D) GP's LDL goal should be less than 100 mg/dL because she is a diabetic.

    Ref: American Diabetes Association. Clinical practice guidelines. *Diabetes Care* 2004;27(S1):S15–S35.

8. (D) Clinical existing CHD is considered a CHD risk equivalent, and GP has a history of a CABG in 2002.

    Ref: National Cholesterol Education Program Adult Treatment Panel III. Washington: National Institutes of Health, National Heart, Lung, and Blood Institute, May 2001.

9. (A) Latanoprost would be most appropriate in GP because of her compliance issues and the once-daily dosing of latanoprost.

    Ref: Package Insert: Xalatan (latanoprost), Pfizer, New York, 2004.

10. (C) Insulin glargine is a peakless insulin with a 24-hour duration in most patients.

    Ref: Package Insert: Lantus (glargine), Aventis Pharmaceuticals, Kansas City, MO, 2004.

PATIENT PROFILE 133
PARKINSON'S DISEASE

ANSWERS

1. (B) The synthetic anticholinergics such as benztropine improve tremor associated with the early stages of Parkinson's disease.

2. (A) Anticholinergics such as benztropine produce peripherally mediated side effects such as dry mouth, blurred vision, constipation, and urinary retention and should be avoided in the care of patients with BPH.

3. (E) Carbidopa, a decarboxylase inhibitor, does not penetrate the blood-brain barrier and is used in combination with levodopa in the formulation Sinemet® to decrease the peripheral conversion of levodopa to dopamine and allow the dose of levodopa to decrease by 80%.

4. (C) Carbidopa and levodopa are available in a 1:10 fixed ratio in the formulations Sinemet® 10/100 and 25/250. Sinemet® 25/100 is available in a 1:4 fixed ratio.

5. (C) The honeymoon phase (favorable response) associated with the initial phase of levodopa therapy usually lasts an average of 2–5 years.

    Ref: Shimomura SK, Fujimoto D. Parkinsonism. In: Herfindal ET, Gourley DR, eds. *Textbook of Therapeutics. Drug and Disease Management.* 6th ed. Baltimore: Williams & Wilkins; 1996: chapter 51.

    Ref; Flaherty JF, Gidal BE. Parkinson's disease. In: Young LY, Koda-Kimbe MA, eds. *Applied Therapeutics: The Clinical Use of Drugs.* 6th ed. Vancouver, Wash: Applied Therapeutics; 1995: chapter 51.

PATIENT PROFILE 134
KIDNEY TRANSPLANTATION

ANSWERS

1. (E) All these may cause an acute rise in serum creatinine. Differentiation is made by clinical presentation and laboratory values.

Ref: Danovitch GM. *Handbook of Kidney Transplantation,* 3d ed. Philadelphia: Lippincott Williams & Wilkins, 2001:182–220.

2. (B) Pulse-dose steroids have and continue to be the treatment of choice for acute cellular rejection. Thymoglobulin, Atgam, and OKT3 may be used to treat rejection but are reserved for steroid-resistant cases. Switching to or optimizing tacrolimus and mycophenolate mofetil is appropriate to slow the progression of chronic rejection.

Ref: Hricik DE, et al. Trends in the use of glucocorticoids in renal transplantation. *Transplantation* 1994;57(7):979–989.

3. (B) Abrupt, high doses of glucocorticoids cause a transient elevation in the WBC count through a process called *demargination.* Glucocorticoids decrease the adherence of granulocytes, resulting in elevated circulating levels.

Ref: Nakagawa M. Glucocorticoid-induced granulocytosis: Contribution of marrow release and demargination of intravascular granulocytes. *Circulation* 1998;98(21):2307–2313.

4. (D) Side effects associated with corticosteroid use include diabetes, cataracts, infection, hypertension, hyperlipidemia, osteoporosis, and psychiatric and cosmetic effects.

Ref: Citteria F, et al. Steroid side effects and their impact on transplantation outcome. *Transplantation* 2001;72(12 suppl):S75–80.

5. (C) Elevated tacrolimus concentrations cause a parallel increase in the serum creatinine concentration. Acute rejection is a possibility but unlikely given the current supratherapeutic tacrolimus levels. This patient does not have any signs or symptoms of dehydration.

Ref: Johnson RG, et al. The clinical impact of nephrotoxicity in renal transplantation. *Transplantation* 2000;69(12 suppl):S14–17.

6. (E) Cyclosporine and tacrolimus are known risks for developing renal dysfunction. The incidence increases with higher exposure, and patients should be titrated carefully and kept at the lowest effective dose throughout therapy. Sirolimus does not cause renal dysfunction and is used commonly to minimize or eliminate calcineurin inhibitor use.

Ref: Danovitch GM. *Handbook of Kidney Transplantation,* 3d ed. Philadelphia: Lippincott Williams & Wilkins, 2001:62–110.

7. (D) Hyperlipidemia is one of the primary adverse effects associated with sirolimus use. A baseline lipid panel should be obtained prior to initiating therapy and should be monitored routinely thereafter.

Ref: Danovitch GM. *Handbook of Kidney Transplantation,* 3d ed. Philadelphia: Lippincott Williams & Wilkins, 2001:79–81.

8. (C) Clarithromycin inhibits the metabolism of tacrolimus. Patients receiving concomitant therapy have elevated tacrolimus levels, resulting in an increased risk of tacrolimus toxicity. This patient has multiple signs and symptoms of tacrolimus toxicity, including an elevated blood level, an elevated serum creatinine, headaches, and tremor.

Ref: Prograf Package Insert, Fujisawa Healthcare, Inc., Deerfield, IL, 2001.

9. (C) Owing to the drug interaction between clarithromycin and tacrolimus, the clarithromycin should be removed from the regimen. Dual therapy with amoxillin and lansoprazole is not sufficient. Metronidazole may be substituted for clarithromycin. Quadruple therapy is indicated for clarithromycin-resistant strains, which is not the case in this patient.

Ref: de Boer WA, et al. Treatment of *Helicobacter pylori* infection (review). *Br Med J* 2000;320(1):31–34.

10. (C) Vaccines may be somewhat less effective in an immunocompromised recipient, but the response is usually sufficient to warrant their use. Live, attenuated vaccines such as OPV, MMR, typhoid, and yellow fever vaccine are not recommended routinely. Killed or inactivated vaccines usually are safe and may be effective. Annual influenza vaccination is strongly recommended for transplant recipients.

Ref: Watson JC, et al. General recommendations on immunization recommendations of the Advisory Committee on Immunization Practices (ACIP). *MMWR* 1994;43:1–38.

PATIENT PROFILE 135
CONGESTIVE HEART FAILURE

ANSWERS

1. (A) NSAIDs can produce salt and water retention.

   Ref: Johnson JA, Parker RB, Geraci SA. Heart failure. In: DiPiro JT, Talbert RL, Yee GC. Matzke GR, Wells BG, Posey LM, eds. *Pharmacotherapy: A Pathophysiologic Approach.* 4th ed. Stamford, Conn: Appleton & Lange; 1999:153–181.

2. (B) Diltiazem is a negative inotrope and reduces cardiac contractility.

   Ref: Johnson JA, Parker RB, Geraci SA. Heart failure. In: DiPiro JT, Talbert RL, Yee GC, Matzke GR, Wells BG, Posey LM, eds. *Pharmacotherapy: A Pathophysiologic Approach.* 4th ed. Stamford, Conn: Appleton & Lange; 1999:153–181.

3. (D) A diuretic is needed to manage acute and chronic fluid overload.

   Ref: Johnson JA, Parker RB, Geraci SA. Heart failure. In: DiPiro JT, Talbert RL, Yee GC, Matzke GR, Wells BG, Posey LM, eds. *Pharmacotherapy: A Pathophysiologic Approach.* 4th ed. Stamford, Conn: Appleton & Lange; 1999:153–181.

4. (C) ACE inhibitor therapy clearly decreases the mortality of CHF. All patients with CHF should take an ACE inhibitor unless such therapy is contraindicated.

   Ref: Johnson JA, Parker RB, Geraci SA. Heart failure. In: DiPiro JT, Talbert RL, Yee GC, Matzke GR, Wells BG, Posey LM, eds. *Pharmacotherapy: A Pathophysiologic Approach.* 4th ed. Stamford, Conn: Appleton & Lange; 1999:153–181.

5. (D) ACE inhibitors can produce renal dysfunction, especially among patients with already compromised renal function.

   Ref: Johnson JA, Parker RB, Geraci SA. Heart failure. In: DiPiro JT, Talbert RL, Yee GC, Matzke GR, Wells BG, Posey LM, eds. *Pharmacotherapy: A Pathophysiologic Approach.* 4th ed. Stamford, Conn: Appleton & Lange; 1999:153–181.

PATIENT PROFILE 136
DIABETES MELLITUS

ANSWERS

1. (A) As people age, their renal function diminishes. Heart failure, diminished renal function, angiotensin-converting enzyme (ACE) inhibitor use, and nonsteroidal anti-inflammatory drug (NSAID) use all can increase the risk of developing renal failure.

   Ref: Mueller BA. Acute renal failure. In: DiPiro JT, Talbert RL, Yee GC, et al, eds. *Pharmacotherapy: A Pathophysiologic Approach,* 5th ed. New York: McGraw-Hill, 2002:157–184.

2. (D) Phenylephrine has the potential to elevate blood pressure. RG's blood pressure is already not controlled.

   Ref: Carter BL, Saseen JJ. Hypertension. In: DiPiro JT, Talbert RL, Yee GC, et al, eds. *Pharmacotherapy: A Pathophysiologic Approach,* 5th ed. New York: McGraw-Hill, 2002:157–184.

3. (B) RG is already maximized on an ACE inhibitor. JNC VII recommends that a diuretic be initiated if the blood pressure goal has not been achieved with multiple-drug therapy. Additionally, because RG has heart failure and diminished renal function, volume overload may be contributing to her elevated blood pressure. Loop diuretics are the most effective diuretics at reducing fluid volume.

   Ref: Carter BL, Saseen JJ. Hypertension. In: DiPiro JT, Talbert RL, Yee GC, et al, eds. *Pharmacotherapy: A Pathophysiologic Approach,* 5th ed. New York: McGraw-Hill, 2002:157–184.

4. (E) Hydrochlorothiazide is known to cause glucose intolerance.

   Ref: Carter BL, Saseen JJ. Hypertension. In: DiPiro JT, Talbert RL, Yee GC, et al, eds. *Pharmacotherapy: A Pathophysiologic Approach,* 5th ed. New York: McGraw-Hill, 2002:157–184.

5. (E) Repaglinide should be taken with each meal. If a meal is skipped, the dose of repaglinide should be skipped as well.

   Ref:Carlisle BA, Kroon LA, Koda-Kimble MA. Diabetes mellitus. In: Koda-Kimble MA, Young LY, Kradjan WA, Guglielmo BJ, eds. *Applied Therapeutics: The Clinical Use of Drugs,* 8th ed. Philadelphia: Lippincott Williams & Wilkins, 2005:50-1–50-80.

6. A Repaglinide is an insulin secretagogue. All insulin secretagogues can cause hypoglycemia.

   Ref: Carlisle BA, Kroon LA, Koda-Kimble MA. Diabetes mellitus. In: Koda-Kimble MA, Young LY, Kradjan WA, Guglielmo BJ, eds. *Applied Therapeutics: The Clinical Use of Drugs,* 8th ed. Philadelphia: Lippincott Williams & Wilkins, 2005:50-1–50-80.

7. (D) Both creatinine and liver function tests should be tested before metformin initiation to ensure that metformin use is not contraindicated owing to an increased risk of lactic acidosis. Metformin use is contraindicated in men with serum creatinine values of 1.5 mg/dL or greater and women with values of 1.4 mg/dL or greater. Metformin use is contraindicated in patients with liver dysfunction.

Ref: Carlisle BA, Kroon LA, Koda-Kimble MA. Diabetes mellitus. In: Koda-Kimble MA, Young LY, Kradjan WA, Guglielmo BJ, eds. *Applied Therapeutics: The Clinical Use of Drugs,* 8th ed. Philadelphia: Lippincott Williams & Wilkins, 2005:50-1–50-80.

8. (D) Metformin is sometimes initiated at 500 mg once daily for a few days before increasing to 500 mg twice daily to decrease the incidence of side effects. The minimal effective dose of metformin is 500 mg twice daily, and of the choices listed, this is the most appropriate.

Ref: Carlisle BA, Kroon LA, Koda-Kimble MA. Diabetes mellitus. In: Koda-Kimble MA, Young LY, Kradjan WA, Guglielmo BJ, eds. *Applied Therapeutics: The Clinical Use of Drugs,* 8th ed. Philadelphia: Lippincott Williams & Wilkins, 2005:50-1–50-80.

9. (C) Ephedra has been associated with hypertension and fatalities.

Ref: United States Food and Drug Administration. FDA fact sheet, February 28, 2003; available from *http://www.fda.gov/bbs/topics/NEWS/ephedra/factsheet.html;* accessed September 2003.

10. (C) Metformin should be held 48 hours after the administration of intravenous radiocontrast agents. If renal function normalizes, then metformin may be resumed.

Ref: Carlisle BA, Kroon LA, Koda-Kimble MA. Diabetes mellitus. In: Koda-Kimble MA, Young LY, Kradjan WA, Guglielmo BJ, eds. *Applied Therapeutics: The Clinical Use of Drugs,* 8th ed. Philadelphia: Lippincott Williams & Wilkins, 2005:50-1–50-80.

PATIENT PROFILE 137
HYPERCHOLESTEROLEMIA

ANSWERS

1. (D) Cholestyramine and pravastatin decrease total cholesterol, whereas gemfibrozil decreases triglycerides. AL's triglyceride level is not elevated, therefore gemfibrozil is not a good choice.

Ref: Expert Panel on Detection, Evaluation, and Treatment of High Blood Cholesterol in Adults. Summary of the second report of the National Cholesterol Education Program (NCEP) Expert Panel on Detection, Evaluation, and Treatment of High Blood Cholesterol in Adults (Adult Treatment Panel II). *JAMA* 1993;269:3015–3023.

2. (E) Flushing that occurs with the use of niacin appears to be mediated with prostaglandins. Prostaglandin inhibitors such as aspirin and ibuprofen taken one-half hour before niacin may reduce flushing. Hot beverages may exacerbate flushing.

Ref: Niacin. In: *American Hospital Formulary Service.* Bethesda, Md: American Society of Health-System Pharmacists; 1999:1560.

3. (B) LDL should be measured 4 to 6 weeks after initiation of pharmacologic therapy for hypercholesterolemia.

Ref: Expert Panel on Detection, Evaluation, and Treatment of High Blood Cholesterol in Adults. Summary of the second report of the National Cholesterol Education Program (NCEP) Expert Panel on Detection, Evaluation, and Treatment of High Blood Cholesterol in Adults (Adult Treatment Panel II). *JAMA* 1993;269:3015–3023.

4. (C) Liver function tests should be performed before initiation of lovastatin therapy, 6 and 12 weeks after initiation of therapy or an increase in dosage, and approximately every 6 months thereafter. Lovastatin therapy should be discontinued if there is persistent elevation (three times the upper limit of normal) of aminotransferase concentration.

Ref: Lovastatin. In: *American Hospital Formulary Service.* Bethesda, Md: American Society of Health-System Pharmacists; 1999:1554.

5. (E) Possible side effects of lovastatin include muscle aches, nausea, headache, abdominal pain, and rash.

Ref: Propranolol. In: *American Hospital Formulary Service.* Bethesda, Md: American Society of Health-System Pharmacists; 1999:1554–1555.

PATIENT PROFILE 138
HYPERLIPIDEMIA

ANSWERS

1. (B) Adults over the age of 20 should be screened for hyperlipidemia every 5 years.

Ref: Expert Panel on Detection, Evaluation, and Treatment of High Blood Cholesterol in Adults. Executive summary of the third report of the National Cholesterol Education Program (NCEP) on detection, evaluation, and treatment of high blood cholesterol in adults (Adult Treatment Panel III). *JAMA* 2001;285(19):2486–2497.

2. (C) Based on the NCEP's ATP III, RF's positive risk factors for heart disease are hypertension and a family history of premature coronary heart disease.

Ref: Expert Panel on Detection, Evaluation, and Treatment of High Blood Cholesterol in Adults. Executive summary of the third report of the National Cholesterol Education Program (NCEP) on detection, evaluation, and treatment of high blood cholesterol in adults (Adult Treatment Panel III). *JAMA* 2001;285(19):2486–2497.

3. (E) RF should institute a limit on daily cholesterol to less than 200 mg, an exercise program of 30 minutes per day, and an increase in soluble fiber intake in his diet.

Ref: Expert Panel on Detection, Evaluation, and Treatment of High Blood Cholesterol in Adults. Executive summary of the third report of the National Cholesterol Education Program (NCEP) on detection, evaluation, and treatment of high blood cholesterol in adults (Adult Treatment Panel III). *JAMA* 2001;285(19):2486–2497.

4. (C) Disagree; his LDL cholesterol goal is less than 100 mg/dL, and follow-up should be in 6 months with a lipoprotein profile.

Ref: Expert Panel on Detection, Evaluation, and Treatment of High Blood Cholesterol in Adults. Executive summary of the third report of the National Cholesterol Education Program (NCEP) on detection, evaluation, and treatment of high blood cholesterol in adults (Adult Treatment Panel III). *JAMA* 2001;285(19):2486–2497.

5. (D) You should not approve the prescription. With LDL cholesterol being the primary target for this patient, this would not be the best option.

Ref: McKenney JM. Dyslipidemias, atherosclerosis, and coronary heart disease. In: Young YL, Koda-Kimble MA, eds. *Applied Therapeutics: The Clinical Use of Drugs*. Vancouver, WA: Applied Therapeutics, 2005:13(1–39).

6. (A) Fibric acid derivatives exert their lipid-lowering effects by blocking lipase.

Ref: McKenney JM. Dyslipidemias, atherosclerosis, and coronary heart disease. In: Young YL, Koda-Kimble MA, eds. *Applied Therapeutics: The Clinical Use of Drugs*. Vancouver, WA: Applied Therapeutics, 2005:13(1–39).

7. (D) The following conditions confer high risk for CHD events: carotid artery disease, peripheral arterial disease, and abdominal aortic aneurysm.

Ref: Expert Panel on Detection, Evaluation, and Treatment of High Blood Cholesterol in Adults. Executive summary of the third report of the National Cholesterol Education Program (NCEP) on detection, evaluation, and treatment of high blood cholesterol in adults (Adult Treatment Panel III). *JAMA* 2001;285(19):2486–2497.

8. (B) Resins, particularly the older resins, are known to cause flatulence.

Ref: McKenney JM. Dyslipidemias, atherosclerosis, and coronary heart disease. In: Young YL, Koda-Kimble MA, eds. *Applied Therapeutics: The Clinical Use of Drugs*. Vancouver, WA: Applied Therapeutics, 2005:13(1–39).

9. (A) Some counseling points that you can offer RF to help minimize the adverse effects associated with this medication include swallowing it without engulfing air (administer it through a straw), maximizing intake of fluids, and mixing the resin in a noncarbonated juice.

Ref: McKenney JM. Dyslipidemias, atherosclerosis, and coronary heart disease. In: Young YL, Koda-Kimble MA, eds. *Applied Therapeutics: The Clinical Use of Drugs*. Vancouver, WA: Applied Therapeutics, 2005:13(1–39).

10. (D) In general, ACE inhibitors such as lisinopril do not have any effect on a lipoprotein profile.

Ref: McKenney JM. Dyslipidemias, atherosclerosis, and coronary heart disease. In: Young YL, Koda-Kimble MA, eds. *Applied Therapeutics: The Clinical Use of Drugs*. Vancouver, WA: Applied Therapeutics, 2005:13(1–39).

PATIENT PROFILE 139

ASTHMA

ANSWERS

1. (C) Short-acting β-agonists are considered the agents of choice for relief of acute bronchospasm because of their prompt onset of action.

Ref: Asthma. In: Young LY, Koda-Kimble MA, eds. *Applied Therapeutics: The Clinical Use of Drugs*. 6th ed. Vancouver, Wash: Applied Therapeutics; 1995: chapter 19.

2. (E) For children who are too young to properly use a metered-dose inhaler, antiasthmatic medications should be administered by means of nebulization. Oral administration usually is associated with more side effects than is the inhalation.

Ref: Asthma. In: Young LY, Koda-Kimble MA, eds. *Applied Therapeutics: The Clinical Use of Drugs*. 6th ed. Vancouver, Wash: Applied Therapeutics; 1995: chapter 19.

3. (D) Because of concern over serious side effects of corticosteroid administration, the antiinflammatory agent cromolyn is used as an alternative in the treatment of children because of its more favorable side effect profile.

Ref: National Asthma Education Panel Prevention Program. Expert Panel Report II. Guidelines for the Diagnosis and Management of Asthma. www.nhlbi.nih.gov/nhlbi/nhlbi.htm

4. (B) Growth suppression is of special concern for children receiving oral corticosteroids, although the data are inconclusive concerning inhaled corticosteroids and growth suppression.

Ref: Asthma. In: Young LY, Koda-Kimble MA, eds. *Applied Therapeutics: The Clinical Use of Drugs.* 6th ed. Vancouver, Wash: Applied Therapeutics; 1995: chapter 19.

5. (C) Because asthma is for the most part a reversible disease, recent guidelines suggest initiating inhaled corticosteroid therapy for mildly and moderately persistent disease to prevent airway remodeling and irreversible changes that occur with uncontrolled asthma.

Ref: National Asthma Education Panel Prevention Program. Expert Panel Report II. Guidelines for the Diagnosis and Management of Asthma. www.nhlbi.nih.gov/nhlbi/nhlbi.htm

---

PATIENT PROFILE 140

ASTHMA

ANSWERS

1. (B) EIA can be triggered by cold, dry air. Warm, humid air actually may prevent exercise-induced bronchospasm. Patients with stable disease who are controlled appropriately are encouraged to exercise.

Ref: Self TH. Asthma. In: Koda-Kimble MA, Young LY, Kradjian WA, Guglielmo BJ, eds. *Applied Therapeutics: The Clinical Use of Drugs.* Philadelphia: Lippincott Williams & Wilkins, 2004: 23-1–23-43.

2. (B) Albuterol is a short-acting β-agonist that is recommended for prevention of bronchospasm if administered 15 minutes prior to exercise and should provide protection for up to 3 hours.

Ref: Self TH. Asthma. In: Koda-Kimble MA, Young LY, Kradjian WA, Guglielmo BJ, eds. *Applied Therapeutics: The Clinical Use of Drugs.* Philadelphia: Lippincott Williams & Wilkins, 2004: 23-1–23-43.

3. (B) For relief of acute bronchospasm, a short-acting β-agonist is recommended.

Ref: Self TH. Asthma. In: Koda-Kimble MA, Young LY, Kradjian WA, Guglielmo BJ, eds. *Applied Therapeutics: The Clinical Use of Drugs.* Philadelphia: Lippincott Williams & Wilkins, 2004: 23-1–23-43.

4. (C) Salmeterol is a long-acting β-agonist and should be administered 30 minutes prior to exercising.

Ref: Self TH. Asthma. In: Koda-Kimble MA, Young LY, Kradjian WA, Guglielmo BJ, eds. *Applied Therapeutics: The Clinical Use of Drugs.* Philadelphia: Lippincott Williams & Wilkins, 2004: 23-1–23-43.

5. (C) Formoterol is a long-acting β-agonist that is an alternative to salmeterol. It should be administered at least 15 minutes prior to exercise.

Ref: Self TH. Asthma. In: Koda-Kimble MA, Young LY, Kradjian WA, Guglielmo BJ, eds. *Applied Therapeutics: The Clinical Use of Drugs.* Philadelphia: Lippincott Williams & Wilkins, 2004: 23-1–23-43.

6. (B) Oral β-agonists may cause cardiovascular side effects, including tachycardia. Hypokalemia is an electrolyte abnormality that may be attributed to β-agonists, not hyperkalemia.

Ref: Self TH. Asthma. In: Koda-Kimble MA, Young LY, Kradjian WA, Guglielmo BJ, eds. *Applied Therapeutics: The Clinical Use of Drugs.* Philadelphia: Lippincott Williams & Wilkins, 2004: 23-1–23-43.

7. (C) All are correct except that when using the open-mouth technique, the inhaler should be positioned 1 to 2 in from the mouth.

Ref: Self TH. Asthma. In: Koda-Kimble MA, Young LY, Kradjian WA, Guglielmo BJ, eds. *Applied Therapeutics: The Clinical Use of Drugs.* Philadelphia: Lippincott Williams & Wilkins, 2004: 23-1–23-43.

8. (B) When using a dry-powder inhaler, patients should be instructed to take a deep, rapid breath. With a metered-dose inhaler, patients should breathe in slowly.

Ref: Self TH. Asthma. In: Koda-Kimble MA, Young LY, Kradjian WA, Guglielmo BJ, eds. *Applied Therapeutics: The Clinical Use of Drugs.* Philadelphia: Lippincott Williams & Wilkins, 2004: 23-1–23-43.

9. (A) Salmeterol is available as a Serevent Diskus dry-powder inhaler.

Ref: Self TH. Asthma. In: Koda-Kimble MA, Young LY, Kradjian WA, Guglielmo BJ, eds. *Applied Therapeutics: The Clinical Use of Drugs.* Philadelphia: Lippincott Williams & Wilkins, 2004: 23-1–23-43.

10. (B) Montelukast, a leukotriene modifier, has been shown to be effective in preventing exercise-induced bronchospasm when administered once a day as chronic therapy.

Ref: Self TH. Asthma. In: Koda-Kimble MA, Young LY, Kradjian WA, Guglielmo BJ, eds. *Applied Therapeutics: The Clinical Use of Drugs.* Philadelphia: Lippincott Williams & Wilkins, 2004: 23-1–23-43.

PATIENT PROFILE 141
COMPOUNDING CAPSULES

ANSWERS

1. (D) Use simple enlargement.

Ref: Stocklosa M, Ansel H. *Pharmaceutical Calculations*. 10th ed. Baltimore: Williams & Wilkins; 1996:79–83.

2. (D) Total milligrams of drug divided by milligrams per tablet would give the number of tablets required.

Ref: Stocklosa M, Ansel H. *Pharmaceutical Calculations*. 10th ed. Baltimore: Williams & Wilkins; 1996:195–197.

3. (C) The amount of diluent required would be the difference between the total powder needed (number of capsules multiplied by total powder per capsule) and the value of the powder generated from the total number of tablets required to produce the desired amount of drug.

Ref: Stocklosa M, Ansel H. *Pharmaceutical Calculations*. 10th ed. Baltimore: Williams & Wilkins; 1996:195–197.

4. (B) The amount of diluent required would be the difference between the total powder needed (number of capsules × total powder per capsule) and the amount of the pure drug powder required.

Ref: Stocklosa M, Ansel H. *Pharmaceutical Calculations*. 10th ed. Baltimore: Williams & Wilkins; 1996:48–52.

5. (C) A less dense powder means that it would take a larger volume than an equivalent weight of aspirin. The first size capsule to try would be the next size larger, a number 2 capsule.

Ref: Ansel H, Popavitch N, Allen L. *Pharmaceutical Dosage Forms and Drug Delivery Systems*. 6th ed. Baltimore: Williams & Wilkins; 1995:169–171.

PATIENT PROFILE 142
ACUTE LEUKEMIA

ANSWERS

1. (C)

Ref: BSA equation from: Lacy CF. *Drug Information Handbook*, 11th ed. Hudson, OH: Lexicomp, 2003:1488.

2. (C)

Ref: Harvey RD III, Valgus JM. Hematologic malignancies. In: Koda-Kimbla MA, Young LY, Kradjan WA, et al, eds. *Applied Therapeutics: The Clinical Use of Drugs,* 8th ed. Philadelphia: Lippincott Williams & Wilkins, 2005:90(5–6).

3. (B)

Ref: Rowinsky EK, Tolcher AW. Antimicrotubule agents. In: Devita VT, Hellman S, Rosenberg SA, eds. *Cancer: Principles and Practice of Oncology,* 6th ed. Philadelphia: Lippincott Williams & Wilkins, 2001:436.

4. (C)

Ref: Lindley C. Adverse effects of chemotherapy. In: Koda-Kimbla MA, Young LY, Kradjan WA, et al, eds. Applied Therapeutics: The Clinical Use of Drugs. Philadelphia: Lippincott Williams & Wilkins, 2005:89(15).

5. (D)

Ref: Rowinsky EK, Tolcher AW. Antimicrotubule agents. In: Devita VT, Hellman S, Rosenberg SA, eds. *Cancer: Principles and Practice of Oncology,* 6th ed. Philadelphia: Lippincott Williams & Wilkins, 2001:437.

6. (A)

Ref: Harvey RD III, Valgus JM. Hematologic malignancies. In: Koda-Kimbla MA, Young LY, Kradjan WA, et al, eds. *Applied Therapeutics: The Clinical Use of Drugs,* 8th ed. Philadelphia: Lippincott Williams & Wilkins, 2005:90(5–6).

7. (A)

Ref: Chu E, Mota AC, Fogarasi MC. Antimetabolites. In: Devita VT, Hellman S, Rosenberg SA, eds. *Cancer: Principles and Practice of Oncology,* 6th ed. Philadelphia: Lippincott Williams & Wilkins, 2001:388.

8. (A)

Ref: Garrison MW, Young LY. Interpretation of clinical laboratory tests. In: Koda-Kimbla MA, Young LY, Kradjan WA, et al, eds. *Applied Therapeutics: The Clinical Use of Drugs,* 8th ed. Philadelphia: Lippincott Williams & Wilkins, 2005:2(18).

9. (D)

Ref: Hughes WT, Armstrong D, Bodey GP, et al. 2002 guidelines for the use od antimicrobial agents in neutropenic patients with cancer. *CID* 2002;34:730–751.

10. (D)

Ref: Cheson BD. Miscellaneous chemotherapeutic agents. In: Devita VT, Hellman S, Rosenberg SA, eds. *Cancer: Principles and Practice of Oncology,* 6th ed. Philadelphia: Lippincott Williams & Wilkins, 2001:455.

PATIENT PROFILE 143

SOFT-TISSUE INFECTION

ANSWERS

1. (C) The most common organisms found on the skin are gram-positive. Infections of the skin most commonly are caused by *Staphylococcus epidermidis, Staphylococcus aureus* (gram-positive cocci in clusters), or streptococci (grampositive cocci in chains) infections.

   Ref: Danziger LH, Fish D. Skin and soft tissue infections. In: DiPiro JT, Talbert RL, Yee GC, Matzke GR, Wells BG, Posey LM, eds. *Pharmacotherapy: A Pathophysiologic Approach.* 4th ed. Stamford, Conn: Appleton & Lange; 1999:1685–1699.

   Ref: McCormack JP, Brown G. Traumatic skin and soft tissue infections. In: Young LY, Koda-Kimble MA, eds. *Applied Therapeutics: The Clinical Use of Drugs.* 6th ed. Vancouver, Wash: Applied Therapeutics; 1995:66-1–66-5.

2. (A) Gram-positive organisms should be the focus in this type of infection. *Staphylococcus aureus* is the only gram-positive organism listed.

   Ref: Danziger LH, Fish D. Skin and soft tissue infections. In: DiPiro JT, Talbert RL, Yee GC, Matzke GR, Wells BG, Posey LM (eds): *Pharmacotherapy: A Pathophysiologic Approach.* 4th ed. Stamford, Conn: Appleton & Lange; 1999:1685–1699.

   Ref: McCormack JP, Brown G. Traumatic skin and soft tissue infections. In: Young LY, Koda-Kimble MA, eds. *Applied Therapeutics: The Clinical Use of Drugs.* 6th ed. Vancouver, Wash: Applied Therapeutics; 1995:66-1–66-5.

3. (D) When it is known that the organism is *Staphylococcus aurcus,* nafcillin is the most likely selection from the choices provided if the patient does not have a penicillin allergy. Nafcillin has the most specific coverage against staphylococci of all the antibiotics listed herein. Clindamycin and erythromycin also provide staphylococcal coverage, but these agents should be considered as second-line therapy in the care of patients with this type of infection.

   Ref: Danziger LH, Fish D. Skin and soft tissue infections. In: DiPiro JT, Talbert RL, Yee GC, Matzke GR, Wells BG, Posey LM (eds): *Pharmacotherapy: A Pathophysiologic Approach.* 4th ed. Stamford, Conn: Appleton & Lange; 1999:1685–1699.

   Ref: McCormack JP, Brown G. Traumatic skin and soft tissue infections. In: Young LY, Koda-Kimble MA, eds. *Applied Therapeutics:*

   The Clinical Use of Drugs. 6th ed. Vancouver, Wash: Applied Therapeutics; 1995:66-1–66-5.

4. (B) Cefazolin, a first-generation cephalosporin, has excellent activity against gram-positive organisms. Patients who have a rash caused by penicillin may be given an appropriate cephalosporin. In this case, a first-generation cephalosporin (cefazolin) would be most appropriate because it is known that there is increased gram-positive activity with first-generation cephalosporins. Aztreonam, a monobactam, and ceftazidime, a third-generation cephalosporin, are not effective against gram-positive infection. There is no clear reason to use imipenem in this instance. An organism has been identified and until proved otherwise it is susceptible to conventional therapy. Azithromycin covers this type of infection, but a first-generation cephalosporin will provide the best coverage (of the selections listed) in this type of infection.

   Ref: Danziger LH, Fish D. Skin and soft tissue infections. In: DiPiro JT, Talbert RL, Yee GC, Matzke GR, Wells BG, Posey LM (eds): *Pharmacotherapy: A Pathophysiologic Approach.* 4th ed. Stamford, Conn: Appleton & Lange; 1999:1685–1699.

   Ref: McCormack JP, Brown G. Traumatic skin and soft tissue infections. In: Young LY, Koda-Kimble MA, eds. *Applied Therapeutics: The Clinical Use of Drugs.* 6th ed. Vancouver, Wash: Applied Therapeutics; 1995:66-1–66-5.

5. (A) Vancomycin is a non–β-lactam antibiotic useful against almost all types of gram-positive infection. Anaphylaxis would exclude the use of any β-lactam antibiotic (penicillin). A single agent with superb gram-positive coverage is preferred. That excludes gentamicin and ciprofloxacin. Rifampin should not be used routinely as a single agent. Although rifampin has excellent gram-positive coverage, organisms become resistant rapidly when this drug is used alone.

   Ref: Danziger LH, Fish D. Skin and soft tissue infections. In: DiPiro JT, Talbert RL, Yee GC, Matzke GR, Wells BG, Posey LM (eds): *Pharmacotherapy: A Pathophysiologic Approach.* 4th ed. Stamford, Conn: Appleton & Lange; 1999:1685–1699.

   Ref: McCormack JP, Brown G. Traumatic skin and soft tissue infections. In: Young LY, Koda-Kimble MA, eds. *Applied Therapeutics: The Clinical Use of Drugs.* 6th ed. Vancouver, Wash: Applied Therapeutics; 1995:66-1–66-5.

PATIENT PROFILE 144

OSTEOARTHRITIS

ANSWERS

1. (E). Obesity, repetitive activities (straining of knees), and advanced age are all risk factors to osteoarthritis.

Ref: Boh LE, Elliot ME. Osteoarthritis. In: Dipiro JT, Talbert RL, Yee GC, et al, eds. *Pharmacotherapy: A Pathophysiologic Approach,* 5th ed. New York: McGraw-Hill, 2002:1639–1658.

2. (C) All the mentioned strategies are nonpharmacologic options to managing osteoarthritis. Acupucture is an invasive procedure; the other two options are not invasive. Trancutaneous electrical nerve stimulation (TENS) involves a small device that sends electrical impulses through the skin to nerves in the painful area. Biofeedback involves an electronic device that provides information regarding muscle contraction to better understand the pain and bodily responses.

Ref: American Pain Society. *Guideline for the Management of Pain in Osteoarthritis, Rheumatoid Arthritis, and Juvenile Chronic Arthritis,* 2d ed. Glenview, IL: APS, 2002:1–184.

3. (C). The effects of glucosamine are seen after 4 weeks of therapy. Since glucosamine comes from shells of crab, shrimp, and lobster, glucosamine should be avoided in patients with shellfish allergy.

Ref: American Pain Society. *Guideline for the Management of Pain in Osteoarthritis, Rheumatoid Arthritis, and Juvenile Chronic Arthritis,* 2d ed. Glenview, IL: APS, 2002:1–184.

4. (D) The effects of chondroitin are seen after 4 weeks of therapy. Side effects of chondroitin include prolonged bleeding time owing to its structure, which is similar to heparin.

Ref: American Pain Society. *Guideline for the Management of Pain in Osteoarthritis, Rheumatoid Arthritis, and Juvenile Chronic Arthritis,* 2d ed. Glenview, IL: APS, 2002:1–184.

5. (E) Advanced age (>65 years), history of peptic ulcer disease, history of upper GI bleeding, anticoagulant use, and use of multiple medications known to cause GI problems are risk factors for GI adverse effects from NSAIDs.

Ref: Boh LE, Elliot ME. Osteoarthritis. In: Dipiro JT, Talbert RL, Yee GC, et al, eds. *Pharmacotherapy: A Pathophysiologic Approach,* 5th ed. New York: McGraw-Hill, 2002:1639–1658.

6. (E) These recommendations all decrease the likelihood of GI toxicity of a nonselective NSAID, in addition to using the lowest possible dose on an as-needed basis.

Ref: Boh LE, Elliot ME. Osteoarthritis. In: Dipiro JT, Talbert RL, Yee GC, et al, eds. *Pharmacotherapy: A Pathophysiologic Approach,* 5th ed. New York: McGraw-Hill, 2002:1639–1658.

7. (E) MN has history of allergy to aspirin and therefore should not take an NSAID. However, if MN were a candidate for an NSAID, multiple-choice selections B and D are appropriate doses to treat osteoarthritis.

Ref: Boh LE, Elliot ME. Osteoarthritis. In: Dipiro JT, Talbert RL, Yee GC, et al, eds. *Pharmacotherapy: A Pathophysiologic Approach,* 5th ed. New York: McGraw-Hill, 2002:1639–1658.

8. (A) Acetaminophen is the optimal drug to use in MN if MN has renal dysfunction. MN should not be started on a nonselective NSAID or COX-2 inhibitor because she has aspirin allergy.

Ref: Boh LE, Elliot ME. Osteoarthritis. In: Dipiro JT, Talbert RL, Yee GC, et al, eds. *Pharmacotherapy: A Pathophysiologic Approach,* 5th ed. New York: McGraw-Hill, 2002:1639–1658.

9. (C) Capsaicin must be applied at least four times daily over 1 to 2 weeks continuously in order to be effective. Capsaicin should not be applied to broken skin. Capsaicin is available over the counter.

Ref: Boh LE, Elliot ME. Osteoarthritis. In: Dipiro JT, Talbert RL, Yee GC, et al, eds. *Pharmacotherapy: A Pathophysiologic Approach,* 5th ed. New York: McGraw-Hill, 2002:1639–1658.

10. (C) Hyaluronate injections are administered intraarticularly.

Ref: Boh LE, Elliot ME. Osteoarthritis. In: Dipiro JT, Talbert RL, Yee GC, et al, eds. *Pharmacotherapy: A Pathophysiologic Approach,* 5th ed. New York: McGraw-Hill, 2002:1639–1658.

PATIENT PROFILE 145

PARKINSON'S DISEASE

ANSWERS

1. (B) Bromocriptine is a semisynthetic ergot alkaloid and may be associated with peripheral vascular side effects because of its α-blocking properties. It may exacerbate Raynaud's phenomenon.

2. (D) The wearing-off effect or end-of-dose effect associated with long-term use of levodopa can be managed with the controlled release (CR) formulation of Sinemet®.

3. (C) Nonselective MAOIs such as phenelzine and tranylcypromine should be avoided by patients taking levodopa because of risk of hypertensive crisis. Tricyclic antidepressants cause gastric degradation of levodopa, delay emptying, and decrease the effect of levodopa.

4. (C) Selegiline may cause insomnia if given at bedtime because its metabolites, L-methamphetamine and L-amphetamine, are associated with excess stimulation.

5. (D) Pyridoxine is a precursor for dopa decarboxylase. It may increase the peripheral metabolism of levodopa, allowing less levodopa to reach the blood brain barrier. The interaction is not clinically significant when the Sinemet® formulation is used.

Ref: Flaherty JF, Gidal BE. Parkinson's disease. In: Young LY, Koda-Kimble MA, eds. *Applied Therapeutics: The Clinical Use of Drugs.* 6th ed. Vancouver, Wash: Applied Therapeutics; 1995: chapter 51.

Ref: Shimomura SK, Fujimoto D. Parkinsonism. In: Herfindal ET, Gourley DR, eds. *Textbook of Therapeutics. Drug and Disease Management.* 6th ed. Baltimore: Williams & Wilkins; 1996: chapter 51.

PATIENT PROFILE 146

DERMATOLOGY: ACNE

ANSWERS

1. (E) Tretinoin, a derivative of vitamin A available in various formulations, increases follicle cell turnover and decreases cohesiveness of cells, resulting in extrusion of existing comedones and inhibition of formation of new comedones.

Ref: Menon M, Ghorbani A, Sloan L, et al. Common skin disorders. In: Herfindal ET, Gourley DR, eds. *Textbook of Therapeutics. Drug and Disease Management.* 6th ed. Baltimore: Williams & Wilkins; 1996:889–921.

2. (E) Tretinoin can cause skin irritation. Patients may notice an exacerbation of acne at initiation of therapy, but the irritation resolves with continued therapy. Long exposure to UV radiation should be avoided.

Ref: Menon M, Ghorbani A, Sloan L, et al. Common skin disorders. In: Herfindal ET, Gourley DR, eds. *Textbook of Therapeutics. Drug and Disease Management.* 6th ed. Baltimore: Williams & Wilkins; 1996:889–921.

3. (E) Isotretinoin, a synthetic derivative of vitamin A, is considered early in the treatment of patients with scars. Prolonged remission can be expected.

Ref: Menon M, Ghorbani A, Sloan L, et al. Common skin disorders. In: Herfindal ET, Gourley DR, eds. *Textbook of Therapeutics. Drug and Disease Management.* 6th ed. Baltimore: Williams & Wilkins; 1996:889–921.

4. (E) Isotretinoin, which is pregnancy category X, should be avoided in pregnancy. The manufacturer provides specific recommendations for women of childbearing age.

Ref: Menon M, Ghorbani A, Sloan L, et al. Common skin disorders. In: Herfindal ET, Gourley DR, eds. *Textbook of Therapeutics. Drug and Disease Management.* 6th ed. Baltimore: Williams & Wilkins; 1996:889–921.

5. (E) Adverse effects if isotretinoin include disturbances in lipid metabolism, mucocutaneous effects, conjunctivitis, and corneal opacity.

Ref: Menon M, Ghorbani A, Sloan L, et al. Common skin disorders. In: Herfindal ET, Gourley DR, eds. *Textbook of Therapeutics. Drug and Disease Management.* 6th ed. Baltimore: Williams & Wilkins; 1996:889–921.

PATIENT PROFILE 147

MEDICINAL CHEMISTRY

ANSWER

1. (C) Spironolactone is a potassium-sparing diuretic clinically useful in avoiding the hypokalemia associated with use of other sulfonamide diuretics, such as hydrochlorothiazide and indapamide. Ethacrynic acid, like furosemide, is a high-ceiling diuretic that also causes hypokalemia. The structural similarity of spironolactone to the hormone aldosterone explains its action in antagonizing the renal action of aldosterone. This action normally causes sodium reabsorption and potassium excretion.

PATIENT PROFILE 148

LACTATION

ANSWERS

1. (B)

Ref: Breitzka RL, et al. Principles of drug transfer into breast milk and drug disposition in the nursing infant. *J Hum Lact* 1997;12:1155.

2. (B)

Ref: Ito S. Drug therapy for breast feeding women. *N Engl J Med* 2000;343:118–126.

3. (A)

Ref: Ito S. Drug therapy for breast feeding women. *N Engl J Med* 2000;343:118–126.

4. (B)

Ref: Tilson B. Mastitis: Plugged ducts and breast infections. *Leaven* 1993;29:91–121.

5. (C)

Ref: Tilson B. Mastitis: Plugged ducts and breast infections. *Leaven* 1993;29:91–121.

6. (C)

Ref: Briggs G, Freeman R, Yaffe Sumner. *A Reference Guide to Fetal and Neonatal Risk: Drugs in Pregnancy and Lactation,* 6th ed. Philadelphia. Lippincott Williams & Wilkins, 2002.

7. (B)

Ref: Briggs G, Freeman R, Yaffe Sumner. *A Reference Guide to Fetal and Neonatal Risk: Drugs in Pregnancy and Lactation,* 6th ed. Philadelphia. Lippincott Williams & Wilkins, 2002.

8. (C)

Ref: Briggs G, Freeman R, Yaffe Sumner. *A Reference Guide to Fetal and Neonatal Risk: Drugs in Pregnancy and Lactation,* 6th ed. Philadelphia. Lippincott Williams & Wilkins, 2002.

9. (B)

Ref: American Academy of Pediatrics Committee on Drugs. Transfer of drugs and other chemicals into human milk. *Pediatrics* 2001;108:776–789.

10. (B)

Ref: American Academy of Pediatrics Committee on Drugs. Transfer of drugs and other chemicals into human milk. *Pediatrics* 2001;108:776–789.

PATIENT PROFILE 149

ONCOLOGY: ADULT CHRONIC MYELOGENOUS LEUKEMIA

ANSWERS

1. (C) If this marker is identified, the diagnosis of CML is essentially confirmed.

Ref: McGuire TR, Kazakoff PW. Chronic leukemias. In: DiPiro JT, Talbert RL, Yee GC, Matzke GR, Wells BG, Posey LM (eds): *Pharmacotherapy: A Pathophysiologic Approach.* 4th ed. Stamford, Conn: Appleton & Lange; 1999:2169–2180.

Ref: Young LY, Koda-Kimble MA, eds. *Applied Therapeutics: The Clinical Use of Drugs.* 6th ed. Vancouver, Wash: Applied Therapeutics; 1995: chapter 92.

2. (D) Drug therapy at this time is directed at maintaining a WBC count <25,000 and minimizing symptoms associated with an increased WBC count.

Ref: McGuire TR, Kazakoff PW. Chronic leukemias. In: DiPiro JT, Talbert RL, Yee GC, Matzke GR, Wells BG, Posey LM (eds):

Pharmacotherapy: A Pathophysiologic Approach. 4th ed. Stamford, Conn: Appleton & Lange; 1999:2169–2180.

Ref: Young LY, Koda-Kimble MA, eds. *Applied Therapeutics: The Clinical Use of Drugs.* 6th ed. Vancouver, Wash: Applied Therapeutics; 1995: chapter 92.

3. (C) The use of hydroxyurea will effectively decrease the WBC count and substantially decrease in the splenomegaly.

Ref: McGuire TR, Kazakoff PW. Chronic leukemias. In: DiPiro JT, Talbert RL, Yee GC, Matzke GR, Wells BG, Posey LM (eds): *Pharmacotherapy: A Pathophysiologic Approach.* 4th ed. Stamford, Conn: Appleton & Lange; 1999:2169–2180.

4. (A) Successful transplantation of marrow from an HLA-matched sibling provides the best chance for long-term survival (>60%).

Ref: McGuire TR, Kazakoff PW. Chronic leukemias. In: DiPiro JT, Talbert RL, Yee GC, Matzke GR, Wells BG, Posey LM (eds): *Pharmacotherapy: A Pathophysiologic Approach.* 4th ed. Stamford, Conn: Appleton & Lange; 1999:2169–2180.

5. (C) The primary purpose of posttransplantation therapy is prevention of recurrence of disease.

Ref: McGuire TR, Kazakoff PW. Chronic leukemias. In: DiPiro JT, Talbert RL, Yee GC, Matzke GR, Wells BG, Posey LM (eds): *Pharmacotherapy: A Pathophysiologic Approach.* 4th ed. Stamford, Conn: Appleton & Lange; 1999:2169– 2180.

PATIENT PROFILE 150

SCHIZOPHRENIA

ANSWERS

1. (A) This is a delusion, and delusions are considered a positive symptom of schizophrenia.

    Ref: Andersson C, Chakos M, Mailman R, et al. Emerging roles for novel antipsychotic medications in the treatment of schizophrenia. *Psychiatr Clin North Am* 1998;21:151–179.

2. (C) Haloperidol does not affect serum levels of carbamazepine. However, persons with schizophrenia have a 50% noncompliance rate, which thereby warrants monitoring serum carbamazepine levels.

    Ref: Marder SR. Facilitating compliance with antipsychotic medication. *J Clin Psychiatry* 1998;59(suppl 3):21–25.

3. (B) The increase in haloperidol has probably caused excessive dopamine blockade and led to the extrapyramidal symptom of dystonia.

Ref: Young LY, Koda-Kimble MA, eds. *Applied Therapeutics: The Clinical Use of Drugs.* 6th ed. Vancouver, Wash: Applied Therapeutics; 1995: chapter 75.

4. (B) Social withdrawal is a negative symptom of schizophrenia, as are anhedonia, psychomotor retardation, and decreased motivation.

    Ref: Andersson C, Chakos M, Mailman R, et al. Emerging roles for novel antipsychotic medications in the treatment of schizophrenia. *Psychiatr Clin North Am* 1998;21:151–179.

5. (E) Olanzapine has been shown to control positive and negative symptoms of schizophrenia. It also has much less risk of causing seizures than the butyrophenones and the phenothiazines.

    Ref: Tollefson GD, Beasley CM, Tran PV, et al. Olanzapine versus haloperidol in the treatment of schizophrenia and schizoaffective and schizopheniform disorders: results of an international collaborative trial. *Am J Psychiatry* 1997; 154:457–465.

PATIENT PROFILE 151

PEPTIC ULCER MEDICATIONS

ANSWERS

1. (E) Ibuprofen for arthritis, lisinopril for hypertension, atorvastatin for high cholesterol, and amitriptyline for depression.

2. (A) Ibuprofen is a prime example of nonsteroidal anti-inflammatory drugs (NSAIDs) that are known to be ulcerogenic.

3. (C) NSAIDs inhibit the enzyme cyclooxygenase (COX) in the stomach. The enzyme catalyzes the synthesis of prostaglandins from the precursor arachidonic acid. Prostaglandins decrease hydrochloric acid production in the stomach and induce the secretion of

mucin, the natural cytoprotective agent for the GI tract linings.

4. (E) All are peptic ulcer drugs, but they act through different mechanisms.

5. (B) Omeprazole is an inhibitor for the H^+,K^+-ATPase pump that is responsible of exchanging protons synthesized in the parietal cells (acid-producing cells) with potassium ions in the stomach.

6. (A) Ranitidine is one of the selective H_2 blockers, a group of drugs that block histamine's stimulatory effects on the parietal cells (acid-producing cells).

7. (E) Sucralfate is an esterified sucrose molecule with sulfuric acid aluminum salts. The drug has gel properties that cover the ulcerated areas and protect it from the harmful effects of HCl and pepsin.

8. (C) Misoprostol is a potent stimulant for uterine smooth muscle contractions and should not be used in pregnancy.

9. (E) Cimetidine is known to be an inhibitor of the cytochrome P450 enzyme system.

10. (B) The cascade leading to stomach acid production involves stimulation of the muscarinic receptors on the endocrine cells. Anticholinergics reduce acid secretion.

PATIENT PROFILE 152
CONGESTIVE HEART FAILURE

ANSWERS

1. (B) IV diuretics should be used in the setting of acute volume overload or acute exacerbation of CHF.

   Ref: Johnson JA, Parker RB, Geraci SA. Heart failure. In: DiPiro JT, Talbert RL, Yee GC, Matzke GR, Wells BG, Posey LM, eds. *Pharmacotherapy: A Pathophysiologic Approach.* 4th ed. Stamford, Conn: Appleton & Lange; 1999:153–181.

2. (D) The addition of a thiazide diuretic is indicated if there is tolerance to large doses of loop diuretics.

   Ref: Johnson JA, Parker RB, Geraci SA. Heart failure. In: DiPiro JT, Talbert RL, Yee GC, Matzke GR, Wells BG, Posey LM, eds. *Pharmacotherapy: A Pathophysiologic Approach.* 4th ed. Stamford, Conn: Appleton & Lange; 1999:153–181.

3. (C) β-Blocker therapy for CHF should not be initiated if a patient has had recent changes in long-term diuretic or ACE inhibitor therapy.

   Ref: Johnson JA, Parker RB, Geraci SA. Heart failure. In: DiPiro JT, Talbert RL, Yee GC, Matzke GR, Wells BG, Posey LM, eds. *Pharmacotherapy: A Pathophysiologic Approach.* 4th ed. Stamford, Conn: Appleton & Lange; 1999:153–181.

4. (E) Loop diuretics can increase uric acid levels and precipitate an attack of gout.

   Ref: AHFS Drug Information, 1998.

5. (D) A long-acting dihydropyridine calcium channel antagonist may be used safely to treat patients with CAD who also have CHF.

   Ref: Talbert RL. Ischemic heart disease. In: DiPiro JT, Talbert RL, Yee GC, Matzke GR, Wells BG, Posey LM, eds. *Pharmacotherapy: A Pathophysiologic Approach.* 4th ed. Stamford, Conn: Appleton & Lange; 1999:182–210.

PATIENT PROFILE 153
CHRONIC RENAL FAILURE

ANSWERS

1. (C) Randomized, controlled studies have shown that ACE inhibitors reduce microalbuminuria or reduce or halt overt proteinuria leading to a reduction in the progression of renal failure, thereby diminishing the increase in serum creatinine over time in type 1 DM.

   Ref: Hudson JQ, Johnson CA. Chronic kidney disease. In: Koda-Kimble MA, Young LY, Kradjan WA, et al, eds. *Applied Therapeutics: The Clinical Use of Drugs,* 8th ed. Philadelphia: Lippincott Williams & Wilkins, 2005:32(1–36).

2. (A) A thiazide diuretic is recommended as add-on therapy to ACE inhibitors as first choice in controlling blood pressure in diabetic patients with good renal function.

   Ref: Chobanian AV, et al. The Seventh Report of the Joint National Committee on Prevention, Detection, Evaluation, and Treatment of High Blood Pressure. *JAMA* 2003;289:2560.

   Ref: Bakris GL, et al. National Kidney Foundation Hypertension and Diabetes Committee Working Group. Preserving renal function in adults with hypertension and diabetes. *Am J Kidney Dis* 2000; 36:646.

3. (C) Strict control of blood pressure and blood glucose has been shown to reduce progression to diabetic nephropathy.

Ref: Hudson JQ, Johnson CA. Chronic kidney disease. In: Koda-Kimble MA, Young LY, Kradjan WA, et al, eds. *Applied Therapeutics: The Clinical Use of Drugs,* 8th ed. Philadelphia: Lippincott Williams & Wilkins, 2005:32(1–36).

4. (D) ACE inhibitors such as lisinopril and loop diuretics such as furosemide should be discontinued 24 hours before and after an imaging study to reduce the potential for contrast medium nephrotoxicity (CMN).

Ref: Hudson JQ, Johnson CA. Chronic kidney disease. In: Koda-Kimble MA, Young LY, Kradjan WA, et al, eds. *Applied Therapeutics: The Clinical Use of Drugs,* 8th ed. Philadelphia: Lippincott Williams & Wilkins, 2005:32(1–36).

5. (C) Intravenous hydration with normal saline 12 hours before and after the imaging study with contrast media has been shown to reduce the incidence of CMN. Oral administration of *N*-acetylcysteine (NAC), a potent antioxidant that scavenges oxygen free radicals, one day before and the same day of the imaging study also has been shown to reduce the incidence of CMN.

Ref: Brophy D. Acute renal failure. In: Koda-Kimble MA, Young LY, Kradjan WA, et al, eds. *Applied Therapeutics: The Clinical Use of Drugs,* 8th ed. Philadelphia: Lippincott Williams & Wilkins, 2005:31(1–22).

6. (C) Vitamin D precursors cannot be hydroxylated to the active form in the presence of renal failure. The active form of active vitamin D, calcitriol, is used to improve calcium absorption and manage secondary hyperparathyroidism in renal failure patients.

Ref: Hudson JQ, Johnson CA. Chronic kidney disease. In: Koda-Kimble MA, Young LY, Kradjan WA, et al, eds. *Applied Therapeutics: The Clinical Use of Drugs,* 8th ed. Philadelphia: Lippincott Williams & Wilkins, 2005:32(1–36).

7. (C) Doxecalciferol and paricalcitol are active vitamin D analogues indicated in secondary hyperparathyroidism when patients become hypercalcemic on conventional therapy.

Ref: Hudson JQ, Johnson CA. Chronic kidney disease. In: Koda-Kimble MA, Young LY, Kradjan WA, et al, eds. *Applied Therapeutics: The Clinical Use of Drugs,* 8th ed. Philadelphia: Lippincott Williams & Wilkins, 2005:32(1–36).

8. (E) NSAIDs inhibit the vasodilatory properties of prostaglandins, which may lead to decreased renal blood flow from afferent arteriole vasoconstriction in patients at risk for developing prerenal azotemia.

Ref: Brophy D. Acute renal failure. In: Koda-Kimble MA, Young LY, Kradjan WA, et al, eds. *Applied Therapeutics: The Clinical Use of Drugs,* 8th ed. Philadelphia: Lippincott Williams & Wilkins, 2005:32(1–36).

9. (D) The patient's response to EPO after 8 weeks of therapy was inadequate despite adequate iron stores. Therefore, the dose of EPO should be increased by 25% because the target Hct has not been reached.

Ref: St. Peter WL, Lewis MJ, Collins A. End-stage renal disease. In: DiPiro JT, Talbert RL, Yee GC, et al, eds. *Pharmacotherapy: A Pathophysiologic Approach,* 5th ed. New York: McGraw-Hill, 2002:815–842.

10. (C) V_d <1 L/kg and $t_{1/2}$ of 3 to 4 hours are two of three pharmacokinetic parameters used to predict the dialyzability of drugs. The third consideration would be PPB <85%.

Ref: Quan DJ, Aweeka FT. Dosing of drugs in renal failure. In: Koda-Kimble MA, Young LY, Kradjan WA, et al, eds. *Applied Therapeutics: The Clinical Use of Drugs,* 8th ed. Philadelphia: Lippincott Williams & Wilkins, 2005:34(1–26).

PATIENT PROFILE 154

THYROID DISEASE

ANSWERS

1. (B) An elevated T4 and a low TSH level indicate hyperthyroidism.

Ref: Dang BJ. Thyroid disorders. In: Young LY, Koda-Kimble MA, eds. *Applied Therapeutics: The Clinical Use of Drugs.* 6th ed. Vancouver, Wash: Applied Therapeutics; 1995:47-1–47-31.

2. (E) Eliminating excess thyroid hormone, minimizing symptoms, and minimizing long-term consequences all are goals of hyperthyroidism therapy.

Ref: Dang BJ. Thyroid disorders. In: Young LY, Koda-Kimble MA, eds. *Applied Therapeutics: The Clinical Use of Drugs.* 6th ed. Vancouver, Wash: Applied Therapeutics; 1995:47-1–47-31.

3. (D) The action of both methimazole and propylthiouracil is to lower thyroid hormone levels. Levothyroxine is thyroid hormone replacement therapy.

Ref: Dang BJ. Thyroid disorders. In: Young LY, Koda-Kimble MA, eds. *Applied Therapeutics: The Clinical Use of Drugs.* 6th ed. Vancouver, Wash: Applied Therapeutics; 1995:47-1–47-31.

4. (A) Increasing propranolol to 80 mg po qid should help to achieve better heart rate control. Preferable treatment is to maximize the drug therapy that the patient is currently taking, if tolerated, before adding other agents.

Ref: Sinder PA, Cooper DS, Levy EG, et al. Treatment guidelines for patients with hyperthyroidism and hypothyroidism. *JAMA* 1995; 273:808–812.

5. (D) Signs and symptoms of hyperthyroidism include tremors, irritability, increased perspiration, diarrhea, soft, moist skin, and weight loss.

Ref: Dang BJ. Thyroid disorders. In: Young LY, Koda-Kimble MA, eds. *Applied Therapeutics: The Clinical Use of Drugs.* 6th ed. Vancouver, Wash: Applied Therapeutics; 1995:47-1–47-31.

PATIENT PROFILE 155

BACTEREMIA AND SEPSIS

ANSWERS

1. (E) Patients treated in ICUs are colonized with gram-negative organisms within the first 24 hours of their stay. Patients in a ward other than an ICU are colonized with gram-negative bacilli within 4 days. Lactose-fermenting gram-negative bacilli include the following species: *Enterobacter, Citrobacter, Klebsiella, Listeria, E. coli, Serratia,* and *Proteus.*

Ref: Toltzis P, Glover ML, Reed MD. Lower respiratory tract infections. DiPiro JT, Talbert RL, Yee GC, et al, eds. *Pharmacotherapy: A Pathophysiologic Approach,* 5th ed. New York: McGraw-Hill, 2002:1857.

2. (A) Of the choices provided, a third-generation cephalosporin such as ceftizoxime has the greatest spectrum of activity against lactose-fermenting gram-negative rods. Vancomyin and penicillin cover only gram-positive organisms. Ampicillin, like cefazolin, has limited gram-negative coverage, but ampicillin is the drug of choice in the treatment of patients with *Listeria* infection.

Ref: Gilbert DN, Moellering RC Jr, Eliopoulos GM, Sande MA, eds. *The Sanford Guide to Antimicrobial Therapy 2004,* 34th ed. Hyde Park, VT: Antimicrobial Therapy, 2004:53.

3. (A) The presence of non-lactose-fermenting gram-negative bacilli should lead one to believe that

Pseudomonas aeruginosa is present. For adequate management of *P. aeruginosa* infection, two drugs with activity against that organism should be used. A is the only combination with that kind of activity. Other non-lactose-fermenting gram-negative bacilli, which are seen less frequently, are *Stenotrophomonas* and *Acinetobacter* species.

Ref: Toltzis P, Glover ML, Reed MD. Lower respiratory tract infections. DiPiro JT, Talbert RL, Yee GC, et al, eds. *Pharmacotherapy: A Pathophysiologic Approach,* 5th ed. New York: McGraw-Hill, 2002:1862.

4. (C) Trimethoprim-sulfamethoxazole (Bactrim) is the drug of choice to manage *Stenotrophomonas* infection. The double gram-negative therapy should be discontinued, and Bactrim should be started.

Ref: Gilbert DN, Moellering RC Jr, Eliopoulos GM, Sande MA, eds. *The Sanford Guide to Antimicrobial Therapy 2004,* 34th ed. Hyde Park, VT: Antimicrobial Therapy, 2004:50.

5. (D) For treatment of patients with infection by resistant *Stenotrophomonas* organisms, piperacillin-tazobactam may be indicated.

Ref: Gilbert DN, Moellering RC Jr, Eliopoulos GM, Sande MA, eds. *The Sanford Guide to Antimicrobial Therapy 2004,* 34th ed. Hyde Park, VT: Antimicrobial Therapy, 2004:50.

PATIENT PROFILE 156

CHRONIC OBSTRUCTIVE LUNG DISEASE

ANSWERS

1. (C) Patients with chronic bronchitis tend to have a long-standing productive cough and are typically more over-

weight and cyanotic (blue bloaters) than patients with emphysema (pink puffers).

Ref: Chronic obstructive airway disease. In: Young LY, Koda-Kimble MA, eds. *Applied Therapeutics: The Clinical Use of*

Drugs. 6th ed. Vancouver, Wash: Applied Therapeutics; 1995: chapter 20.

2. (D) Side effects such as nausea, mouth and throat irritation, light-headedness, and hiccups are more likely if the patient chews nicotine gum too rapidly.

Ref: Chronic obstructive airway disease. In: Young LY, Koda-Kimble MA, eds. *Applied Therapeutics: The Clinical Use of Drugs.* 6th ed. Vancouver, Wash: Applied Therapeutics; 1995: chapter 20.

3. (C) In theory the 8-hour nicotine-free period of Nicotrol® may be associated with fewer sleep disturbances.

Ref: Chronic obstructive airway disease. In: Young LY, Koda-Kimble MA, eds. *Applied Therapeutics: The Clinical Use of Drugs.* 6th ed. Vancouver, Wash: Applied Therapeutics; 1995: chapter 20.

4. (B) Use of nicotine patches commonly causes skin irritation, which can be reduced by means of rotating the sites of application.

Ref: Chronic obstructive airway disease. In: Young LY, Koda-Kimble MA, eds. *Applied Therapeutics: The Clinical Use of Drugs.* 6th ed. Vancouver, Wash: Applied Therapeutics; 1995: chapter 20.

5. (D) Patients should be advised that if they continue to smoke while using nicotine replacement products, cardiovascular complications such as angina and arrhythmias may occur.

Ref: Chronic obstructive airway disease. In: Young LY, Koda-Kimble MA, eds. *Applied Therapeutics: The Clinical Use of Drugs.* 6th ed. Vancouver, Wash: Applied Therapeutics; 1995: chapter 20.

PATIENT PROFILE 157
URINARY TRACT INFECTION

ANSWERS

1. (C) Dipstick tests are rapid screening tests. The presence of nitrite in the urine (formed by bacteria that reduce nitrate) often indicates gram-negative pathogens. Positive leukocyte esterase (found in neutrophils) indicates the presence of WBC (>10 WBC/mm^3).

Ref: Coyle EA, Prince RA. Urinary tract infections and prostatitis. In Dipiro JT, Talbert RL, Yee GC, et al., eds. Pharmacotherapy: A Pathophysiologic Approach, 5th edition. New York: McGraw-Hill, 2002:1981–1996.

Ref: Fish DN. Urinary tract infections. In Koda-Kimble MA, Young LY, Kradian WA, et al., eds. *Applied Therapeutics: The Clinical Use of Drugs,* 8th edition. Philadelphia: Lippincott Williams & Wilkins, 2004:64(1–22).

2. (C) Seventy-five to ninety percent of community-acquired acute uncomplicated UTIs are caused by *E. coli.*

Ref: Coyle EA, Prince RA. Urinary tract infections and prostatitis. In Dipiro JT, Talbert RL, Yee GC, et al., eds. *Pharmacotherapy: A Pathophysiologic Approach,* 5th edition. New York: McGraw-Hill, 2002:1981–1996.

Ref: Fihn SD. Acute uncomplicated urinary tract infection in women. *NEJM* 2003;349(3):259–266.

3. (B) A 3-day course is currently recommended for uncomplicated cystitis because single-dose regimens have been associated with higher rates of recurrences and less effective eradication of bacteriuria (about 87% of patients compared to 94% with 3-day regimens). PL had two recent UTIs and is not a suitable candidate for single-dose UTI treatment.

Ref: Fihn SD. Acute uncomplicated urinary tract infection in women. *NEJM* 2003;349(3):259–266.

Ref: Fish DN. Urinary tract infections. In Koda-Kimble MA, Young LY, Kradian WA, et al., eds. *Applied Therapeutics: The Clinical Use of Drugs,* 8th edition. Philadelphia: Lippincott Williams & Wilkins, 2004:64(1–22).

4. (C) Trimethoprim-sulfamethoxazole (TMP-SMX; Bactrim®) is considered the drug of choice for un complicated cystitis as long as the geographic incidence of resistance to the drug is below 15% to 20%. However, PL has severe sulfa allergy and should not be treated with this drug. Fluoroquinolones are as effective as TMP-SMX, and norfloxacin is an appropriate choice for PL. Nitrofurantoin is less active against several gram-negative pathogens and needs to be given for 7 days. Doxycycline is not recommended, and fosfomycin is approved as a single dose.

Ref: Fihn SD. Acute uncomplicated urinary tract infection in women. *NEJM* 2003;349(3):259–266.

Ref: Fish DN. Urinary tract infections. In Koda-Kimble MA, Young LY, Kradian WA, et al., eds. *Applied Therapeutics: The Clinical Use of Drugs,* 8th edition. Philadelphia: Lippincott Williams & Wilkins, 2004:64(1–22).

5. (D) TMP-SMX has been associated with hemolytic anemia (especially in G6PD-deficient patients), thrombocytopenia, and neutropenia. A wide variety of drug eruptions (e.g., photosensitivity, exfoliate dermatitis, erythema multiforme, or Stevens-Johnson syndrome) can occur with TMP-SMX.

Ref: Ellsworth A, Smith RE. Dermatotherapy and drug induced skin disorders. In Koda-Kimble MA, Young LY, Kradian WA, et al., eds. *Applied Therapeutics: The Clinical Use of Drugs,* 8th edition. Philadelphia: Lippincott Williams & Wilkins, 2004: 38(1–19).

Ref: Fish DN. Urinary tract infections. In Koda-Kimble MA, Young LY, Kradian WA, et al., eds. *Applied Therapeutics: The Clinical Use of Drugs,* 8th edition. Philadelphia: Lippincott Williams & Wilkins, 2004:64(1–22).

6. (C) Fluoroquinolones may cause photosensitivity reactions that differ in their incidence rate according to the agent used (e.g., up to 2.4% with ciprofloxacin or norfloxacin). They also interact with products containing divalent and trivalent cations (Al^{2+}, Mg^{2+}, Ca^{2+}, Zn^{2+}, Fe^{3+}) resulting in significantly decreased fluoroquinolone absorption (20% to 70%). This may lead to therapeutic failure. PL should be instructed to best avoid intake of ferrous sulfate while taking ciprofloxacin, or to take the drug at least 2 hours before or 4 to 6 hours after the antibiotic dose.

Ref: Fihn SD. Acute uncomplicated urinary tract infection in women. *NEJM* 2003;349(3):259–266.

Ref: Fish DN. Urinary tract infections. In Koda-Kimble MA, Young LY, Kradian WA, et al., eds. *Applied Therapeutics: The Clinical Use of Drugs,* 8th edition. Philadelphia: Lippincott Williams & Wilkins, 2004:64(1–22).

Ref: Itokazu GS, Bearden DT, Danziger LH. Infectious diarrhea. In Koda-Kimble MA, Young LY, Kradian WA, et al., eds. *Applied Therapeutics: The Clinical Use of Drugs,* 8th edition. Philadelphia: Lippincott Williams & Wilkins, 2004:62(1–23).

7. (E) Recurrent urinary infections develop in about 20% of women with cystitis. 80% are reinfections occurring weeks to months after the previous UTI. Risk factors for recurrent infections include sexual intercourse and the use of a diaphragm, especially with a spermicide, for contraception. Reinfections are not a failure of the previous therapy and should be treated like a new infection using the same antibiotics as before. Prophylaxis should be instituted in patients who have more than three episodes per year, and this is considered more cost effective than treating each individual infection.

Ref: Coyle EA, Prince RA. Urinary tract infections and prostatitis. In Dipiro JT, Talbert RL, Yee GC, et al., eds. *Pharmacotherapy: A Pathophysiologic Approach,* 5th edition. New York: McGraw-Hill, 2002:1981–1996.

Ref: Fihn SD. Acute uncomplicated urinary tract infection in women. *NEJM* 2003;349(3):259–266.

Ref: Fish DN. Urinary tract infections. In Koda-Kimble MA, Young LY, Kradian WA, et al., eds. *Applied Therapeutics: The Clinical Use of Drugs,* 8th edition. Philadelphia: Lippincott Williams & Wilkins, 2004:64(1–22).

8. (A) Patients who develop reinfections associated with sexual activity benefit significantly from postcoital prophylactic antibiotic therapy. Both nitrofurantoin and trimethoprim are convenient and cost-effective options for PL.

Ref: Fihn SD. Acute uncomplicated urinary tract infection in women. *NEJM* 2003;349(3):259–266.

Ref: Fish DN. Urinary tract infections. In Koda-Kimble MA, Young LY, Kradian WA, et al., eds. *Applied Therapeutics: The Clinical Use of Drugs,* 8th edition. Philadelphia: Lippincott Williams & Wilkins, 2004:64(1–22).

9. (E) Food slows the absorption rate of nitrofurantoin and decrease peak serum concentration, thereby decreasing nausea and vomiting. The macrocrystalline preparation has a larger particle size, leading to slower dissolution rate, absorption, and lower blood levels. Doses less than 7 mg/kg also seem to cause fewer gastrointestinal side effects.

Ref: Fish DN. Urinary tract infections. In Koda-Kimble MA, Young LY, Kradian WA, et al., eds. *Applied Therapeutics: The Clinical Use of Drugs,* 8th edition. Philadelphia: Lippincott Williams & Wilkins, 2004:64(1–22).

10. (D) Four to seven percent of pregnant patients have asymptomatic bacteriuria that may progress to acute pyelonephritis in 20% to 40%. Untreated asymptomatic bacteriuria has been associated with premature birth, low birth weight, and stillbirth; therefore, treatment is recommended. Penicillins and cephalosporins appear to be relatively safe for use during pregnancy, and treatment should continue for 7 to 10 days.

Ref: Coyle EA, Prince RA. Urinary tract infections and prostatitis. In Dipiro JT, Talbert RL, Yee GC, et al., eds. *Pharmacotherapy: A Pathophysiologic Approach,* 5th edition. New York: McGraw-Hill, 2002:1981–1996.

Ref: Fish DN. Urinary tract infections. In Koda-Kimble MA, Young LY, Kradian WA, et al., eds. *Applied Therapeutics: The Clinical Use of Drugs,* 8th edition. Philadelphia: Lippincott Williams & Wilkins, 2004:64(1–22).

PATIENT PROFILE 158

PARENTERAL NUTRITION

ANSWERS

1. (C) The RME equation is solved with the patient's metric system equivalent values for height and weight.

   Ref: Stocklosa M, Ansel H. *Pharmaceutical Calculations*. 10th ed. Baltimore: Williams & Wilkins; 1996:177.

2. (E) The stressed value is the nonstressed daily requirement multiplied by the stress factor.

   Ref: Stocklosa M, Ansel H. *Pharmaceutical Calculations*. 10th ed. Baltimore: Williams & Wilkins; 1996:177, 180.

3. (A) Sixty percent of the stressed value would be supplied from a fat source. The number of kilocalories then is converted to grams and the volume of emulsion determined.

   Ref: Stocklosa M, Ansel H. *Pharmaceutical Calculations*. 10th ed. Baltimore: Williams & Wilkins; 1996:177–178.

4. (A) Grams of protein needed is found by means of multiplying kilograms body weight by allowed protein per kilogram. The volume of solution needed to provide that amount of protein as amino acid then is determined.

   Ref: Stocklosa M, Ansel H. *Pharmaceutical Calculations*. 10th ed. Baltimore: Williams & Wilkins; 1996:177, 180.

5. (A) Subtract the number of kilocalories of fat and protein (grams required multiplied by 4 kcal/g) used in the TPN solution from the stressed value of kilocalories. Convert the kilocalorie value to grams and determine the volume of dextrose solution needed.

   Ref: Stocklosa M, Ansel H. *Pharmaceutical Calculations*. 10th ed. Baltimore: Williams & Wilkins; 1996:177.

PATIENT PROFILE 159

SEXUALLY TRANSMITTED DISEASES

ANSWERS

1. (A) Coinfection with *Chlamydia trachomatis* often occurs among patients with gonococcal infection, and dual therapy is warranted. In the care of patients with a history of noncompliance, azithromycin is an appropriate option for chlamydial coverage, and ceftriaxone is an appropriate option for uncomplicated gonococcal infection.

   Ref: Centers for Disease Control and Prevention. 1998 guidelines for treatment of sexually transmitted diseases. MMWR Morb *Mortal Wkly Rep* 1998;47(RR-1):49–70.

2. (B) Quinolones and tetracycline should e avoided in pregnancy. A regimen of ceftriaxone for gonococcal coverage and erythromycin base for chlamydial coverage is the most appropriate regimen during pregnancy.

   Ref: Centers for Disease Control and Prevention. 1998 guidelines for treatment of sexually transmitted diseases. MMWR Morb *Mortal Wkly Rep* 1998;47(RR-1):49–70.

3. (B) Doxycycline is not adequate coverage for trichomoniasis or gonorrhea. Widespread resistance now prevents clinical use of this agent to manage gonorrhea.

   Ref: Centers for Disease Control and Prevention. 1998 guidelines for treatment of sexually transmitted diseases. *MMWR Morb Mortal Wkly Rep* 1998;47(RR-1):49–70.

4. (D) Ceftriaxone is approved for intramuscular administration and provides adequate coverage for gonorrhea but not for chlamydia or trichomoniasis.

   Ref: Centers for Disease Control and Prevention. 1998 guidelines for treatment of sexually transmitted diseases. *MMWR Morb Mortal Wkly Rep* 1998;47(RR-1):49–70.

5. (E) BT should be offered HIV counseling, HIV testing, and education on prevention strategies. Her sex partner(s) should be referred for evaluation.

   Ref: Centers for Disease Control and Prevention. 1998 guidelines for treatment of sexually transmitted diseases. *MMWR Morb Mortal Wkly Rep* 1998;47(RR-1):49–70.

6. (C) Oral metronidazole is the therapy of choice for trichomoniasis for both men and women.

   Ref: Centers for Disease Control and Prevention. 1998 guidelines for treatment of sexually transmitted diseases. *MMWR Morb Mortal Wkly Rep* 1998;47(RR-1):49–70.

7. (C) Metronidazole interacts with the metabolism of alcohol and can cause a disulfiramlike reaction.

8. (D) Both famciclovir and valacyclovir are both prodrugs; ganciclovir is not a prodrug.

Ref: Centers for Disease Control and Prevention. *USPHS/IDSA Guidelines for the Prevention of Opportunistic Infections in Persons with Human Immunodeficiency Virus*, 2001.

9. (E) Acyclovir, famciclovir, and valacyclovir all require careful monitoring in patients with renal impairment.

10. (C) Parental penicillin G is the drug of choice for the management of all stages of syphilis.

Ref: Centers for Disease Control and Prevention. 1998 guidelines for treatment of sexually transmitted diseases. *MMWR Morb Mortal Wkly Rep* 1998;47(RR-1):49–70.

PATIENT PROFILE 160
SOFT-TISSUE INFECTION

ANSWERS

1. (C) Diabetic foot infections typically are mixed infections. Many organisms may be present. Impairment of host defenses, poor blood circulation, and neuropathy caused by diabetes mellitus make it difficult for patients to ward off infection. Foot infections can have many organisms present. Daily events such as showering can carry many organisms from other parts of the body and deposit them in an open wound in the foot. Adding host impairment makes severe infection possible. Fastidious foot care is essential for persons with diabetes.

Ref: Danziger LH, Fish D. Skin and soft tissue infections. In: DiPiro JT, Talbert RL, Yee GC, Matzke GR, Wells BG, Posey LM, eds. *Pharmacotherapy: A Pathophysiologic Approach*. 4th ed. Stamford, Conn: Appleton & Lange; 1999:1685–1699.

Ref: McCormack JP, Brown G. Traumatic skin and soft tissue infections. In: Young LY, Koda-Kimble MA, eds. *Applied Therapeutics: The Clinical Use of Drugs*. 6th ed. Vancouver, Wash: Applied Therapeutics; 1995:66-5-66-7.

Ref: Gilbert DN, Moellering RC Jr, Sande MA, eds. *The Sanford Guide to Antimicrobial Therapy 1998*. 28th ed. Vienna, Va: Antimicrobial Therapy; 1998:11.

2. (A) Broad-spectrum antibiotics, including fluoroquinolones, allow adequate management of infections from osteomyelitis. These infections are severe and may necessitate hospitalization.

Ref: Danziger LH, Fish D. Skin and soft tissue infections. In: DiPiro JT, Talbert RL, Yee GC, Matzke GR, Wells BG, Posey LM, eds. *Pharmacotherapy: A Pathophysiologic Approach*. 4th ed. Stamford, Conn: Appleton & Lange; 1999:1685–1699.

Ref: McCormack JP, Brown G. Traumatic skin and soft tissue infections. In: Young LY, Koda-Kimble MA, eds. *Applied Therapeutics: The Clinical Use of Drugs*. 6th ed. Vancouver, Wash: Applied Therapeutics; 1995:66–5–66–7.

Ref: Gilbert DN, Moellering RC Jr, Sande MA, eds. *The Sanford Guide to Antimicrobial Therapy 1998*. 28th ed. Vienna, Va: Antimicrobial Therapy; 1998:11.

3. (D) Of the selections listed, piperacillin-tazobactam has the broadest spectrum of coverage. Diabetic foot infections often are polymicrobial. Until a definitive organism is cultured with proper technique, a broad-spectrum antibiotic directed at gram-positive organisms, including enterococci and gram-negative organisms, and at anaerobic organisms, including Bacteroides fragilis, should be considered. Ampicillin-sulbactam is another antibiotic frequently selected for its spectrum of coverage of this type of infection.

Ref: Danziger LH, Fish D. Skin and soft tissue infections. In: DiPiro JT, Talbert RL, Yee GC, Matzke GR, Wells BG, Posey LM, eds. *Pharmacotherapy: A Pathophysiologic Approach*. 4th ed. Stamford, Conn: Appleton & Lange; 1999:1685–1699.

Ref: McCormack JP, Brown G. Traumatic skin and soft tissue infections. In: Young LY, Koda-Kimble MA, eds. *Applied Therapeutics: The Clinical Use of Drugs*. 6th ed. Vancouver, Wash: Applied Therapeutics; 1995:66–5–66–7.

Ref: Gilbert DN, Moellering RC Jr, Sande MA, eds. *The Sanford Guide to Antimicrobial Therapy 1998*. 28th ed. Vienna, Va: Antimicrobial Therapy; 1998:11.

4. (C) Although piperacillin-tazobactam has activity against *Pseudomonas aeruginosa*, single agents should be avoided when treating patients with this type of infection. Adding a second agent such as an aminoglycoside or a fluoroquinolone with activity against *P. aeruginosa* would be useful to this patient. P. aeruginosa is the only deficiency in antibiotic coverage in this patient.

Ref: Danziger LH, Fish D. Skin and soft tissue infections. In: DiPiro JT. Talbert RL, Yee GC, Matzke GR, Wells BG, Posey LM, eds. *Pharmacotherapy: A Pathophysiologic Approach*. 4th ed. Stamford, Conn: Appleton & Lange; 1999:1685–1699.

Ref: McCormack JP, Brown G. Traumatic skin and soft tissue infections. In: Young LY, Koda-Kimble MA, eds. *Applied Therapeutics: The Clinical Use of Drugs*. 6th ed. Vancouver, Wash: Applied Therapeutics; 1995:66–5–66–7.

Ref: Gilbert DN, Moellering RC Jr, Sande MA, eds. *The Sanford Guide to Antimicrobial Therapy 1998*. 28th ed. Vienna, Va: Antimicrobial Therapy; 1998:11.

5. (E) Proper foot care is paramount in preventing diabetic foot infections. Avoidance truly is the best treatment in this case. Once an infection is present, poor circulation, impaired nerve responses, and

maintenance of foot care become difficult and often necessitate hospitalization.

Ref: Danziger LH, Fish D. Skin and soft tissue infections. In: DiPiro JT. Talbert RL, Yee GC, Matzke GR, Wells BG, Posey LM, eds.: *Pharmacotherapy: A Pathophysiologic Approach.* 4th ed. Stamford, Conn: Appleton & Lange; 1999:1685–1699.

Ref: McCormack JP, Brown G. Traumatic skin and soft tissue infections. In: Young LY, Koda-Kimble MA, eds. *Applied Therapeutics: The Clinical Use of Drugs.* 6th ed. Vancouver, Wash: Applied Therapeutics; 1995:66-5–66-7.

Ref: Gilbert DN, Moellering RC Jr, Sande MA, eds. *The Sanford Guide to Antimicrobial Therapy* 1998. 28th ed. Vienna, Va: Antimicrobial Therapy; 1998:11.

PATIENT PROFILE 161

ASTHMA

ANSWERS

1. (E) All of the above; indoor mold, cockroach allergen, and house dust mite allergen all are potential triggers for JJ.

   Ref: National Asthma Education and Prevention Program, Expert Panel Report 2. *Guidelines for the Diagnosis and Management of Asthma.* NIH Publication No. 97-4051. Bethesda, MD: US Department of health and Human Services, 1997.

2. (B) Gastroesophageal reflux disease has been known to exacerbate asthma symptoms in some patients.

   Ref: National Asthma Education and Prevention Program, Expert Panel Report 2. *Guidelines for the Diagnosis and Management of Asthma.* NIH Publication No. 97-4051. Bethesda, MD: US Department of health and Human Services, 1997.

3. (D) Step 3: moderate persistent asthma caused by nightly symptoms two times a week.

   Ref: National Asthma Education and Prevention Program, Expert Panel Report 2. *Guidelines for the Diagnosis and Management of Asthma.* NIH Publication No. 97-4051. Bethesda, MD: US Department of health and Human Services, 1997.

4. (E) Low-dose inhaled corticosteroid and long-acting β_2 agonist because of the proven efficacy of the two agents when used in combination in Step 2.

   Ref: National Asthma Education and Prevention Program, Expert Panel Report 2. *Guidelines for the Diagnosis and Management of Asthma.* NIH Publication No. 97-4051. Bethesda, MD: US Department of health and Human Services, 1997.

5. (D) Recommend that JJ discontinue his Primatene Mist® use and obtain a new prescription for his albuterol to use on an as-needed basis because of the efficacy of albuterol and safety concerns with Primatene Mist®.

Ref: National Asthma Education and Prevention Program, Expert Panel Report 2. *Guidelines for the Diagnosis and Management of Asthma.* NIH Publication No. 97-4051. Bethesda, MD: US Department of health and Human Services, 1997.

6. (B) Smoking one pack per day because of smoking impact on theophylline levels.

   Ref: National Asthma Education and Prevention Program, Expert Panel Report 2. *Guidelines for the Diagnosis and Management of Asthma.* NIH Publication No. 97-4051. Bethesda, MD: US Department of health and Human Services, 1997.

7. (B) Improves lung function when used with a long-acting β_2-agonist and is usually a first-line agent in the treatment of asthma.

   Ref: National Asthma Education and Prevention Program, Expert Panel Report 2. *Guidelines for the Diagnosis and Management of Asthma.* NIH Publication No. 97-4051. Bethesda, MD: US Department of health and Human Services, 1997.

8. (C) Cough and pharyngitis.

   Ref: National Asthma Education and Prevention Program, Expert Panel Report 2. *Guidelines for the Diagnosis and Management of Asthma.* NIH Publication No. 97-4051. Bethesda, MD: US Department of health and Human Services, 1997.

9. (B) Leukotriene modifier.

   Ref: National Asthma Education and Prevention Program, Expert Panel Report 2. *Guidelines for the Diagnosis and Management of Asthma.* NIH Publication No. 97-4051. Bethesda, MD: US Department of health and Human Services, 1997.

10. (C) Zileuton and Zafirlukast.

    Ref: National Asthma Education and Prevention Program, Expert Panel Report 2. *Guidelines for the Diagnosis and Management of Asthma.* NIH Publication No. 97-4051. Bethesda, MD: US Department of health and Human Services, 1997.

PATIENT PROFILE 162

OSTEOPOROSIS

ANSWERS

1. (E) Estrogen supplementation, the single most effective measure for preventing postmenopausal osteoporosis, provides other benefits, including cardiovascular and relief of vasomotor symptoms associated with menopause. The daily dose shown to preserve bone mineral density is equivalent to 0.625 mg conjugated estrogen.

   Ref: Prevost RR. Osteoporosis and osteomalacia. In: Herfindal ET, Gourley DR, eds. *Textbook of Therapeutics. Drug and Disease Management.* 6th ed. Baltimore: Williams & Wilkins; 1996: 639–649.

2. (B) Concomitant progesterone therapy can prevent endometrial tissue buildup in women with intact uteri. Women who have undergone hysterectomy do not need concomitant progesterone therapy.

   Ref: Prevost RR. Osteoporosis and osteomalacia. In: Herfindal ET, Gourley DR, eds. *Textbook of Therapeutics. Drug and Disease Management.* 6th ed. Baltimore: Williams & Wilkins; 1996:639–649.

3. (D) Adequate calcium intake (1000 mg elemental calcium daily for women older than 50 years who are taking estrogen supplementation) and vitamin D optimize osteoporosis therapy and decrease the incidence of hip fracture among elderly women.

   Ref: Prevost RR. Osteoporosis and osteomalacia. In: Herfindal ET, Gourley DR, eds. *Textbook of Therapeutics. Drug and Disease Management.* 6th ed. Baltimore: Williams & Wilkins; 1996: 639–649.

4. (A) The intranasal dose of calcitonin-salmon solution (Miacalcin® Nasal Spray) is 200 IU daily, alternating nares.

   Ref: O'Connell MB. Osteoporosis and osteomalacia. In: DiPiro JT, Talbert RL, Yee GC, Matzke GR, Wells BG, Posey LM, eds. *Pharmacotherapy. A Pathophysiologic Approach.* 4th ed. Stamford, Conn: Appleton & Lange; 1999:1406–1426.

5. (E) Various studies have reported that excessive caffeine consumption, excessive alcohol consumption, and smoking are risk factors for fracture and contribute to bone loss.

   Ref: Ross PD. Osteoporosis: frequency, consequences, and risk factors. *Arch Intern Med* 1996;156:1399–1411.

PATIENT PROFILE 163

ISOTONIC SOLUTIONS (PHARMACEUTICS)

ANSWERS

1. E

   Ref: Zatz, J. *Pharmaceutical Calculations.* 3rd ed. New York: John Wiley & Sons; 1995:273.

2. B

   Ref: Zatz, J. *Pharmaceutical Calculations.* 3rd ed. New York: John Wiley & Sons; 1995:274–275.

3. A

   Ref: Zatz, J. *Pharmaceutical Calculations.* 3rd ed. New York: John Wiley & Sons; 1995:271.

4. B

   Ref: Shargel L, Mutnick AH, Souney PF, et al. *Comprehensive Pharmacy Review.* 4th ed. Philadelphia: Lippincott Williams and Wilkins; 2001:14.

5. C

   Ref: Zatz, J. *Pharmaceutical Calculations.* 3rd ed. New York: John Wiley & Sons; 1995:252.

6. E

   Ref: Zatz, J. *Pharmaceutical Calculations.* 3rd ed. New York: John Wiley & Sons; 1995:258.

7. D

   Ref: Shargel L, Mutnick AH, Souney PF, et al. *Comprehensive Pharmacy Review.* 4th ed. Philadelphia: Lippincott Williams and Wilkins; 2001:14.

8. E

   Ref: Shargel L, Mutnick AH, Souney PF, et al. *Comprehensive Pharmacy Review.* 4th ed. Philadelphia: Lippincott Williams and Wilkins; 2001:14.

9. C

   Ref: Allen LV, Popovich NG, Ansel HC. *Ansel's Pharmaceutical Dosage Forms and Drug Delivery Systems.* 8th ed. Philadelphia: Lippincott Williams and Wilkins; 2005:543.

10. A

    Ref: Zatz, J. *Pharmaceutical Calculations.* 3rd ed. New York: John Wiley & Sons; 1995:267.

ONCOLOGY: NAUSEA AND VOMITING CONTROL

ANSWERS

1. (C) The increased GI motility associated with metoclopramide use decreases nausea and vomiting but increases the risk of diarrhea.

   Ref: AHFS 1998

2. (B) Highly emetogenic antineoplastic agents included in the regimen necessitate use of a 5-HT3 antiemetic agent with addition of a steroid.

   Ref: Taylor AT. Nausea and vomiting. In: DiPiro JT, Talbert RL, Yee GC, Matzke GR, Wells BG, Posey LM, eds. *Pharmacotherapy: A Pathophysiologic Approach.* 4th ed. Stamford, Conn: Appleton & Lange; 1999:586–598.

   Ref: In: Herfindal ET, Gourley DR, eds. *Textbook of Therapeutics. Drug and Disease Management.* 6th ed. Baltimore: Williams & Wilkins; 1996: chapter 25.

3. (E) Emesis that occurs more than 24 hours after administration of an antineoplastic agent is categorized as delayed.

   Ref: Taylor AT. Nausea and vomiting. In: DiPiro JT, Talbert RL, Yee GC, Matzke GR, Wells BG, Posey LM, eds. *Pharmacotherapy: A Pathophysiologic Approach.* 4th ed. Stamford, Conn: Appleton & Lange; 1999:586–598.

   Ref: In: Herfindal ET, Gourley DR, eds. *Textbook of Therapeutics. Drug and Disease Management.* 6th ed. Baltimore: Williams & Wilkins; 1996: chapter 25.

4. (A) Vomiting before receiving antineoplastic agents is categorized as anticipatory and usually responds to therapy with benzodiazepines.

   Ref: Taylor AT. Nausea and vomiting. In: DiPiro JT, Talbert RL, Yee GC, Matzke GR, Wells BG, Posey LM, eds. *Pharmacotherapy: A Pathophysiologic Approach.* 4th ed. Stamford, Conn: Appleton & Lange; 1999:586–598.

   Ref: In: Herfindal ET, Gourley DR, eds. *Textbook of Therapeutics. Drug and Disease Management.* 6th ed. Baltimore: Williams & Wilkins; 1996: chapter 25.

5. (E) The prochlorperazine dose ordered is the maximum recommended daily dose. VT should be aware of possible extrapyramidal symptoms.

   Ref: Taylor AT. Nausea and vomiting. In: DiPiro JT, Talbert RL, Yee GC, Matzke GR, Wells BG, Posey LM, eds. *Pharmacotherapy: A Pathophysiologic Approach.* 4th ed. Stamford, Conn: Appleton & Lange; 1999:586–598.

   Ref: In: Herfindal ET, Gourley DR, eds. *Textbook of Therapeutics. Drug and Disease Management.* 6th ed. Baltimore: Williams & Wilkins; 1996: chapter 25.

OPIOID OVERDOSE AND DEPENDENCE

ANSWERS

1. (C) Immediate treatment of opioid overdose includes airway management, cardiorespiratory support (advanced cardiac life support [ACLS] if indicated), and opioid reversal with an opioid antagonist. Naloxone is a full opioid antagonist that rapidly reverses the respiratory depression and hypotension associated with overdose. Benzodiazepines are not used in the treatment of opioid overdose.

   Ref: Zizzo WO, Zizzo PV. Drug abuse. In: Koda-Kimble MA, Young LY, Kradjan WA, Guglielmo BJ, eds. *Applied Therapeutics: The Clinical Use of Drugs,* 8th edition. Baltimore, MD: Lippincott Williams & Wilkins, 2005:1–24.

2. (D) Symptoms of opioid withdrawal include anxiety, hyperactivity, restlessness, insomnia with yawning, sialorrhea, rhinorrhea, lacrimation, diaphoresis, gooseflesh, anorexia, nausea, vomiting, abdominal cramps, and diarrhea. Auditory hallucinations are associated with alcohol withdrawal.

   Ref: Zizzo WO, Zizzo PV. Drug abuse. In: Koda-Kimble MA, Young LY, Kradjan WA, Guglielmo BJ, eds. *Applied Therapeutics: The Clinical Use of Drugs,* 8th edition. Baltimore, MD: Lippincott Williams & Wilkins, 2005:1–24.

3. (B) The onset, severity, and time course of opioid withdrawal symptoms are dependent on many factors, including the particular opioid, total daily dose, interval

between doses, duration of use, and the health and personality of the user. Physiologic withdrawal symptoms from all opioid drugs are qualitatively similar but quantitatively different in onset, duration, and severity. Symptoms of heroin withdrawal subside after 5 to 10 days of abstinence. A return to complete physiologic equilibrium may take months or longer.

Ref: Zizzo WO, Zizzo PV. Drug abuse. In: Koda-Kimble MA, Young LY, Kradjan WA, Guglielmo BJ, eds. *Applied Therapeutics: The Clinical Use of Drugs,* 8th edition. Baltimore, MD: Lippincott Williams & Wilkins, 2005:1–24.

4. (C) Narcan is the brand name for naloxone, a potent opioid antagonist.

Ref: Zizzo WO, Zizzo PV. Drug abuse. In: Koda-Kimble MA, Young LY, Kradjan WA, Guglielmo BJ, eds. *Applied Therapeutics: The Clinical Use of Drugs,* 8th edition. Baltimore, MD: Lippincott Williams & Wilkins, 2005:1–24.

5. (D) Currently, buprenorphine, a Schedule III medication, is the only medication approved for the treatment of opioid dependence in an office setting under the Drug Addiction Treatment Act of 2000.

Ref: Zizzo WO, Zizzo PV. Drug abuse. In: Koda-Kimble MA, Young LY, Kradjan WA, Guglielmo BJ, eds. *Applied Therapeutics: The Clinical Use of Drugs,* 8th edition. Baltimore, MD: Lippincott Williams & Wilkins, 2005:1–24.

6. (B) Buprenorphine is a partial opioid agonist at the μ-receptors. Methadone is a full opioid agonist at the μ-receptor. Naloxone is a μ-opioid receptor antagonist.

Ref: Zizzo WO, Zizzo PV. Drug abuse. In: Koda-Kimble MA, Young LY, Kradjan WA, Guglielmo BJ, eds. *Applied Therapeutics: The Clinical Use of Drugs,* 8th edition. Baltimore, MD: Lippincott Williams & Wilkins, 2005:1–24.

7. (E) Methadone does not appear to be teratogenic or have an adverse effect on mental development. Methadone

does cross the placental barrier and can cause central nervous system and respiratory depression as well as signs and symptoms of withdrawal in the infant after birth. These withdrawal symptoms (twitching and irritability) may be delayed for up to 3 days.

Ref: Zizzo WO, Zizzo PV. Drug abuse. In: Koda-Kimble MA, Young LY, Kradjan WA, Guglielmo BJ, eds. *Applied Therapeutics: The Clinical Use of Drugs,* 8th edition. Baltimore, MD: Lippincott Williams & Wilkins, 2005:1–24.

8. (A) Clonidine, a central α_2-adrenergic agonist, inhibits locus ceruleus noradrenergic outflow during opioid withdrawal and can significantly reduce anxiety. Clonidine is less effective in treating other target symptoms and is best used as part of a multidrug regimen.

Ref: Zizzo WO, Zizzo PV. Drug abuse. In: Koda-Kimble MA, Young LY, Kradjan WA, Guglielmo BJ, eds. *Applied Therapeutics: The Clinical Use of Drugs,* 8th edition. Baltimore, MD: Lippincott Williams & Wilkins, 2005:1–24.

9. (C) Naloxone, a μ-opioid receptor antagonist, is poorly absorbed orally. Its use in combination with buprenorphine sublingual tablets is to discourage the intravenous abuse of buprenorphine.

Ref: Zizzo WO, Zizzo PV. Drug abuse. In: Koda-Kimble MA, Young LY, Kradjan WA, Guglielmo BJ, eds. *Applied Therapeutics: The Clinical Use of Drugs,* 8th edition. Baltimore, MD: Lippincott Williams & Wilkins, 2005:1–24.

10. (C) Currently, methadone and buprenorphine are FDA approved for use as substitution therapy for detoxification and maintenance therapy for opioid dependence. Methadone is a synthetic, orally acting μ-opioid receptor agonist with a duration of action of 12 to 24 hours.

Ref: Zizzo WO, Zizzo PV. Drug abuse. In: Koda-Kimble MA, Young LY, Kradjan WA, Guglielmo BJ, eds. *Applied Therapeutics: The Clinical Use of Drugs,* 8th edition. Baltimore, MD: Lippincott Williams & Wilkins, 2005:1–24.

PATIENT PROFILE 166
MEDICINAL CHEMISTRY

ANSWER

1. (E) There is a serious pharmacologic drug-drug interaction between carbachol and triflupromazine. Carbachol is a cholinergic agonist, and triflupromazine, with structural features indicating anticholinergic proper-

ties, may antagonize the action of carbachol. A switch to an antipsychotic agent with little or no anticholinergic effects, such as haloperidol, or to another class of antiglaucoma drug, such as β-blockers, is appropriate.

PATIENT PROFILE 167

HYPERCHOLESTEROLEMIA

ANSWERS

1. (D) A 3-month trial of TLC is advised before starting drug therapy in most patients.

   Ref: Third Report of the National Cholesterol Education Program Expert Panel on Detection, Evaluation, and Treatment of High Blood Cholesterol in Adults (Adult Treatment Panel III). Final report. *Circulation* 2002;106:3143–3421.

2. (C) Based on GK's two risk factors other than elevated LDL (age and low HDL) his LDL goal is <130 mg/dL.

   Ref: Third Report of the National Cholesterol Education Program Expert Panel on Detection, Evaluation, and Treatment of High Blood Cholesterol in Adults (Adult Treatment Panel III). Final report. *Circulation* 2002;106:3143–3421.

3. (C) Non-HDL cholesterol is calculated as total cholesterol minus HDL cholesterol.

   Ref: Third Report of the National Cholesterol Education Program Expert Panel on Detection, Evaluation, and Treatment of High Blood Cholesterol in Adults (Adult Treatment Panel III). Final report. *Circulation* 2002;106:3143–3421.

4. (E) Based on GK's number of risk factors his non-HDL goal is <160 mg/dL.

   Ref: Third Report of the National Cholesterol Education Program Expert Panel on Detection, Evaluation, and Treatment of High Blood Cholesterol in Adults (Adult Treatment Panel III). Final report. *Circulation* 2002;106:3143–3421.

5. (E) Secondary causes of dyslipidemia include hypothyroidism, diabetes, chronic renal failure, obstructive liver disease, as well as drugs that increase LDL cholesterol and decrease HDL cholesterol (progestins, anabolic steroids, and corticosteroids).

   Ref: Third Report of the National Cholesterol Education Program Expert Panel on Detection, Evaluation, and Treatment of High Blood

Cholesterol in Adults (Adult Treatment Panel III). Final report. *Circulation* 2002;106:3143–3421.

6. (C) The usual starting dose of simvastatin is 20 mg once daily.

   Ref: Third Report of the National Cholesterol Education Program Expert Panel on Detection, Evaluation, and Treatment of High Blood Cholesterol in Adults (Adult Treatment Panel III). Final report. *Circulation* 2002;106:3143–3421.

7. (A) Nicotinamide only has vitamin functions and does not affect lipid and lipoprotein levels.

   Ref: Third Report of the National Cholesterol Education Program Expert Panel on Detection, Evaluation, and Treatment of High Blood Cholesterol in Adults (Adult Treatment Panel III). Final report. *Circulation* 2002;106:3143–3421.

8. (A) The usual daily dose of Niaspan® is 1 to 2 g once daily at bedtime.

   Ref: Third Report of the National Cholesterol Education Program Expert Panel on Detection, Evaluation, and Treatment of High Blood Cholesterol in Adults (Adult Treatment Panel III). Final report. *Circulation* 2002;106:3143–3421.

9. (D) Simvastatin is a substrate for cytochrome P450 3A4 and azithromycin does not inhibit the CYP3A4 system.

   Ref: Gruer PJK, Vega JM, Mercuri MF, Dobrinska MR, Tobert JA. Concomitant use of cytochrome P450 3A4 inhibitors and simvastatin. *Am J Cardiol* 1999;84:811–815.

10. (A) Statins display dose-dependent and log-linear reductions in LDL-cholesterol so that LDL falls by about 6% for each doubling of the dose of statin.

    Ref: Third Report of the National Cholesterol Education Program Expert Panel on Detection, Evaluation, and Treatment of High Blood Cholesterol in Adults (Adult Treatment Panel III). Final report. *Circulation* 2002;106:3143–3421.

PATIENT PROFILE 168

OPIATE ABUSE

ANSWERS

1. (D) IV drug users have a higher rate of HIV infection and hepatitis than the general population.

   Ref: In: Young LY, Koda-Kimble MA, eds. *Applied Therapeutics: The Clinical Use of Drugs.* 6th ed. Vancouver, Wash: Applied Therapeutics; 1995: chapter 83.

2. (C) Methadone is metabolized by means of N demethylation through CYP450 3A4.

   Ref: Moody DE, Alburges ME, Parker RJ, et al. The involvement of cytochrome P450 3A4 in the N-demethylation of L-alpha-acetylmethadol (LAAM), norLAAM, and methadone. *Drug Metab Dispos* 1997:25;1347–1353.

3. (A) Nefazodone is a potent inhibitor of CYP450 3A4. Methadone is metabolized almost exclusively through this system and would likely be inhibited by the addition of nefazodone to such an extent that clinical intervention is necessary.

Ref: Nefazodone [package insert]. Bristol-Myers Squibb Co.

Ref: Moody DE, Alburges ME, Parker RJ, et. al. The involvement of cytochrome P450 3A4 in the N-demethylation of L-alpha-acetylmethadol (LAAM), norLAAM, and methadone. Drug Metab Dispos 1997:25;1347–1353.

4. (A) To convert a patient from methadone to LAAM you multiply the daily methadone dose by 1.2 and dispense that on Monday and Wednesday. The Friday dose of LAAM is the daily methadone dose multiplied by 1.3, or 5–10 mg more than the Monday and Wednesday dose.

Ref: Ling W, Rawson RA, Compton MA. Substitution pharmacotherapies for opioid addiction: from methadone to LAAM and buprenorphine. J Psychosom Drugs 1994; 26:119–128.

5. (C) Naltrexone is an opiate receptor antagonist that blocks the euphoric effect associated with opiate abuse.

Ref: Best SE, Oliveto AH, Kosten TR. Opioid addiction: recent advances in detoxification and maintenance therapy. CNS Drugs 1996;6:301–314.

PATIENT PROFILE 169

OSTEOPOROSIS

ANSWERS

1. (D) There are many factors that increase the risk for the development of osteoporosis, including genetics (female, Caucasian or Asian ethnicity, small body frame); lifestyle (sedentary, smoking, minimal sun exposure); diet (high caffeine or phosphorus intake, low calcium intake); Ob/Gyn history (nulliparity, late menarche, early menopause); chronic illnesses (hyperthyroidism, diabetes mellitus, falls); medications (glucocorticoids, long-term heparin, anticonvulsants); and fall-related conditions (decreased visual acuity, use of walking aids, medications that cause dizziness).

Ref: O'Connell MB, Elliott ME. Osteoporosis and osteomalacia. In: DiPiro JT, Talbert RL, Yee GC, et al., eds. Pharmacotherapy: A Pathophysiologic Approach, 5th edition. New York: McGraw-Hill, 2002:1599–1621.

2. (D) The World Health Organization's definition of osteoporosis is based on t-scores, the number of standard deviations away from the mean bone mineral density for the young normal population. A t-score of <-2.5 defines osteoporosis. A t-score of -1 to -2.5 defines osteopenia.

Ref: AACE Osteoporosis Task Force. American Association of Clinical Endocrinologists medical guidelines for clinical practice for the prevention and treatment of postmenopausal osteoporosis: 2001 edition, with selected updates for 2003. Endocr Pract 2003;9:544–564.

3. (D) In individuals aged 51 to 70 years, daily calcium and vitamin D requirements are 1200 mg and 400 IU, respectively. In adults aged 19 to 50 years, 1000 mg and 200 IU, respectively, and in adults aged greater than or equal to 71 years, 1200 mg and 600 IU, respectively.

Ref: O'Connell MB, Elliott ME. Osteoporosis and osteomalacia. In: DiPiro JT, Talbert RL, Yee GC, et al., eds. Pharmacotherapy: A Pathophysiologic Approach, 5th edition. New York: McGraw-Hill, 2002:1599–1621.

4. (A) Calcium carbonate contains 40% elemental calcium, which is a greater percentage than the other calcium salts.

Ref: O'Connell MB, Elliott ME. Osteoporosis and osteomalacia. In: DiPiro JT, Talbert RL, Yee GC, et al., eds. Pharmacotherapy: A Pathophysiologic Approach, 5th edition. New York: McGraw-Hill, 2002:1599–1621.

5. (E) At calcium carbonate doses greater than 500 to 600 mg, divided doses are recommended. The fraction of calcium absorption decreases with dose.

Ref: O'Connell MB, Elliott ME. Osteoporosis and osteomalacia. In: DiPiro JT, Talbert RL, Yee GC, et al., eds. Pharmacotherapy: A Pathophysiologic Approach, 5th edition. New York: McGraw-Hill, 2002:1599–1621.

6. (B) For the treatment of osteoporosis, alendronate 10 mg po daily or 70 mg po weekly is appropriate dosing. Osteoporosis prevention doses are 5 mg po daily or 35 mg po qd.

Ref: AACE Osteoporosis Task Force. American Association of Clinical Endocrinologists medical guidelines for clinical practice for the prevention and treatment of postmenopausal osteoporosis: 2001 edition, with selected updates for 2003. Endocr Pract 2003; 9:544–564.

7. (C) Alendronate should be taken at least one-half hour before breakfast with 8 oz. of water. Administration with food would reduce the bioavailability. Individuals taking alendronate should remain upright for at least 30 minutes to reduce irritation of the esophagus.

Ref: AACE Osteoporosis Task Force. American Association of Clinical Endocrinologists medical guidelines for clinical practice for the prevention and treatment of postmenopausal osteoporosis: 2001 edition, with selected updates for 2003. *Endocr Pract* 2003; 9:544–564.

8. (D) In addition to esophagitis and hypocalcemia, contraindications of alendronate include the inability to follow administration directions and hypersensitivity to alendronate.

Ref: AACE Osteoporosis Task Force. American Association of Clinical Endocrinologists medical guidelines for clinical practice for the prevention and treatment of postmenopausal osteoporosis: 2001 edition, with selected updates for 2003. *Endocr Pract* 2003; 9:544–564.

9. (E) Abdominal pain, dyspepsia, and esophagitis are all potential adverse effects of alendronate.

Ref: AACE Osteoporosis Task Force. American Association of Clinical Endocrinologists medical guidelines for clinical practice for the prevention and treatment of postmenopausal osteoporosis: 2001 edition, with selected updates for 2003. *Endocr Pract* 2003; 9:544–564.

10. (A) Bisphosphonates, alendronate and risedronate, have been shown to decrease the incidence of hip fractures in prospective controlled trials. Calcitonin and raloxifene reduce the risk of vertebral fractures and teriparatide has been shown to decrease the risk of vertebral and nonvertebral fractures in prospective trials.

Ref: AACE Osteoporosis Task Force. American Association of Clinical Endocrinologists medical guidelines for clinical practice for the prevention and treatment of postmenopausal osteoporosis: 2001 edition, with selected updates for 2003. *Endocr Pract* 2003; 9:544–564.

PATIENT PROFILE 170
PARKINSON'S DISEASE

ANSWERS

1. (E) Immobility during a drug holiday may lead to serious psychological manifestations, DVT, aspiration pneumonia, and decubitus ulcer formation.

2. (A) Long-term use of levodopa may lead to "down-regulation" of dopamine receptors. The drug holiday may allow dopamine receptors to be resensitized and provide a beneficial effect with lower doses of levodopa.

3. (E) Ferrous sulfate forms a chelation complex with levodopa, causing a 50% decrease in levodopa absorption. To avoid this clinically significant drug interaction, the drugs should not be administered concomitantly.

4. (A) SSRIs such as fluoxetine taken concomitantly with selegiline have been reported to cause hypomania.

5. (E) Selegiline 10 mg/d usually is well tolerated and may be used in combination with levodopa or Sinemet® (carbidopa-levodopa) and has been reported to slow the progress of Parkinson's disease.

Ref: Flaherty JF, Gidal BE. Parkinson's disease. In: Young LY, Koda-Kimble MA, eds. *Applied Therapeutics: The Clinical Use of Drugs.* 6th ed. Vancouver, Wash: Applied Therapeutics; 1995: chapter 51.

Ref: Shimomura SK, Fujimoto D. Parkinsonism. In: Herfindal ET, Gourley DR, eds. *Textbook of Therapeutics. Drug and Disease Management.* 6th ed. Baltimore: Williams & Wilkins; 1996: chapter 51.

PATIENT PROFILE 171
PARKINSON'S DISEASE

ANSWERS

1. (B) Wearing off is characterized by increased symptoms toward the end of the dose of carbidopa/ levodopa. The use of the controlled release formulation enhances the drug therapy by prolonging the time of levodopa transport to the brain. Reliance on stored levodopa in the presynaptic neurons is lessened.

Ref: Nelson MV, Berchou, RC, LeWitt PA. Parkinson's disease. In: DiPiro JT, Talbert RL, Yee GC, et al., eds. *Pharmacotherapy: A Pathophysiologic Approach,* 5th edition. New York: McGraw-Hill, 2002:1089–1102.

2. (C) When switching to controlled-release carbidopa/levodopa, the dosing regimen should be decreased from qid to tid. The bioavailability of levodopa is decreased and patients may require an increase in levodopa dose.

Ref: Nelson MV, Berchou, RC, LeWitt PA. Parkinson's disease. In: DiPiro JT, Talbert RL, Yee GC, et al., eds. *Pharmacotherapy: A Pathophysiologic Approach,* 5th edition. New York: McGraw-Hill, 2002:1089–1102.

3. (A) Carbidopa is a potent inhibitor of dopa decarboxylase. It is necessary to include with levodopa to prevent the peripheral breakdown, thereby decreasing side effects such as nausea, vomiting, and orthostatic hypotension and also increasing the concentration of levodopa in the central nervous system.

Ref: Nelson MV, Berchou, RC, LeWitt PA. Parkinson's disease. In: DiPiro JT, Talbert RL, Yee GC, et al., eds. *Pharmacotherapy: A Pathophysiologic Approach,* 5th edition. New York: McGraw-Hill, 2002:1089–1102.

4. (D) A dose of immediate-acting carbidopa/levodopa taken one-half hour before arising will enable BB to rise out of bed in the morning with minimal difficulty. Taking the controlled release formation at bedtime also may help minimize early morning dystonias.

Ref: Nelson MV, Berchou, RC, LeWitt PA. Parkinson's disease. In: DiPiro JT, Talbert RL, Yee GC, et al., eds. *Pharmacotherapy: A Pathophysiologic Approach,* 5th edition. New York: McGraw-Hill, 2002:1089–1102.

5. (B) Selegiline is an MAO-B inhibitor. MAO-B is responsible for the breakdown of dopamine so selegiline can be used to augment the actions of levodopa.

Ref: Nelson MV, Berchou, RC, LeWitt PA. Parkinson's disease. In: DiPiro JT, Talbert RL, Yee GC, et al., eds. *Pharmacotherapy: A Pathophysiologic Approach,* 5th edition. New York: McGraw-Hill, 2002:1089–1102.

6. (C) The controlled release formulation of carbidopa/ levodopa should be taken with food, which increases the bioavailability by slowing down absorption. Dizziness (orthostatic systolic hypotension [OSHT]) is a common side effect of carbidopa/ levodopa.

Ref: Nelson MV, Berchou, RC, LeWitt PA. Parkinson's disease. In: DiPiro JT, Talbert RL, Yee GC, et al., eds. *Pharmacotherapy: A Pathophysiologic Approach,* 5th edition. New York: McGraw-Hill, 2002:1089–1102.

7. (A) Many antipsychotics can cause side effects such as tardive dyskinesias. These would not be preferred in Parkinson's disease patients. The atypical antipsychotics, such as quetiapine and clozapine, are preferred for Parkinson-induced psychosis because of their side-effect profile. Clozapine does require monitoring for leukopenia.

Ref: Nelson MV, Berchou, RC, LeWitt PA. Parkinson's disease. In: DiPiro JT, Talbert RL, Yee GC, et al., eds. *Pharmacotherapy: A Pathophysiologic Approach,* 5th edition. New York: McGraw-Hill, 2002:1089–1102.

8. C. Entacapone has a short half life and must be taken with each dose of carbidopa/levodopa. It cannot be used as monotherapy and its mechanism of action involves peripheral COMT inhibition.

Ref: Nelson MV, Berchou, RC, LeWitt PA. Parkinson's disease. In: DiPiro JT, Talbert RL, Yee GC, et al., eds. *Pharmacotherapy: A Pathophysiologic Approach,* 5th edition. New York: McGraw-Hill, 2002:1089–1102.

9. (B) Dopamine agonists are not a good choice for BB because of their propensity to cause psychosis. This is true in elderly patients in general.

Ref: Nelson MV, Berchou, RC, LeWitt PA. Parkinson's disease. In: DiPiro JT, Talbert RL, Yee GC, et al., eds. *Pharmacotherapy: A Pathophysiologic Approach,* 5th edition. New York: McGraw-Hill, 2002:1089–1102.

10. A. The selective serotonin reuptake inhibitors are the preferred therapy for depression in patients with Parkinson's disease. The rule is to start with a low dose and increase gradually if necessary. Other antidepressants also can be used but their side-effect profiles can become problematic, especially in elderly people.

Ref: Ernst M, Gottwald MD, Gidal BE. Parkinson's disease. In: Koda-Kimble MA, Young LY, Kradjan WA, et al., eds. *Applied Therapeutics: The Clinical Use of Drugs,* 8th edition. Philadelphia: Lippincott Williams & Wilkins, 2005:1–30.

PATIENT PROFILE 172

ARRHYTHMIAS

ANSWERS

1. (E) The patient needs an agent to provide acute ventricular rate control and cannot take a β-blocker because of a history of asthma.

Ref: Bauman JL, Schoen MD. Arrhythmias. In: DiPiro JT, Talbert RL, Yee GC, Matzke GR, Wells BG, Posey LM, eds. *Pharmacotherapy: A Pathophysiologic Approach.* 4th ed. Stamford, Conn: Appleton & Lange; 1999:232–264.

2. (D) The patient needs long-term oral antiarrhythmic therapy and cannot use sotalol because of its β-blocking properties.

Ref: Bauman JL, Schoen MD. Arrhythmias. In: DiPiro JT, Talbert RL, Yee GC, Matzke GR, Wells BG, Posey LM, eds. *Pharmacotherapy: A Pathophysiologic Approach.* 4th ed. Stamford, Conn: Appleton & Lange; 1999:232–264.

3. (C) There is no reported interaction between amiodarone and allopurinol.

Ref: Drug Interaction Facts. St. Louis: Facts and Comparisons; 1999.

4. (C) The patient is younger than 65 years and has no other risk factors for stroke.

Ref: Bauman JL, Schoen MD. Arrhythmias. In: DiPiro JT, Talbert RL, Yee GC, Matzke GR, Wells BG, Posey LM, eds. *Pharmacotherapy: A Pathophysiologic Approach.* 4th ed. Stamford, Conn: Appleton & Lange; 1999:232–264.

Ref: Drug Interaction Facts. St. Louis: Facts and Comparisons; 1999.

5. (A) The target INR range for atrial fibrillation is 2.0–3.0.

Ref: Bauman JL, Schoen MD. Arrhythmias. In: DiPiro JT, Talbert RL, Yee GC, Matzke GR, Wells BG, Posey LM, eds. *Pharmacotherapy: A Pathophysiologic Approach.* 4th ed. Stamford, Conn: Appleton & Lange; 1999:232–264.

Ref: AHFS Drug Information, 1998.

Ref: *Drug Interaction Facts.* St. Louis: Facts and Comparisons; 1999.

PATIENT   PROFILE   173

OSTEOPOROSIS

ANSWERS

1. (B) A t-score is the number of standard deviations away from the mean BMD for the young normal population. Normal bone mass is a t-score greater than –1, osteopenia is a t-score of –1 to –2.5, and a t-score of less than –2.5 is classified as osteoporosis.

Ref: O'Connell MB, Elliot ME. Osteoporosis and osteomalacia. In: Dipiro JT, Talbert RL, Yee GC, et al., eds. *Pharmacotherapy: A Pathophysiologic Approach,* 5th edition. New York: McGraw-Hill, 2002:1599–1621.

2. (A) Risk factors for the development of osteoporosis include increased age, female gender, Caucasian or Asian heritage, family history, small stature, low weight, early menopause or oophorectomy, sedentary lifestyle, decreased mobility, low calcium intake, excessive alcohol intake, and cigarette smoking.

Ref: Parent-Stevens L, Sagraves R. Gynecologic and other disorders of women. In: Koda-Kimble MA, Young LY, Kradjan WA, et al., eds. *Applied Therapeutics: The Clinical Use of Drugs,* 8th edition. Baltimore: Lippincott Williams & Wilkins, 2005:1–47.

3. (E) Drugs such as corticosteroids, anticonvulsants, excessive use of aluminum-containing antacids, long-term high-dose heparin, furosemide, and excessive levothyroxine therapy are associated with osteoporotic bone loss and osteoporosis.

Ref: Parent-Stevens L, Sagraves R. Gynecologic and other disorders of women. In: Koda-Kimble MA, Young LY, Kradjan WA, et al., eds. *Applied Therapeutics: The Clinical Use of Drugs,* 8th edition. Baltimore: Lippincott Williams & Wilkins, 2005:1–47.

4. (E) The National Institute of Health Consensus Development Panel on Optimal Calcium Intake recommends that postmenopausal women who do not receive estrogen-progestin therapy should have a daily elemental calcium intake of 1500 mg/day.

Ref: Parent-Stevens L, Sagraves R. Gynecologic and other disorders of women. In: Koda-Kimble MA, Young LY, Kradjan WA, et al., eds. *Applied Therapeutics: The Clinical Use of Drugs,* 8th edition. Baltimore: Lippincott Williams & Wilkins, 2005:1–47.

5. (A) Calcium carbonate contains the highest percentage of elemental calcium (40%).

Ref: Parent-Stevens L, Sagraves R. Gynecologic and other disorders of women. In: Koda-Kimble MA, Young LY, Kradjan WA, et al., eds. *Applied Therapeutics: The Clinical Use of Drugs,* 8th edition. Baltimore: Lippincott Williams & Wilkins, 2005:1–47.

6. (C) When taken concomitantly, calcium can decrease the absorption of many drugs and medications such as tetracyclines, fluoroquinolones, and atenolol. Calcium should be separated from these medications by at least 2 hours.

Ref: Parent-Stevens L, Sagraves R. Gynecologic and other disorders of women. In: Koda-Kimble MA, Young LY, Kradjan WA, et al., eds. *Applied Therapeutics: The Clinical Use of Drugs,* 8th edition. Baltimore: Lippincott Williams & Wilkins, 2005:1–47.

7. (A) Alendronate, a bisphosphonate, adsorb to bone apatite and are permanently incorporated into bone, inhibiting the binding of osteoclasts to bone surface.

Ref: O'Connell MB, Elliot ME. Osteoporosis and osteomalacia. In: Dipiro JT, Talbert RL, Yee GC, et al., eds. *Pharmacotherapy: A Pathophysiologic Approach,* 5th edition. New York: McGraw-Hill, 2002:1599–1621.

8. (D) Contraindications to bisphosphonate therapy include patients with significant renal insufficiency (Cr Cl < 35 mL/min), hypocalcemia, upper gastrointestinal problems such as esophageal disease (including strictures), dysphagia, duodenitis, or ulcer, and patients who cannot sit upright for 30 consecutive minutes after ingestion of the drug.

Ref: Parent-Stevens L, Sagraves R. Gynecologic and other disorders of women. In: Koda-Kimble MA, Young LY, Kradjan WA, et al., eds. *Applied Therapeutics: The Clinical Use of Drugs,* 8th edition. Baltimore: Lippincott Williams & Wilkins, 2005:1–47.

9. (A) In May 2002, the estrogen-progestin therapy (specifically patients receiving Prempro® 0.625/ 2.5 mg) arm of the Women's Health Initiative was stopped prematurely after 5.2 years because overall cardiovascular risks for individuals enrolled in the treatment group exceed the benefits and a coronary heart disease hazard ratio of 1.29 was determined.

Ref: Parent-Stevens L, Sagraves R. Gynecologic and other disorders of women. In: Koda-Kimble MA, Young LY, Kradjan WA, et al., eds. *Applied Therapeutics: The Clinical Use of Drugs,* 8th edition. Baltimore: Lippincott Williams & Wilkins, 2005:1–47.

10. (C) Thiazide diuretics increase urinary calcium reabsorption. A 10-year study of 83,728 women demonstrated fewer fractures among women taking thiazides. Prescribing thiazides solely for the treatment osteoporosis is not recommended but it is reasonable choice for patients with osteoporosis who require a diuretic.

Ref: O'Connell MB, Elliot ME. Osteoporosis and osteomalacia. In: Dipiro JT, Talbert RL, Yee GC, et al., eds. *Pharmacotherapy: A Pathophysiologic Approach,* 5th edition. New York: McGraw-Hill, 2002:1599–1621.

PATIENT PROFILE 174

THYROID DISEASE

ANSWERS

1. (D) Baseline thyroid function tests should be performed before therapy is initiated because hypothyroidism due to amiodarone therapy is not rare.

Ref: Dang BJ. Thyroid disorders. In: Young LY, Koda-Kimble MA, eds. *Applied Therapeutics: The Clinical Use of Drugs.* 6th ed. Vancouver, Wash: Applied Therapeutics; 1995: 47-1–47-31.

2. (C) Levothyroxine is hormone replacement therapy and is therefore appropriate in the management of hypothyroidism caused by amiodarone.

Ref: Dang BJ. Thyroid disorders. In: Young LY, Koda-Kimble MA, eds. *Applied Therapeutics: The Clinical Use of Drugs.* 6th ed. Vancouver, Wash: Applied Therapeutics; 1995: 47-1–47-31.

3. (C) It may take 6–8 weeks for the pituitary gland to secrete TSH at normal capacity. It is recommended that TSH be measured 6–8 weeks after levothyroxine therapy is initiated to assess response to therapy.

Ref: Dang BJ. Thyroid disorders. In: Young LY, Koda-Kimble MA, eds. *Applied Therapeutics: The Clinical Use of Drugs.* 6th ed. Vancouver, Wash: Applied Therapeutics; 1995: 47-1–47-31.

4. (E) Signs and symptoms of hypothyroidism include cold intolerance, dry skin, weight gain, constipation, and lethargy.

Ref: Dang BJ. Thyroid disorders. In: Young LY, Koda-Kimble MA, eds. *Applied Therapeutics: The Clinical Use of Drugs.* 6th ed. Vancouver, Wash: Applied Therapeutics; 1995:47-1–47-31.

PATIENT PROFILE 175

OBESITY

ANSWERS

1. (C) Body mass index is calculated by dividing a patient's weight in kilograms by height in meters squared. PJ weighs 253 pounds; this should be divided by 2.2 to calculate her weight in kilograms; the result is 115 kg. Her height is 4'11", which is equivalent to 1.499 meters; this should then be squared; the result is 2.247 m^2. The final calculation is 115 kg divided by 2.246 m^2, which equals 51.3 kg/m^2.

Ref: St. Peter JV, Khan MA. Obesity. In: DiPiro JT, Talbert RL, Yee GC, et al., eds. *Pharmacotherapy: A Pathophysiologic Approach,* 5th edition. New York: McGraw-Hill, 2002: 2543–2563.

2. (E) BMI is used as a tool to classify obesity. A BMI less than 18.5 kg/m^2 is classified as underweight. BMI 18.5 to 24.9 kg/m^2 is considered normal weight. Overweight is associated with BMI 25.0 to 29.9 kg/m^2. Obesity is defined as a BMI greater than 30 kg/m^2. Morbid or extreme obesity is defined as BMI greater than 40 kg/m^2.

Ref: Fankhauser MP, Lee KC. Eating disorders. In: Koda-Kimble MA, Young LY, Kradjan WA, et al., editors. *Applied Therapeutics: The Clinical Use of Drugs,* 8th edition. Philadelphia: Lippincott Williams & Wilkins, 2005:82.1–28.

3. (B) Sibutramine may increase blood pressure and should be avoided in patients with uncontrolled hypertension (despite treatment with lisinopril, PJ's blood pressure remains elevated at 142/88). The other statements are not true; it would not interact with her atorvastatin, nor would it be expected to increase her cholesterol.

Ref: St. Peter JV, Khan MA. Obesity. In: DiPiro JT, Talbert RL, Yee GC, et al., eds. *Pharmacotherapy: A Pathophysiologic Approach,* 5th edition. New York: McGraw-Hill, 2002: 2543–2563.

4. (B) A reasonable 6-month weight loss goal for PJ is 25 pounds; this represents 10% of her current weight. Although PJ would still be considered obese after losing 25 pounds, it should improve her obesity-related conditions.

Ref: Wood AJJ, Yanovski SZ, Yanovski JA. Obesity. *N Engl J Med* 2002;346:591–602.

5. (B) A reasonable weight loss rate is 1 to 2 pounds (0.5 to 1 kg) over 6 months. Rapid weight loss is associated with a higher rate of regain.

Ref: *The Practical Guide: Identification, Evaluation, and Treatment of Overweight and Obesity in Adults.* (NIH publication no. 00-4084). Bethesda, MD: National Heart, Lung, and Blood Institute, North American Association for the Study of Obesity, 2000.

6. (D) Orlistat reduces the absorption of fat by binding to and inhibiting gastric lipases. Orlistat has no effect on neurotransmitters; in fact, very little is actually absorbed.

Ref: St. Peter JV, Khan MA. Obesity. In: DiPiro JT, Talbert RL, Yee GC, et al., eds. *Pharmacotherapy: A Pathophysiologic Approach,* 5th edition. New York: McGraw-Hill, 2002: 2543–2563.

7. (E) The brand name of orlistat is Xenical®. Adipex-P® (phentermine), Didrex® (benzphetamine), and Fastin® (phentermine), are noradrenergic agents approved for the short-term treatment of obesity. Meridia® is a mixed noradrenergic and serotonergic agent for obesity.

Ref: Wood AJJ, Yanovski SZ, Yanovski JA. Obesity. *N Engl J Med* 2002;346:591–602.

8. (A) Common side effects of orlistat include flatulence with discharge, fecal incontinence, steatorrhea, oily spotting, and increased frequency of defecation. These symptoms typically resolve within 1 to 2 months of therapy. Orlistat impairs the absorption of fat-soluble vitamins (A, D, E, and K) and a supplement is recommended, but should not be taken at the same time as orlistat, it should be spaced at least 2 hours apart. Diet and exercise is an essential component to any weight loss program.

Ref: Fankhauser MP, Lee KC. Eating disorders. In: Koda-Kimble MA, Young LY, Kradjan WA, et al., eds. *Applied Therapeutics: The Clinical Use of Drugs,* 8th edition. Philadelphia: Lippincott Williams & Wilkins, 2005:82.1–28.

Ref: St. Peter JV, Khan MA. Obesity. In: DiPiro JT, Talbert RL, Yee GC, et al., eds. *Pharmacotherapy: A Pathophysiologic Approach,* 5th edition. New York: McGraw-Hill, 2002: 2543– 2563.

9. (E) All three statements are correct.

Ref: Fankhauser MP, Lee KC. Eating disorders. In: Koda-Kimble MA, Young LY, Kradjan WA, et al., eds. *Applied Therapeutics: The Clinical Use of Drugs,* 8th edition. Philadelphia: Lippincott Williams & Wilkins, 2005:82.82.1–28.

10. (E) All three products may produce stimulant-like effects. Citrus aurantii is a "thermogenic agent," it is reported to "burn fat" by increasing energy expenditure. Citrus aurantii contains synephrine, which has a-adrenergic activity and may increase blood pressure and heart rate. The active ingredient in guarana is caffeine; the guarana seed may contain up to 5.8% caffeine. Green tea also contains a significant amount of caffeine.

Ref: Preuss HG, DeFerdinando D, Bagchi M, et al. Citrus aurantii as a thermogenic, weight-reduction replacement for ephedra: an overview. *J Med* 2002;33:247–264.

Ref: St. Peter JV, Khan MA. Obesity. In: DiPiro JT, Talbert RL, Yee GC, et al., eds. *Pharmacotherapy: A Pathophysiologic Approach,* 5th edition. New York: McGraw-Hill, 2002: 2543–2563.

PATIENT PROFILE 176
CHRONIC OBSTRUCTIVE LUNG DISEASE

ANSWERS

1. (D) Both ciprofloxacin and erythromycin inhibit the metabolism of theophylline. This can cause toxicity if the theophylline dosage is not reduced.

    Ref: Chronic obstructive airway disease. In: Young LY, Koda-Kimble MA, eds. *Applied Therapeutics: The Clinical Use of Drugs*. 6th ed. Vancouver, Wash: Applied Therapeutics; 1995: chapter 20.

2. (E) Theophylline is a methylxanthine derivative. Side effects related to serum concentration include CNS effects ranging from sleep disturbances to seizures as well as cardiac arrhythmias.

    Ref: Chronic obstructive airway disease. In: Young LY, Koda-Kimble MA, eds. *Applied Therapeutics: The Clinical Use of Drugs*. 6th ed. Vancouver, Wash: Applied Therapeutics; 1995: chapter 20.

3. (C) Because cigarette smoke induces the hepatic metabolism of theophylline, smokers may need higher doses of theophylline to maintain therapeutic serum concentrations.

    Ref: Chronic obstructive airway disease. In: Young LY, Koda-Kimble MA, eds. *Applied Therapeutics: The Clinical Use of Drugs*. 6th ed. Vancouver, Wash: Applied Therapeutics; 1995: chapter 20.

4. (A) Because the parasympathetic nervous system is important in maintenance of airway tone among patients with COPD, the anticholinergic agent ipratropium is the drug of choice for long-term management of COPD.

    Ref: Chronic obstructive airway disease. In: Young LY, Koda-Kimble MA, eds. *Applied Therapeutics: The Clinical Use of Drugs*. 6th ed. Vancouver, Wash: Applied Therapeutics; 1995: chapter 20.

5. (B) The evidence seems to indicate that for COPD, the combination of a sympathomimetic and an anticholinergic agent provides additive effects with long-term but not short-term use. Combivent® contains the combination of ipratropium and albuterol.

    Ref: Chronic obstructive pulmonary disease. In: Herfindal ET, Gourley DR, eds. *Textbook of Therapeutics, Drug and Disease Management*. 6th ed. Baltimore: Williams & Wilkins; 1996: chapter 36.

PATIENT PROFILE 177
SMALLPOX

ANSWERS

1. (A) Category A. The CDC has determined that agents in category A are easy to disseminate, have a high rate of contagiousness, and require special public health preparedness.

    Ref: CDC. *Evaluating patients for smallpox*. www.cdc.gov/nip/smallpox, Accessed 10/26/2004.

    Ref: Weinstein R, Alibek K. *Biological and Chemical Terrorism: A Guide for Healthcare Providers and First Responders*. New York: Thieme Medical Publishers, 2003.

2. (E) B, C, and D are correct. Smallpox is caused by the orthopox viruses' variola major (30% fatality rate) or variola minor (1% fatality rate).

    Ref: CDC. *Evaluating patients for smallpox*. www.cdc.gov/nip/smallpox, Accessed 10/26/2004.

    Ref: Weinstein R, Alibek K. *Biological and Chemical Terrorism: A Guide for Healthcare Providers and First Responders*. New York: Thieme Medical Publishers, 2003.

3. (B) Lesions are superficial. The lesions for smallpox are deep and leave pitted scars, unlike the superficial lesions of chickenpox. The lesions of smallpox always appear at the same stage of development. Chickenpox appears in clusters at varying stages of development. Smallpox always begins on the face and forearms working in. Chickenpox begins in the trunk working their way outward.

    Ref: CDC. *Evaluating patients for smallpox*. www.cdc.gov/nip/smallpox, Accessed 10/26/2004.

    Ref: Weinstein R, Alibek K. *Biological and Chemical Terrorism: A Guide for Healthcare Providers and First Responders*. New York: Thieme Medical Publishers, 2003.

4. (C) 7 to 17 days. The typical incubation period is considered 7 to 17 days, with most people showing signs in 10 to 12 days.

Ref: CDC. *Evaluating patients for smallpox. www.cdc.gov/nip/smallpox*, Accessed 10/26/2004.

Ref: Weinstein R, Alibek K. *Biological and Chemical Terrorism: A Guide for Healthcare Providers and First Responders*. New York: Thieme Medical Publishers, 2003.

5. (D) All of the above. Smallpox is the most contagious disease known, needing only 5 to 10 virions to cause an infection. The virus can be spread via droplets, aerosols, and fomites (contaminated clothing).

Ref: CDC. *Evaluating patients for smallpox. www.cdc.gov/nip/smallpox*, Accessed 10/26/2004.

Ref: Weinstein R, Alibek K. *Biological and Chemical Terrorism: A Guide for Healthcare Providers and First Responders*. New York: Thieme Medical Publishers, 2003.

6. (A) True. The last naturally occurring disease occurred in 1977 in Somalia, the last case in the United States occurred in 1949. Eradication was accomplished by "ring immunizations." The WHO declared the disease eradicated and immunizations were stopped in the early 1980s worldwide.

Ref: Centers for Disease Control and Prevention, *www.cdc.gov*.

7. (D) All of the above. Smallpox vaccines have not been routinely administered in the United States for approximately 30 years. The vaccine requires knowledge of bifurcated needles. The vaccine requires multiple punctures in the deltoid area of the upper arm. The vaccine is a live virus that proliferate on the skin requiring special education to the vaccinee to prevent transmission to others.

Ref: CDC. *Evaluating patients for smallpox. www.cdc.gov/nip/smallpox*, Accessed 10/26/2004.

Ref: Weinstein R, Alibek K. *Biological and Chemical Terrorism: A Guide for Healthcare Providers and First Responders*. New York: Thieme Medical Publishers, 2003.

8. (E) All of the above. DryVax™ manufactured by Wyeth and Aventis contains polymyxin B, streptomycin sulfate, chlortetracycline HCl, and neomycin sulfate. In the event of a smallpox outbreak, those who have a contraindication, such as pregnancy, eczema, and immunosuppressive conditions, should be offered the vaccine.

Ref: CDC. Evaluating patients for smallpox. *www.cdc.gov/nip/smallpox*. Accessed 10/26/2004.

9. (B) Accidental implantation (extensive lesions). VIG is stored at the CDC and is indicated for the following conditions:
   1. Accidental implantations (extensive lesions)
   2. Eczema vaccinatum
   3. Generalized vaccine (if severe or recurrent)
   4. Progressive vaccinia

Ref: CDC. *Evaluating patients for smallpox. www.cdc.gov/nip/smallpox*, Accessed 10/26/2004.

10. (D) A and B. If a smallpox vaccine is administered within 2 to 3 days one can gain enough immunization to protect against smallpox. If administered within 4 to 5 days after exposure there is a reduction in a fatal outcome.

Ref: CDC. *Evaluating patients for smallpox. www.cdc.gov/ nip/smallpox*, Accessed 10/26/2004.

Ref: Weinstein R, Alibek K. *Biological and Chemical Terrorism: A Guide for Healthcare Providers and First Responders*. New York: Thieme Medical Publishers, 2003.

PATIENT PROFILE 178

EYE DROPS

ANSWERS

1. (B) $(0.1 \text{ g} = 100 \text{ mg}/5 \text{ mL})/(20 \text{ drops/mL}) = 1$ mg/drop

Ref: Stocklosa M, Ansel H. *Pharmaceutical Calculations*. 10th ed. Baltimore: Williams & Wilkins; 1996:61–65.

2. (B) The patient uses 8 drops per day (4 drops per dose): $5 \text{ mL} \times (20 \text{ drops/mL})/(8 \text{ drops/day}) = 12.5$ days supply.

Ref: Stocklosa M, Ansel H. *Pharmaceutical Calculations*. 10th ed. Baltimore: Williams & Wilkins; 1996:61–65.

3. (D) The sodium chloride would be used to effect isotonicity.

Ref: Stocklosa M, Ansel H. *Pharmaceutical Calculations*. 10th ed. Baltimore: Williams & Wilkins; 1996:144–147.

4. (E) If the solution were only saline, 5 mL would require 0.045 g sodium chloride. The amount of drug multiplied by the sodium chloride equivalent value gives the equivalent of drug in sodium chloride. The difference between the two would be the amount of sodium chloride needed.

Ref: Stocklosa M, Ansel H. *Pharmaceutical Calculations*. 10th ed. Baltimore: Williams & Wilkins; 1996:147–148.

5. (B) To determine the amount of boric acid needed, the amount of sodium chloride needed is divided by the sodium chloride equivalent of boric acid.

Ref: Stocklosa M, Ansel H. *Pharmaceutical Calculations*. 10th ed. Baltimore: Williams & Wilkins; 1996:147–148.

PATIENT PROFILE 179

GENERALIZED ANXIETY DISORDER

ANSWERS

1. (A) Lorazepam is metabolized by glucuronidation, which is less impacted by hepatic dysfunction than the cytochrome P450 system that the other choices require for metabolism.

   Ref: AF Schatzberg, CB Nemeroff, eds. *Essentials of Clinical Psychopharmacology*. Washington, DC: American Psychiatric Publishing, 2001.

2. (A) Although all the choices could initially worsen a person's anxiety if dosed too high, only bupropion remains anxiogenic. Nefazodone, desipramine, and fluoxetine all can treat anxiety symptoms.

   Ref: AF Schatzberg, CB Nemeroff, eds. *Essentials of Clinical Psychopharmacology*. Washington, DC: American Psychiatric Publishing, 2001.

3. (A) Nefazodone has been shown to cause hepatotoxicity in rare instances. It has a black box warning for this event.

   Ref: MICROMEDEX. Accessed 2004.

4. (A) Lorazepam can reduce anxiety within 40 minutes of ingestion. The other choices all take 4 to 8 weeks to have a significant impact on anxiety.

   Ref: AF Schatzberg, CB Nemeroff, eds. *Essentials of Clinical Psychopharmacology*. Washington, DC: American Psychiatric Publishing, 2001.

5. (B) Citalopram is metabolized via the cytochrome P450 system. Therefore, it has a longer elimination half-life in persons whose hepatic functioning is decreased.

   Ref: MICROMEDEX. Accessed 2004.

PATIENT PROFILE 180

SOFT-TISSUE INFECTION

ANSWERS

1. (B) Whenever an animal bite has occurred, one needs to consider the oropharyngeal pathogens of the animal. In general, animal bites are less severe than bites from humans, but infection by Pasteurella multocida with its delayed onset and high acuity should be considered.

   Ref: Danziger LH, Fish D. Skin and soft tissue infections. In: DiPiro JT, Talbert RL, Yee GC, Matzke GR, Wells BG, Posey LM, eds. *Pharmacotherapy: A Pathophysiologic Approach*. 4th ed. Stamford, Conn: Appleton & Lange; 1999:1685–1699.

   Ref: McCormack JP, Brown G. Traumatic skin and soft tissue infections. In: Young LY, Koda-Kimble MA, eds. *Applied Therapeutics: The Clinical Use of Drugs*. 6th ed. Vancouver, Wash: Applied Therapeutics; 1995:66-8–66-10.

   Ref: Gilbert DN, Moellering RC Jr, Sande MA, eds. *The Sanford Guide to Antimicrobial Therapy* 1998. 28th ed. Vienna, Va: Antimicrobial Therapy; 1998:36.

2. (D) Rabies and tetanus vaccinations should be considered after all animal bites, especially if the animal is not

captured. If the animal is domestic, it usually is captured, and rabies vaccination becomes unnecessary. Hepatitis treatment is not indicated in the management of animal bites.

Ref: Danziger LH, Fish D. Skin and soft tissue infections. In: DiPiro JT, Talbert RL, Yee GC, Matzke GR, Wells BG, Posey LM, eds. *Pharmacotherapy: A Pathophysiologic Approach*. 4th ed. Stamford, Conn: Appleton & Lange; 1999:1685–1699.

Ref: McCormack JP, Brown G. Traumatic skin and soft tissue infections. In: Young LY, Koda-Kimble MA, eds. *Applied Therapeutics: The Clinical Use of Drugs*. 6th ed. Vancouver, Wash: Applied Therapeutics; 1995:66-8–66-10.

Ref: Gilbert DN, Moellering RC Jr, Sande MA, eds. *The Sanford Guide to Antimicrobial, Therapy* 1998. 28th ed. Vienna, Va: Antimicrobial Therapy; 1998:36.

3. (C) A mild infection from a dog bite can be easily managed with amoxicillin–clavulanate (Augmentin®). This agent covers most gram-positive organisms, yet has a limited gram-negative spectrum and good anaerobic

coverage. This broad spectrum is needed to cover organisms that live on the skin and may have been introduced with the bite. It also covers organisms present in the dog's mouth and between its teeth that may have infectious potential.

Ref: Danziger LH, Fish D. Skin and soft tissue infections. In: DiPiro JT, Talbert RL, Yee GC, Matzke GR, Wells BG, Posey LM, eds. *Pharmacotherapy: A Pathophysiologic Approach.* 4th ed. Stamford, Conn: Appleton & Lange; 1999:1685–1699.

Ref: McCormack JP, Brown G. Traumatic skin and soft tissue infections. In: Young LY, Koda-Kimble MA, eds. *Applied Therapeutics: The Clinical Use of Drugs.* 6th ed. Vancouver, Wash: Applied Therapeutics; 1995:66-8–66-10.

Ref: Gilbert DN, Moellering RC Jr, Sande MA, eds. *The Sanford Guide to Antimicrobial Therapy 1998.* 28th ed. Vienna, Va: Antimicrobial Therapy; 1998:36.

4. (A) Patients who are unable to tolerate β-lactam therapy still need antimicrobial therapy similar to that provided by amoxicillin-clavulanate. Combining clindamycin and levofloxacin provides a similar spectrum of coverage. Clindamycin covers gram-positive organisms and anaerobic organisms including Bacteroides fragilis. Levofloxacin adds additional gram-positive coverage, but its focus is on the gram-negative spectrum. This regimen is not as convenient to take; the twice daily Augmentin® regimen may lead to adherence difficulties.

Ref: Danziger LH, Fish D. Skin and soft tissue infections. In: DiPiro JT, Talbert RL, Yee GC, Matzke GR, Wells BG, Posey LM, eds. *Pharmacotherapy: A Pathophysiologic Approach.* 4th ed. Stamford, Conn: Appleton & Lange; 1999:1685–1699.

Ref: McCormack JP, Brown G. Traumatic skin and soft tissue infections. In: Young LY, Koda-Kimble MA, eds. *Applied Therapeutics: The Clinical Use of Drugs.* 6th ed. Vancouver, Wash: Applied Therapeutics; 1995:66-8–66-10.

Ref: Gilbert DN, Moellering RC Jr, Sande MA, eds. *The Sanford Guide to Antimicrobial Therapy 1998.* 28th ed. Vienna, Va: Antimicrobial Therapy; 1998:36.

5. (E) The key is prophylaxis. Three days has not been shown to be long enough because of the incubation period of the infection. Treatment duration greater than 5 days increases the risk of an antibiotic-related adverse reaction.

Ref: Danziger LH, Fish D. Skin and soft tissue infections. In: DiPiro JT, Talbert RL, Yee GC, Matzke GR, Wells BG, Posey LM, eds. *Pharmacotherapy: A Pathophysiologic Approach.* 4th ed. Stamford, Conn: Appleton & Lange; 1999:1685–1699.

Ref: McCormack JP, Brown G. Traumatic skin and soft tissue infections. In: Young LY, Koda-Kimble MA, eds. *Applied Therapeutics: The Clinical Use of Drugs.* 6th ed. Vancouver, Wash: Applied Therapeutics; 1995:66-8–66-10.

Ref: Gilbert DN, Moellering RC Jr, Sande MA, eds. *The Sanford Guide to Antimicrobial Therapy 1998.* 28th ed. Vienna, Va: Antimicrobial Therapy; 1998:36.

PATIENT PROFILE 181

DIABETES

ANSWERS

1. (D) Strong data exist to suggest that ACEIs, ARBs, thiazide diuretics, and β-blockers are superior to placebo for the management of hypertension. Patients with diabetes require at least two agents and most require three or more agents to achieve BP goals. The American Diabetes Associates recommends all patients with diabetes achieve a minimum blood pressure goal of ≤130/80 mm Hg in the absence of nephropathy and optimal pressures should be ≤120/70 mm Hg. The pharmacist can help prevent microvascular and macrovascular complications stemming from hypertension in patients with diabetes through aggressive monitoring, education, and making therapeutic recommendations when appropriate. SN has diabetes and hypertension, which require attention to potential metabolic consequences from new antihypertensive therapy. Thiazide diuretics are not benign in regard to the metabolic profile. Thiazides can exacerbate hyperglycemia and contribute to insulin resistance and the metabolic syndrome as well as increase serum lipids,

uric acid, and homocysteine. Atenolol also is associated with exacerbating hyperglycemia, weight gain, and insulin resistance, especially at higher doses. Felodipine, a dihydropyridine calcium-channel blocker, may be appropriate adjunctive therapy but an ACEI, ARB, or β-blocker would be considered first. Enalapril is an ACEI requiring bid dosing for optimal blood pressure control; this frequently results in skipped doses and patient nonadherence. Ramipril is a long-acting ACEI that reduces the progression to proteinuria in diabetes and more importantly reduces the occurrence of death, myocardial infarction, or stroke in patients with diabetes.

Ref: American Diabetes Association. Hypertension management in adults with diabetes. *Diabetes Care* 2004;27:S65–67.

2. (C) Short-term sulfonylurea therapy decreases microvascular complications, reduces HbA1c by 1% to 2%, and fasting plasma glucose by 60 to 70 mg/dL. However, longer-term sulfonylurea use is associated with hyperinsulinemia, hypoglycemia, weight gain (typically, 2 to

5 kg), and worsening insulin resistance. Additionally, most patients receiving sulfonylurea therapy require a second and third agent for glycemic control because of ß-islet cell exhaustion. It is unclear if the ß-islet exhaustion results from the underlying progression of diabetes or it may be accelerated by sulfonylureas. In all likelihood, the reason most patients need three oral hypoglycemics for glucose control may be partially explained by both of these reasons. Repaglinide is a nonsulfonylurea secretagogue that should not be used for monotherapy because it requires complex TID dosing before each meal and is associated with hypoglycemia taken without a meal, weight gain, hyperinsulinemia, and long-term reductions in diabetes complications have not been documented. α-Glucosidase inhibitors are associated with 0.6% to 1.3% reduction in HbA1c and have the greatest effect on postprandial hyperglycemia and reduction in postprandial hyperglycemia is associated with reductions in cardiovascular mortality. However, α-glucosidase inhibitors require TID dosing, produce much flatulence, diarrhea, and abdominal discomfort leading to a high rate of discontinuation. Thiazolidinediones increase insulin sensitivity, lower HbA1c, and fasting glucose. However, thiazolidinediones are associated with increased plasma volume expansion, fluid retention, edema, and weight gain (2 to 3 kg per 1% reduction in HbA1c) and expansion of subcutaneous fat tissue stores. Metformin remains the best choice for SN because he has no contraindications, has extensive documentation for the UKPDS establishing decrease of microvascular risk, macrovascular risk along with weight loss or weight maintenance, reduction of hyperinsulinemia, and improvement of metabolic syndrome. Additionally, metformin is inexpensive, comes in an XL dosage form, and is approved for use for monotherapy and in combination with sulfonylureas or thiazolidinediones.

Ref: Inzucchi SE. Oral antihyperglycemic therapy for type 2 diabetes: scientific review. *JAMA* 2002;287:360–372.

3. (A) Moderate-intensity HMG-CoA reductase inhibitor therapy (statins) is the recommended starting point for managing hypercholesterolemia in patients with type 2 diabetes. Moderate-intensity therapy with statin should reduce LDL-C by approximately 40%; thus, select doses that can achieve at minimum of 40% reduction of LDL-C to start in patients with type 2 diabetes. Atorvastatin 40 mg qd is the best choice because it can reduce LDL-C up to 51% and should reduce SN's LDL-C to approximately 85 mg/dL and further with diet and exercise. Lovastatin 40 mg can reduce his LDL-C by 31%, pravastatin 40 mg can reduce his LDL-C by 35%, and fluvastatin 40 mg can reduce his LDL-C by 25%. Rosuvastatin 40 mg is considered high-intensity therapy and is best reserved for patients who fail to achieve LDL-C goals with moderate intensity therapy.

Ref: Vijan S, Hayward RA. Pharmacologic lipid-lowering therapy in type 2 diabetes mellitus: background paper for the American College of Physicians. *Ann Intern Med* 2004;140:650–658.

4. (B) Patients with diabetes and hypertension require at least two drugs and most require three or more drugs to achieve optimal control. SN will eventually need two+ agents, but every effort should be made to maximize the doses of ACEI therapy before adding new agents. The most reasonable option is to double his ramipril dose from 5 to 10 mg and follow-up within 2 weeks to assess his blood pressure. If this is not tolerated, then other agents should be explored. At this time there is no compelling reason to discontinue his current therapy and switch to an ARB or dihydropyridine CCB.

Ref: Chobanian AV, Bakris GL, Black HR, et al. Seventh report of the joint national committee on prevention, detection, evaluation and treatment of high blood pressure. *Hypertension* 2003;42: 1206–1252.

5. (F) Cough is reported in up to 20% of patients who receive ACEI therapy. However, cough is not entirely predictable with each ACEI, and patients who can gain the most benefit from ACEIs (patients with DM, CAD) should be advised to try at least two and optimally three different ACEIs before abandoning this class because of cough. Patients who are unwilling to try another ACEI should be switched at this time.

Ref: Chobanian AV, Bakris GL, Black HR, et al. Seventh report of the joint national committee on prevention, detection, evaluation and treatment of high blood pressure. *Hypertension* 2003;42: 1206–1252.

6. (A) Maximizing metformin therapy is the most appropriate option for SN because he has been receiving therapy for a relatively short period (<1 year). The optimal dose of metformin is 2 g/day. Doses of metformin >2 g provide little additional benefit in HbA1c reduction (≤0.5%), and it can take 3 months before the effect of metformin is maximized. SN will likely need additional oral agents within 3 years (50% achieve control within first 3 years).

Ref: Inzucchi SE. Oral antihyperglycemic therapy for type 2 diabetes: scientific review. *JAMA* 2002;287:360–372.

7. (E) Serum creatinine ≥1.5 mg/dL (or ≥1.4 mg/dL in women), hepatic dysfunction, metabolic acidosis, dehydration, congestive heart failure, and alcoholism are contraindications to metformin therapy.

Ref: Inzucchi SE. Oral antihyperglycemic therapy for type 2 diabetes: scientific review. *JAMA* 2002;287:360–372.

8. (E) SN has diabetes that is not under adequate control, hypertension, and features consistent with the metabolic syndrome. These characterize SN as "high risk"

for developing coronary disease in the future. New updates to the ATP III issued in 2004 summarize and provide new evidence that LDL-C levels ≤70 mg/dL are the ideal therapeutic target in patients with diabetes.

Ref: Grundy SM, Cleeman JI, Merz CNB, et al. Implications of recent clinical trials for the National Cholesterol Education Program Adult Treatment Panel III Guidelines. *Circulation* 2004;110: 227–239.

9. (C) SN needs a 10% reduction in his LDL-C to meet the new ATP III LDL-C target for patients with diabetes. Also, he needs a 50% reduction of his triglycerides, which is the secondary target when HDL-C is >40 mg/dL. Gemfibrozil can decrease LDL-C by 10% and decrease triglycerides by 35%. The combination of gemfibrozil and atorvastatin may increase the likelihood of new myalgia, arthralgia, or muscle enzymes and liver function test elevations. Thus, it is warranted to check LFTs and CPK initially and periodically when starting a statin-gemfibrozil combination. Doubling the dose of atorvastatin may not be the best choice because it will not reduce triglycerides to goal and is associated with a greater likelihood of myalgia and LFT changes. Reducing the dose is not warranted unless SN begins experiencing troublesome adverse effects and would compromise LDL-C control, which is important for diabetic patients with hypercholesterolemia.

Ref: Grundy SM, Cleeman JI, Merz CNB, et al. Implications of recent clinical trials for the National Cholesterol Education Program Adult Treatment Panel III Guidelines. *Circulation* 2004; 110:227–239.

10. (B) Substantial evidence suggests that antiplatelet therapy with aspirin should be a primary prevention strategy for men and women with diabetes who are at high risk of cardiovascular events. Despite proven efficacy, aspirin therapy is often overlooked or underused. Current estimates suggest that less than one-half of all patients who could benefit from aspirin therapy receive it. ADA guidelines recommend low-dose aspirin (81 to 162 mg of aspirin) therapy daily as a primary prevention strategy in all patients with diabetes without a contraindication to aspirin (aspirin hypersensitivity, active bleeding, concurrent anticoagulant therapy, recent gastrointestinal bleeding, and clinically active hepatic disease). Low-dose aspirin is equally as effective as full-strength aspirin (325 mg) and is associated with less risk of bleeding; thus, it should be the first choice in antiplatelet therapy. Clopidogrel was marginally more effective than aspirin for the reduction of stroke, myocardial infarction, or vascular death among patients with diabetes and peripheral artery disease (PAD) in the CAPRIE study. However, clopidogrel should remain second-line therapy for patients who are unable to tolerate aspirin therapy.

Ref: American Diabetes Association. Hypertension management in adults with diabetes. *Diabetes Care* 2004; 27:S65–67.

PATIENT PROFILE 182

OSTEOPOROSIS

ANSWERS

1. (C) Alendronate should be taken first thing in the morning with a full glass of plain water and at least 30 minutes before the first food or beverage of the day.

Ref: De Groen PC, Lubbe DF, Hirsch LJ, et al. Esophagitis associated with the use of alendronate. *N Engl J Med* 1996;335: 1016–1021.

2. (A) Alendronate should be taken first thing in the morning, and the patient should remain in the upright position for at least 30 minutes after swallowing the tablet.

Ref: De Groen PC, Lubbe DF, Hirsch LJ, et al. Esophagitis associated with the use of alendronate. *N Engl J Med* 1996; 335:1016–1021.

3. (D) Alendronate is not recommended for use by patients with ulcer disease or severe renal insufficiency.

Ref: Alendronate (Fosamax®) [product information]. Merck Laboratories.

4. (B) Raloxifene is a selective estrogen receptor modulator (SERM) that can be administered with our without food and at any time of the day. This agent, which is currently FDA approved for the prevention of osteoporosis among postmenopausal women, can cause hot flashes.

Ref: O'Connell MB. Osteoporosis and osteomalacia. In: DiPiro JT, Talbert RL, Yee GC, Matzke GR, Wells BG, Posey LM, eds. *Pharmacotherapy: A Pathophysiologic Approach.* 4th ed. Stamford, Conn: Appleton & Lange; 1999:1406–1426.

5. (B) Raloxifene is pregnancy category X.

Ref: Raloxifene (Evista®) [product information]. Lilly.

HUMAN IMMUNODEFICIENCY VIRUS

ANSWERS

1. (D) Because of this patient's sulfonamide allergy, Bactrim (trimethoprim/sulfamethoxazole) should not be administered unless the patient undergoes sulfonamide desensitization. However, desensitization takes time and this patient likely needs antibiotic therapy now because of the severity of his illness. Atovaquone can be used for milder cases of PCP. Dapsone has activity against PCP but is typically combined with TMP to treat acute episodes of PCP (especially if severe disease). Pentamidine IV is considered appropriate for severe PCP (pO_2 <70 mm Hg or A-a gradient >35 mm Hg).

Ref: Goldschmidt RH, Dong B. Treatment of AIDS and HIV-related conditions: 2001. *J Am Board Fam Pract* 2001;14:283-309.

2. (C) Patients with severe respiratory decompensation caused by PCP (pO_2 <70 mm Hg or A-a gradient >35 mmg Hg) also should receive corticosteroids to attenuate the vigorous inflammatory response that occurs in the lung with PCP. When used in this setting, corticosteroids decrease mortality, respiratory failure, and further deterioration in oxygenation. A 21-day tapering regimen of prednisone is recommended. Equivalent doses of methylprednisone may be used for patients who require intravenous therapy.

Ref: Consensus statement on the use of corticosteroids as adjunctive therapy for *Pneumocystis* pneumonia in the acquired immunodeficiency syndrome. *N Engl J Med* 1990;323:1500–1504.

3. (C) Dapsone therapy can cause a dose-related hemolytic anemia and methemoglobinemia. These adverse effects are observed in patients with or without glucose-6-phosphate dehydrogenase (G-6-PD) deficiency. However, they tend to be most severe in patients with G-6-PD deficiency.

Ref: McEnvoy GK, ed. *AHFS Drug Information*. Bethesda, MD: American Society of Health-System Pharmacists, 2004.

4. (B) This patient should receive both *Pneumocystis* (secondary prophylaxis) and toxoplasmosis prophylaxis (antibody-positive patient, CD4 count <100 cells/mm³). Aerosolized pentamidine provides protection against *Pneumocystis* but not toxoplasmosis. TMP-SMX provides protection against these pathogens but should not be used unless the patient is desensitized to sulfonamides. Although atovaquone is an option, it should only be used for toxoplasmosis prevention when first-line options (e.g., option B) cannot be used.

Ref: Centers for Disease Control and Prevention. Guidelines for preventing opportunistic infections among HIV-infected persons—2002 recommendations of the U.S. Public Health Service and the Infectious Diseases Society of America. *MMWR Morbid Mortal Wkly Rep* 2002;51(RR-8):1–46.

5. (A) This patient may be a candidate for MAC primary prophylaxis because his last measured CD4 count was <50 cells/mm³. Options A, B, and C can be used to provide MAC prophylaxis. However, clarithromycin and rifabutin may interact with protease inhibitors such as ritonavir. Although the significance of the interaction with clarithromycin is not clear, the rifabutin interaction would require a reduction in the rifabutin dose to 150 mg three times per week.

Ref: Centers for Disease Control and Prevention. Guidelines for preventing opportunistic infections among HIV-infected persons—2002 recommendations of the U.S. Public Health Service and the Infectious Diseases Society of America. *MMWR Morbid Mortal Wkly Rep* 2002;51(RR-8):1–46.

6. (A) Each of these pieces of information can help determine whether and what type of CMV prophylaxis should be started. Patients at greatest risk of CMV retinitis are those who are CMV-seropositive and have a CD4 cell count <50 cells/mm³. Although primary prophylaxis is not routinely indicated because of cost and toxicity, some clinicians may elect to initiate CMV prophylaxis for such patients. Patients with a history of CMV retinitis should be continued on chronic maintenance to prevent recurrence. Because the agents used to prevent CMV retinitis can cause significant adverse effects, the risk for experiencing these drug-related toxicities also must be considered.

Ref: Centers for Disease Control and Prevention. Guidelines for preventing opportunistic infections among HIV-infected persons—2002 recommendations of the U.S. Public Health Service and the Infectious Diseases Society of America. *MMWR Morbid Mortal Wkly Rep* 2002;51(RR-8):1–46.

7. (A) Stavudine (d4T) therapy is associated with the development of peripheral neuropathy. Patients may complain of numbness, tingling, or pain in the distal extremities. Stavudine-related peripheral neuropathy appears to be dose related. It is reported most often in patients with advanced HIV, patients with a history of peripheral neuropathy, and those who are receiving concomitant therapy with other neurotoxic drugs (i.e., ddC or ddI). Symptoms typically resolve with drug discontinuation.

Ref: McEnvoy GK, ed. *AHFS Drug Information*. Bethesda, MD: American Society of Health-System Pharmacists, 2004.

8. (D) Ritonavir is a potent inhibitor of the CYP 3A4 hepatic enzymes. Because lopinavir is a substrate of these enzymes, coadministration causes the serum levels of lopinavir to be increased. Lopinavir/ritonavir 400 mg/100 mg twice daily provides steady-state lopinavir plasma concentrations 15- to 20-fold higher than those of ritonavir. The antiviral activity of this product results from its lopinavir content.

   Ref: Corbett AH, Lim ML, Kashuba ADM. Kaletra (lopinavir/ritonavir). *Ann Pharmacother* 2002;36:1193–1203.

9. (C) Ritonavir is a potent inhibitor of the CYP 3A4 hepatic enzymes. Lovastatin, simvastatin, and atorvastatin are substrates of these enzymes. Coadministration may increase the concentration of these HMG-CoA enzyme inhibitors and place patients at risk for rhabdomyolysis. The majority of pravastatin metabolism is not dependent on CYP hepatic enzymes. Interaction studies with ritonavir show that pravastatin concentrations actually may decrease. Subsequently, patients may need higher doses to achieve cholesterol targets.

   Ref: Dube MP, Stein JH, Aberg JA, et al. Guidelines for the evaluation and management of dyslipidemia in human immunodeficiency virus (HIV)-infected adults receiving antiretroviral therapy: recommendations of the HIV Medicine Association of the Infectious Disease Society of America and the Adult AIDS Clinical Trials Group. *Clin Infect Dis* 2003;37:613–617.

10. (C) Enfuvirtide is a fusion inhibitor. It targets a portion of gp41, a viral envelope protein that changes its conformation to bring the viral and CD4+ cell membranes close together for fusion of the cell and virion. Options A, B, and D describe the mechanism of action for nucleoside-reverse transcriptase inhibitors, nonnucleoside reverse transcriptase inhibitors, and protease inhibitors, respectively.

   Ref: Duffalo ML, James CW. Enfuvirtide: a novel agent for the treatment of HIV-1 infection. *Ann Pharmacother* 2003;37: 1448–1456.

PATIENT PROFILE 184

ONCOLOGY: PAIN CONTROL

ANSWERS

1. (B) Pain of long duration with no discernible end point would be classified as chronic.

   Ref: In: Young LY, Koda-Kimble MA, eds. *Applied Therapeutics: The Clinical Use of Drugs*. 6th ed. Vancouver, Wash: Applied Therapeutics; 1995: chapter 7.

2. (B) LB can take oral agents and has reasonable control of pain with oxycodone. Changing the oxycodone to a longer acting dosage form and adding a NSAID for bone-specific pain should provide better pain control and longer intervals without medication.

   Ref: In: Young LY, Koda-Kimble MA, eds. *Applied Therapeutics: The Clinical Use of Drugs*. 6th ed. Vancouver, Wash: Applied Therapeutics; 1995: chapter 7.

   Ref: In: Herfindal ET, Gourley DR, eds. *Textbook of Therapeutics. Drug and Disease Management*. 6th ed. Baltimore: Williams & Wilkins; 1996: chapter 52.

3. (C) The use of a stimulant laxative should prevent constipation.

   Ref: In: Young LY, Koda-Kimble MA, eds. *Applied Therapeutics: The Clinical Use of Drugs*. 6th ed. Vancouver, Wash: Applied Therapeutics; 1995: chapter 7.

   Ref: In: Herfindal ET, Gourley DR, eds. *Textbook of Therapeutics. Drug and Disease Management*. 6th ed. Baltimore: Williams & Wilkins; 1996: chapter 52.

4. (D) The effective use of tricyclic antidepressants has been documented in the management of neuropathic pain.

   Ref: In: Young LY, Koda-Kimble MA, eds. *Applied Therapeutics: The Clinical Use of Drugs*. 6th ed. Vancouver, Wash: Applied Therapeutics; 1995: chapter 7.

   Ref: In: Herfindal ET, Gourley DR, eds. *Textbook of Therapeutics. Drug and Disease Management*. 6th ed. Baltimore: Williams & Wilkins; 1996: chapter 52.

5. (C) LB will become tolerant to previously effective doses of opiates as the pain increases.

   Ref: In: Young LY, Koda-Kimble MA, eds. *Applied Therapeutics: The Clinical Use of Drugs*. 6th ed. Vancouver, Wash: Applied Therapeutics; 1995: chapter 7.

PATIENT PROFILE 185

ACUTE OTITIS MEDIA

ANSWERS

1. (B) *S. pneumoniae, H. influenzae,* and *M. catarrhalis* are the three organisms that most commonly cause acute otitis media.

   Ref: Richer M, Deschenes M. Upper respiratory tract infections. In: DiPiro JT, Talbert RL, Yee GC, eds. *Pharmacotherapy: A Pathophysiologic Approach,* 5th ed. New York: McGraw-Hill, 2002:1870.

2. (D) Risk factors for the presence of a bacterial species resistant to amoxicillin include attendance at day care, recent receipt (<30 days) of antibacterial treatment, and age younger than 2 years.

   Ref: American Academy of Pediatrics and American Academy of Family Physicians. Clinical Practice Guideline: Diagnosis and Management of Acute Otitis Media. *Pediatrics* 2004;113(5): 1457.

3. (B) High-dose amoxicillin–lavulanic acid. JS has risk factors for potential resistance to amoxicillin (age younger than 2 and attendance in day care). Clindamycin will only cover *S. pneumoniae* (not *H. influenzae* and *M. catarrhalis*). Azithromycin should be reserved for patients with severe penicillin allergies. Recent pneumococcal surveillance studies indicate that resistance to trimethoprim-sulfamethoxazole is substantial.

   Ref: American Academy of Pediatrics and American Academy of Family Physicians. Clinical Practice Guideline: Diagnosis and Management of Acute Otitis Media. *Pediatrics* 2004;113(5): 1457–1458.

4. (C) A single dose of ceftriaxone (50 mg/kg IM) has been shown to be effective for the initial treatment of AOM.

   Ref: American Academy of Pediatrics and American Academy of Family Physicians. Clinical Practice Guideline: Diagnosis and Management of Acute Otitis Media. *Pediatrics* 2004;113(5): 1458.

5. (D) Meningitis is an infrequent intracranial complication of AOM.

   Ref: Richer M, Deschenes M. Upper respiratory tract infections. In: DiPiro JT, Talbert RL, Yee GC, eds. *Pharmacotherapy: A Pathophysiologic Approach,* 5th ed. New York: McGraw-Hill, 2002:1870.

6. (E) Adding clavulanic acid (a β-lactamase inhibitor) to amoxicillin increases the spectrum of activity.

   Ref: Amoxicillin–clavulanic acid. In: *American Hospital Formulary Service Drug Information.* Washington: ASHP, 2001:383.

7. (A) The eustachian tube lies at a 45° angle to the horizontal plane in adults and at a 10° angle in infants. The difference in angulation may cause improper drainage of the middle ear in infants.

   Ref: Richer M, Deschenes M. Upper respiratory tract infections. In: DiPiro JT, Talbert RL, Yee GC, eds. *Pharmacotherapy: A Pathophysiologic Approach,* 5th ed. New York: McGraw-Hill, 2002:1870.

8. (D) Supportive therapy with analgesics and antipyretics is beneficial in the comfort of the child. Antihistamines and decongestants are not efficacious in resolution of the effusion or relief of the symptoms in AOM.

   Ref: Richer M, Deschenes M. Upper respiratory tract infections. In: DiPiro JT, Talbert RL, Yee GC, eds. *Pharmacotherapy: A Pathophysiologic Approach,* 5th ed. New York: McGraw-Hill, 2002:1871.

9. (E) Children younger than 1 year of age should not be given nonprescription cold medicines except under the direction of a primary care provider.

   Ref: Tietze KJ. Disorders related to cold and allergy. In: *Handbook of Nonprescription Drugs,* 14th ed. Washington: American Pharmacists Association, 2004:248.

10. (D) A 10-day course of antibiotics is recommended for younger children and for children with severe disease. For children 6 years of age and older with mild to moderate disease, a 5- to 7-day course is appropriate.

    Ref: American Academy of Pediatrics and American Academy of Family Physicians. Clinical Practice Guideline: Diagnosis and Management of Acute Otitis Media. *Pediatrics* 2004;113(5): 1458.

PATIENT PROFILE 186

MEDICINAL CHEMISTRY

ANSWER

1. (B) C is incorrect because clonidine has a very basic sites for hydrochloride salt formation. **D** is incorrect because clonidine is a direct α_2 agonist that acts centrally by inhibiting so-called sympathetic outflow (responsible for increasing the blood pressure). If given by injection, clonidine may cause sudden vasoconstriction through the peripheral α_2 receptors.

PATIENT PROFILE 187
IRRITABLE BOWEL SYNDROME

ANSWERS

1. (D) The Rome II criteria for the diagnosis of IBS include the presence of symptoms for more than 3 months, abdominal pain, pain associated with a change in stool frequency, and pain associated with a change in stool appearance.

   Ref: Wall GC. Lower gastrointestinal disorders. In: Young YL, Koda-Kimble MA, eds. *Applied Therapeutics: The Clinical Use of Drugs.* Vancouver, WA: Applied Therapeutics, 2005:28-17–28-21.

2. (C) The gastrointestinal (GI) tract contains more than 95 percent of the body's serotonin.

   Ref: Wall GC. Lower gastrointestinal disorders. In: Young YL, Koda-Kimble MA, eds. *Applied Therapeutics: The Clinical Use of Drugs.* Vancouver, WA: Applied Therapeutics, 2005:28-17–28-21.

3. (D) IBS is prevalent in patients with psychiatric conditions, particularly depression and generalized anxiety. A family history of colon cancer may warrant a more extensive GI workup. Eating habits can contribute to IBS symptoms.

   Ref: Wall GC. Lower gastrointestinal disorders. In: Young YL, Koda-Kimble MA, eds. *Applied Therapeutics: The Clinical Use of Drugs.* Vancouver, WA: Applied Therapeutics, 2005: 28-17–28-21.

4. (C) According to the guidelines for the management of constipation-predominant IBS, gradually increasing dietary fiber intake to 20 mg/day is appropriate first-line therapy. Patients also should complete a food diary to determine if there are food intolerances that can be identified. Antimotility agents such as loperamide can worsen DK's clinical condition. Lactulose therapy should be used if the patient is unable to achieve relief with the increase in dietary fiber. Alosetron is used only for diarrhea-predominant IBS.

   Ref: Wall GC. Lower gastrointestinal disorders. In: Young YL, Koda-Kimble MA, eds. *Applied Therapeutics: The Clinical Use of Drugs.* Vancouver, WA: Applied Therapeutics, 2005: 28-17–28-21.

5. (D) Gradual increases in fiber intake can increase patient tolerance.

   Ref: Wall GC. Lower gastrointestinal disorders. In: Young YL, Koda-Kimble MA, eds. *Applied Therapeutics: The Clinical Use of Drugs.* Vancouver, WA: Applied Therapeutics, 2005: 28-17–28-21.

6. (D) DK may be experiencing increasing abdominal pain from her fiber intake. It is reasonable to recommend the use of laxatives such as lactulose, milk of magnesia, or polyethylene glycol.

   Ref: Wall GC. Lower gastrointestinal disorders. In: Young YL, Koda-Kimble MA, eds. *Applied Therapeutics: The Clinical Use of Drugs.* Vancouver, WA: Applied Therapeutics, 2005: 28-17–28-21.

7. (B) Osmotic laxatives, such as lactulose, can cause hypernatremia and hypokalemia. Other more common side effects include bloating, cramping, epigastric pain, and flatulence.

   Ref: Wall GC. Lower gastrointestinal disorders. In: Young YL, Koda-Kimble MA, eds. *Applied Therapeutics: The Clinical Use of Drugs.* Vancouver, WA: Applied Therapeutics, 2005:28-17–28-21.

8. (C) Laxative abuse is a serious limitation to long-term use. Patients who do become dependent on laxatives can develop severe conditions such as dehydration, electrolyte abnormalities, and bowel ulceration.

   Ref: Wall GC. Lower gastrointestinal disorders. In: Young YL, Koda-Kimble MA, eds. *Applied Therapeutics: The Clinical Use of Drugs.* Vancouver, WA: Applied Therapeutics, 2005:28-17–28-21.

9. (A) Tegaserod is considered a third-line treatment option in patients who are refractory to standard therapy. Clinical trials evaluating tegaserod report modest improvements in abdominal pain and bloating. Tegaserod is not approved for use in men.

   Ref: Wall GC. Lower gastrointestinal disorders. In: Young YL, Koda-Kimble MA, eds. *Applied Therapeutics: The Clinical Use of Drugs.* Vancouver, WA: Applied Therapeutics, 2005:28-17–28-21.

10. (D) Morphine is not a reasonable option because of the high incidence of constipation associated with opioid use. Hyoscyamine and amitriptyline both have demonstrated efficacy in patients with pain-predominant IBS; however, their anticholinergic properties could exacerbate DK's constipation.

    Ref: Wall GC. Lower gastrointestinal disorders. In: Young YL, Koda-Kimble MA, eds. *Applied Therapeutics: The Clinical Use of Drugs.* Vancouver, WA: Applied Therapeutics, 2005:28-17–28-21.

P A T I E N T   P R O F I L E   1 8 8

ALCOHOL ABUSE

ANSWERS

1. (A) Acute alcohol ingestion usually results in transient increases in AST, ALT, and alkaline phosphatase levels.

   Ref: *Basic Skills in Interpreting Lab Data*. 2nd ed. Bethesda, Md: American Society of Health-Systems Pharmacists; 1996: chapter 11.

2. (A) By mimicking the effect of alcohol on the GABA receptor, benzodiazepines can lessen alcohol withdrawal symptoms.

   Ref: Saitz R, O'Malley SS. Pharmacotherapies for alcohol abuse: withdrawal and treatment. *Med Clin North Am* 1997;4: 881–907.

3. (C) The tachycardia that occurs with alcohol withdrawal is caused by an increase in sympathetic stimulation. Because β_1 receptors in the heart respond to sympathetic stimulation by increasing heart rate, any medication that blocks β_1 stimulation will help to prevent tachycardia.

   Ref: Saitz R, O'Malley SS. Pharmacotherapies for alcohol abuse: withdrawal and treatment. *Med Clin North Am* 1997;4: 881–907.

4. (A) There are four stages of alcohol withdrawal. Stage 1 is autonomic hyper-activity. Stage 2 is auditory and visual hallucinations. Stage 3 is grand mal seizures. Stage 4 is delirium tremens.

   Ref: In: Young LY, Koda-Kimble MA, eds. *Applied Therapeutics: The Clinical Use of Drugs*. 6th ed. Vancouver, Wash: Applied Therapeutics; 1995: chapter 82.

5. (D) Benzodiazepines are the drugs of choice for the management of alcohol withdrawal because they are relatively safe, decrease autonomic hyperactivity and protect against seizures.

   Ref: Saitz R, O'Malley SS. Pharmacotherapies for alcohol abuse: withdrawal and treatment. *Med Clin North Am* 1997;4: 881–907.

P A T I E N T   P R O F I L E   1 8 9

OBESITY

ANSWERS

1. (B) HJ's BMI is 30.

   Ref: NHLBI Clinical Guidelines on the Identification, Evaluation, and Treatment of Overweight and Obesity in Adults. Washington: National Institutes of Health, National Heart, Lung, and Blood Institute, September 1998.

2. (C) HJ is classified as obese.

   Ref: NHLBI Clinical Guidelines on the Identification, Evaluation, and Treatment of Overweight and Obesity in Adults. Washington: National Institutes of Health, National Heart, Lung, and Blood Institute; September 1998.

3. (D) Both sleep apnea and osteoarthritis are weight-related diseases, both of which HJ is experiencing.

   Ref: NHLBI Clinical Guidelines on the Identification, Evaluation, and Treatment of Overweight and Obesity in Adults. Washington: National Institutes of Health, National Heart, Lung, and Blood Institute, September 1998.

4. (C) HJ has hypertension, hypertriglyceridemia, and type 2 diabetes.

   Ref: National Cholesterol Education Program Adult Treatment Panel III. Washington: National Institutes of Health, National Heart, Lung, and Blood Institute, May 2001.

5. (B) HJ has a BMI of greater than 30, which makes her a candidate for drug therapy, after failing 6 months of diet and exercise.

   Ref: NHLBI Clinical Guidelines on the Identification, Evaluation, and Treatment of Overweight and Obesity in Adults. Washington: National Institutes of Health, National Heart, Lung, and Blood Institute, September 1998.

6. (A) Based on her history of hypertension and the lack of data for topiramate, orlistat would be the best first-line treatment for HJ.

   Ref: Yanovski S, Yanovski J. Obesity. *N Eng J Med* 2002;346(8): 591–602.

   Ref: Williamson DF. Pharmacotherapy for obesity. *JAMA* 1999; 281(3): 278–280.

7. (D) Sibutramine may increase blood pressure and should not be used in patients with hypertension.

   Ref: Wirth A, Krause J. Long-term weight loss with sibutramine: A randomized, controlled trial. *JAMA* 2001;286(11): 1331–1339.

8. (D) Orlistat and sibutramine have been studied for long-term use in weight loss (up to 2 years).

Ref: Yanovski S, Yanovski J. Obesity. *N Eng J Med* 2002; 346(8):591–602.

Ref: Williamson DF. Pharmacotherapy for obesity. *JAMA* 1999; 281(3):278–280.

Ref: Wirth A, Krause J. Long-term weight loss with sibutramine: A randomized, controlled trial. *JAMA* 2001;286(11): 1331–1339.

9. (A) Orlistat has been shown to decrease the absorption of fat-soluble vitamins, and some patients may benefit from supplementation of these vitamins.

Ref: Yanovski S, Yanovski J. Obesity. *N Eng J Med* 2002; 346(8):591–602.

Ref: Williamson DF. Pharmacotherapy for obesity. *JAMA* 1999;281(3):278–280.

10. (D) Both BMI >35 with comorbid disease and BMI >40 with no comorbid disease are appropriate cut points for weight-loss surgery.

Ref: *NHLBI Clinical Guidelines on the Identification, Evaluation, and Treatment of Overweight and Obesity in Adults.* Washington: National Institutes of Health, National Heart, Lung, and Blood Institute, September 1998.

PATIENT PROFILE 190

CONGESTIVE HEART FAILURE, ARRHYTHMIAS

ANSWERS

1. (A) Nitrate therapy for only 24 hours will produce tolerance to the drug. A nitrate-free interval is necessary to maintain efficacy of the nitrate preparation.

Ref: Talbert RL. Ischemic heart disease. In: DiPiro JT, Talbert RL, Yee GC, Matzke GR, Wells BG, Posey LM, eds. *Pharmacotherapy: A Pathophysiologic Approach.* 4th ed. Stamford, Conn: Appleton & Lange; 1999:182–210.

2. (E) Goal INR range for venous thromboembolism is 2.0–3.0.

Ref: Bauman JL, Schoen MD. Arrhythmias. In: DiPiro JT, Talbert RL, Yee GC, Matzke GR, Wells BG, Posey LM, eds. *Pharmacotherapy: A Pathophysiologic Approach.* 4th ed. Stamford, Conn: Appleton & Lange; 1999:232–264.

Ref: Talbert RL. Ischemic heart disease. In: DiPiro JT, Talbert RL, Yee GC, Matzke GR, Wells BG, Posey LM, eds. *Pharmacotherapy: A Pathophysiologic Approach.* 4th ed. Stamford, Conn: Appleton & Lange; 1999:182–210.

Ref: Talbert RL. Hyperlipidemia. In: DiPiro JT, Talbert RL, Yee GC, Matzke GR, Wells BG, Posey LM, eds. *Pharmacotherapy: A*

Pathophysiologic Approach. 4th ed. Stamford, Conn: Appleton & Lange; 1999:350–373.

3. (D) The combination of hydralazine and nitrates is an appropriate alternative to ACE inhibitors in the management of CHF.

Ref: Johnson JA, Parker RB, Geraci SA. Heart failure. In: DiPiro JT, Talbert RL, Yee GC, Matzke GR, Wells BG, Posey LM, eds. *Pharmacotherapy: A Pathophysiologic Approach.* 4th ed. Stamford, Conn: Appleton & Lange; 1999:153–181.

4. (A) The use of carvedilol has been demonstrated to lower mortality among patients with CHF.

Ref: Johnson JA, Parker RB, Geraci SA. Heart failure. In: DiPiro JT, Talbert RL, Yee GC, Matzke GR, Wells BG, Posey LM, eds. *Pharmacotherapy: A Pathophysiologic Approach.* 4th ed. Stamford, Conn: Appleton & Lange; 1999:153–181.

5. (B) Goal blood pressure is less than 140/90 mm Hg.

Ref: Talbert RL. Ischemic heart disease. In: DiPiro JT, Talbert RL, Yee GC, Matzke GR, Wells BG, Posey LM, eds. *Pharmacotherapy: A Pathophysiologic Approach.* 4th ed. Stamford, Conn: Appleton & Lange; 1999:182–210.

PATIENT PROFILE 191

HEPATIC CIRRHOSIS

ANSWERS

1. (D) Propranolol is the correct choice. β-Blockers are the class of choice because they are able to decrease splanchnic blood flow and portal hypertension. A non-

selective β-blocker is mandatory, and both propranolol and nadolol have demonstrated therapeutic efficacy.

Ref: Talwalkar JA, et al. An evidence-based medicine approach to beta-blocker therapy in patients with cirrhosis. *Am J Med* 2004;116(11):759–766.

2. (C) Variceal hemorrhage is the most immediate life-threatening complication of portal hypertension. β-Blockers are not very effective in managing ascites, especially when compared with appropriate diuretic therapy. Decreasing portal hypertension does not affect hepatic encephalopathy.

Ref: Talwalkar JA, et al. An evidence-based medicine approach to beta-blocker therapy in patients with cirrhosis. *Am J Med* 2004;116(11):759–766.

3. (C) Lactulose is indicated for hepatic encephalopathy and works by acidifying the colon and reducing blood ammonia levels. This patient's ascites are being treated with furosemide and spironolactone. Portal hypertension and esophageal varices should be managed with a nonselective β-blocker.

Ref: Gerber T, et al. Hepatic encephalopathy in liver cirrhosis: Pathogenesis, diagnosis and management. *Drugs* 2000;60(6): 1353–1370.

4. (B) When using lactulose for hepatic encephalopathy, the drug should be initiated at 20 to 30 g three to four times daily and adjusted every couple of days to achieve a target of two to three soft formed stools daily.

Ref: Gerber T, et al. Hepatic encephalopathy in liver cirrhosis: Pathogenesis, diagnosis and management. *Drugs* 2000;60(6): 1353–1370.

5. (A) The exact etiology of pruritus is not well understood, and more than one factor may be at play. From these options, the most likely culprit is the elevated bilirubin because pruritus has been associated with impaired secretion of bile.

Ref: Mela M, et al. Review article: Pruritis in cholestatic and other liver diseases. *Aliment Pharmacol Ther* 2003;17(7):857–870.

6. (E) All these agents have demonstrated a therapeutic benefit in managing pruritus associated with liver disease.

Ref: Mela M, et al. Review article: Pruritis in cholestatic and other liver diseases. *Aliment Pharmacol Ther* 2003;17(7):857–870.

7. (E) All these events can result in worsening ascites. Salt restriction facilitates the elimination of ascites and delays the reaccumulation of fluid. Diuretics hasten the loss of ascitic fluid.

Ref: Gines P, et al. Management of cirrhosis and ascites. *New Engl J Med* 2004;350(16):1646–1654.

8. (A) Albumin acts as a plasma expander and minimizes the risk of circulatory dysfunction after large-volume paracentesis or aggressive diuresis. Albumin is not used to treat hypoalbuminemia and is not cost-effective for use in all patients with ascites.

Ref: Gines P, et al. Management of cirrhosis and ascites. *New Engl J Med* 2004;350(16):1646–1654.

9. (B) Recurrence of spontaneous bacterial peritonitis is common, and long-term antibiotic prophylaxis is indicated after treatment of the initial episode is complete. Quinolones traditionally have been the drug of choice, with sulfamethoxazole-trimethoprim as an alternative.

Ref: Gines P, et al. Management of cirrhosis and ascites. *New Engl J Med* 2004;350(16):1646–1654.

10. (E) Ursodiol generally is very well tolerated. It does not affect lipid levels, liver function, renal function, nor blood counts.

Ref: Ursodiol Drug Information, Micromedex, Thompson Healthcare, Inc., March 2004. Available at *http://micromedex.com*.

PATIENT PROFILE 192

THYROID DISEASE

ANSWERS

1. (D) The recommended duration of therapy with propylthiouracil is 6 to 24 months, although some patients continue therapy indefinitely.

Ref: Sinder PA, Cooper DS, Levy EG, et al. Treatment guidelines for patients with hyper-thyroidism and hypothyroidism. *JAMA* 1995;273:808–812.

2. (E) Side effects of propylthiouracil include gastrointestinal intolerance, agranulocytosis, benign transient leukopenia, hair loss, rash, and headache.

Ref: Propylthiouracil. American Hospital Formulary Service. Bethesda, Md: American Society of Health-System Pharmacists; 1999:2801.

3. (C) The average starting dose of levothyroxine is 1.7 μg/kg/day once daily.

Ref: Sinder PA, Cooper DS, Levy EG, et al. Treatment guidelines for patients with hyperthyroidism and hypothyroidism. *JAMA* 1995;273:808–812.

4. (A) Phenytoin may increase the metabolism of levothyroxine. This may cause a decreased effect of levothyroxine and make a higher dose of levothyroxine necessary to achieve the desired effect.

Ref: Dang BJ. Thyroid disorders. In: Young LY, Koda-Kimble MA, eds. *Applied Therapeutics: The Clinical Use of Drugs.* 6th ed. Vancouver, Wash: Applied Therapeutics; 1995: 47-1–47-31.

PATIENT PROFILE 193

DIABETES MELLITUS

ANSWERS

1. (A) An adverse effect of angiotensin-converting enzyme (ACE) inhibitors is angioedema.

   Ref: Kradjan W. Heart failure. In: Koda-Kimble MA, Young LY, Kradjan WA, Guglielmo BJ, eds. *Applied Therapeutics: The Clinical Use of Drugs,* 8th ed. Philadelphia: Lippincott Williams & Wilkins, 2005:19-1–19-64.

2. (A) The doses for acarbose and rosiglitazone are inappropriate. GF's morning blood sugar is at goal, but her pre-evening meal blood sugars are elevated. Both adding bedtime insulin and 10 mg glipizide in the evening would decrease the morning blood sugar value

   Ref: Carlisle BA, Kroon LA, Koda-Kimble MA. Diabetes mellitus. In: Koda-Kimble MA, Young LY, Kradjan WA, Guglielmo BJ, eds. *Applied Therapeutics: The Clinical Use of Drugs,* 8th ed. Philadelphia: Lippincott Williams & Wilkins, 2005:50-1–50-80.

3. (A) Only insulin is indicated for treatment of women who are pregnant.

   Ref: Oki JC. Diabetes mellitus. In: DiPiro JT, Talbert RL, Yee GC, et al, eds. *Pharmacotherapy: A Pathophysiologic Approach,* 5th ed. New York: McGraw-Hill, 2002:1335–1358.

4. (E) Increasing the bedtime insulin is the most effective way of lowering fasting blood sugar of the choices presented.

   Ref: Carlisle BA, Kroon LA, Koda-Kimble MA. Diabetes mellitus. In: Koda-Kimble MA, Young LY, Kradjan WA, Guglielmo BJ, eds. *Applied Therapeutics: The Clinical Use of Drugs,* 8th ed. Philadelphia: Lippincott Williams & Wilkins, 2005:50-1–50-80.

5. (C) For patients using greater than 10 cigarettes per day, the 21 mg/24 h patch should be initiated.

   Ref: Nicoderm CQ Web site: *http://nicodermcq.quit.com/default. aspx;* accessed September 2004.

6. (A) Nicotine patch use is associated with insomnia.

   Ref: Doering P. Substance-related disorders: Alcohol, nicotine and caffeine. In: DiPiro JT, Talbert RL, Yee GC, et al, eds. *Pharmacotherapy: A Pathophysiologic Approach,* 5th ed. New York: McGraw-Hill, 2002:1203–1218.

7. (B) Nicotine gum should be chewed until a taste emerges and then parked between gum and cheek until the taste disappears repeatedly over approximately a half hour.

   Ref: Doering P. Substance-related disorders: Alcohol, nicotine and caffeine. In: DiPiro JT, Talbert RL, Yee GC, et al, eds. *Pharmacotherapy: A Pathophysiologic Approach,* 5th ed. New York: McGraw-Hill, 2002:1203–1218.

8. (A) Cilostazol is indicated for intermittent claudication.

   Ref: Talbert RL. Peripheral vascular disease. In: DiPiro JT, Talbert RL, Yee GC, et al, eds. *Pharmacotherapy: A Pathophysiologic Approach,* 5th ed. New York: McGraw-Hill, 2002: 419–434.

9. (D) Both ibuprofen and cilostazol increase bleeding risk, particularly gastrointestinal bleeding.

   Ref: Talbert RL. Peripheral vascular disease. In: DiPiro JT, Talbert RL, Yee GC, et al, eds. *Pharmacotherapy: A Pathophysiologic Approach,* 5th ed. New York: McGraw-Hill, 2002: 419–434.

10. (A) Niacin is associated with glucose intolerance. It does not interact with metformin or lisinopril. Niacin lowers LDL, lowers triglycerides, and increases HDL.

    Ref: McKenney JM. Dyslipidemias, atherosclerosis and coronary heart disease. In: Koda-Kimble MA, Young LY, Kradjan WA, Guglielmo BJ, eds. *Applied Therapeutics: The Clinical Use of Drugs,* 8th ed. Philadelphia: Lippincott Williams & Wilkins, 2005:13-1–13-39.

PATIENT PROFILE 194

CHRONIC OBSTRUCTIVE LUNG DISEASE

ANSWERS

1. (B) Because of the potential for serious side effects associated with high concentrations of theophylline and because there is minimal added benefit, recent recommendations have lowered the target therapeutic concentration from 10–20mg/L to 10–15mg/L.

   Ref: Chronic obstructive pulmonary disease. In: Herfindal ET, Gourley DR, eds. *Textbook of Therapeutics, Drug and Disease Management,* 6th ed. Baltimore: Williams & Wilkinds; 1996: Chapter 36.

2. (B) Because of the pharmacokinetics of aminophylline, the drug should be given as a loading dose over

30 minutes to achieve a desired target serum concentration, followed a continuous infusion to maintain the concentration.

Ref: Chronic obstructive pulmonary disease. In: Herfindal ET, Gourley DR, eds. *Textbook of Therapeutics, Drug and Disease Management.* 6th ed. Baltimore: Williams & Wilkins; 1996: chapter 36.

3. (C) Aminophylline is approximately 80% theophylline. For conversion to oral theophylline, the total daily IV aminophylline dose should be multiplied by 0.8 to obtain an equivalent total daily theophylline dose.

Ref: Konzem SL, Stratton MA. Chronic obstructive lung disease. In: DiPiro JT, Talbert RL, Yee GC, Matzke GR, Wells BG, Posey LM, eds. *Pharmacotherapy: A Pathophysiologic Approach.* 4th ed. Stamford, Conn: Appleton & Lange; 1999:460–477.

4. (C) Because the efficacy of corticosteroid therapy among patients with COPD is unpredictable, patients should be examined within 2 weeks to assess response to treatment.

Ref: Konzem SL, Stratton MA. Chronic obstructive lung disease. In: DiPiro JT, Talbert RL, Yee GC, Matzke GR, Wells BG, Posey LM, eds. *Pharmacotherapy: A Pathophysiologic Approach.* 4th ed. Stamford, Conn: Appleton & Lange; 1999: 460–477.

5. (C) Acetylcysteine is given by means of nebulization for the specific purpose of decreasing mucous viscosity.

Ref: Konzem SL, Stratton MA. Chronic obstructive lung disease. In: DiPiro JT, Talbert RL, Yee GC, Matzke GR, Wells BG, Posey LM, eds. *Pharmacotherapy: A Pathophysiologic Approach.* 4th ed. Stamford, Conn: Appleton & Lange; 1999:460–477.

PATIENT PROFILE 195

GOUT

ANSWERS

1. (C) Disagree; probenecid would not be an appropriate suggestion at this time, and the patient should be started on an indomethacin regimen for the acute attack.

Ref: Russell TM, Young LL. Gout and hyperuricemia. In: Young YL, Koda-Kimble MA, eds. *Applied Therapeutics: The Clinical Use of Drugs.* Vancouver, WA: Applied Therapeutics, 2005:42(1–17).

2. (B) Aspiration and analysis of joint synovial fluid is necessary to make a definitive diagnosis of gout.

Ref: Russell TM, Young LL. Gout and hyperuricemia. In: Young YL, Koda-Kimble MA, eds. *Applied Therapeutics: The Clinical Use of Drugs.* Vancouver, WA: Applied Therapeutics, 2005:42(1–17).

3. (A) Hydrochlorothizaide has been associated with reduced uric acid excretion and precipitation of acute gouty arthritis.

Ref: Russell TM, Young LL. Gout and hyperuricemia. In: Young YL, Koda-Kimble MA, eds. *Applied Therapeutics: The Clinical Use of Drugs.* Vancouver, WA: Applied Therapeutics, 2005:42(1–17).

4. (E) RM's risk factors for acute gouty attacks are obesity, his uric acid level, and his renal function.

Ref: Russell TM, Young LL. Gout and hyperuricemia. In: Young YL, Koda-Kimble MA, eds. *Applied Therapeutics: The Clinical Use of Drugs.* Vancouver, WA: Applied Therapeutics, 2005:42(1–17).

5. (A) A potential complication of gout is deposition of sodium urate in tissues.

Ref: Russell TM, Young LL. Gout and hyperuricemia. In: Young YL, Koda-Kimble MA, eds. *Applied Therapeutics: The Clinical Use of Drugs.* Vancouver, WA: Applied Therapeutics, 2005:42(1–17).

6. (C) A common adverse effect of indomethacin when used for acute attacks of gouty arthritis is headache.

Ref: Russell TM, Young LL. Gout and hyperuricemia. In: Young YL, Koda-Kimble MA, eds. *Applied Therapeutics: The Clinical Use of Drugs.* Vancouver, WA: Applied Therapeutics, 2005:42(1–17).

7. (D) As an overproducer and with a creatinine clearance of 66 mL/min, the patient should be started on allopurinol 100 mg PO qd.

Ref: Russell TM, Young LL. Gout and hyperuricemia. In: Young YL, Koda-Kimble MA, eds. *Applied Therapeutics: The Clinical Use of Drugs.* Vancouver, WA: Applied Therapeutics, 2005:42(1–17).

8. (B) A source of uric acid in the human body is a breakdown of dietary and tissue purines.

Ref: Russell TM, Young LL. Gout and hyperuricemia. In: Young YL, Koda-Kimble MA, eds. *Applied Therapeutics: The Clinical Use of Drugs.* Vancouver, WA: Applied Therapeutics, 2005:42(1–17).

9. (D) Corticosteroids would be used to treat an acute attack of gouty arthritis in patients with severe renal impairment, patients who are resistant to NSAIDs and colchicines, and patients with prior NSAID intolerance.

Ref: Russell TM, Young LL. Gout and hyperuricemia. In: Young YL, Koda-Kimble MA, eds. *Applied Therapeutics: The Clinical Use of Drugs.* Vancouver, WA: Applied Therapeutics, 2005:42(1–17).

10. (C) Allopurinol is a xanthine oxidase inhibitor and prevents production of uric acid.

Ref: Russell TM, Young LL. Gout and hyperuricemia. In: Young YL, Koda-Kimble MA, eds. *Applied Therapeutics: The Clinical Use of Drugs.* Vancouver, WA: Applied Therapeutics, 2005:42(1–17).

PATIENT PROFILE 196

ARRHYTHMIAS

ANSWERS

1. (B) Intravenous Lasix® (furosemide) is indicated in the setting of acute volume overload.

   Ref: Johnson JA, Parker RB, Geraci SA. Heart failure. In: DiPiro JT, Talbert RL, Yee GC, Matzke GR, Wells BG, Posey LM, eds. *Pharmacotherapy: A Pathophysiologic Approach.* 4th ed. Stamford, Conn: Appleton & Lange; 1999:153–181.

2. (C) Both verapamil, a negative inotrope, and naproxen, an NSAID that can lead to sodium and water retention, can exacerbate CHF.

   Ref: Johnson JA, Parker RB, Geraci SA. Heart failure. In: DiPiro JT, Talbert RL, Yee GC, Matzke GR, Wells BG, Posey LM, eds. *Pharmacotherapy: A Pathophysiologic Approach.* 4th ed. Stamford, Conn: Appleton & Lange; 1999:153–181.

3. (A) The patient currently has a therapeutic serum digoxin concentration.

   Ref: Johnson JA, Parker RB, Geraci SA. Heart failure. In: DiPiro JT, Talbert RL, Yee GC, Matzke GR, Wells BG, Posey LM, eds. *Pharmacotherapy: A Pathophysiologic Approach.* 4th ed. Stamford, Conn: Appleton & Lange; 1999:153–181.

4. (E) Amiodarone is the best choice because of its superior efficacy and lack of disease state interactions in this patient

   Ref: Bauman JL, Schoen MD. Arrhythmias. In: DiPiro JT, Talbert RL, Yee GC, Matzke GR, Wells BG, Posey LM, eds. *Pharmacotherapy: A Pathophysiologic Approach.* 4th ed. Stamford, Conn: Appleton & Lange; 1999:232–264.

5. (E) Procainamide can cause several types of arrhythmias, such as bradycardia or torsade de pointes.

   Ref: Bauman JL, Schoen MD. Arrhythmias. In: DiPiro JT, Talbert RL, Yee GC, Matzke GR, Wells BG, Posey LM, eds. *Pharmacotherapy: A Pathophysiologic Approach.* 4th ed. Stamford, Conn: Appleton & Lange; 1999:232–264.

   Ref: AHFS Drug Information, 1998.

PATIENT PROFILE 197

CHRONIC OBSTRUCTIVE PULMONARY DISEASE

ANSWERS

1. (D) Pack-year history refers to the number of packs of cigarettes smoked per day times the number of years smoked.

   Ref: Williams DM, Kradjan WA. Chronic obstructive pulmonary disease. In: Koda-Kimble MA, Young LY, Kradjian WA, Guglielmo BJ, eds. *Applied Therapeutics: The Clinical Use of Drugs.* Philadelphia: Lippincott Williams & Wilkins, 2004:24-1–24-28.

2. (B) The chronic productive cough and lack of significant improvement after administration of an inhaled β-agonist are consistent with chronic bronchitis.

   Ref: Williams DM, Kradjan WA. Chronic obstructive pulmonary disease. In: Koda-Kimble MA, Young LY, Kradjian WA, Guglielmo BJ, eds. *Applied Therapeutics: The Clinical Use of Drugs.* Philadelphia: Lippincott Williams & Wilkins, 2004:24-1–24-28.

3. (E) Currently none of the therapies for COPD alter the natural course of the disease. They only provide symptomatic improvement.

   Ref: Williams DM, Kradjan WA. Chronic obstructive pulmonary disease. In: Koda-Kimble MA, Young LY, Kradjian WA, Guglielmo BJ, eds. *Applied Therapeutics: The Clinical Use of Drugs.* Philadelphia: Lippincott Williams & Wilkins, 2004:24-1–24-28.

4. (D) Both ipratropium and tiotropium are anticholinergics. The cholinergic nervous system plays a major role in controlling airway tone in patients with COPD; therefore, these agents are effective bronchodilators.

   Ref: Williams DM, Kradjan WA. Chronic obstructive pulmonary disease. In: Koda-Kimble MA, Young LY, Kradjian WA, Guglielmo BJ, eds. *Applied Therapeutics: The Clinical Use of Drugs.* Philadelphia: Lippincott Williams & Wilkins, 2004:24-1–24-28.

5. (C) These agents should be prescribed twice daily. They are not intended for immediate relief of symptoms.

   Ref: Williams DM, Kradjan WA. Chronic obstructive pulmonary disease. In: Koda-Kimble MA, Young LY, Kradjian WA, Guglielmo

BJ, eds. *Applied Therapeutics: The Clinical Use of Drugs.* Philadelphia: Lippincott Williams & Wilkins, 2004:24-1-24-28.

6. (D) As compared with atropine, ipratropium is relatively free of systemic side effects.

    Ref: Williams DM, Kradjan WA. Chronic obstructive pulmonary disease. In: Koda-Kimble MA, Young LY, Kradjian WA, Guglielmo BJ, eds. *Applied Therapeutics: The Clinical Use of Drugs.* Philadelphia: Lippincott Williams & Wilkins, 2004:24-1-24-28.

7. (C) Patients should be advised to rinse their mouth out after using steroid inhalers to avoid oral candidiasis, hoarseness, and throat irritation.

    Ref: USP DI System: Klasco RK, ed. *USP DI Advice for the Patient.* Greenwood Village, CO: Thomson Micromedex; edition expires 12/2004.

8. (D) Ciprofloxacin inhibits the hepatic metabolism of theophylline and can result in increased serum concentrations. The other agents have not been reported to alter theophylline pharmacokinetics.

Ref: Hendeles L, Ingrim N. Theophylline. In: Klasco RK, ed. *DRUGDEX System.* Greenwood Village, CO: Thomson Micromedex; edition expires 12/2004.

9. (E) All these side effects are associated with elevated theophylline levels.

    Ref: Williams DM, Kradjan WA. Chronic obstructive pulmonary disease. In: Koda-Kimble MA, Young LY, Kradjian WA, Guglielmo BJ, eds. *Applied Therapeutics: The Clinical Use of Drugs.* Philadelphia: Lippincott Williams & Wilkins, 2004:24-1-24-28.

10. (B) If GG stops smoking, a lower dose of theophylline may be necessary. Smoking increases the clearance of theophylline, which means that higher doses may be required to maintain appropriate levels in smokers.

    Ref: Konzem SL, Stratton MA. Chronic obstructive lung disease. In: Dipiro JT, Talbert RL, Yee GC, et al, eds. *Pharmacotherapy: A Pathophysiologic Approach.* New York: McGraw-Hill, 2002: 511–529.

PATIENT PROFILE 198

HYPERTENSION

ANSWERS

1. (E) All stages of hypertension including isolated systolic hypertension (ISH) have significant rates of morbidity and mortality related to target organ involvement.

    Ref: Carter BL, et al. Essential Hypertension. In: Young YL, Koda-Kimble MA, eds. *Applied Therapeutics: The Clinical Use of Drugs.* Vancouver, WA: Applied Therapeutics; 1995: 10-8–10-11.

2. (C) LL's high blood pressure is not drug or disease induced and it does not meet the definition of ISH.

    Ref: Carter BL, et al. Essential Hypertension. In: Young YL, Koda-Kimble MA, eds. *Applied Therapeutics: The Clinical Use of Drugs.* Vancouver, WA: Applied Therapeutics; 1995: 10-2–10-3.

3. (D) Caffeine may cause a transient elevation in blood pressure but it is not a cardiovascular risk factor.

    Ref: Carter BL, et al. Essential Hypertension. In: Young YL, Koda-Kimble MA, eds. *Applied Therapeutics: The Clinical Use of Drugs.* Vancouver, WA: Applied Therapeutics; 1995: 10-7–10-8, 10–11.

4. (B) HCTZ has been reported to cause hypokalemia, hypercalcemia, hypo-magnesemia, hyponatremia, hyperuricemia, hyperglycemia, and hypercholesterolemia.

    Ref: Carter BL, et al. Essential Hypertension. In: Young YL, Koda-Kimble MA, eds. *Applied Therapeutics: The Clinical Use of Drugs.* Vancouver, WA: Applied Therapeutics; 1995:10–13, 10–17.

5. (D) Increasing the dose of HCTZ beyond 50 mg per day produces no real added response. Therefore, adding the ACEI to the regimen is a best choice since LL has diabetes and ACEIs have renal protective effects in this patient population.

    Ref: Carter BL, et al. Essential Hypertension. In: Young YL, Koda-Kimble MA, eds. *Applied Therapeutics: The Clinical Use of Drugs.* Vancouver, WA: Applied Therapeutics; 1995: 10-18–10-23.

6. (E) All are appropriate monitoring parameters to evaluate the effectiveness of LL's treatment plan.

    Ref: Carter BL, et al. Essential Hypertension. In: Young YL, Koda-Kimble MA, eds. *Applied Therapeutics: The Clinical Use of Drugs.* Vancouver, WA: Applied Therapeutics; 1995: Chapter 10.

COLON CANCER

ANSWERS

1. (B)

Ref: Chu E, Mota AC, Fogarasi MC. Antimetabolites. In: Devita VT, Hellman S, Rosenberg SA, eds. *Cancer: Principles and Practice of Oncology,* 6th ed. Philadelphia: Lippincott Williams & Wilkins, 2001:393.

2. (A)

Ref: Chu E, Mota AC, Fogarasi MC. Antimetabolites. In: Devita VT, Hellman S, Rosenberg SA, eds. *Cancer: Principles and Practice of Oncology,* 6th ed. Philadelphia: Lippincott Williams & Wilkins, 2001:397.

3. (B)

Ref: Skibber JM, Minske BD, Hoff PM. Cancer of the colon. In: Devita VT, Hellman S, Rosenberg SA, eds. *Cancer: Principles and Practice of Oncology,* 6th ed. Philadelphia: Lippincott Williams & Wilkins, 2001:1257.

4. (C)

Ref: Davis L, Lindley C. Neoplastic disorders and their treatment: general principles. In Koda-Kimbla MA, Young LY, Kradjan WA, et al, eds. *Applied Therapeutics: The Clinical Use of Drugs,* 8th ed. Philadelphia: Lippincott Williams & Wilkins, 2005:88(16–22).

5. (B)

Ref: BSA equation from Lacy CF. *Drug Information Handbook,* 11th ed. Hudson, OH: Lexicomp, 2003:1488.

6. (C)

Ref: Stewart CF, Ratain MJ. Topoisomerase interactive agents. In: Devita VT, Hellman S, Rosenberg SA, eds. *Cancer: Principles and Practice of Oncology,* 6th ed. Philadelphia: Lippincott Williams & Wilkins, 2001:424.

7. (D)

Ref: Stewart CF, Ratain MJ. Topoisomerase interactive agents. In: Devita VT, Hellman S, Rosenberg SA, eds. *Cancer: Principles and Practice of Oncology,* 6th ed. Philadelphia: Lippincott Williams & Wilkins, 2001:416–418.

8. (D)

Ref: Davis L, Lindley C. Neoplastic disorders and their treatment: general principles. In Koda-Kimbla MA, Young LY, Kradjan WA, et al, eds. *Applied Therapeutics: The Clinical Use of Drugs,* 8th ed. Philadelphia: Lippincott Williams & Wilkins, 2005:88(7).

9. (D)

Ref: Lindley C. Adverse effects of chemotherapy. In Koda-Kimbla MA, Young LY, Kradjan WA, et al, eds. *Applied Therapeutics: The Clinical Use of Drugs,* 8th ed. Philadelphia: Lippincott Williams & Wilkins, 2005:89(8).

10. (A) The patient is receiving 90 mg oral morphine per day. The equianalgesic dose of IV hydromorphone is 4.5 mg. Since we are changing to a new agent and cross-tolerance between the opiates is not 100%, the dose of the new agent can be 75% of the equianalgesic dose, which is approximately 3.4 mg. This will be divided every 4 hours.

Ref: Reisner L, Koo PJS. Pain and its management. In Koda-Kimbla MA, Young LY, Kradjan WA, et al, eds. *Applied Therapeutics: The Clinical Use of Drugs,* 8th ed. Philadelphia: Lippincott Williams & Wilkins, 2005:9(12–16).

HYPERTENSION

ANSWERS

1. (A) ACEIs have been reported to cause hyperkalemia.

Ref: Carter BL, et al. Essential Hypertension. In: Young YL, Koda-Kimble MA, eds. *Applied Therapeutics: The Clinical Use of Drugs.* Vancouver, WA: Applied Therapeutics; 1995: 10–14.

2. (D) Angioneurotic edema can be life threatening and has been reported to occur from 1 hour up to 1 week after starting therapy with an ACEI.

Ref: Beringer PM, et al. Anaphylaxis and Drug Allergies. In: Young YL, Koda-Kimble MA, eds. *Applied Therapeutics: The Clinical Use of Drugs.* Vancouver, WA: Applied Therapeutics; 1995:6–16.

3. (B) First-dose syncope (profound hypotension, dizziness, and possible fainting) can be minimized by starting at a low dose at bedtime.

Ref: Carter BL, et al. Essential Hypertension. In: Young YL, Koda-Kimble MA, eds. *Applied Therapeutics: The Clinical Use of Drugs.* Vancouver, WA: Applied Therapeutics; 1995: 10–24.

4. (E) All are possible adverse effects of prazosin.

Ref: Carter BL, et al. Essential Hypertension. In: Young YL, Koda-Kimble MA, eds. *Applied Therapeutics: The Clinical Use of Drugs.* Vancouver, WA: Applied Therapeutics; 1995: 10-14–10-24.

5. (C) Rising slowly from a seated or supine position helps to minimize the postural hypotensive effects of prazosin.

Ref: Carter BL, et al. Essential Hypertension. In: Young YL, Koda-Kimble MA, eds. *Applied Therapeutics: The Clinical Use of Drugs.* Vancouver, WA: Applied Therapeutics; 1995: 10-24–10-25.

6. (A) Minipress® is the brand name product for prazosin.

Ref: Carter BL, et al. Essential Hypertension. In: Young YL, Koda-Kimble MA, eds. *Applied Therapeutics: The Clinical Use of Drugs.* Vancouver, WA: Applied Therapeutics; 1995: 10–24.

7. (D) Finasteride can be added to the alpha blocker to induce atrophy of the prostate gland and halt progression of the disease until JW undergoes the TURP procedure.

Ref: Thompson JF. Geriatric Urological Disorders. In: Young YL, Koda-Kimble MA, eds. *Applied Therapeutics: The Clinical Use of Drugs.* Vancouver, WA: Applied Therapeutics; 1995: 103–15.

PATIENT PROFILE 201
ERECTILE DYSFUNCTION

ANSWERS

1. (D) Diabetes mellitus is a risk factor for erectile dysfunction. Other risk factors for erectile dysfunction include age greater than 40 years, hypertension, hypogonadism (low testosterone levels), and smoking. These are not current risk factors for JS because he is 38 years old, does not have high blood pressure (lisinopril used to prevent microvascular complications of nephropathy), has normal testosterone levels, and quit smoking 10 years ago. Although JS's diabetes is under control, he is still at risk for erectile dysfunction.

Ref: Impotence. NIH Consensus Statement Online, December 7–9, 1992 (October 15, 2004), 10(4);1–31.

2. (C) Antihistamines (e.g., benadryl) and cimetidine are examples of medications that may cause drug-induced erectile dysfunction. Other drugs that may cause erectile dysfunction include β-blockers, thiazide diuretics, tricyclic antidepressants, etc. Angiotensin-converting enzyme (ACE) inhibitors (i.e., lisinopril) often are used as alternatives to β-blockers in erectile dysfunction induced by β-blockers.

Ref: Lee M. Erectile dysfunction. In: Dipiro JT, Talbert RL, Yee GC, et al, eds. *Pharmacotherapy: A Pathophysiologic Approach,* 5th ed. New York: McGraw-Hill, 2002:1511–1531.

3. (C) Antidepressant therapy reported to cause erectile dysfunction includes selective serotonin reuptake inhibitors (SSRIs), tricyclic antidepressants, and monoamine oxidase (MAO) inhibitors. Alternatives that do not cause erectile dysfunction include buproprion, nefazodone, and mirtazapine.

Ref: Lee M. Erectile dysfunction. In: Dipiro JT, Talbert RL, Yee GC, et al, eds. *Pharmacotherapy: A Pathophysiologic Approach,* 5th ed. New York: McGraw-Hill, 2002:1511–1531.

Ref: AACE Male Sexual Dysfunction Task Force. Medical guidelines for clinical practice for the evaluation and treatment of male sexual dysfunction: A couple's problem—2003 update. *Endocr Pract* 2003;9(1):77–95.

4. (D) All the mentioned actions may be taken for antidepressants, with the exception that remission and tolerance to erectile dysfunction symptoms do not occur with TCA therapy.

Ref: Keene LC, Davies P. Drug-related erectile dysfunction. *Adverse Drug React Toxicol Rev* 1999;18:5–24.

5. (B) History of unstable angina is a contraindication to initiating phosphodiesterase inhibitor therapy. Other contraindications include myocardial infarction, stroke, and life-threatening arrythmias within the last 6 months; resting hypotension or severe hypertension; unstable angina; and retinitis pigmentosa.

Ref: Lee M. Erectile dysfunction. In: Dipiro JT, Talbert RL, Yee GC, et al, eds. *Pharmacotherapy: A Pathophysiologic Approach,* 5th ed. New York: McGraw-Hill, 2002:1511–1531.

6. (E) Testosterone supplementation should be initiated only if testosterone levels fall below normal (300–1100 ng/dL). Since testosterone directly stimulates androgen receptors, testosterone supplementation worsens and should be avoided in BPH and prostate cancer.

Ref: AACE Male Sexual Dysfunction Task Force. Medical guidelines for clinical practice for the evaluation and treatment of male sexual dysfunction: A couple's problem—2003 update. *Endocr Pract* 2003;9(1):77–95.

7. (D) Striant must be removed if it does not dissolve after 12 hours of administration. Striant is not affected by food, gum chewing, tooth brushing, or alcoholic

beverages. Striant should never be chewed or swallowed.

Ref: Package insert: Striant, Columbia Laboratories, Inc., Linvingtsont, New Jersey. 2003.

8. (E) Testosterone is available in the following formulations: buccal, IM, pellet, patch, and gel. Testosterone administered intravascularly has been discontinued owing to severe liver toxicity.

Ref: Lee M. Erectile dysfunction. In: Dipiro JT, Talbert RL, Yee GC, et al, eds. *Pharmacotherapy: A Pathophysiologic Approach,* 5th ed. New York: McGraw-Hill, 2002:1511–1531.

9. (E) All the listed are disadvantages of pellet administration.

Ref: Package insert, Testopel, Bartor Pharmacal Co., New York. 1992.

10. (B) Vacuum device is a noninvasive pump for erectile dysfunction. Alprostadil is an intracavernosal or intraurethral injection. Phentolamine/papaverine typically is administered as a combination intracavernosal injection. Vascular surgery and insertion of penile prostheses are highly invasive procedures.

Ref: Lee M. Erectile dysfunction. In: Dipiro JT, Talbert RL, Yee GC, et al, eds. *Pharmacotherapy: A Pathophysiologic Approach,* 5th ed. New York: McGraw-Hill, 2002:1511–1531.

PATIENT PROFILE 202
ANTICOAGULATION

ANSWERS

1. (A) Additional necessary baseline data includes a platelet count, hemoglobin, and hemocrit which can be obtained by a complete blood count.

Ref: Wittkowsky AK. Thrombosis. In: Young YL, Koda-Kimble MA, eds. *Applied Therapeutics: The Clinical Use of Drugs.* Vancouver, WA: Applied Therapeutics; 1995:12–7.

2. (D) Initial heparin loading doses are usually 70 to 100 units/kg with most practitioners starting mid-range with 80 units/kg which is commonly used in heparin protocols.

Ref: Wittkowsky AK. Thrombosis. In: Young YL, Koda-Kimble MA, eds. *Applied Therapeutics: The Clinical Use of Drugs.* Vancouver, WA: Applied Therapeutics; 1995:12–9.

3. (D) The continuous infusion rate ranges from 15–25 units/kg/hr with most practitioners starting mid-range with 18 units/kg/hr rounded to the nearest 100 units. This starting rate is also commonly used in heparin protocols.

Ref: Wittkowsky AK. Thrombosis. In: Young YL, Koda-Kimble MA, eds. *Applied Therapeutics: The Clinical Use of Drugs.* Vancouver, WA: Applied Therapeutics; 1995:12–9.

4. (C) The aPTT should be checked 6 hours after the loading dose and 6 hours after making any changes in the infusion rate.

Ref: Wittkowsky AK. Thrombosis. In: Young YL, Koda-Kimble MA, eds. *Applied Therapeutics: The Clinical Use of Drugs.* Vancouver, WA: Applied Therapeutics; 1995:12–9.

5. (C) The aPTT goal is 1.5-2.5X mean control. Therefore, AQ's aPTT is 2X mean control which is therapeutic and warrants no change in therapy at this time.

Ref: Wittkowsky AK. Thrombosis. In: Young YL, Koda-Kimble MA, eds. *Applied Therapeutics: The Clinical Use of Drugs.* Vancouver, WA: Applied Therapeutics; 1995:12–9.

6. (D) Heparin may cause a Type 1 or Type II drug-induced thrombocytopenia.

Ref: Wittkowsky AK. Thrombosis. In: Young YL, Koda-Kimble MA, eds. *Applied Therapeutics: The Clinical Use of Drugs.* Vancouver, WA: Applied Therapeutics; 1995:12–8–12–9.

PATIENT PROFILE 203
MENOPAUSE

ANSWERS

1. (A)

Ref: North American Menopause Society. Estrogen and progesterone use in peri- and postmenopausal women: September 2003

position statement of The North American Menopause Society. *Menopause* 2003;10(6):497–506.

2. (B)

Ref: Package insert: Estroven (menopause monitor), Amerifit Nutrition, Bloomfield CT, 2002.

3. (D)

   Ref: Writing Group for the Women's Health Initiative Investigators. Risks and benefits of estrogen plus progestin in healthy post-menopausal women: Principal results from the Women's Health Initiative Randomized Controlled Trial. *JAMA* 2002;288: 321–333.

4. (B)

   Ref: Parent-Stevens L, Sagraves R. Gynecologic and other disorders of women. In: Koda-Kimbla MA, Young LY, Kradjan WA, et al, eds. *Applied Therapeutics: The Clinical Use of Drugs,* 8th ed. Philadelphia: Lippincott Williams & Wilkins, 2005:48(23–28).

5. (C)

   Ref: Micromedex Healthcare Series Online, Micromedex, Inc., Greenwood Village, CO, 2004.

6. (C)

   Ref: Micromedex Healthcare Series Online, Micromedex, Inc., Greenwood Village, CO, 2004.

7. (D)

Ref: Writing Group for the Women's Health Initiative Investigators. Risks and benefits of estrogen plus progestin in healthy postmenopausal women: Principal results from the Women's Health Initiative Randomized Controlled Trial. *JAMA* 2002;288: 321–333.

8. (A)

   Ref: North American Menopause Society. Estrogen and progesterone use in peri- and postmenopausal women: September 2003 position statement of The North American Menopause Society. *Menopause* 2003;10(6):497–506.

9. (B)

   Ref: Micromedex Healthcare Series Online, Micromedex, Inc., Greenwood Village, CO, 2004.

10. (C)

   Ref: Writing Group for the Women's Health Initiative Investigators. Risks and benefits of estrogen plus progestin in healthy postmenopausal women: Principal results from the Women's Health Initiative Randomized Controlled Trial. *JAMA* 2002;288: 321–333.

PATIENT   PROFILE   204

ANGINA AND BLOOD CLOTTING

ANSWERS

1. (D) Nitroglycerin is a fast-acting vasodilator for all arteries and veins. It decreases both preload and afterload and consequently decreases cardiac tissues oxygen demand. Nitroglycerin is a not long-acting vasodilator owing to deactivation by ester hydrolysis into inactive products.

2. (D) Nitroglycerin structure indicates neither acidic nor basic functional groups. The drug is manufactured for IV infusion as solution in a mixture of water and organic solvent (propylene glycol).

3. (E) All the three agents reduce blood clotting via different mechanisms.

4. (D) Aspirin and clopedogril act by inhibiting platelet aggregation.

5. (C) Warfarin is the only drug among the three that acts by enzyme-inhibitory mechanism.

6. (B) The similarity in chemical structures between warfarin and vitamin K is the key for warfarin's inhibitory effects on the enzyme vitamine K reductase. The enzyme is responsible for regeneration of the reduced form of vitamin K from its oxidized form. Reduced vitamin K is essential for prothrombin activation from descarboxy prothrombin.

7. (D) Both clofibrate and atorvastatin are antihyperlipproteinemic agents, but they act via different mechanisms.

8. (B) Atorvastatin is a member of the statin family of cholesterol-lowering agents. Drugs belonging to this class inhibit cholesterol biosynthesis via enzyme-inhibitory mechanism.

9. (C) HMG-CoA reductase is the enzyme responsible of converting hydroxymethylglutaric acid into mevalonic acid, an important intermediate in cholesterol biosynthesis.

10. (E) All numbers and statements are correct.

PARKINSON'S DISEASE

ANSWERS

1. (C) The initiation of a dopamine agonist such as pramipexole as a first-line agent is a strategy used to delay the introduction of levodopa in younger patients (65 years of age) with mild PD.

   Ref: Ernst ME, Gottwald MD, Gidal BE. Parkinson's disease. In: Koda-Kimble MA, Young LY, Kradjan WA, et al, eds. *Applied Therapeutics: The Clinical Use of Drugs,* 8th ed. Philadelphia: Lippincott Williams & Wilkins, 2005:53(1–30).

2. (D) The honeymoon period related to levodopa therapy usually lasts approximately 5 years.

   Ref: Ernst ME, Gottwald MD, Gidal BE. Parkinson's disease. In: Koda-Kimble MA, Young LY, Kradjan WA, et al, eds. *Applied Therapeutics: The Clinical Use of Drugs,* 8th ed. Philadelphia: Lippincott Williams & Wilkins, 2005:53(1–30).

3. (A) Patients receiving levodopa-carbidopa who experience a "wearing off" effect may benefit from the addition of a catechol-*O*-methyltransferase (COMT) inhibitor. The agent inhibits the metabolic pathways in the brain that degrade levodopa and its metabolites.

   Ref: Ernst ME, Gottwald MD, Gidal BE. Parkinson's disease. In: Koda-Kimble MA, Young LY, Kradjan WA, et al, eds. *Applied Therapeutics: The Clinical Use of Drugs,* 8th ed. Philadelphia: Lippincott Williams & Wilkins, 2005:53(1–30).

4. (B) Anticholinergics such as trihexyphenidyl help to control tremor in early PD by blocking the excitatory neurotransmitter acetylcholine in the striatum, minimizing the effect of a relative increase in cholinergic sensitivity.

   Ref: Ernst ME, Gottwald MD, Gidal BE. Parkinson's disease. In: Koda-Kimble MA, Young LY, Kradjan WA, et al, eds. *Applied Therapeutics: The Clinical Use of Drugs,* 8th ed. Philadelphia: Lippincott Williams & Wilkins, 2005:53(1–30).

5. (A) Anticholinergics such as trihexyphenidyl commonly cause peripherally mediated side effects such as urinary retention. The agent should be avoided in this patient because he has BPH, which could result in urinary retention if exacerbated by anticholinergics.

   Ref: Ernst ME, Gottwald MD, Gidal BE. Parkinson's disease. In: Koda-Kimble MA, Young LY, Kradjan WA, et al, eds. *Applied Therapeutics: The Clinical Use of Drugs,* 8th ed. Philadelphia: Lippincott Williams & Wilkins, 2005:53(1–30).

6. (E) The dopamine agonist ropinirole has shown efficacy in improving motor scores in patients with advanced PD and likely would be recommended in this case.

   Ref: Ernst ME, Gottwald MD, Gidal BE. Parkinson's disease. In: Koda-Kimble MA, Young LY, Kradjan WA, et al, eds. *Applied Therapeutics: The Clinical Use of Drugs,* 8th ed. Philadelphia: Lippincott Williams & Wilkins, 2005:53(1–30).

7. (a) Hypertension rather than hypotension is one of the side effects of levodopa.

   Ref: Ernst ME, Gottwald MD, Gidal BE. Parkinson's disease. In: Koda-Kimble MA, Young LY, Kradjan WA, et al, eds. *Applied Therapeutics: The Clinical Use of Drugs,* 8th ed. Philadelphia: Lippincott Williams & Wilkins, 2005:53(1–30).

8. (E) Carbidopa in doses of 75 to 100 mg effectively inhibits the peripheral conversion of levodopa to dopamine, allowing a reduction in levodopa dose and thereby improving efficacy and minimizing potential side effects.

   Ref: Ernst ME, Gottwald MD, Gidal BE. Parkinson's disease. In: Koda-Kimble MA, Young LY, Kradjan WA, et al, eds. *Applied Therapeutics: The Clinical Use of Drugs,* 8th ed. Philadelphia: Lippincott Williams & Wilkins, 2005:53(1–30).

9. (E) Slow-release levodopa-carbidopa (Sinemet CR) allows a smooth, sustained delivery of drug and may be beneficial in patients taking the immediate-release form who experience the "wearing off" effect. The bioavailability of Sinemet CR is 30% less than the immediate-release product, and it is more costly. Compliance may improve because of its twice-daily dosing

   Ref: Ernst ME, Gottwald MD, Gidal BE. Parkinson's disease. In: Koda-Kimble MA, Young LY, Kradjan WA, et al, eds. *Applied Therapeutics: The Clinical Use of Drugs,* 8th ed. Philadelphia: Lippincott Williams & Wilkins, 2005:53(1–30).

10. (D) Ferrous sulfate 325 mg may reduce levodopa absorption by 50% through chelation of iron by levodopa.

    Ref: Ernst ME, Gottwald MD, Gidal BE. Parkinson's disease. In: Koda-Kimble MA, Young LY, Kradjan WA, et al, eds. *Applied Therapeutics: The Clinical Use of Drugs,* 8th ed. Philadelphia: Lippincott Williams & Wilkins, 2005:53(1–30).

PATIENT PROFILE 206
ANTICOAGULATION

ANSWERS

1. (E) JF may have been discharged from the hospital on a maintenance dose that was too high because he had not reached steady state by his discharge date. He is also taking lovastatin, which has been reported to increase INRs in patients receiving warfarin.

   Ref: Wittkowsky AK. Thrombosis. In: Young YL, Koda-Kimble MA, eds. *Applied Therapeutics: The Clinical Use of Drugs.* Vancouver, WA: Applied Therapeutics; 1995:12-12–12-17, 12–20.

2. (B) Vitamin K administration is not necessary because JF has no bleeding complications.

   Ref: Wittkowsky AK. Thrombosis. In: Young YL, Koda-Kimble MA, eds. *Applied Therapeutics: The Clinical Use of Drugs.* Vancouver, WA: Applied Therapeutics; 1995:12–16.

3. (C) JF's total weekly dose should be decreased by 10–15%. Anytime a change in warfarin dosing occurs,

the INR should be checked to 1–2 weeks in order to reevaluate the patient's clinical response.

   Ref: Wittkowsky AK. Thrombosis. In: Young YL, Koda-Kimble MA, eds. *Applied Therapeutics: The Clinical Use of Drugs.* Vancouver, WA: Applied Therapeutics; 1995:12–16.

4. (C) The INR goal for treatment of a first occurrence DVT is 2–3.

   Ref: Wittkowsky AK. Thrombosis. In: Young YL, Koda-Kimble MA, eds. *Applied Therapeutics: The Clinical Use of Drugs.* Vancouver, WA: Applied Therapeutics; 1995:12–6.

5. (B) The length of treatment for a first occurrence DVT is 3–6 months. Three months is appropriate in patients who have an identifiable cause.

   Ref: Wittkowsky AK. Thrombosis. In: Young YL, Koda-Kimble MA, eds. *Applied Therapeutics: The Clinical Use of Drugs.* Vancouver, WA: Applied Therapeutics; 1995:12–6.

PATIENT PROFILE 207
PARENTERAL NUTRITION

ANSWERS

1. (A) Subtract the number of kilocalories of fat and protein (grams required multiplied by 4 kcal/g) used in the total parenteral nutrition (TPN) solution from the stressed value of kilocalories. Convert the kilocalorie value to grams, and determine the volume of dextrose solution needed.

   Ref: Stocklosa M, Ansel H. *Pharmaceutical Calculations.* 11th ed. Baltimore: Lippincott Williams & Wilkins; 2001:195.

2. (C) The RME equation is solved with the patient's metric system equivalent values for height and weight.

   Ref: Stocklosa M, Ansel H. *Pharmaceutical Calculations.* 11th ed. Baltimore: Lippincott Williams & Wilkins; 2001:195.

3. (E) The stressed value is the nonstressed daily requirement multiplied by the stress factor.

   Ref: Stocklosa M, Ansel H. *Pharmaceutical Calculations.* 11th ed. Baltimore: Lippincott Williams & Wilkins; 2001:195.

4. (A) Sixty percent of the stressed value would be supplied from a fat source. The number of kilocalories then is converted to grams, and the volume of emulsion is determined.

   Ref: Stocklosa M, Ansel H. *Pharmaceutical Calculations.* 11th ed. Baltimore: Lippincott Williams & Wilkins; 2001:195.

5. (A) Grams of protein needed is found by means of multiplying kilograms of body weight by allowed protein per kilogram. The volume of solution needed to provide that amount of protein as amino acid then is determined.

   Ref: Stocklosa M, Ansel H. *Pharmaceutical Calculations.* 11th ed. Baltimore: Lippincott Williams & Wilkins; 2001:195.

PATIENT PROFILE 208

GASTROINTESTINAL INFECTIONS

ANSWERS

1. (A) Depending on the species involved *Salmonella* infections can present in four different ways: acute gastroenteritis, bacteremia, extraintestinal localized infection, and enteric fever. The salmonella serotypes have a broad range of invasive potential often leading to dysentery diarrhea with bloody appearance and fecal leucocytes. Ingestion of contaminated water or food (poultry or poultry products) is the major cause for *Salmonella* infections.

   Ref: Anderson JD, Lemke TD, Odell LJ, et al. Gastrointestinal infections and enterotoxigenic poisonings. In: Dipiro JT, Talbert RL, Yee GC, et al., eds. *Pharmacotherapy: A Pathophysiologic Approach,* 5th edition. New York: McGraw-Hill. 2002: 1939–1954.

   Ref: Itokazu GS, Bearden DT, Danziger LH. Infectious diarrhea. In: Koda-Kimble MA, Young LY, Kradian WA, et al., eds. *Applied Therapeutics: The Clinical Use of Drugs,* 8th edition. Philadelphia: Lippincott Williams & Wilkins, 2004:62(1–23).

2. (D) The patient presents with nausea and vomiting, dry mucous membranes, and dry skin and is most likely dehydrated. Metoprolol may mask the physiologic response to this (e.g., tachycardia). He needs rehydration with IV fluids such as normal saline or Ringer's lactate, with the addition of potassium and bicarbonate to replenish low electrolytes. For otherwise healthy patients, Salmonella gastroenteritis may be self-limiting, and antibiotic therapy may not be necessary. However, MM is elderly and has other risk factors that could predispose him to bacteremia and more severe complications; therefore, antibiotics are indicated.

   Ref: Anderson JD, Lemke TD, Odell LJ, et al. Gastrointestinal infections and enterotoxigenic poisonings. In: Dipiro JT, Talbert RL, Yee GC, et al., eds. *Pharmacotherapy: A Pathophysiologic Approach,* 5th edition. New York: McGraw-Hill. 2002:1939–1954.

   Ref: Itokazu GS, Bearden DT, Danziger LH. Infectious diarrhea. In: Koda-Kimble MA, Young LY, Kradian WA, et al., eds. *Applied Therapeutics: The Clinical Use of Drugs,* 8th edition. Philadelphia: Lippincott Williams & Wilkins, 2004:62(1–23).

3. (E) Older age (>65 years), gastric surgery, and use of acid-suppressive drugs such as proton-pump inhibitors, antacids, and H_2-blockers, lead to decreased gastric acidity allowing gastrointestinal pathogens such as *Salmonella* to become more invasive. Malignancy (immunodeficiency) is another risk factor for bacteremia.

   Ref: Itokazu GS, Bearden DT, Danziger LH. Infectious diarrhea. In: Koda-Kimble MA, Young LY, Kradian WA, et al., eds. *Applied Therapeutics: The Clinical Use of Drugs,* 8th edition. Philadelphia: Lippincott Williams & Wilkins, 2004:62(1–23).

4. (E) Ampicillin, amoxicillin, Bactrim, fluoroquinolones, third-generation cephalosporins, and azithromycin are effective against *Salmonella* sp. As empiric therapy third-generation cephalosporins (e.g., ceftriaxone or cefotaxime) or fluoroquinolones are recommended to prevent treatment failure because of potentially prevalent multidrug-resistant *Salmonella* sp. However, microbial resistance to the latter agents is emerging, too.

   Ref: Anderson JD, Lemke TD, Odell LJ, et al. Gastrointestinal infections and enterotoxigenic poisonings. In: Dipiro JT, Talbert RL, Yee GC, et al., eds. *Pharmacotherapy: A Pathophysiologic Approach,* 5th edition. New York: McGraw-Hill. 2002: 1939–1954.

   Ref: Itokazu GS, Bearden DT, Danziger LH. Infectious diarrhea. In: Koda-Kimble MA, Young LY, Kradian WA, et al., eds. *Applied Therapeutics: The Clinical Use of Drugs,* 8th edition. Philadelphia: Lippincott Williams & Wilkins, 2004:62(1–23).

5. (B) *Clostridium difficile*-associated diarrhea is a common nosocomial infection, and a major risk factor is prior antibiotic use (within the last few days up to the last 2 months). Clindamycin, ampicillin, and cephalosporins are frequently associated with the development of C-DAD.

   Ref: Anderson JD, Lemke TD, Odell LJ, et al. Gastrointestinal infections and enterotoxigenic poisonings. In: Dipiro JT, Talbert RL, Yee GC, et al., eds. *Pharmacotherapy: A Pathophysiologic Approach,* 5th edition. New York: McGraw-Hill. 2002:1939–1954.

   Ref: Itokazu GS, Bearden DT, Danziger LH. Infectious diarrhea. In: Koda-Kimble MA, Young LY, Kradian WA, et al., eds. *Applied Therapeutics: The Clinical Use of Drugs,* 8th edition. Philadelphia: Lippincott Williams & Wilkins, 2004:62(1–23).

6. (C) Both oral metronidazole and vancomycin are highly effective for C-DAD (>95% response rate). Metronidazole is the drug of choice because it is much less expensive than vancomycin, and vancomycin resistance is of concern.

   Ref: Anderson JD, Lemke TD, Odell LJ, et al. Gastrointestinal infections and enterotoxigenic poisonings. In: Dipiro JT, Talbert RL, Yee GC, et al., eds. *Pharmacotherapy: A Pathophysiologic Approach,* 5th edition. New York: McGraw-Hill. 2002:1939–1954.

   Ref: Itokazu GS, Bearden DT, Danziger LH. Infectious diarrhea. In: Koda-Kimble MA, Young LY, Kradian WA, et al., eds. *Applied Therapeutics: The Clinical Use of Drugs,* 8th edition. Philadelphia: Lippincott Williams & Wilkins, 2004:62(1–23).

7. (C) Metronidazole is known to cause an unpleasant metallic taste and central nervous system reactions such as headaches, dizziness and confusion. It also interacts with alcohol and alcohol-containing medications (Disulfiram-like reaction).

Ref: Itokazu GS, Bearden DT, Danziger LH. Infectious diarrhea. In: Koda-Kimble MA, Young LY, Kradian WA, et al., eds. *Applied Therapeutics: The Clinical Use of Drugs,* 8th edition. Philadelphia: Lippincott Williams & Wilkins, 2004:62(1–23).

8. (B) The best way to prevent TD is to avoid consumption of potentially contaminated food (especially uncooked or raw meat or seafood, and unpeeled fruits or vegetables) and drinks such as unbottled water or ice cubes. The Centers for Disease Control does not recommend routine prophylaxis with antibiotics in patients without major risk factors (e.g., immunocompromised patients, or those with decreased gastric acidity or inflammatory bowel disease). Prophylaxis with bismuth subsalicylate (for a maximum of 3 weeks) is a potential option with a protective efficacy of about 65%.

    Ref: Anderson JD, Lemke TD, Odell LJ, et al. Gastrointestinal infections and enterotoxigenic poisonings. In: Dipiro JT, Talbert RL, Yee GC, et al., eds. *Pharmacotherapy: A Pathophysiologic Approach,* 5th edition. New York: McGraw-Hill. 2002:1939–1954.

    Ref: Itokazu GS, Bearden DT, Danziger LH. Infectious diarrhea. In: Koda-Kimble MA, Young LY, Kradian WA, et al., eds. *Applied Ther-*

apeutics: The Clinical Use of Drugs, 8th edition. Philadelphia: Lippincott Williams & Wilkins, 2004:62(1–23).

9. (E) The significant amount of salicylate in Bismuth subsalicylate (Pepto-Bismol®) may contribute to salicylate toxicity in older patients, people who take aspirin products, and those with bleeding disorders or renal dysfunction.

    Ref: Itokazu GS, Bearden DT, Danziger LH. Infectious diarrhea. In: Koda-Kimble MA, Young LY, Kradian WA, et al., eds. *Applied Therapeutics: The Clinical Use of Drugs,* 8th edition. Philadelphia: Lippincott Williams & Wilkins, 2004:62(1–23).

10. (D) Both Bactrim and fluoroquinolones have been shown to shorten the duration and severity of TD. Fluoroquinolones are preferred because of the worldwide increasing antimicrobial resistance of enteropathogens against Bactrim.

    Ref: Itokazu GS, Bearden DT, Danziger LH. Infectious diarrhea. In: Koda-Kimble MA, Young LY, Kradian WA, et al., eds. *Applied Therapeutics: The Clinical Use of Drugs,* 8th edition. Philadelphia: Lippincott Williams & Wilkins, 2004:62(1–23).

PATIENT   PROFILE   209

ANTICOAGULATION

ANSWERS

1. (E) All three of these factors are risk factors for developing a post-surgical DVT.

    Ref: Wittkowsky AK. Thrombosis. In: Young YL, Koda-Kimble MA, eds. *Applied Therapeutics: The Clinical Use of Drugs.* Vancouver, WA: Applied Therapeutics; 1995:12–7, 12–11.

2. (D) Possible interventions would include low-dose subcutaneous heparin, intermittent pneumatic compression, or low intensity warfarin.

    Ref: Wittkowsky AK. Thrombosis. In: Young YL, Koda-Kimble MA, eds. *Applied Therapeutics: The Clinical Use of Drugs.* Vancouver, WA: Applied Therapeutics; 1995:12–11.

3. (E) Low-dose heparin prophylaxis does not warrant laboratory monitoring like treatment with heparin.

    Ref: Wittkowsky AK. Thrombosis. In: Young YL, Koda-Kimble MA, eds. *Applied Therapeutics: The Clinical Use of Drugs.* Vancouver, WA: Applied Therapeutics; 1995:12–11.

4. (D) In order to evaluate the effectiveness of the prophylactic heparin, MS should be monitored for signs and symptoms of a DVT and a PE because a dislodged DVT can cause a PE.

    Ref: Wittkowsky AK. Thrombosis. In: Young YL, Koda-Kimble MA, eds. *Applied Therapeutics: The Clinical Use of Drugs.* Vancouver, WA: Applied Therapeutics; 1995:12–7, 12–11.

PATIENT   PROFILE   210

TUBERCULOSIS

ANSWERS

1. (B) Tuberculosis is acquired through inhalation of infectious airborne pathogens.

Ref: Official Joint Statement of the American Thoracic Society, Centers for Disease Control and Prevention and the Infectious Diseases Society of America. Treatment of tuberculosis. *Am J Resp Crit Care Med* 2003;167:603–662.

2. (D) The Mantoux tuberculin skin test is an intradermal injection of 5 tuberculin units of PPD of killed tubercula bacilli. The test usually is administered on the inner forearm. The area tested is examined induration and the result interpreted by a trained health care provider 48 to 72 hours after injection.

Ref: Official Joint Statement of the American Thoracic Society, Centers for Disease Control and Prevention and the Infectious Diseases Society of America. Treatment of tuberculosis. *Am J Resp Crit Care Med* 2003;167:603–662.

3. (A) Pyridoxine (vitamin B_6) should be given with isoniazid to persons who have conditions in which neuropathy is common. It also should be given to pregnant patients and persons with a history of seizure disorders.

Ref: Official Joint Statement of the American Thoracic Society, Centers for Disease Control and Prevention and the Infectious Diseases Society of America. Treatment of tuberculosis. *Am J Resp Crit Care Med* 2003;167:603–662.

4. (D) Optic neuritis is most toxic effect of ethambutol.

Ref: Official Joint Statement of the American Thoracic Society, Centers for Disease Control and Prevention and the Infectious Diseases Society of America. Treatment of tuberculosis. *Am J Resp Crit Care Med* 2003;167:603–662.

5. (D) Rifabutin belongs to the rifamycin B class and can potentially cause hematologic toxicity.

Ref: Official Joint Statement of the American Thoracic Society, Centers for Disease Control and Prevention and the Infectious Diseases Society of America. Treatment of tuberculosis. *Am J Resp Crit Care Med* 2003;167:603–662.

6. (B) The addition of rifampin, which is a potent inducer of CYP450, may decrease phenytoin serum concentrations.

7. (A) Hepatoxicity is the most toxic effect of pyrazinamide.

Ref: Official Joint Statement of the American Thoracic Society, Centers for Disease Control and Prevention and the Infectious Diseases Society of America. Treatment of tuberculosis. *Am J Resp Crit Care Med* 2003;167:603–662.

8. (B) Although rare, progressive liver dysfunction, jaundice, bilirubinuria, and severe and sometimes fatal hepatitis have been associated with the use of isoniazid.

Ref: Official Joint Statement of the American Thoracic Society, Centers for Disease Control and Prevention and the Infectious Diseases Society of America. Treatment of tuberculosis. *Am J Resp Crit Care Med* 2003;167:603–662.

9. (D) The main toxicities associated with streptomycin, an aminoglycoside, are nephrotoxicity and ototoxicity.

Ref: Official Joint Statement of the American Thoracic Society, Centers for Disease Control and Prevention and the Infectious Diseases Society of America. Treatment of tuberculosis. *Am J Resp Crit Care Med* 2003;167:603–662.

10. (D) Rifampin, a potent inducer of hepatic microsomal enzymes, may decrease the efficacy of oral contraceptives. This agent may impart an orange discoloration to the urine, feces, sputum, tears, and sweat and may permanently discolor soft contact lenses.

Ref: Official Joint Statement of the American Thoracic Society, Centers for Disease Control and Prevention and the Infectious Diseases Society of America. Treatment of tuberculosis. *Am J Resp Crit Care Med* 2003;167:603–662.

PATIENT PROFILE 211

CHRONIC OBSTRUCTIVE PULMONARY DISEASE

ANSWERS

1. (C) Stage II moderate COPD owing to his FEV_1/FVC is <70% and FEV_1 is 75% of personnel best

Ref: Global Initiative for Chronic Obstructive Lung Disease. Global strategy for the diagnosis management, and prevention of chronic obstructive pulmonary disease. Updated 2003. Available at: *http://www.goldcopd.com.* Accessed November 1, 2004.

2. (E) Albuterol as needed, Ipratropium inhaler two puffs by mouth three times a day, and rehabilitation. Albuterol for as needed use, Ipratropium is the first-line chronic agent, and rehabilitation is recommended for all patients.

Ref: Global Initiative for Chronic Obstructive Lung Disease. Global strategy for the diagnosis management, and prevention of chronic obstructive pulmonary disease. Updated 2003. Available at: *http://www.goldcopd.com.* Accessed November 1, 2004.

3. (B) AP's goal of therapy is attain an SaO_2 of at least 90%.

Ref: Global Initiative for Chronic Obstructive Lung Disease. Global strategy for the diagnosis management, and prevention of chronic obstructive pulmonary disease. Updated 2003. Available at: *http://www.goldcopd.com.* Accessed November 1, 2004.

4. (A) Antitussives, because it is beneficial for COPD patients to cough up mucus.

Ref: Global Initiative for Chronic Obstructive Lung Disease. Global strategy for the diagnosis management, and prevention of chronic obstructive pulmonary disease. Updated 2003. Available at: *http://www.goldcopd.com*. Accessed November 1, 2004.

5. (D) Ipratropium because of the propellant's having a soy component in the inhaler.

Ref: Global Initiative for Chronic Obstructive Lung Disease. Global strategy for the diagnosis management, and prevention of chronic obstructive pulmonary disease. Updated 2003. Available at: *http://www.goldcopd.com*. Accessed November 1, 2004.

6. (A) Daily prophylactic antibiotic therapy is not justified because of the risk of resistance.

Ref: Global Initiative for Chronic Obstructive Lung Disease. Global strategy for the diagnosis management, and prevention of chronic obstructive pulmonary disease. Updated 2003. Available at: *http://www.goldcopd.com*. Accessed November 1, 2004.

7. (A) Regular treatment with inhaled corticosteroids is appropriate when AP's FEV$_1$ <50% predicted because of benefit being seen with these medications used at this stage of COPD.

Ref: Global Initiative for Chronic Obstructive Lung Disease. Global strategy for the diagnosis management, and prevention of chronic obstructive pulmonary disease. Updated 2003. Available at: *http://www.goldcopd.com*. Accessed November 1, 2004.

8. (C) Flunisolide inhaler two puffs by mouth twice daily. This is the only option with appropriate dosing of the product.

Ref: Global Initiative for Chronic Obstructive Lung Disease. Global strategy for the diagnosis management, and prevention of chronic obstructive pulmonary disease. Updated 2003. Available at: *http://www.goldcopd.com*. Accessed November 1, 2004.

9. (D) Nicotine lozenge and nicotine sublingual tablet

Ref: Global Initiative for Chronic Obstructive Lung Disease. Global strategy for the diagnosis management, and prevention of chronic obstructive pulmonary disease. Updated 2003. Available at: *http://www.goldcopd.com*. Accessed November 1, 2004.

10. (E) Zyban®, nortriptyline, and clonidine have all been used to some extent for smoking cessation.

Ref: Global Initiative for Chronic Obstructive Lung Disease. Global strategy for the diagnosis management, and prevention of chronic obstructive pulmonary disease. Updated 2003. Available at: *http://www.goldcopd.com*. Accessed November 1, 2004.

PATIENT PROFILE 212
HYPERCHOLESTEROLEMIA

ANSWERS

1. (B) Identidex is the preferred database to identify a drug based on tablet characteristics.

Ref: Rumack BH, Bird PE, Gelman CR, et al (eds): Identidex ® System. Micromedex, Inc., Englewood, Colorado.

2. (A) HH's has no positive cardiovascular risk factors besides hypercholesterolemia.

Ref: McKenney JM. Dyslipidemias. In: Young YL, Koda-Kimble MA, eds. *Applied Therapeutics: The Clinical Use of Drugs.* Vancouver, WA: Applied Therapeutics; 1995:9–11.

3. (C) Since HH has no cardiovascular risk factors and no history of CVD, her LDL goal is <160 mg/dL.

Ref: McKenney JM. Dyslipidemias. In: Young YL, Koda-Kimble MA, eds. *Applied Therapeutics: The Clinical Use of Drugs.* Vancouver, WA: Applied Therapeutics; 1995:9–14.

4. (B) Niacin would be contraindicated due to HH's history of PUD.

Ref: McKenney JM. Dyslipidemias. In: Young YL, Koda-Kimble MA, eds. *Applied Therapeutics: The Clinical Use of Drugs.* Vancouver, WA: Applied Therapeutics; 1995:9–17.

5. (A) Estrogens have the following positive effects on lipoprotein profiles: decreases LDL and increases HDL. They may also increase triglycerides but this is a negative effect.

Ref: McKenney JM. Dyslipidemias. In: Young YL, Koda-Kimble MA, eds. *Applied Therapeutics: The Clinical Use of Drugs.* Vancouver, WA: Applied Therapeutics; 1995:9-17–9-18.

6. (B) The benefits of estrogen therapy (relief of menopausal symptoms, prevention of osteoporosis, and cardioprotective effects) outweigh the risk of breast cancer especially in a patients without a family history of breast cancer. Since HH's uterus is not intact, she does not need the addition of progestins to her estrogen.

Ref: McKenney JM. Dyslipidemias. In: Young YL, Koda-Kimble MA, eds. *Applied Therapeutics: The Clinical Use of Drugs.* Vancouver, WA: Applied Therapeutics; 1995:9–18.

PATIENT PROFILE 213
99MTC-MAA CONSIDERATIONS

ANSWERS

1. A

Ref: Saha GB. *Fundamentals of Nuclear Pharmacy*, 4th edition. New York: Springer-Verlag, 1997:252–253.

2. C

Ref: Saha GB. *Fundamentals of Nuclear Pharmacy*, 4th edition. New York: Springer-Verlag, 1997:153–158.

3. E

Ref: Saha GB. *Fundamentals of Nuclear Pharmacy*, 4th edition. New York: Springer-Verlag, 1997:113.

4. A

Ref: Saha GB. *Fundamentals of Nuclear Pharmacy*, 4th edition. New York: Springer-Verlag, 1997:43–45.

5. D

Ref: Saha GB. *Fundamentals of Nuclear Pharmacy*, 4th edition. New York: Springer-Verlag, 1997:16.

6. E

Ref: Saha GB. *Fundamentals of Nuclear Pharmacy*, 4th edition. New York: Springer-Verlag, 1997:9.

7. C

Ref: Zatz. *J. Pharmaceutical Calculations*, 3rd edition. New York: John Wiley & Sons, 1995:311.

8. A

Ref: Saha GB. *Fundamentals of Nuclear Pharmacy*, 4th edition. New York: Springer-Verlag, 1997:13.

9. D

Ref: Saha GB. *Fundamentals of Nuclear Pharmacy*, 4th edition. New York: Springer-Verlag, 1997:113.

10. B

Ref: Saha GB. *Fundamentals of Nuclear Pharmacy*, 4th edition. New York: Springer-Verlag, 1997:11.

PATIENT PROFILE 214
POST-TRAUMATIC STRESS DISORDER

ANSWERS

1. (D) Most people who are exposed to a traumatic event do not develop PTSD. Post-traumatic stress disorder occurs in individuals who have experienced a traumatic event and it involves re-experiencing the event (e.g., dreams, nightmares, flashbacks, recurrent thoughts or images) or intense distress associated with the traumatic event. Significant impairment in some aspect of daily functioning can result.

Ref: Augustin SG. Anxiety disorders. In: Koda-Kimble MA, Young LY, Kradjan WA, Guglielmo BJ, eds. *Applied Therapeutics: The Clinical Use of Drugs,* 8th edition. Baltimore, MD: Lippincott Williams & Wilkins, 2005:1–47.

2. (B) PTSD is twice as common in women than in men, although overall, men are exposed to trauma more often than women. In general, people who experience traumas involving personal assault (rape, combat) are associated with much higher conditional risks of developing PTSD than other types of trauma.

Ref: Augustin SG. Anxiety disorders. In: Koda-Kimble MA, Young LY, Kradjan WA, Guglielmo BJ, eds. *Applied Therapeutics: The Clinical Use of Drugs,* 8th edition. Baltimore, MD: Lippincott Williams & Wilkins, 2005:1–47.

3. (E) SSRIs are considered first-line medications in the treatment of patients with PTSD. Benzodiazepines are generally ineffective in treating patients with PTSD. They may be useful in managing sleep disturbances during the early weeks after trauma but chronic use may be detrimental. Atypical antipsychotic agents can be used to treat PTSD-related psychotic symptoms and sleep disturbances but are not useful for treating core PTSD symptoms.

Ref: Augustin SG. Anxiety disorders. In: Koda-Kimble MA, Young LY, Kradjan WA, Guglielmo BJ, eds. *Applied Therapeutics: The Clinical Use of Drugs,* 8th edition. Baltimore, MD: Lippincott Williams & Wilkins, 2005:1–47.

4. (A) Sertraline is an SSRI and is FDA approved for the treatment of PTSD. All other statements are false.

Ref: Augustin SG. Anxiety disorders. In: Koda-Kimble MA, Young LY, Kradjan WA, Guglielmo BJ, eds. *Applied Therapeutics: The Clinical Use of Drugs,* 8th edition. Baltimore, MD: Lippincott Williams & Wilkins, 2005:1–47.

5. (A) Low initial doses of an SSRI are recommended in PTSD. Sertraline should be started at 25 mg per day and gradually increased to a target dosage range of 100 to 150 mg per day, based on patient response and tolerance.

Ref: Augustin SG. Anxiety disorders. In: Koda-Kimble MA, Young LY, Kradjan WA, Guglielmo BJ, eds. *Applied Therapeutics: The Clinical Use of Drugs,* 8th edition. Baltimore, MD: Lippincott Williams & Wilkins, 2005:1–47.

6. (D) The brand name for sertraline is Zoloft (Prozac = fluoxetine; Celexa = citalopram; Geodon = ziprasidone; Effexor = venlafaxine).

Ref: Augustin SG. Anxiety disorders. In: Koda-Kimble MA, Young LY, Kradjan WA, Guglielmo BJ, eds. *Applied Therapeutics: The Clinical Use of Drugs,* 8th edition. Baltimore, MD: Lippincott Williams & Wilkins, 2005:1–47.

7. (E) Diazepam is a benzodiazepine. The other medications are SSRIs. See answer to Question 3.

Ref: Augustin SG. Anxiety disorders. In: Koda-Kimble MA, Young LY, Kradjan WA, Guglielmo BJ, eds. *Applied Therapeutics: The Clinical Use of Drugs,* 8th edition. Baltimore, MD: Lippincott Williams & Wilkins, 2005:1–47.

8. (D) Response of PTSD symptoms to pharmacotherapy occurs gradually and may take 8 to 12 weeks or longer. Partial response at 12 weeks of treatment may be followed by full remission after several more months of therapy. An adequate time period should be allowed to fully determine the response to a particular medication before it is discontinued or other medications are added to the regimen.

Ref: Augustin SG. Anxiety disorders. In: Koda-Kimble MA, Young LY, Kradjan WA, Guglielmo BJ, eds. *Applied Therapeutics: The Clinical Use of Drugs,* 8th edition. Baltimore, MD: Lippincott Williams & Wilkins, 2005:1–47.

9. (D) Nonpharmacologic therapies (e.g., CBT) alone may be appropriate for the initial treatment of mild symptoms of PTSD. Pharmacotherapy, either alone or in combination with CBT, is usually recommended for patients with moderate to severe symptoms of PTSD.

Ref: Augustin SG. Anxiety disorders. In: Koda-Kimble MA, Young LY, Kradjan WA, Guglielmo BJ, eds. *Applied Therapeutics: The Clinical Use of Drugs,* 8th edition. Baltimore, MD: Lippincott Williams & Wilkins, 2005:1–47.

10. (E) For patients who respond to pharmacologic treatment, the medication should be continued for an additional 6 to 12 months for acute cases (when symptoms were present <3 months before treatment) and 12 to 24 months for chronic cases (when symptoms lasted >3 months before treatment). GN had been experiencing his symptoms for 2 months prior to treatment and should continue an additional 6 to 12 months after response. Long-term SSRI treatment can prevent relapse of PTSD, especially in those who show good response during the first 3 months of therapy.

Ref: Augustin SG. Anxiety disorders. In: Koda-Kimble MA, Young LY, Kradjan WA, Guglielmo BJ, eds. *Applied Therapeutics: The Clinical Use of Drugs,* 8th edition. Baltimore, MD: Lippincott Williams & Wilkins, 2005:1–47.

PATIENT PROFILE 215
HYPERCHOLESTEROLEMIA

ANSWERS

1. (C) Martindale is the preferred reference to use to identify foreign drugs.

Ref: Martindale: The Complete Drug Reference. 32nd ed. Parfitt, K, ed. London, England: The Pharmaceutical Press, 1999.

2. (A) Since TA has a history of CVD, his LDL goal in <100 mg/dL.

Ref: McKenney JM. Dyslipidemias. In: Young YL, Koda-Kimble MA, eds. *Applied Therapeutics: The Clinical Use of Drugs.* Vancouver, WA: Applied Therapeutics; 1995:9–14.

3. (B) Smoking increases free fatty acids as well as VLDL and decreases HDL.

Ref: DeSimone EM et al. Nicotine and Caffeine Abuse. In: Young YL, Koda-Kimble MA, eds. *Applied Therapeutics: The Clinical Use of Drugs.* Vancouver, WA: Applied Therapeutics; 1995: 85–4.

4. (D) Alpha blockers may decrease total cholesterol and triglycerides.

Ref: McKenney JM. Dyslipidemias. In: Young YL, Koda-Kimble MA, eds. *Applied Therapeutics: The Clinical Use of Drugs.* Vancouver, WA: Applied Therapeutics; 1995:9–12.

5. (D) Routine monitoring of CPK is unnecessary. A baseline CPK should be obtained prior to initiation of therapy and repeated if the patient has unexplained symptoms of myopathy (muscle aches, soreness, or weakness).

Ref: McKenney JM. Dyslipidemias. In: Young YL, Koda-Kimble MA, eds. *Applied Therapeutics: The Clinical Use of Drugs.* Vancouver, WA: Applied Therapeutics; 1995:9-16–9-17.

6. (A) The "statins" may cause hepatotoxicity manifested as elevations in liver function tests and other clinical findings.

Ref: McKenney JM. Dyslipidemias. In: Young YL, Koda-Kimble MA, eds. *Applied Therapeutics: The Clinical Use of Drugs.* Vancouver, WA: Applied Therapeutics; 1995:9–16.

7. (C) The dose of lovastatin is maximized; therefore, a second agent such as a bile acid resin must be added.

Ref: McKenney JM. Dyslipidemias. In: Young YL, Koda-Kimble MA, eds. *Applied Therapeutics: The Clinical Use of Drugs.* Vancouver, WA: Applied Therapeutics; 1995:9–16, 9–18.

8. (B) If a change in therapy occurs, the lipid profile should be rechecked every 4–8 weeks until control is achieved.

Ref: McKenney JM. Dyslipidemias. In: Young YL, Koda-Kimble MA, eds. *Applied Therapeutics: The Clinical Use of Drugs.* Vancouver, WA: Applied Therapeutics; 1995:9–17.

9. (E) All are benefits of smoking cessation.

    Ref: DeSimone EM et al. Nicotine and Caffeine Abuse. In: Young YL, Koda-Kimble MA, eds. *Applied Therapeutics: The Clinical Use of Drugs.* Vancouver, WA: Applied Therapeutics; 1995:85-4–85-5.

10. (A) Patients who have a history of CVD should be started on a lower strength patch such as 14 mg/day versus 21 mg/day.

Ref: DeSimone EM et al. Nicotine and Caffeine Abuse. In: Young YL, Koda-Kimble MA, eds. *Applied Therapeutics: The Clinical Use of Drugs.* Vancouver, WA: Applied Therapeutics; 1995: 85–6.

11. (E) All are important components of a smoking cessation counseling session.

    Ref: DeSimone EM et al. Nicotine and Caffeine Abuse. In: Young YL, Koda-Kimble MA, eds. *Applied Therapeutics: The Clinical Use of Drugs.* Vancouver, WA: Applied Therapeutics; 1995:85-6–85-7.

PATIENT PROFILE 216

METABOLIC SYNDROME

ANSWERS

1. (A) A patient with type 2 diabetes mellitus is considered to be at the same risk as a patient with documented coronary heart disease; thus, the LDL goal is <100 mg/dL.

    Ref: Third Report of the National Cholesterol Education Program (NCEP) Expert Panel on Detection, Evaluation, and Treatment of High Blood Cholesterol in Adults (Adult Treatment Panel III) final report. *Circulation* 2002;106:343–421.

2. (E) MJ exhibits five risk factors for metabolic syndrome: triglycerides >150 mg/dL, waist circumference >40 inches, HDL <40 mg/dL, BP >130/>85 mm Hg, and a fasting glucose >110 mg/dL.

    Ref: Third Report of the National Cholesterol Education Program (NCEP) Expert Panel on Detection, Evaluation, and Treatment of High Blood Cholesterol in Adults (Adult Treatment Panel III) final report. *Circulation* 2002;106:343–421.

3. (C) A patience must exhibit at least three risk factors for metabolic syndrome to be diagnosed as having metabolic syndrome.

    Ref: Third Report of the National Cholesterol Education Program (NCEP) Expert Panel on Detection, Evaluation, and Treatment of High Blood Cholesterol in Adults (Adult Treatment Panel III) final report. *Circulation* 2002;106:343–421.

4. (D) Rosuvastatin has the ability to lower serum LDL levels and elevate serum HDL levels greater than the other statins.

    Ref: Implications of Recent Clinical Trials for the National Cholesterol Education Program Adult Treatment Panel III Guidelines. *Circulation* 2004;110:227–239.

5. (E) Niacin is associated with causing hyperglycemia; thus, it may worsen MJ's diabetes.

    Ref: Third Report of the National Cholesterol Education Program (NCEP) Expert Panel on Detection, Evaluation, and Treatment of

High Blood Cholesterol in Adults (Adult Treatment Panel III) final report. *Circulation* 2002;106:343–421.

6. (A) Fenofibrate would be the best choice because it will help lower MJ's serum LDL and also may help elevate his HDL.

    Ref: Third Report of the National Cholesterol Education Program (NCEP) Expert Panel on Detection, Evaluation, and Treatment of High Blood Cholesterol in Adults (Adult Treatment Panel III) final report. *Circulation* 2002;106:343–421.

7. (D) The maximum daily dose of fenofibrate is 200 mg.

    Ref: Third Report of the National Cholesterol Education Program (NCEP) Expert Panel on Detection, Evaluation, and Treatment of High Blood Cholesterol in Adults (Adult Treatment Panel III) final report. *Circulation* 2002;106:343–421.

8. (A) Both fibrates and statins may cause myopathy; thus, when used together they may increase the risk of myopathy.

    Ref: Third Report of the National Cholesterol Education Program (NCEP) Expert Panel on Detection, Evaluation, and Treatment of High Blood Cholesterol in Adults (Adult Treatment Panel III) final report. *Circulation* 2002;106:343–421.

9. (C) MJ needs to add aspirin to his regimen to help decrease the risk of having AMI.

    Ref: Third Report of the National Cholesterol Education Program (NCEP) Expert Panel on Detection, Evaluation, and Treatment of High Blood Cholesterol in Adults (Adult Treatment Panel III) final report. *Circulation* 2002;106:343–421.

10. (B) Fluvastatin has been shown to lower serum LDL levels the least when given in standard daily doses.

    Ref: Third Report of the National Cholesterol Education Program (NCEP) Expert Panel on Detection, Evaluation, and Treatment of High Blood Cholesterol in Adults (Adult Treatment Panel III) final report. *Circulation* 2002;106:343–421.

OSTEOPOROSIS

ANSWERS

1. (A) DEXA is considered the "gold standard" for osteoporosis diagnosis. Magnetic resonance imaging is not practical and the others are appropriate for screening purposes.

    Ref: O'Connell MB, Elliott ME. Osteoporosis and osteomalacia. In: DiPiro JT, Talbert RL, Yee GC, et al., eds. *Pharmacotherapy: A Pathophysiologic Approach,* 5th edition. New York: McGraw-Hill; 2002:1599–1621.

2. (E) TH's age, family history, and thyroid replacement therapy are all risk factors for the development of osteoporosis.

    Ref: O'Connell MB, Elliott ME. Osteoporosis and osteomalacia. In: DiPiro JT, Talbert RL, Yee GC, et al., eds. *Pharmacotherapy: A Pathophysiologic Approach,* 5th edition. New York: McGraw-Hill;2002:1599–1621.

3. (E) Chronic back pain, DEXA results, and loss of height all indicate the presence or severity of osteoporosis in TH.

    Ref: O'Connell MB, Elliott ME. Osteoporosis and osteomalacia. In: DiPiro JT, Talbert RL, Yee GC, et al., eds. *Pharmacotherapy: A Pathophysiologic Approach,* 5th edition. New York: McGraw-Hill;2002:1599–1621.

4. (E) Goals of osteoporosis treatment include prevent fractures, optimize physical function, relieve symptoms, and stabilize or increase bone mineral density.

    Ref: AACE Osteoporosis Task Force. American association of clinical endocrinologists medical guidelines for clinical practice for the prevention and treatment of postmenopausal osteoporosis: 2001 edition, with selected updates for 2003. *Endocr Pract* 2003;9: 544–564.

5. (E) TH's daily calcium requirement is 1200 mg because her age is greater than or equal to 50 years.

    Ref: O'Connell MB, Elliott ME. Osteoporosis and osteomalacia. In: DiPiro JT, Talbert RL, Yee GC, et al., eds. *Pharmacotherapy: A Pathophysiologic Approach,* 5th edition. New York: McGraw-Hill; 2002:1599–1621.

6. (E) TH's daily vitamin D requirement is 600 IU because her age is greater than or equal to 71 years.

    Ref: O'Connell MB, Elliott ME. Osteoporosis and osteomalacia. In: DiPiro JT, Talbert RL, Yee GC, et al., eds. *Pharmacotherapy: A Pathophysiologic Approach,* 5th edition. New York: McGraw-Hill; 2002:1599–1621.

7. (D) Raloxifene is the best therapeutic option for TH. Alendronate is contraindicated because TH has an esophageal stricture; calcitonin decreases the risk of vertebral fractures less than raloxifene; estrogen therapy is not recommended for osteoporosis treatment; and teriparatide is given subcutaneously and the experience of its use is limited.

    Ref: AACE Osteoporosis Task Force. American association of clinical endocrinologists medical guidelines for clinical practice for the prevention and treatment of postmenopausal osteoporosis: 2001 edition, with selected updates for 2003. *Endocr Pract* 2003;9: 544–564.

8. (D) Calcitonin is derived from salmon calcitonin.

    Ref: Calcitonins (Drug Monograph). In: Klasco RK, ed. DRUGDEX® System. Thomson MICROMEDEX®, Greenwood Village, CO (Edition expires 9/2004).

9. (D) Thromboembolism may occur with raloxifene therapy as so can hot flashes, leg cramps, and peripheral edema.

    Ref: AACE Osteoporosis Task Force. American association of clinical endocrinologists medical guidelines for clinical practice for the prevention and treatment of postmenopausal osteoporosis: 2001 edition, with selected updates for 2003. *Endocr Pract* 2003;9: 544–564.

10. (D) For individuals on therapy, the AACE recommendation for bone mineral density follow-up is a measurement every year for the first 2 years. Yearly follow-up should occur until stable bone mass is observed, at which time testing every 2 years should occur.

    Ref: AACE Osteoporosis Task Force. American association of clinical endocrinologists medical guidelines for clinical practice for the prevention and treatment of postmenopausal osteoporosis: 2001 edition, with selected updates for 2003. *Endocr Pract* 2003;9: 544–564.

PATIENT PROFILE 218
ALZHEIMER'S DISEASE

ANSWERS

1. (D) The diagnostic criteria for Alzheimer's disease include progressive cognitive decline, as reported by the patient or family members, and the onset must not be related to any other type of central nervous system disorder. The cognitive deficits must include memory loss and at least one of the following: aphasia, agnosia, or apraxia. Other diagnostic tests may include computed tomography, positron emission tomography, mini mental status examinations (MMSE), hematology, magnetic resonance imaging, and B$_{12}$, folate, and thyroid function tests.

Ref: Difilippi JL, Crismon ML, Clark WR. Alzheimer's disease. In: DiPiro JT, Talbert RL, Yee GC, et al., eds. *Pharmacotherapy: A Pathophysiologic Approach,* 5th edition. New York: McGraw-Hill, 2002:1165–1182.

2. (B) The loss of cholinergic cells is believed to be the result of Alzheimer's disease. Drug therapy with acetylcholinesterase inhibitors is believed to slow the progression of the disease only and minimize or improve symptoms.

Ref: Difilippi JL, Crismon ML, Clark WR. Alzheimer's disease. In: DiPiro JT, Talbert RL, Yee GC, et al., eds. *Pharmacotherapy: A Pathophysiologic Approach,* 5th edition. New York: McGraw-Hill, 2002:1165–1182.

3. (A) The starting dose of donepezil is 5 mg by mouth in the morning; the dose may be increased to 10 mg after 4 to 6 weeks if the side effects are tolerated.

Ref: Difilippi JL, Crismon ML, Clark WR. Alzheimer's disease. In: DiPiro JT, Talbert RL, Yee GC, et al., eds. *Pharmacotherapy: A Pathophysiologic Approach,* 5th edition. New York: McGraw-Hill, 2002:1165–1182.

4. (D) Donepezil is a reversible inhibitor of acetylcholinesterase, thereby decreasing the breakdown of acetylcholine. The cholinesterase inhibitors are the first-line treatment for Alzheimer's disease. They have shown improvement of cognitive function in patients with mild to moderately severe Alzheimer's disease.

Ref: Difilippi JL, Crismon ML, Clark WR. Alzheimer's disease. In: DiPiro JT, Talbert RL, Yee GC, et al., eds. *Pharmacotherapy: A Pathophysiologic Approach,* 5th edition. New York: McGraw-Hill, 2002:1165–1182.

5. (A) The common side effects of donepezil include nausea, vomiting, and diarrhea. Other side effects include headache, dizziness, and insomnia. The insomnia necessitates the administration of donepezil in the morning.

Ref: Difilippi JL, Crismon ML, Clark WR. Alzheimer's disease. In: DiPiro JT, Talbert RL, Yee GC, et al., eds. *Pharmacotherapy: A Pathophysiologic Approach,* 5th edition. New York: McGraw-Hill, 2002:1165–1182.

6. (B) MS has been forgetting to take her furosemide. She also did not refill the furosemide prescription between 7/2/04 and 8/21/04. This is an indication of inadvertent noncompliance, most likely resulting from her memory loss.

Ref: Difilippi JL, Crismon ML, Clark WR. Alzheimer's disease. In: DiPiro JT, Talbert RL, Yee GC, et al., eds. *Pharmacotherapy: A Pathophysiologic Approach,* 5th edition. New York: McGraw-Hill, 2002:1165–1182.

7. (D) There is currently no cure for Alzheimer's disease. Drug therapy can be effective in slowing the progression and maintaining a degree of independence. Because of MS's age and other medical conditions, she needs her daughter's assistance and must give up her independent living arrangement.

Ref: Difilippi JL, Crismon ML, Clark WR. Alzheimer's disease. In: DiPiro JT, Talbert RL, Yee GC, et al., eds. *Pharmacotherapy: A Pathophysiologic Approach,* 5th edition. New York: McGraw-Hill, 2002:1165–1182.

8. (C) Donepezil therapy should be continued for 3 months and family members and caretakers should monitor the patient for improvement in cognitive function. If there is no improvement after 3 months the patient may be switched to an alternative cholinesterase inhibitor.

Ref: Williams BR. Geriatric dementias. In: Koda-Kimble MA, Young LY, Kradjan WA, Guglielmo BJ, et al., eds. *Applied Therapeutics: The Clinical Use of Drugs,* 8th edition. Philadelphia: Lippincott Williams & Wilkins, 2005:1–20.

9. (D) Namenda® was recently approved as an adjunctive therapy for Alzheimer's disease. Its mechanism as an NMDA receptor antagonist is believed to decrease levels of glutamate in the central nervous system decreasing cell death.

Ref: Williams BR. Geriatric dementias. In: Koda-Kimble MA, Young LY, Kradjan WA, Guglielmo BJ, et al., eds. *Applied Therapeutics: The Clinical Use of Drugs,* 8th edition. Philadelphia: Lippincott Williams & Wilkins, 2005:1–20.

10. (B) Gingko biloba is an herbal product that is proposed to improve the memory by functioning as an antioxidant. Unfortunately because herbal products are not

Food and Drug Administration approved, gingko biloba cannot be recommended for patients with Alzheimer's disease.

Ref: Difilippi JL, Crismon ML, Clark WR. Alzheimer's disease. In: DiPiro JT, Talbert RL, Yee GC, et al., eds. *Pharmacotherapy: A Pathophysiologic Approach,* 5th edition. New York: McGraw-Hill, 2002:1165–1182.

PATIENT PROFILE 219

TYPE 1 DIABETES

ANSWERS

1. (C) Within days or weeks after initial diagnosis, many patients with type 1 diabetes experience an apparent remission, which is reflected by decreased blood glucose concentrations and markedly decreased insulin requirements. This is called the honeymoon phase.

   Ref: Carlisle BA, Kroon LA, Koda-Kimble MA. Diabetes mellitus. In: Koda-Kimble MA, Young LY, Kradjan WA, et al., eds. *Applied Therapeutics: The Clinical Use of Drugs,* 8th edition. Baltimore: Lippincott Williams & Wilkins, 2005:1–86.

2. (B) A diagnosis of diabetes can be made when one of the following is present: classic signs and symptoms of diabetes combined with a random plasma glucose ≥200 mg/dL, a fasting plasma glucose (FPG) ≥126 mg/dL, a venous plasma glucose concentration >200 mg/dL at 2 hours and >200 mg/d at least one other time (0.5, 1, 1.5 hours) after a standard oral glucose challenge (75 mg glucose).

   Ref: Carlisle BA, Kroon LA, Koda-Kimble MA. Diabetes mellitus. In: Koda-Kimble MA, Young LY, Kradjan WA, et al., eds. *Applied Therapeutics: The Clinical Use of Drugs,* 8th edition. Baltimore: Lippincott Williams & Wilkins, 2005:1–86.

3. (A) Urine ketones should be evaluated when glucose concentrations consistently exceed 300 mg/dL or during acute illness to check for the presence of ketoacidosis.

   Ref: Carlisle BA, Kroon LA, Koda-Kimble MA. Diabetes mellitus. In: Koda-Kimble MA, Young LY, Kradjan WA, et al., eds. *Applied Therapeutics: The Clinical Use of Drugs,* 8th edition. Baltimore: Lippincott Williams & Wilkins, 2005:1–86.

4. (A) The rate-limiting step of insulin activity after subcutaneous administration is the absorption of insulin from the injection site, which depends on the type of insulin administered, as well as a multitude of other factors, including inter-patient variability.

   Ref: Carlisle BA, Kroon LA, Koda-Kimble MA. Diabetes mellitus. In: Koda-Kimble MA, Young LY, Kradjan WA, et al., eds. *Applied Therapeutics: The Clinical Use of Drugs,* 8th edition. Baltimore: Lippincott Williams & Wilkins, 2005:1–86.

5. (C) Lispro is a rapid-acting insulin analog with an onset of 15 minutes, peak action in 30 to 90 minutes, and a duration of action of 4 to 5 hours.

Ref: Carlisle BA, Kroon LA, Koda-Kimble MA. Diabetes mellitus. In: Koda-Kimble MA, Young LY, Kradjan WA, et al., eds. *Applied Therapeutics: The Clinical Use of Drugs,* 8th edition. Baltimore: Lippincott Williams & Wilkins, 2005:1–86.

6. (C) Insulin glargine is an insulin analogue with glargine in the A21 position instead of asparagines and two arginines added to the C-terminus of the ß chain. These changes shift the isoelectric point from pH 5.4 to 6.7, making it more soluble at an acidic pH. Once injected, it precipitates at physiologic pH, forming a depot that releases insulin slowly over 24 hours, allowing for a basal level of insulin. Zinc is added to further prolong the duration of action. Insulin glargine cannot be mixed with other insulin formulations.

   Ref: Carlisle BA, Kroon LA, Koda-Kimble MA. Diabetes mellitus. In: Koda-Kimble MA, Young LY, Kradjan WA, et al., eds. *Applied Therapeutics: The Clinical Use of Drugs,* 8th edition. Baltimore: Lippincott Williams & Wilkins, 2005:1–86.

7. (B) Insulin pump systems are designed to deliver various basal amounts of insulin throughout the day as well as meal-related boluses proved by regular insulin, insulin lispro, or insulin aspartate.

   Ref: Carlisle BA, Kroon LA, Koda-Kimble MA. Diabetes mellitus. In: Koda-Kimble MA, Young LY, Kradjan WA, et al., eds. *Applied Therapeutics: The Clinical Use of Drugs,* 8th edition. Baltimore: Lippincott Williams & Wilkins, 2005:1–86.

8. (B) It is not necessary to use alcohol to clean the injection site. When drawing insulin into a syringe, the patient should withdraw the plunger to the level of insulin he or she intends to inject and then insert the needle into the vial and inject that amount of air into the vial to prevent creation of a vacuum within the vial. The vial should be inverted with the syringe inserted, and the amount of insulin desired should be withdrawn. Previously, patients were advised to rotate injection sites among the arms, thighs, abdomen, and buttocks. However, the rate of insulin absorption from these sites results in altered glucose control. The American Diabetes Association recommends that injections be rotated within the same anatomical region to avoid this effect.

   Ref: Carlisle BA, Kroon LA, Koda-Kimble MA. Diabetes mellitus. In: Koda-Kimble MA, Young LY, Kradjan WA, et al., eds. *Applied*

Therapeutics: The Clinical Use of Drugs, 8th edition. Baltimore: Lippincott Williams & Wilkins, 2005:1–86.

9. (C) The most common adverse effect of insulin is hypoglycemia.

    Ref: Oki JC, Isley WL. Diabetes mellitus. In: Dipiro JT, Talbert RL, Yee GC, et al., eds. *Pharmacotherapy: A Pathophysiologic Approach,* 5th edition. New York: McGraw-Hill, 2002:1335–1358.

10. (C) Oral administration of glucose (10 to 15 g) is the recommended treatment for hypoglycemia. Individuals who have lost consciousness may require intravenous dextrose.

    Ref: Oki JC, Isley WL. Diabetes mellitus. In: Dipiro JT, Talbert RL, Yee GC, et al., eds. *Pharmacotherapy: A Pathophysiologic Approach,* 5th edition. New York: McGraw-Hill, 2002:1335–1358.

PATIENT PROFILE 220

OBESITY

ANSWERS

1. (D) The calculation for ideal body weight (IBW) for men is 50 + 2.3 kg for every inch over 5 feet tall. EL is 5'10" tall; therefore, the calculation to determine EL's IBW is 50 + 23 kg = 73 kg.

    Ref: Chessman KH, Teasley-Strausburg KM. Assessment of nutrition status and nutrition requirements. In: DiPiro JT, Talbert RL, Yee GC, et al., eds. *Pharmacotherapy: A Pathophysiologic Approach,* 5th edition. New York: McGraw-Hill, 2002:2445–2463.

2. (E) A reasonable 6-month goal for EL is 317.3 lbs; this represents a 10% weight loss. Although EL still would be classified as obese, a 5% to 10% weight loss is associated with improving obesity-related health conditions. Once EL reaches this goal, he should be encouraged to continue to lose 5% to 10% of his excess body weight every 6 months. The ultimate goal will depend on improvement of his comorbid conditions and his ability to maintain the reduction in weight.

    Ref: *The practical guide: identification, evaluation, and treatment of overweight and obesity in adults.* Bethesda, MD: National Heart, Lung, and Blood Institute, North American Association for the Study of Obesity, 2000. (NIH publication no. 00-4084).

3. (E) Depression, GERD, and hypertension are all comorbid conditions associated with obesity. EL's obesity contributes to several of his health conditions, such as type 2 diabetes, hypercholesterolemia, and osteoarthritis. These conditions are expected to improve with gradual weight loss. Obesity is associated with many conditions, such as left ventricular hypertrophy, congestive heart failure, coronary artery disease, stroke, sleep apnea, pulmonary hypertension, hypertriglyceridemia, low serum HDL, glucose intolerance, hyperinsulinemia, degenerative joint disease, cholelithiasis, hiatal hernia, breast cancer, endometrial cancer, colon cancer, and prostate cancer.

    Ref: St. Peter JV, Khan MA. Obesity In: DiPiro JT, Talbert RL, Yee GC, et al., eds. *Pharmacotherapy: A Pathophysiologic Approach,* 5th edition. New York: McGraw-Hill, 2002:2543–2563.

4. (D) Weight Watchers® promotes a nutritionally balanced diet plan low in fat and high in fiber to reduce body weight and maintain loss. Weight Watchers® is most successful for patients who desire a structured program with weekly meetings and group support. The Atkins diet is high in fat and prohibits all carbohydrates (even fruits and vegetables). Although this plan does cause rapid weight loss, it is typically short-term. Rapid weight loss typically is associated with regain once the diet is discontinued. The South Beach diet is a spin off of the Atkins diet. It does not prohibit all carbohydrates; it classifies carbohydrates as "good" or "bad." There is no credible evidence that supports this diet for long-term weight loss maintenance. The Pritikin and Ornish diets promote low fat intake but monounsaturated and polyunsaturated fats are currently considered beneficial. The Zone diet is based on the 40-30-30 rule (40% carbohydrates, 30% protein, and 30% fat); this plan is very complicated to follow. The theory that this proportion of carbohydrates, protein, and fat will result in less storage of fat has not been proved.

    Ref: Scott GN. Diets and supplements for weight loss In: *Pharmacist's Letter/Prescriber's Letter.* Stockton, CA: Therapeutic Research Center, 2004. No. 200110.

5. (B) A reduction in caloric intake by 500 to 1000 calories per day is associated with a 1- to 2-lb weight loss per week. Although it is true that dietary fat is high in calories, reduction in calories must involve total daily caloric intake, not just one source. EL should consume 1200 to 1600 calories per day. Less than 800 calories per day is not appropriate and has not been associated with weight loss.

    Ref: *The practical guide: identification, evaluation, and treatment of overweight and obesity in adults.* Bethesda, MD: National Heart, Lung, and Blood Institute, North American Association for the Study of Obesity, 2000. (NIH publication no. 00-4084).

6. (A) Obesity is considered a chronic disease that is not "cured" once goals are met; rather, it requires lifelong effort to maintain the goal weight. Weight loss should be slow and steady, averaging 1 to 2 lbs per week.

Ref: *The practical guide: identification, evaluation, and treatment of overweight and obesity in adults.* Bethesda, MD: National Heart, Lung, and Blood Institute, North American Association for the Study of Obesity, 2000. (NIH publication no. 00-4084).

7. (D) Bupropion has been associated with a small weight reduction. Bupropion is an antidepressant; it weakly inhibits the reuptake of norepinephrine, serotonin, and dopamine. Bupropion is structurally similar to diethylpropion (a noradrenergic agent approved for short-term treatment of obesity). All selective serotonin reuptake inhibitors have been associated with weight gain. Paroxetine has been implicated as causing the most. There is no interaction between paroxetine and lisinopril. Mirtazapine also has been associated with significant weight gain.

Ref: Finley PR, Laird LK, Benefield WH. Mood disorders I. major depressive disorders. In: Koda-Kimble MA, Young LY, Kradjan WA, et al., eds. *Applied Therapeutics: The Clinical Use of Drugs,* 8th edition. Baltimore: Lippincott Williams & Wilkins, 2005:1–37.

8. (C) The brand name of sibutramine is Meridia®. Adipex-P® (phentermine), Didrex® (benzphetamine), and Fastin® (phentermine) are noradrenergic agents approved for the short-term treatment of obesity. Xenical® is the brand name of orlistat.

Ref: Yanovski SZ, Yanovski JA. Obesity. *N Engl J Med* 2002; 346:591–602.

9. (E) All three statements are true. Sibutramine is approved for weight loss and maintenance in conjunction with reduction of caloric intake. The starting dose of sibutramine is 10 mg qd, based on response the dose may be increased to 15 mg/day after 4 weeks. If no response (<1 lb/wk) in 4 weeks, the dose of sibutramine may be increased to 15 mg/day. Sibutramine inhibits the reuptake of norepinephrine and serotonin, and weakly dopamine; when taken in combination with dextromethorphan it may cause serotonin syndrome (characterized by mental status and behavioral changes).

Ref: Yanovski SZ, Yanovski JA. Obesity. *N Engl J Med* 2002; 346:591–602.

10. (D) Phentermine has a potential for abuse and as such has been scheduled by the DEA (C-IV). Phentermine may increase blood pressure and heart rate; therefore, it should be avoided in patients with hypertension. Other side effects of phentermine include insomnia, dry mouth, constipation, euphoria, and palpitations. Phentermine is only approved by the FDA for short-term (<12-wk) treatment of obesity, it should not be used as maintenance therapy for weight loss.

Ref: Yanovski SZ, Yanovski JA. Obesity. *N Engl J Med* 2002; 346:591–602.

PATIENT   PROFILE   221

PLAGUE

ANSWERS

1. (C) *Yersinia pestis* is a gram-negative rod-shaped bacterium. Variola is the causative organism of smallpox, *Bacillus anthracis* is the causative organism of anthrax, and *Francisella tularensis* is the causative organism of tularemia.

Ref: Inglesby T, Dennis D, Henderson D, et al. Plague as a biological weapon: medical and public health management. *JAMA* 2000;283(17):2281–2290.

Ref: Weinstein R, Alibek K. *Biological and Chemical Terrorism: A Guide for Healthcare Providers and First Responders.* New York: Thieme, 2003:80–81.

2. (A) Bubonic plague is the most common form produced by the bite of an infected flea. It occurs throughout the world, including the United States.

Ref: Inglesby T, Dennis D, Henderson D, et al. Plague as a biological weapon: medical and public health management. *JAMA* 2000;283(17):2281–2290.

Ref: Weinstein R, Alibek K. *Biological and Chemical Terrorism: A Guide for Healthcare Providers and First Responders.* New York: Thieme, 2003:80–81.

3. (B) Bubonic plague has a typical incubation period of 2 to 10 days; pneumonic plague has a quicker incubation period of 1 to 6 days.

Ref: Inglesby T, Dennis D, Henderson D, et al. Plague as a biological weapon: medical and public health management. *JAMA* 2000;283(17):2281–2290.

Ref: Weinstein R, Alibek K. *Biological and Chemical Terrorism: A Guide for Healthcare Providers and First Responders.* New York: Thieme, 2003:80–81.

4. (E) Streptomycin is the drug of choice but its availability is limited in the United States. Gentamicin is an acceptable alternative if streptomycin is unavailable per CDC guidelines.

Ref: Inglesby T, Dennis D, Henderson D, et al. Plague as a biological weapon: medical and public health management. *JAMA* 2000;283(17):2281–2290.

Ref: Weinstein R, Alibek K. *Biological and Chemical Terrorism: A Guide for Healthcare Providers and First Responders*. New York: Thieme, 2003:80–81.

5. (C) 10 days.

Ref: Inglesby T, Dennis D, Henderson D, et al. Plague as a biological weapon: medical and public health management. *JAMA* 2000;283(17):2281–2290.

Ref: Weinstein R, Alibek K. *Biological and Chemical Terrorism: A Guide for Healthcare Providers and First Responders*. New York: Thieme, 2003:80–81.

6. (B) Aminoglycosides.

Ref: *AHFS DI Bioterrorism Resource Manual*. Bethesda, MD: American Society of Health-System Pharmacists 2002;120:313.

7. (E) Aminoglycosides have been associated with the adverse effects of both nephrotoxicity and ototoxicity. Patients need to be monitored carefully while on these medications.

Ref: Lacy C, Armstrong L, Goldman M, et al. *Drug Information Handbook-Pocket*. Hudson, NY: Lexi-Comp, 2000:407.

8. (B) Blood dyscrasias, such as aplastic anemia, thrombocytopenia, and granulocytopenia, may occur because of bone marrow suppression. Hematologic tests should be performed before therapy is started and approximately every 2 days while on chloramphenicol.

Ref: *AHFS DI Bioterrorism Resource Manual*. Bethesda, MD: American Society of Health-System Pharmacists 2002:13.

9. (A) Tetracycline could be used but would not be a bid regimen; it would be qid. Erythromycin and amoxicillin are not recommended for prophylaxis therapy.

Ref: Weinstein R, Alibek K. *Biological and Chemical Terrorism: A Guide for Healthcare Providers and First Responders*. New York: Thieme, 2003:80–81.

10. (C) If outdated or degraded, tetracyclines may cause Fanconi's syndrome, which leads to renal tubular dysfunction and eventual renal failure.

Ref: Thomson MicroMedex.. Micromedex® Healthcare Series Vol. 121. Expires 12/2004.*http://micromedex/ciprofloxacin/overview*.Accessed 10/26/2004.

PATIENT PROFILE 222

SCHIZOPHRENIA

ANSWERS

1. (D) Long-acting medications have about twice better compliance than administration by mouth.

Ref: Gaebel W. Towards the improvement of compliance: the significance of psycho-education and new antipsychotic drugs. *Int Clin Psychopharmacol* 1997;12(suppl 1):S37–42.

2. (A) Clozapine has the highest risk of weight gain amongst the atypical antipsychotics.

Ref: Allison, et al. Antipsychotic induce weight gain: A comprehensive research synthesis. *Am J Psychiatry* 1999,156:1686–1696.

3. (B) Chlorpromazine has a higher risk of tardive dyskinesia than any of the atypical antipsychotics.

Ref: AF Schatzberg, CB Nemeroff, eds. *Essentials of Clinical Psychopharmacology*. Washington, DC: American Psychiatric Publishing, 2001.

4. (D) Thioridazine has the highest risk of QT prolongation and has a black box warning for this event.

Ref: US Food and Drug Administration Advisory Committee. Zeldox capsules. *Summary of Efficacy and Safety and Overall Benefit Risk Relationship*. Study O54. Bethesda, MD: US FDA, 2000.

5. (D) Olanzapine is metabolized via cytochrome P450 1A. This pathway is induced by cigarette smoking. If a person were to stop smoking, then the induction would stop and the olanzapine serum levels subsequently would increase.

Ref: Product information. Zyprexa. Eli Lilly and Company.

PATIENT PROFILE 223

DIABETES

ANSWERS

1. (C) Thiazolidinediones (rosiglitazone, pioglitazone) are associated with fluid retention and plasma volume expansion leading to peripheral edema, increased body weight, and new heart failure. Edema is two to three times more likely (4% to 6% of patients) when receiving

a thiazolidinedione compared with other oral hypoglycemic therapies (1% to 2% of patients). The incidence of new heart failure is greater in patients treated with a combination thiazolidinedione and insulin compared with thiazolidinedione alone. The Food and Drug Administration has recently included this warning in the prescription information for rosiglitazone and pioglitazone.

Ref: Yki-Järvinen H. Thiazolidinediones. *N Engl J Med* 2004; 351:1106–1118.

2. (A) Thiazolidinediones are only approved for use in patients with diabetes who are in NYHA stage I or II heart failure. Pioglitazone is known to result in fluid retention and edema; it is rational to discontinue given the side effects noted. Pioglitazone's parent drug has a half-life of elimination of 3 to 7 hours. The total half-life of pioglitazone, including parent drug, hydroxymetabolites and ketometabolites, is up to 24 hours. Thus, it may take 3.3 half-lives of elimination or 72 hours to remove 90% of pioglitazone parent drug and metabolites. RG's symptoms are causing concern but are not severely limiting her daily activities; thus, admission to urgent care or a visit to the emergency department may not be necessary yet. Additionally, RG is receiving a thiazide and loop diuretic that work synergistically. Because she is already receiving this combination she will continue to have diuresis while pioglitazone and metabolites are being eliminated. Excessive diuresis can disrupt RG's electrolyte status and result in hospitalization.

Ref: Pioglitazone (Actos® [product information]. Takeda Pharmaceuticals & Eli Lilly and Company.

3. (E) The American Diabetes Association recommends that all patients with diabetes receive therapy to achieve an HbA1c goal of ≤7%. An HbA1c of 7% correlates with a mean plasma glucose of 170 mg/dL.

Ref: The American Diabetes Association. Standards of medical care in diabetes. *Diabetes Care* 2004;27(Suppl 1):S15–35.

4. (B) Patients in NYHA functional class II are considered to have mild limitations in physical activity. Patients are comfortable at rest but normal physical activity can result in fatigue, dyspnea, or palpitations. Patients in NYHA functional class II still can be treated with a metformin-glimeperide combination to maximize oral therapy with careful monitoring. Nateglinide therapy in combination with glimeperide is not an approved combination and can result in hypoglycemia. Insulin-sulfonylurea combination should be reserved for when the insulin-metformin combination fails because of comparatively more fluid retention, weight gain, hyperinsulinemia, and insulin resistance. Note that an insulin-sulfonylurea combination results in less fluid retention and weight gain than insulin alone.

Ref: Nesto RW, Bell D, Bonow RO, et al. Thiazolidinedione use, fluid retention, and congestive heart failure: a consensus statement from the American Heart Association and American Diabetes Association. *Circulation* 2003;108:2941–2948.

5. (D) Metformin is contraindicated when serum creatinine is ≥1.4 mg/dL in women or 1.5 mg/dL in men and should be stopped. Patients with a serum creatinine values higher than these cutoffs are at risk for the rare but potentially fatal adverse effect of metformin-induced lactic acidosis.

Ref: The American Diabetes Association. Standards of medical care in diabetes. *Diabetes Care* 2004;27(Suppl 1):S15–35.

6. (E) RG's most recent HbA1c was 8% despite various oral hypoglycemic strategies. Because her most recent oral anti-hypoglycemic medication was discontinued she will need additional therapy for glycemic control. The addition of insulin is an appropriate consideration. Goals of therapy when beginning insulin include patient education and empowerment to facilitate aggressive glucose control, achieving HbA1c goals, and the reduction of microvascular and macrovascular complications. It is important to adjust insulin doses upward as necessary to achieve tighter glycemic control rather than to minimize insulin doses to prevent hypoglycemia because tight glucose control is crucial to preventing chronic complications of hyperglycemia. Pharmacist-delivered education should be a first-line defense against the complications of poorly controlled glucose and potential hypoglycemia.

Ref: DeWitt DE, Hirsch IB. Outpatient insulin therapy in type 1 and type 2 diabetes mellitus: scientific review. *JAMA* 2003;289: 2254–2264.

7. (D) Patients receiving insulin glargine report greater satisfaction over insulin NPH and insulin glargine is associated with fewer instances of hypoglycemia, better postprandial glucose control, and less weight gain.

Ref: Rosenstock J, Schwartz SL, Clarck CM, et al. Basal insulin therapy in type 2 diabetes. *Diabetes Care* 2001;24:631–636.

Ref: Yki-Jarvinen H, Dressler A, Ziemen M. Less nocturnal hypoglycemia and better post-dinner glucose control with bedtime insulin glargine compared with bedtime NPH insulin during insulin combination therapy in type 2 diabetes. *Diabetes Care* 2000; 23:113–136.

8. (A) Insulin glargine is intended to be administered once daily. The initial dose of insulin glargine can be calculated as: 0.1 to 0.2 U/kg per day or 10 to 20 U/day in 1 sq injection. RG weighs 170 lbs or 77.3 kg. 77.3 kg × 0.2 U/kg per day = 15.46 U/day.

Ref: DeWitt DE, Dugdale DC. Using new insulin strategies in the outpatient treatment of diabetes: clinical applications. *JAMA* 2003; 289:2265–2269.

9. (C) Adjustment of basal insulin can be performed by following the following standardized procedure: Increase by 4 U (insulin glargine or insulin NPH) if fasting capillary blood glucose is >140 mg/dL on three consecutive measures. Increase by 2 U (insulin glargine or insulin NPH) if fasting capillary blood glucose is 110 to 140 mg/dL on three consecutive measures. Most patients with type 2 diabetes require basal insulin and a prandial insulin combination with 50% of the daily insulin requirement from basal insulin and 50% coming from prandial insulin to maintain tight control (HbA1c ≤7%). This is likely to require basal insulin (glargine/NPH) doses of 0.5 to 0.6 U/kg per day and prandial insulin (lispro/aspart) doses of 0.5 to 0.6 U/kg per day.

Ref: DeWitt DE, Dugdale DC. Using new insulin strategies in the outpatient treatment of diabetes: clinical applications. *JAMA* 2003;289:2265–2269.

10. (B) RG is using 20 U/day of insulin glargine. Insulin glargine is available in 10-mL vials with a concentration of 100 U/mL. Each vial contains 1000 U. 1000 U/20 units per day = 50 days.

Ref: Insulin glargine (Lantus® [product information]. Aventis Pharmaceuticals.

PATIENT PROFILE 224

HUMAN IMMUNODEFICIENCY VIRUS

ANSWERS

1. (B) Because of concerns with the rapid emergence of resistance, flucytosine is not used as single-agent therapy. Clinical trials have shown that combination therapy with flucytosine is superior to either amphotericin B or fluconazole monotherapy. Amphotericin B–containing regimens may allow for faster cerebrospinal fluid clearing and the addition of flucytosine may reduce the risk of relapses. Clinical guidelines recommend the amphotericin B/flucytosine combination as the induction therapy of choice.

Ref: Saag MS, Graybill RJ, Larsen RA, et al. Practice guidelines for the management of cryptococcal disease. *Clin Infect Dis* 2000; 30:710–718.

2. (B) Fluconazole maintenance therapy has a lower risk for relapse than maintenance with weekly amphotericin B, itraconazole, or ketoconazole.

Ref: Saag MS, Graybill RJ, Larsen RA, et al. Practice guidelines for the management of cryptococcal disease. *Clin Infect Dis* 2000; 30:710–718.

3. (D) Nephrotoxicity is a major therapy-limiting toxicity with conventional intravenous amphotericin B. It occurs to some degree in the majority of patients receiving this drug. There are reports of agranulocytosis with amphotericin B therapy, but this is considered a rare effect.

Ref: McEnvoy GK, ed. *AHFS Drug Information*. Bethesda, MD: American Society of Health-System Pharmacists, 2004.

4. (A) The most frequent adverse effects with flucytosine therapy are related to the drug's effect on rapidly growing tissues, particularly the bone marrow and lining of the GI tract. Patients receiving this drug may experience bone marrow hypoplasia, resulting in anemia, leukopenia, pancytopenia, thrombocytopenia, or agranulocytosis.

Ref: McEnvoy GK, ed. *AHFS Drug Information*. Bethesda, MD: American Society of Health-System Pharmacists, 2004.

5. (B) Normal saline boluses administered before or after amphotericin B infusions appear to reduce the risk for nephrotoxicity associated with administration of this drug. Options A, C, and D are interventions that sometimes are used to prevent the acute infusion-related reactions associated with amphotericin B administration.

Ref: Gardner ML, Godley PJ, Wasan SM. Sodium loading treatment for amphotericin B-induced nephrotoxicity. *Drug Intell Clin Pharm* 1990;24:940–946.

6. (A) Hyperglycemia, new-onset diabetes mellitus, and exacerbation of pre-existing diabetes mellitus have been reported in patients receiving antiretroviral therapy. However, theses metabolic alterations have a strong association with protease inhibitor use.

Ref: US Department of Health and Human Services. Guidelines for the use of antiretroviral agents in HIV-1–infected adults and adolescents. 2004 Mar 24 [cited 2004 Oct 12]:1–97. *http://www.aidsinfo.nih.gov/guidelines/adult/AA_032304.pdf.*

7. (D) The decision to start postexposure prophylaxis and the intensity of that prophylaxis (two versus three antiretrovirals) depends on the degree of exposure and the likelihood that the source will transmit HIV. Factors I to IV must be taken into account because each of them plays a role in determining the degree of exposure and the likelihood that the source will transmit HIV.

Ref: Centers for Disease Control and Prevention. Updated US Public Service guidelines for the management of occupational exposures to HBV, HCV, and HIV and recommendations for postexposure prophylaxis. *MMWR Morbid Mortal Wkly Rep* 2001;50 (RR-11):1–54.

8. (D) Results from a retrospective case-controlled study involving health care workers who received percutaneous injuries indicate that zidovudine PEP reduces the risk of HIV transmission by 81%. There are no data published that addresses the efficacy of the currently recommended two- and three-drug PEP regimens.

    Ref: Centers for Disease Control and Prevention. Updated US Public Service guidelines for the management of occupational exposures to HBV, HCV, and HIV and recommendations for postexposure prophylaxis. *MMWR Morbid Mortal Wkly Rep* 2001;50 (RR-11):1–54.

9. (A) Nucleoside reverse transcriptase inhibitors act as viral DNA chain terminators. After being triphosphorylated by cellular enzymes, these agents compete with nucleotides for incorporation into the growing viral DNA chain. After incorporation into the chain, DNA elongation is terminated.

    Ref: Raffanti S, Haas DW. Antimicrobial agents: antiretroviral agents. In: Hardman JG, Limbird LE, eds. *Goodman & Gilman's the Pharmacologic Basis of Therapeutics,* 10th edition. New York: McGraw-Hill, 2001:1349–1380.

10. (C) Abacavir is the nucleoside reverse transcriptase inhibitor most commonly associated with rash. It may be a manifestation of an abacavir hypersensitivity syndrome. Other symptoms associated with this syndrome are fever, malaise, fatigue, and gastrointestinal complaints. Patients who experience this syndrome should have their abacavir discontinued and an alternative agent administered to replace it.

    Ref: Centers for Disease Control and Prevention. Updated US Public Service guidelines for the management of occupational exposures to HBV, HCV, and HIV and recommendations for postexposure prophylaxis. *MMWR Morbid Mortal Wkly Rep* 2001;50 (RR-11):1–54.

PATIENT PROFILE 225
SEROTONIN SYNDROME

ANSWERS

1. (D) Rosiglitazone is a thiazolidinedione antidiabetic agent that lowers blood glucose by improving target-cell response to insulin. It has no known effect on 5-HT receptors.

    Ref: Oki JC, Isley WL. Diabetes mellitus. In: DiPiro JT, Talbert RL, Yee GC, ed. *Pharmacotherapy: A Pathophysiologic Approach,* 5th ed. New York: McGraw-Hill, 2002:1335–1358.

2. (B) Overstimulation of 5-HT receptors is responsible for causing the signs and symptoms associated with serotonin syndrome.

    Ref: Chyka PA. Clinical toxicology. In: DiPiro JT, Talbert RL, Yee GC, ed. *Pharmacotherapy: A Pathophysiologic Approach,* 5th ed. New York: McGraw-Hill, 2002:116.

3. (E) Phenelzine (Nardil) is a monoamine oxidase inhibitor (MAOI) and inhibits the enzyme responsible for the breakdown of serotonin.

    Ref: Kando JC, Wells BG, Hayes PE. Depressive disorders. In: DiPiro JT, Talbert RL, Yee GC, ed. *Pharmacotherapy: A Pathophysiologic Approach,* 5th ed. New York: McGraw-Hill, 2002:1248.

4. (B) Fluoxetine's active metabolite is norfluoxetine, which significantly increases the half-life of the drug, up to 16 days.

    Ref: Kando JC, Wells BG, Hayes PE. Depressive disorders. In: DiPiro JT, Talbert RL, Yee GC, ed. *Pharmacotherapy: A Pathophysiologic Approach,* 5th ed. New York: McGraw-Hill, 2002:1253.

5. (A) Clomiphene is an ovulation stimulator and has no known effect on serotonin receptors. In each of the other options, both drugs have effects at the 5-HT receptors.

    Ref: Lieu CL, Yoshida T. Infertility. In: DiPiro JT, Talbert RL, Yee GC, ed. *Pharmacotherapy: A Pathophysiologic Approach,* 5th ed. New York: McGraw-Hill, 2002:1435.

6. (B) The active ingredient in both Wellbutrin and Zyban is bupropion.

    Ref: Doering PL. Substance-related disorders: alcohol, nicotine, and caffeine. In: DiPiro JT, Talbert RL, Yee GC, ed. *Pharmacotherapy: A Pathophysiologic Approach,* 5th ed. New York: McGraw-Hill, 2002:1214.

    Ref: Kando JC, Wells BG, Hayes PE. Depressive disorders. In: DiPiro JT, Talbert RL, Yee GC, ed. *Pharmacotherapy: A Pathophysiologic Approach,* 5th ed. New York: McGraw-Hill, 2002:1248.

7. (E) Ultracet contains tramadol and acetaminophen. Tramadol not only has been shown to have effects at the opioid receptors but also can inhibit the reuptake of norepinephrine and serotonin.

    Ref: Gutstein HB, Akil H. Opioid analgesics. In: Gilman A, Hardman JG, Limbird LE, eds. *Goodman & Gilman's The Pharmacological Basis of Therapeutics.* New York: McGraw-Hill, 2001: 590.

8. (C) Answers I and II are correct for the reasons stated. Nefazodone can increase the risk of liver toxicity.

Ref: *Drug Facts and Comparisons,* 2003 ed. St. Louis: Facts and Comparisons, 2002.

9. (B) Effexor may cause a dose-related increase in diastolic blood pressure.

Ref: Kando JC, Wells BG, Hayes PE. Depressive disorders. In: DiPiro JT, Talbert RL, Yee GC, ed. *Pharmacotherapy: A Pathophysiologic Approach,* 5th ed. New York: McGraw-Hill, 2002:1251.

10. (D) Lithium influences the reuptake of serotonin.

Ref:Fankhauser MP. Bipolar disorder. In: DiPiro JT, Talbert RL, Yee GC, ed. *Pharmacotherapy: A Pathophysiologic Approach,* 5th ed. New York: McGraw-Hill, 2002:1265.

PATIENT PROFILE 226
CHRONIC HEPATITIS C

ANSWERS

1. (D) Modes of transmission for the hepatitis C virus (HCV) are categorized as percutaneous, nonpercutaneous, or sporadic. Percutaneous transmission arises from IV drug abuse, body piercing, tattooing, hemodialysis, and health care worker needle sticks. Transmission between sexual partners and mother to child are considered nonpercutaneous. *Sporadic transmission* is defined as the acquisition of HCV without known risk factors.

Ref: Holt CD. Viral hepatitis. In: Young YL, Koda-Kimble MA, eds. *Applied Therapeutics: The Clinical Use of Drugs.* Vancouver, WA: Applied Therapeutics, 2005:73-29–73-41.

2. (B) Most patients with chronic hepatitis C infection can be considered for therapy. Treatment is highly recommended in patients considered to be at risk for the development of cirrhosis. These patients will have the presence of liver fibrosis and inflammation, as well as an HCV RNA level of more than 50 IU/mL.

Ref: Holt CD. Viral hepatitis. In: Young YL, Koda-Kimble MA, eds. *Applied Therapeutics: The Clinical Use of Drugs.* Vancouver, WA: Applied Therapeutics, 2005:73-29–73-41.

Ref: National Institutes of Health. Consensus Statement on the Management of Hepatitis C: 2002; available at *http://www.consensus.nih.gov.*

3. (D) Other goals of therapy include improvement in clinical symptoms, prevention of the spread of disease, prevention of the progression to cirrhosis and hepatocellular carcinoma, and prevention of end-stage liver disease and its manifestations.

Ref: Holt CD. Viral hepatitis. In: Young YL, Koda-Kimble MA, eds. *Applied Therapeutics: The Clinical Use of Drugs.* Vancouver, WA: Applied Therapeutics, 2005:73-29–73-41.

4. (C) Interferon-β-1A and -β-1B are approved for use in patients with multiple sclerosis. Interferon-γ is approved for use in osteopetrosis and chronic granulomatous disease.

Ref: Holt CD. Viral hepatitis. In: Young YL, Koda-Kimble MA, eds. *Applied Therapeutics: The Clinical Use of Drugs.* Vancouver, WA: Applied Therapeutics, 2005:73-29–73-41.

5. (D) Additional side effects associated with the use of interferon include hypotension, depression, alterations in thyroid function, and retinal hemorrhage.

Ref: Product information: Intron A, interferon-α-2B, Schering.

6. (A) Interferon-α-2B should be stored in the refrigerator. Additionally, the vial should not be shaken prior to use.

Ref: Product information: Intron A, interferon=α-2B, Schering.

7. (A) Additional side effects associated with the use of ribavirin include insomnia, fatigue, irritability, nephrolithiasis, increased uric acid levels, and dyspnea. Changes in thyroid function and retinal hemorrhage have been associated with interferon use.

Ref: Product information: Rebetol, ribavirin, Schering.

8. (A) Pegylated interferon offers a longer duration of action, allowing for once weekly dosing. However, it has been associated with a higher incidence of adverse effects.

Ref: Holt CD. Viral hepatitis. In: Young YL, Koda-Kimble MA, eds. *Applied Therapeutics: The Clinical Use of Drugs.* Vancouver, WA: Applied Therapeutics, 2005:73-29–73-41.

Ref: Product information: Pegasys, peginterferon alpha-2B, Roche.

9. (B) Its higher incidence of adverse effects is due to its long half-life.

Ref: Holt CD. Viral hepatitis. In: Young YL, Koda-Kimble MA, eds. *Applied Therapeutics: The Clinical Use of Drugs.* Vancouver, WA: Applied Therapeutics, 2005:73-29–73-41.

Ref: Product information: Pegasys, peginterferon-α-2B, Roche.

10. (B) Selective serotonin reuptake inhibitors have been used effectively to manage depression induced by the use of pegylated interferon.

Ref: Holt CD. Viral hepatitis. In: Young YL, Koda-Kimble MA, eds. *Applied Therapeutics: The Clinical Use of Drugs*. Vancouver, WA: Applied Therapeutics, 2005:73-29–73-41.

Ref: National Institutes of Health. Consensus Statement on the Management of Hepatitis C: 2002: available at: *http://www.consensus.nih.gov*.

PATIENT PROFILE 227

HYPERTENSION

ANSWERS

1. (D) FD's blood pressure goal is less than 140/90 mm Hg.

Ref: Chobanian AV, Bakris GL, Black HR, et al. The Seventh Report of the Joint National Committee on Prevention, Detection, Evaluation, and Treatment of High Blood Pressure. *Hypertension* 2003;42:1206–1252.

2. (C) Prehypertension is categorized as blood pressure of 120–139 mm Hg systolic and/or 80–89 mm Hg diastolic.

Ref: Chobanian AV, Bakris GL, Black HR, et al. The Seventh Report of the Joint National Committee on Prevention, Detection, Evaluation, and Treatment of High Blood Pressure. *Hypertension* 2003;42:1206–1252.

3. (C) FD has stage 2 hypertension according to current guidelines.

Ref: Chobanian AV, Bakris GL, Black HR, et al. The Seventh Report of the Joint National Committee on Prevention, Detection, Evaluation, and Treatment of High Blood Pressure. *Hypertension* 2003;42:1206–1252.

4. (D) FD has a family history of premature cardiovascular disease (father had an MI at age 50).

Ref: Chobanian AV, Bakris GL, Black HR, et al. The Seventh Report of the Joint National Committee on Prevention, Detection, Evaluation, and Treatment of High Blood Pressure. *Hypertension* 2003;42:1206–1252.

5. (D) In otherwise healthy adults, thiazide diuretics are considered first-line treatment for uncomplicated hypertension.

Ref: Chobanian AV, Bakris GL, Black HR, et al. The Seventh Report of the Joint National Committee on Prevention, Detection, Evaluation, and Treatment of High Blood Pressure. *Hypertension* 2003;42:1206–1252.

6. (C) FD is a diabetic; therefore, it is beneficial to begin therapy with an ACE inhibitor. Increasing the atenolol dose will not have any further effect on his blood pressure, and diabetes is considered a compelling indication for blood pressure therapy with an ACE inhibitor.

Ref: Chobanian AV, Bakris GL, Black HR, et al. The Seventh Report of the Joint National Committee on Prevention, Detection, Evaluation, and Treatment of High Blood Pressure. *Hypertension* 2003;42:1206–1252.

7. (D) Orthostatic hypotension is defined as a decrease in systolic blood pressure by greater than 20 mm Hg.

Ref: Chobanian AV, Bakris GL, Black HR, et al. The Seventh Report of the Joint National Committee on Prevention, Detection, Evaluation, and Treatment of High Blood Pressure. *Hypertension* 2003;42:1206–1252.

8. (D) FD's overactive bladder may be causing him to become dehydrated. Dehydration can contribute to orthostatic hypotension.

Ref: Chobanian AV, Bakris GL, Black HR, et al. The Seventh Report of the Joint National Committee on Prevention, Detection, Evaluation, and Treatment of High Blood Pressure. *Hypertension* 2003;42:1206–1252.

9. (D) BPH is a compelling indication for blood pressure treatment with an α-blocker.

Ref: Chobanian AV, Bakris GL, Black HR, et al. The Seventh Report of the Joint National Committee on Prevention, Detection, Evaluation, and Treatment of High Blood Pressure. *Hypertension* 2003;42:1206–1252.

10. (D) A common side effect of ACE inhibitors is persistent dry cough. Patients should be counseled on this adverse effect when starting on therapy with ACE inhibitors.

Ref: Chobanian AV, Bakris GL, Black HR, et al. The Seventh Report of the Joint National Committee on Prevention, Detection, Evaluation, and Treatment of High Blood Pressure. *Hypertension* 2003;42:1206–1252.

PATIENT PROFILE 228

LIVER TRANSPLANTATION

ANSWERS

1. (C) Methylprednisolone, tacrolimus, and mycophenolate mofetil together comprise BU's immunosuppressive regimen. Ursodiol does not have immunosuppressive properties.

   Ref: Cohen SM. Current immunosuppression in liver transplantation. *Am J Ther* 2002;9(2):119–125.

2. (D) Mycophenolate mofetil blocks de novo synthesis of purines and results in the selective inhibition of lymphocyte proliferation.

   Ref: Cellcept Package Insert, Roche Laboratories, Inc., Nutley, NJ, 2003.

3. (D) Mycophenolate mofetil and azathioprine are both antiproliferative agents. Sirolimus inhibits cell cycle progression; cyclosporine blocks IL-2 production; daclizumab is an IL-2 receptor antagonist; and thymoglobulin is a polyclonal antibody that causes a rapid and profound depletion of peripheral lymphocytes.

   Ref: Cohen SM. Current immunosuppression in liver transplantation. *Am J Ther* 2002;9(2):119–125.

4. (D) Hypoalbuminemia is the most common cause of hypocalcemia, and serum calcium levels must be corrected in patients with a low albumin. Adjusted calcium = serum calcium − serum albumin + 4. In BU's case, 8.1 mg/dL − 2 g/dL + 4 = 10.1 mg/dL.

   Ref: Bakerman S. *ABC's of Interpretive Laboratory Data,* 4th ed. Scottsdale, AZ: Interpretive Laboratory Data, Inc., 2002:121–123.

5. (A) Even though the CMV status of the donor is unknown, this recipient is at risk for CMV disease because he was seropositive prior to transplant and is a candidate for prophylaxis. BU does not have a clinical picture consistent with active disease. Ganciclovir has activity against the herpes simplex virus, but that is not the primary indication for therapy in this patient.

   Ref: Schnitzler MA. Costs and consequences of cytomegalovirus disease. *Am J Health Syst Pharm* 2003;60(suppl 8):S5–8.

6. (C) Ganciclovir must be dose adjusted in patients with renal insufficiency, but renal insufficiency does not affect dose requirements of the other medications.

   Ref: Cytovene Package Insert, Roche Laboratories, Inc., Nutley, NJ, 2000.

7. (C) HCV reinfection occurs universally in patients with pretransplant viremia. Early HCV recurrence, infection with genotype 1b, high HCV RNA, induction immunosuppression, and treatment of rejection are associated with a poor prognosis. Once hepatitis recurs after transplantation, typically it has a more rapid and aggressive progression to advanced disease owing to the immunosuppression.

   Ref: Curry MP. Hepatitis B and hepatitis C viruses in liver transplantation. *Transplantation* 2004;78(7):955–963.

8. (E) Induction immunosuppression and treatment of rejection (particularly with OKT3 or high-dose methylprednisolone) are associated with HCV recurrence. Cumulative steroid exposure may be associated with HCV recurrence rates, but an association has not been shown with low, chronic, oral steroid use. Pulse doses of 2 g or more of IV methylprednisolone are associated with a greater incidence of recurrence and a more aggressive hepatitis course.

   Ref: Curry MP. Hepatitis B and hepatitis C viruses in liver transplantation. *Transplantation* 2004;78(7):955–963.

9. (E) The treatment of choice is pegylated interferon-alfa and ribavirin combination therapy, although it is a difficult regimen to tolerate. At optimal doses, pegylated interferon offers a greater efficacy with similar tolerability compared with unmodified interferon-alfa. Interferon or ribavirin monotherapy is ineffective.

   Ref: Curry MP. Hepatitis B and hepatitis C viruses in liver transplantation. *Transplantation* 2004;78(7):955–963.

10. (B) Common side effects include flulike symptoms, injection-site inflammation, headache, alopecia, pruritus, and rash. Hemolytic anemia (related to ribavirin) occurs in approximately 10% of patients. Depression and suidicidal ideation are not uncommon and have prompted many practitioners to initiate a selective serotonin reuptake inhibitor (SSRI) when planning to use this combination.

    Ref: Ribavirin/Interferon alfa Drug Information, Micromedex, Thompson Healthcare, Inc., June 2003. Available at *http://www.micromedex.com*

PATIENT PROFILE 229

DIABETES MELLITUS

ANSWERS

1. (B) Oral or intravenous antibiotics that will cover a wide spectrum of both aerobic and anaerobic bacteria are required for treatment of diabetic foot infections. Intravenous antibiotics are only used for severe infections. Intravenous vancomycin does not cover anaerobes, so it would not be appropriate for use as monotherapy.

Ref: Danziger LH, Fish DN, Pendland SL. Skin and soft tissue infections. In: DiPiro JT, Talbert RL, Yee GC, et al, eds. *Pharmacotherapy: A Pathophysiologic Approach,* 5th ed. New York: McGraw-Hill, 2002:1885–1898.

2. (C) Clindamycin is associated with causing diarrhea. Severe cramping, blood stools, and/or persistent diarrhea are associated with *Clostridium difficile* colitis. Patients should contact their provider immediately if these symptoms occur.

Ref: Spruill WJ, Wade WE. Diarrhea, constipation and irritable bowel syndrome. In: DiPiro JT, Talbert RL, Yee GC, et al, eds. *Pharmacotherapy: A Pathophysiologic Approach,* 5th ed. New York: McGraw-Hill, 2002:655–670.

3. (E) Valproic acid is associated with significant weight gain in some individuals.

Ref: Gidal BE, Garnett WR, Graves N. Epilepsy. In: DiPiro JT, Talbert RL, Yee GC, et al, eds. *Pharmacotherapy: A Pathophysiologic Approach,* 5th ed. New York: McGraw-Hill, 2002:1031–1060.

4. (C) JH's prelunch blood sugars are elevated. The rest of his blood sugars are close to goal. His prebreakfast Novolog affects his prelunch values the most and should be increased.

Ref: Carlisle BA, Kroon LA, Koda-Kimble MA. Diabetes mellitus. In: Koda-Kimble MA, Young LY, Kradjan WA, Guglielmo BJ, eds. *Applied Therapeutics: The Clinical Use of Drugs,* 8th ed. Philadelphia:: Lippincott Williams & Wilkins, 2005:50-1–50-80.

5. (B) Binge drinking inhibits hepatic gluconeogenesis, which is one of the ways the body responds to hypoglycemia.

Ref: Oki JC. Diabetes mellitus. In: DiPiro JT, Talbert RL, Yee GC, et al, eds. *Pharmacotherapy: A Pathophysiologic Approach,* 5th ed. New York: McGraw-Hill, 2002:1335–1358.

6. (E) Gemfibrozil has the greatest effect on lowering triglycerides.

Ref: McKenney JM. Dyslipidemias, atherosclerosis and coronary heart disease. In: Koda-Kimble MA, Young LY, Kradjan WA, Guglielmo BJ, eds. *Applied Therapeutics: The Clinical Use of Drugs,* 8th ed. Philadelphia: Lippincott Williams & Wilkins, 2005:13-1–13-39.

7. (B) Statins rarely cause hepatitis.

Ref: McKenney JM. Dyslipidemias, atherosclerosis and coronary heart disease. In: Koda-Kimble MA, Young LY, Kradjan WA, Guglielmo BJ, eds. *Applied Therapeutics: The Clinical Use of Drugs,* 8th ed. Philadelphia: Lippincott Williams & Wilkins, 2005:13-1–13-39.

8. (E) Both statins and fibrates can cause muscle degradation and rhabdomyolysis. The combination increases the risk of experiencing the adverse event.

Ref: McKenney JM. Dyslipidemias, atherosclerosis and coronary heart disease. In: Koda-Kimble MA, Young LY, Kradjan WA, Guglielmo BJ, eds. *Applied Therapeutics: The Clinical Use of Drugs,* 8th ed. Philadelphia: Lippincott Williams & Wilkins, 2005:13-1–13-39.

9. (E) His blood sugars are elevated, so he needs more medication. The only option that will decrease both morning and evening blood sugars is increasing metformin to 1000 mg twice daily.

Ref: Carlisle BA, Kroon LA, Koda-Kimble MA. Diabetes mellitus. In: Koda-Kimble MA, Young LY, Kradjan WA, Guglielmo BJ, eds. *Applied Therapeutics: The Clinical Use of Drugs,* 8th ed. Philadelphia:: Lippincott Williams & Wilkins, 2005:50-1–50-80.

10. (A) Epoetin therapy is associated with elevations in diastolic blood pressure. This is theorized to occur because of an increase in peripheral vascular resistance.

Ref: Waddelow TA, Sproat TT. Anemias. In: DiPiro JT, Talbert RL, Yee GC, et al, eds. *Pharmacotherapy: A Pathophysiologic Approach,* 5th ed. New York: McGraw-Hill, 2002:1729–1746.

PATIENT PROFILE 230

GOUT

ANSWERS

1. (E) Probenecid is a uricosuric; it decreases uric acid reabsorption, and it requires a 24-hour urine collection.

   Ref: Russell TM, Young LL. Gout and hyperuricemia. In: Young YL, Koda-Kimble MA, eds. *Applied Therapeutics: The Clinical Use of Drugs.* Vancouver, WA: Applied Therapeutics, 2005:42(1–17).

2. (B) If LF's physician decides to start her on probenecid therapy, you should recommend an increase in fluid intake in order to prevent uric acid stone formation.

   Ref: Russell TM, Young LL. Gout and hyperuricemia. In: Young YL, Koda-Kimble MA, eds. *Applied Therapeutics: The Clinical Use of Drugs.* Vancouver, WA: Applied Therapeutics, 2005:42(1–17).

3. (C) Colchicine is a useful option in patients that are fluid restricted.

   Ref: Russell TM, Young LL. Gout and hyperuricemia. In: Young YL, Koda-Kimble MA, eds. *Applied Therapeutics: The Clinical Use of Drugs.* Vancouver, WA: Applied Therapeutics, 2005:42(1–17).

4. (C) Identidex is the preferred database to identify a drug based on tablet characteristics.

   Ref: Rumack BH, Bird PE, Gelman CR, et al, eds. *Identidex System.* Englewood, CO: Micromedex, Inc., 2005.

5. (A) Allopurinol is an appropriate treatment of patients who are classified as overproducers of uric acid.

   Ref: Russell TM, Young LL. Gout and hyperuricemia. In: Young YL, Koda-Kimble MA, eds. *Applied Therapeutics: The Clinical Use of Drugs.* Vancouver, WA: Applied Therapeutics, 2005: 42(1–17).

6. (D) Allopurinol and probenecid can be appropriate treatments for patients who are classified as having decreased renal clearance of uric acid.

   Ref: Russell TM, Young LL. Gout and hyperuricemia. In: Young YL, Koda-Kimble MA, eds. *Applied Therapeutics: The Clinical Use of Drugs.* Vancouver, WA: Applied Therapeutics, 2005:42(1–17).

7. (E) In a case such as LF's, where there is a history of chronic attacks of gout, prophylactic therapy may be initiated in patients with a serum uric acid level greater than 10 mg/dL, in very severe attacks, and in patients with hyperuricemia from medications that are essential to treatment.

   Ref: Russell TM, Young LL. Gout and hyperuricemia. In: Young YL, Koda-Kimble MA, eds. *Applied Therapeutics: The Clinical Use of Drugs.* Vancouver, WA: Applied Therapeutics, 2005:42(1–17).

8. (B) Based on LF's 24-hour urine collection for uric acid, she is considered an overproducer of uric acid.

   Ref: Russell TM, Young LL. Gout and hyperuricemia. In: Young YL, Koda-Kimble MA, eds. *Applied Therapeutics: The Clinical Use of Drugs.* Vancouver, WA: Applied Therapeutics, 2005:42(1–17).

9. (D) Probenecid's brand name (trademark name) is Benemid.

   Ref: Cada DE, Covington TI, Generali, JO, et al, eds. *Facts and Comparisons.* St. Louis: Facts and Comparisons, 2002.

10. (E) When initiating probenecid therapy in LF, colchicine should be added to LF's regimen.

    Ref: Russell TM, Young LL. Gout and hyperuricemia. In: Young YL, Koda-Kimble MA, eds. *Applied Therapeutics: The Clinical Use of Drugs.* Vancouver, WA: Applied Therapeutics, 2005:42(1–17).

PATIENT PROFILE 231

SEIZURES

ANSWERS

1. (D) Zonisamide is a sulfonamide derivative and is contraindicated in patients allergic to sulfonamides.

   Ref: McAuley JW, Lott RS. Seizure disorders. In: Koda-Kimble MA, Young LY, Kradjian WA, Guglielmo BJ, eds. *Applied Therapeutics: The Clinical Use of Drugs.* Philadelphia: Lippincott Williams & Wilkins, 2004:54-1–54-42.

2. (A) Carbarmazepine is thought to cause hyponatremia as a result of the release of antidiuretic hormone and may be associated with the syndrome of inappropriate antidiuretic hormone (SIADH).

   Ref: McAuley JW, Lott RS. Seizure disorders. In: Koda-Kimble MA, Young LY, Kradjian WA, Guglielmo BJ, eds. *Applied Therapeutics: The Clinical Use of Drugs.* Philadelphia: Lippincott Williams & Wilkins, 2004:54-1–54-42.

3. (E) Oxcarbazepine is a prodrug of carbamazepine and does not have the autoinduction properties of carbamazepine. Because it not converted to the epoxide metabolite, it may be better tolerated.

Ref: McAuley JW, Lott RS. Seizure disorders. In: Koda-Kimble MA, Young LY, Kradjian WA, Guglielmo BJ, eds. *Applied Therapeutics: The Clinical Use of Drugs.* Philadelphia: Lippincott Williams & Wilkins, 2004:54-1–54-42.

4. (D) One of the concerns with phenobarbital is its effect on cognition. The other side effects are not attributed to this AED.

Ref: McAuley JW, Lott RS. Seizure disorders. In: Koda-Kimble MA, Young LY, Kradjian WA, Guglielmo BJ, eds. *Applied Therapeutics: The Clinical Use of Drugs.* Philadelphia: Lippincott Williams & Wilkins, 2004:54-1–54-42.

5. (B) Primidone is metabolized to phenobarbital, which accounts for most of the antiepileptic effects of the drug.

Ref: McAuley JW, Lott RS. Seizure disorders. In: Koda-Kimble MA, Young LY, Kradjian WA, Guglielmo BJ, eds. *Applied Therapeutics: The Clinical Use of Drugs.* Philadelphia: Lippincott Williams & Wilkins, 2004:54-1-54–42.

6. (D) Hepatotoxicity is associated with valproate therapy and is most likely due to accumulation of hepatotoxic metabolites in some individuals.

Ref: McAuley JW, Lott RS. Seizure disorders. In: Koda-Kimble MA, Young LY, Kradjian WA, Guglielmo BJ, eds. *Applied Therapeutics: The Clinical Use of Drugs.* Philadelphia: Lippincott Williams & Wilkins, 2004:54-1–54-42.

7. (E) Both may be dosed twice a day, Tegretol XR uses an Oros tablet (osmotic pump) extended-dosage form, and the empty tablet shell can be observed in the stool. Carbatrol consists of enteric beads that can be sprinkled on food or administered through a feeding tube.

Ref: McAuley JW, Lott RS. Seizure disorders. In: Koda-Kimble MA, Young LY, Kradjian WA, Guglielmo BJ, eds. *Applied Therapeutics: The Clinical Use of Drugs,* Philadelphia: Lippincott Williams & Wilkins, 2004:54-1–54-42.

8. (C) Accumulation of the epoxide metabolite can result in a paradoxical increase in seizures at higher doses of carbamazepine even at normal serum concentrations of the parent drug.

Ref: McAuley JW, Lott RS, Seizure disorders. In: Koda-Kimble MA, Young LY, Kradjian WA, Guglielmo BJ, eds. *Applied Therapeutics: The Clinical Use of Drugs.* Philadelphia: Lippincott Williams & Wilkins, 2004:54-1–54-42.

9. (C) Erythromycin inhibits cytochrome P450 3A4 and can cause significant elevations in carbamazepine serum concentrations.

Ref: McAuley JW, Lott RS. Seizure disorders. In: Koda-Kimble MA, Young LY, Kradjian WA, Guglielmo BJ, eds. *Applied Therapeutics: The Clinical Use of Drugs.* Philadelphia: Lippincott Williams & Wilkins, 2004:54-1–54-42.

10. (A) Phenytoin exhibits dose-dependent kinetics, where the half life changes with the dose and serum concentration. Small increases in doses that exceed the maximum rate of elimination from the body (V_{max}) can result in disproportionately high serum concentrations.

Ref: McAuley JW, Lott RS. Seizure disorders. In: Koda-Kimble MA, Young LY, Kradjian WA, Guglielmo BJ, eds. *Applied Therapeutics: The Clinical Use of Drugs.* Philadelphia: Lippincott Williams & Wilkins, 2004:54-1–54-42.

PATIENT PROFILE 232

LUNG CANCER

ANSWERS

1. (A)

Ref: Davis L, Lindley C. Neoplastic disorders and their treatment: general principles. In Koda-Kimbla MA, Young LY, Kradjan WA, et al, eds. *Applied Therapeutics: The Clinical Use of Drugs,* 8th ed. Philadelphia: Lippincott Williams & Wilkins, 2005:88(17).

2. (D)

Ref: Johnson SW, Stevenson JP, O'Dwyer PJ. Cisplatin and its analogues. In: Devita VT, Hellman S, Rosenberg SA, eds. *Cancer:* *Principles and Practice of Oncology,* 6th ed. Philadelphia: Lippincott Williams & Wilkins, 2001:385.

3. (C)

Ref: Gralla RJ, Osoba D, Kris MG, et al. Recommendations for the use of antiemetics: Evidence-based clinical practice guidelines. *J Clin Oncol* 1999;17:2971.

4. (A)

Ref: Davis L, Lindley C. Neoplastic disorders and their treatment: general principles. In Koda-Kimbla MA, Young LY, Kradjan WA, et al, eds. *Applied Therapeutics: The Clinical Use of Drugs,* 8th ed. Philadelphia: Lippincott Williams & Wilkins, 2005:88(16–22).

5. (B)

Ref: BSA equation from Lacy CF. *Drug Information Handbook,* 11th ed. Hudson, OH: Lexicomp, 2003:1488.

6. (B)

Ref: Goodin S. Solid tumors. In Koda-Kimbla MA, Young LY, Kradjan WA, et al, eds. *Applied Therapeutics: The Clinical Use of Drugs,* 8th ed. Philadelphia: Lippincott Williams & Wilkins, 2005:91(13).

7. (C)

Ref: Stewart CF, Ratain MJ. Topoisomerase interactive agents. In: Devita VT, Hellman S, Rosenberg SA, eds. *Cancer: Principles and Practice of Oncology,* 6th ed. Philadelphia: Lippincott Williams & Wilkins, 2001:421.

8. (B)

Ref: Lindley C. Adverse effects of chemotherapy. In Koda-Kimbla MA, Young LY, Kradjan WA, et al, eds. *Applied Therapeutics: The Clinical Use of Drugs,* 8th ed. Philadelphia: Lippincott Williams & Wilkins, 2005:89(25).

9. (A)

Ref: Lindley C. Adverse effects of chemotherapy. In Koda-Kimbla MA, Young LY, Kradjan WA, et al, eds. *Applied Therapeutics: The Clinical Use of Drugs,* 8th ed. Philadelphia: Lippincott Williams & Wilkins, 2005:89(25).

10. (B)

Ref: Stewart CF, Ratain MJ. Topoisomerase interactive agents. In: Devita VT, Hellman S, Rosenberg SA, eds. *Cancer: Principles and Practice of Oncology,* 6th ed. Philadelphia: Lippincott Williams & Wilkins, 2001:416–418.

PATIENT   PROFILE   233

ERECTILE DYSFUNCTION

ANSWERS

1. (C) For PK, anxiety and depression are risk factors for erectile dysfunction. PK's cholesterol levels are at goal and do not pose a risk for erectile dysfunction at this time.

   Ref: Lee M. Erectile dysfunction. In: Dipiro JT, Talbert RL, Yee GC, et al, eds. *Pharmacotherapy: A Pathophysiologic Approach,* 5th ed. New York: McGraw-Hill, 2002:1511–1531.

2. (E) All the mentioned are potential risk factors for erectile dysfunction. Over-the-counter antihistamines and cimetidine also may cause erectile dysfunction; note that PK has seasonal allergies and likely may use over-the-counter products for symptom relief.

   Ref: Lee M. Erectile dysfunction. In: Dipiro JT, Talbert RL, Yee GC, et al, eds. *Pharmacotherapy: A Pathophysiologic Approach,* 5th ed. New York: McGraw-Hill, 2002:1511–1531.

3. (D) Phosphodiesterase inhibitors work by decreasing the breakdown of cGMP, a vasodilatory neurotransmitter in the corporal tissue. Thus this medication class works by maintaining adequate blood volume in the penis, thereby maintaining an erection. These medications do not help increase testosterone levels, as needed in hypogonadism, and do not relieve anxiety or distress. cGMP is only produced during sexual stimulation. Therefore, a patient without an intact neurologic pathway will not experience sexual stimulation, and as a result, this medication class will prove ineffective.

   Ref: Lee M. Erectile dysfunction. In: Dipiro JT, Talbert RL, Yee GC, et al, eds. *Pharmacotherapy: A Pathophysiologic Approach,* 5th ed. New York: McGraw-Hill, 2002:1511–1531.

4. (D) Viagra (sildenafil) lasts between 4 to 6 hours and should be taken without food because absorption is decreased with the presence of food. Viagra must be taken at least 30 minutes prior to sexual activity.

   Ref: Package insert: Viagra, Pfizer, Inc., New York. 2002.

5. (A) Cialis (tadalafil) may be taken 15 minutes prior to sexual activity. Cialis works over a 72-hour period; food does not affect the absorption of Cialis.

   Ref: Package insert: Cialis, Lilly ICOS, LLC, Indianapolis, IN, 2004.

6. (D) Levitra (vardenafil) lasts between 4 to 6 hours and should be taken without food because absorption is decreased in the presence of food. Levitra must be taken at least 30 minutes prior to sexual activity.

   Ref: Package insert: Levitra, Bayer Pharmaceuticals Corporation, West Haven, CT, 2003.

7. (E) Renal/hepatic dysfunction and CYP3A4 inhibitor use will cause increased levels of all phosphodiesterase inhibitors.

   Ref: Lee M. Erectile dysfunction. In: Dipiro JT, Talbert RL, Yee GC, et al, eds. *Pharmacotherapy: A Pathophysiologic Approach,* 5th ed. New York: McGraw-Hill, 2002:1511–1531.

8. (D) Sildenafil and trazodone both may cause the complication of prolonged erection known as priapism.

   Ref: Lee M. Erectile dysfunction. In: Dipiro JT, Talbert RL, Yee GC, et al, eds. *Pharmacotherapy: A Pathophysiologic Approach,* 5th ed. New York: McGraw-Hill, 2002:1511–1531.

9. (C) Caverject should be administered with an injection at 2 o'clock and 10 o'clock angles. The patient must wait 24 hours between injections. The patient should apply pressure at the site of injection for 5 minutes or until bleeding stops.

   Ref: Package insert: Caverjet, Pharmacia Corporation, Kalamazoo, MI, 2003.

10. (E) Muse should be injected 1/2 in into the urethra. Rather than applying pressure, the patient should massage the penis for 10 seconds or until burning subsides.

    Ref: Package insert: Muse, Vivus, Inc., Mountain View, CA, 1998.

PATIENT PROFILE 234
PREGNANCY

ANSWERS

1. (C)

   Ref: Young V. Teratogenicity and drugs in breast milk. In: Koda-Kimbla MA, Young LY, Kradjan WA, et al, eds. *Applied Therapeutics: The Clinical Use of Drugs,* 8th ed. Philadelphia: Lippincott Williams & Wilkins, 2005:47(1–32).

2. (A)

   Ref: Berardi RR. DeSimone EM, et al. *Handbook of Nonprescription Drugs,* 13th ed. Washington: American Pharmaceutical Association, 2002:1019–1021.

3. (B)

   Ref: JAMA patient page. Spina bifida. *JAMA* 2001;285(23):3050.

4. (D)

   Ref: Young V. Teratogenicity and drugs in breast milk. In: Koda-Kimbla MA, Young LY, Kradjan WA, et al, eds. *Applied Therapeutics: The Clinical Use of Drugs,* 8th ed. Philadelphia: Lippincott Williams & Wilkins, 2005:47(1–32).

5. (C)

   Ref: *N Engl J Med* 2003;338:1128–1137.

6. (B)

   Ref: Centers for Disease Control and Prevention. U.S. Public Health Service Task Force recommendations for the use of antiretroviral drugs in pregnant HIV-1-infected women for maternal health and interventions to reduce perinatal HIV-1 transmission in the United States. *MMWR* 2002;51(No RR-18):1–38.

7. (B)

   Ref: Centers for Disease Control and Prevention. U.S. Public Health Service Task Force recommendations for the use of antiretroviral drugs in pregnant HIV-1-infected women for maternal health and interventions to reduce perinatal HIV-1 transmission in the United States. *MMWR* 2002;51(No RR-18):1–38.

8. (D)

   Ref: Gardner MO, Doyle NM. Asthma in pregnancy. *Obstet Gynecol Clin North Am* 2004;31(2):385–413.

9. (D)

   Ref: Rampono J, Proud S, Hackett LP, et al. A pilot study of newer antidepressant concentrations in cord and maternal serum and possible effects in the neonate. *Int J Neuropsychopharmacol* 2004;7(3):329–334.

   Ref: Bonari L, Bennett H, Einarson A. Risks of untreated depression during pregnancy. *Can Fam Phys* 2004;50:37–39.

10. (B)

    Ref: Briggs GG, Freeman RK, Yaffe SJ, eds. *A Reference Guide to Fetal and Neonatal Risk: Drugs in Pregnancy and Lactation,* 6th ed. Philadelphia: Lippincott Williams & Wilkins, 2002.

ANTI-PARKINSON MEDICATIONS

ANSWERS

1. (E) All are facts about Parkinson's disease.

2. (E) Dopamine is very polar molecule with very poor absorption through biologic membranes. It does not cross the blood-brain barrier to reach the site of action.

3. (B) Levodopa has an amino acid structure; therefore, it is transported through biomembranes by active transport mechanism independent of lipophilicity.

4. (E) All are correct statements.

5. (C) Carbidopa is an inhibitor of the enzymes dopa decarboxylase that converts levodopa into its active form, dopamine. The inhibitor does not cross the blood-brain barrier, so only peripheral conversion is inhibited. This leads to less levodopa dose and less dopamine peripheral side effects.

6. (E) Carbidopa is a polar molecule with a hydrazine group replacing the amino group of levodopa, so the molecule is not an amino acid and is not transported to the brain by the active transport mechanism.

7. (C) Both agents are direct dopamine agonists.

8. (C) The catechol structure of tolcapone explains its mechanism of action as a COMT inhibitor. The drug is used as adjunct therapy to limit levodopa and dopamine deactivation.

9. (A) Parkinson's disease is an imbalance between the concentrations of dopamine and acetylcholine in the brain toward high cholinergic and low dopaminergic effects. Anticholinergic agent help to restore the balance.

10. (C) Both atropine and benzotropine are anticholinergic agents. Benzotropine is more lipophilic than atropine and crosses the blood-brain barrier easier. In addition, benzotropine has an ether group, which is metabolically more stable than the ester function of atropine.

BACTEREMIA AND SEPSIS

ANSWERS

1. (A) Endocarditis can be caused by a variety of organisms. The most common are *S. aureus* and *S. viridans*. Nafcillin with gentamicin is the only choice that provides adequate coverage against these organisms. Nafcillin, a cell-wall antibiotic, retains excellent activity against *S. aureus* and will cover most strains of *Streptococcus*. The synergistic combination with gentamicin in low doses is indicated for the initial treatment of patients with this life-threatening infection.

Ref: Taubert KA, Dajani AS. Optimisation of the prevention and treatment of bacterial endocarditis. *Drugs Aging* 2001;18(6): 415–424.

Ref: Gilbert DN, Moellering RC Jr, Eliopoulos GM, Sande MA, eds. *The Sanford Guide to Antimicrobial Therapy 2004,* 34th ed. Hyde Park, VT: Antimicrobial Therapy, 2004:20.

2. (E) Rifampin has excellent activity against gram-positive organisms. Rifampin always should be used in combination with other antibiotics because it is susceptible to resistance fairly rapidly. When rifampin is used in combination with vancomycin, however, to treat patients with endocarditis, the synergistic benefits prevail.

Ref: Taubert KA, Dajani AS. Optimisation of the prevention and treatment of bacterial endocarditis. *Drugs Aging* 2001;18(6): 415–424.

Ref: Gilbert DN, Moellering RC Jr, Eliopoulos GM, Sande MA, eds. *The Sanford Guide to Antimicrobial Therapy 2004,* 34th ed. Hyde Park, VT: Antimicrobial Therapy, 2004:20.

3. (E) All these effects should be monitored when a patient receives IV nafcillin.

Ref: Gilbert DN, Moellering RC Jr, Eliopoulos GM, Sande MA, eds. *The Sanford Guide to Antimicrobial Therapy 2004,* 34th ed. Hyde Park, VT: Antimicrobial Therapy, 2004:20.

4. (A) According to current guidelines for endocarditis pro-phylaxis before dental procedures, amoxicillin is the drug of choice because of its good bioavailability and low side effect profile.

Ref: Taubert KA, Dajani AS. Optimisation of the prevention and treatment of bacterial endocarditis. *Drugs Aging* 2001;18(6): 415–424.

Ref: Gilbert DN, Moellering RC Jr, Eliopoulos GM, Sande MA, eds. *The Sanford Guide to Antimicrobial Therapy 2004,* 34th ed. Hyde Park, VT: Antimicrobial Therapy, 2004:20.

5. (B) The presence of organisms that are resistant to peni-cillin does not preclude the use of penicillins, provided that the resistance is low or of intermediate level. In this instance, however, the dose of penicillin should be in-creased to overcome the resistance.

Ref: Taubert KA, Dajani AS. Optimisation of the prevention and treat-ment of bacterial endocarditis. *Drugs Aging* 2001;18(6): 415–424.

PATIENT PROFILE 237

NOSOCOMIAL URINARY TRACT INFECTIONS

ANSWERS

1. (A) Although elderly patients often have asymptomatic bacteriuria, treatment is not recommended. Studies have shown no beneficial outcome with antibiotic therapy com-pared to untreated patients. In addition, the high adverse drug reaction rate in elderly people, costs, and the poten-tial for resistant organisms should be considered. Sympto-matic patients need to be treated.

Ref: Coyle EA, Prince RA. Urinary tract infections and prostatitis. In: Dipiro JT, Talbert RL, Yee GC, et al., eds. *Pharmacotherapy: A Pathophysiologic Approach,* 5th edition. New York: McGraw-Hill, 2002::1981–1996.

Ref: Fish DN. Urinary tract infections. In: Koda-Kimble MA, Young LY, Kradian WA, et al., eds. *Applied Therapeutics: The Clinical Use of Drugs,* 8th edition. Philadelphia: Lippincott Williams & Wilkins, 2004:64(1–22).

2. (D) Nosocomial UTIs are commonly associated with the use of indwelling catheters. Because the sensitivity of nosocomial urinary pathogens differs from community-acquired ones, the microbiology lab of the hospital should be consulted to provide current antimicrobial sus-ceptibility data. *E. coli* is still the predominant organism but other gram-negative and -positive pathogens, less sensitive to routinely used antibiotics, may play a signifi-cant role in nosocomial UTIs.

Ref: Fish DN. Urinary tract infections. In: Koda-Kimble MA, Young LY, Kradian WA, et al., eds. *Applied Therapeutics: The Clinical Use of Drugs,* 8th edition. Philadelphia: Lippincott Williams & Wilkins, 2004:64(1–22).

3. (D) Either vancomycin or ampicillin, with or without gen-tamicin, is an appropriate choice against *Enterococcus faecalis.*

Ref: Fish DN. Urinary tract infections. In: Koda-Kimble MA, Young LY, Kradian WA, et al., eds. *Applied Therapeutics: The Clinical Use of Drugs,* 8th edition. Philadelphia: Lippincott Williams & Wilkins, 2004:64(1–22).

4. (B) 1.5 to 2 mg/kg is the usual loading dose of gentamicin regardless of the patient's renal function. The patient's IBW should be used to calculate the loading dose. If a pa-tient's weight is more than 30% of IBW, then the dosing weight (DW = IBW + 0.4 [TBW-IBW]) should be used. WA weighs 68 kg and is 5'5" tall.

IBW: 45.5 kg + 2.3 ((inch >5')
45.5 + 2.3 × 5
45.5 + 11.5 = 57 kg
57 kg × 2 mg = 114 mg, rounded to 120 mg

Ref: Bauer LA. Clinical pharmacokinetics and pharmacodynamics. In: Dipiro JT, Talbert RL, Yee GC, et al., eds. *Pharmacotherapy: A Pathophysiologic Approach,* 5th edition. New York: McGraw-Hill, 2002:4(33–54).

Ref: Qan DJ, Aweeka FT. Dosing of drugs in renal failure. In: Koda-Kimble MA, Young LY, Kradian WA, et al., eds. *Applied Therapeu-tics: The Clinical Use of Drugs,* 8th edition. Philadelphia: Lippin-cott Williams & Wilkins, 2004:34(1–26).

5. (A) Gentamicin is eliminated through the kidneys. Main-tenance doses of gentamicin need to be adjusted (as percentage of loading dose) based on the patient's renal function and desired dosing interval to minimize toxic-ity. The trough level should be less than 2 µg/mL. Based on the Scr level of 1.4 mg/dL, WA's CrCl is cal-culated as 28.8 mL/min. Using the Hull and Sarrubi nomogram, her maintenance dose should have been 63% of the loading dose (75.6 mg rounded to 80 mg) given q 12h.

Ref: Bauer LA. Clinical pharmacokinetics and pharmacodynamics. In: Dipiro JT, Talbert RL, Yee GC, et al., eds. *Pharmacotherapy: A Pathophysiologic Approach,* 5th edition. New York: McGraw-Hill, 2002:33–54.

Ref: Qan DJ, Aweeka FT. Dosing of drugs in renal failure. In: Koda-Kimble MA, Young LY, Kradian WA, et al., eds. *Applied Therapeutics: The Clinical Use of Drugs,* 8th edition. Philadelphia: Lippincott Williams & Wilkins, 2004:34(1–26).

6. (D) Nephrotoxicity and ototoxicity are known adverse reactions of aminoglycosides. Risk factors include high drug concentrations, duration of therapy, dehydration, age, and concomitant nephrotoxins.

Ref: Gugliemo BJ. Principles of infectious diseases. In: Koda-Kimble MA, Young LY, Kradian WA, et al., eds. *Applied Therapeutics: The Clinical Use of Drugs,* 8th edition. Philadelphia: Lippincott Williams & Wilkins, 2004:56(1–25).

7. (D) Gentamicin's postantibiotic effect (delayed bacterial regrowth after antibiotic exposure) and its concentration-dependent killing (higher peak concentration results in increased clinical response) allow for qd dosing. Patients with renal disease need individualized gentamicin dosing.

Ref: Bauer LA. Clinical pharmacokinetics and pharmacodynamics. In: Dipiro JT, Talbert RL, Yee GC, et al., eds. *Pharmacotherapy: A Pathophysiologic Approach,* 5th edition. New York: McGraw-Hill, 2002:33–54.

Ref: Gugliemo BJ. Principles of infectious diseases. In: Koda-Kimble MA, Young LY, Kradian WA, et al., eds. *Applied Therapeutics: The Clinical Use of Drugs,* 8th edition. Philadelphia: Lippincott Williams & Wilkins, 2004:56(1–25).

8. (A) Piperacillin-tazobactam has a broad spectrum of gram-negative coverage similar to aminoglycosides. Amoxicillin does not cover many gram-negative pathogens, whereas cefazolin, quinupristin-dalfopristin, and oxacillin cover primarily or exclusively gram-positive organisms.

Ref: Fish DN. Urinary tract infections. In: Koda-Kimble In: Koda-Kimble MA, Young LY, Kradian WA, et al., eds. *Applied Therapeutics: The Clinical Use of Drugs,* 8th edition. Philadelphia: Lippincott Williams & Wilkins, 2004:64(1–22).

9. (D) Fluconazole given for 7 to 14 days is recommended for urinary candidiasis in symptomatic patients. Amphotericin B is an alternative (especially in immunocompromised patients) but the drug can only be administered IV (0.3 to 1 mg/kg per day) or may be used as bladder irrigation.

Ref: Carver PL. Invasive fungal infections. In: Dipiro JT, Talbert RL, Yee GC, et al., eds. *Pharmacotherapy: A Pathophysiologic Approach,* 5th edition. New York: McGraw-Hill, 2002:2059–2088.

Ref: Cleary JD, Chapman SW, Pearson M. Fungal infections. In: Koda-Kimble MA, Young LY, Kradian WA, et al., eds. *Applied Therapeutics: The Clinical Use of Drugs,* 8th edition. Philadelphia: Lippincott Williams & Wilkins, 2004:71(1–28).

10. (E) Fluconazole can substantially increase phenytoin levels. It may also increase the risk of bleeding by interfering with warfarin's metabolism by the liver (cytochrome P450 alteration) leading to increased warfarin concentrations. Because fluconazole is excreted primarily unchanged in the urine, doses need to be adjusted according to renal function.

Ref: Carver PL. Invasive fungal infections. In: Dipiro JT, Talbert RL, Yee GC, et al., eds. *Pharmacotherapy: A Pathophysiologic Approach,* 5th edition. New York: McGraw-Hill, 2002:2059–2088.

Ref: Cleary JD, Chapman SW, Pearson M. Fungal infections. In: Koda-Kimble MA, Young LY, Kradian WA, et al., eds. *Applied Therapeutics: The Clinical Use of Drugs,* 8th edition. Philadelphia: Lippincott Williams & Wilkins, 2004:71(1–28).

PATIENT PROFILE 238

DERMATOLOGY

ANSWERS

1. (E) At initiation of benzoyl peroxide therapy, application once daily (apply sparingly and avoid the periorbital, perinasal, and perioral skin) minimizes irritation. If the medication is applied at bedtime, erythema should be minimal by the next morning.

Ref: Seaton TL. Acne. In: Koda-Kimble MA, Young LY, Kradjan WA, et al., eds. *Applied Therapeutics: The Clinical Use of Drugs,* 8th edition. Philadelphia: Lippincott Williams & Wilkins, 2004: 1–10.

2. (D) Tolerance to adverse effects occurs at therapy continues. The full therapeutic benefit may not be experienced for 4 to 8 weeks. Benzoyl peroxide can bleach hair and clothes.

Ref: Seaton TL. Acne. In: Koda-Kimble MA, Young LY, Kradjan WA, et al., eds. *Applied Therapeutics: The Clinical Use of Drugs,* 8th edition. Philadelphia: Lippincott Williams & Wilkins, 2004:1–10.

3. (D) Minocycline may cause vestibular toxicity and esophagitis from reflux, so it should not be taken just

before retiring. Minocycline belongs to the class of tetra-cyclines and should be avoided in pregnancy.

Ref: Seaton TL. Acne. In: Koda-Kimble MA, Young LY, Kradjan WA, et al., eds. *Applied Therapeutics: The Clinical Use of Drugs,* 8th edition. Philadelphia: Lippincott Williams & Wilkins, 2004:1–10.

4. (E) Photosensitivity can occur with use of tetracyclines, as can vaginal yeast infections. Patients should separate administration of tetracyclines with that of dairy products, antacids, iron products, and bismuth salts.

Ref: Seaton TL. Acne. In: Koda-Kimble MA, Young LY, Kradjan WA, et al., eds. *Applied Therapeutics: The Clinical Use of Drugs,* 8th edition. Philadelphia: Lippincott Williams & Wilkins, 2004:1–10.

5. (E) Tretinoin, a derivative of vitamin A available in various formulations, increases follicle cell turnover and decreases cohesiveness of cells, resulting in extrusion of existing comedones and inhibition of formation of new comedones.

Ref: Seaton TL. Acne. In: Koda-Kimble MA, Young LY, Kradjan WA, et al., eds. *Applied Therapeutics: The Clinical Use of Drugs,* 8th edition. Philadelphia: Lippincott Williams & Wilkins, 2004:1–10.

6. (E) Tretinoin can cause skin irritation. Patients may notice an exacerbation of acne at initiation of therapy, but the irritation resolves with continued therapy. Long exposure to ultraviolet radiation should be avoided.

Ref: Seaton TL. Acne. In: Koda-Kimble MA, Young LY, Kradjan WA, et al., eds. *Applied Therapeutics: The Clinical Use of Drugs,* 8th edition. Philadelphia: Lippincott Williams & Wilkins, 2004:1-10.

7. (B) Isotretinoin, a synthetic derivative of vitamin A, is considered for patients with severe acne and early in the treatment of patients with scars. Prolonged remission can be expected.

Ref: Seaton TL. Acne. In: Koda-Kimble MA, Young LY, Kradjan WA, et al., eds. *Applied Therapeutics; The Clinical Use of Drugs,* 8th edition. Philadelphia: Lippincott Williams & Wilkins, 2004:1–10.

8. (C) Isotretinoin, which is pregnancy category X, should be avoided in pregnancy. The manufacturer provides specific recommendations for women of child-bearing age. The patient should not become pregnant for at least 1 month after stopping isotretinoin therapy.

Ref: Seaton TL. Acne. In: Koda-Kimble MA, Young LY, Kradjan WA, et al., eds. *Applied Therapeutics: The Clinical Use of Drugs,* 8th edition. Philadelphia: Lippincott Williams & Wilkins, 2004:1–10.

9. (E) Adverse effects if isotretinoin include disturbances in lipid metabolism, mucocutaneous effects, conjunctivitis, and corneal capacity.

Ref: Seaton TL. Acne. In: Koda-Kimble MA, Young LY, Kradjan WA, et al., eds. *Applied Therapeutics: The Clinical Use of Drugs,* 8th edition. Philadelphia: Lippincott Williams & Wilkins, 2004:1–10.

10. (D) A baseline liver panel that includes serum transaminases and bilirubin, as well as a baseline, a fractionated lipid panel should be obtained before initiation of isotretinoin.

Ref: Seaton TL. Acne. In: Koda-Kimble MA, Young LY, Kradjan WA, et al., eds. *Applied Therapeutics: The Clinical Use of Drugs,* 8th edition. Philadelphia: Lippincott Williams & Wilkins, 2004:1-10.

PATIENT PROFILE 239

CHRONIC OBSTRUCTIVE PULMONARY DISEASE

ANSWERS

1. (D) Stage III severe COPD caused by her FEV_1 of 45% of predicted.

Ref: Global Initiative for Chronic Obstructive Lung Disease. Global strategy for the diagnosis management, and prevention of chronic obstructive pulmonary disease. Updated 2003. Available at: *http://www.goldcopd.com.* Accessed November 1, 2004.

2. (D) Albuterol as needed, Ipratropium inhaler two puffs by mouth three times a day, rehabilitation, and fluticasone inhaler two puffs by mouth two times a day.

Ref: Global Initiative for Chronic Obstructive Lung Disease. Global strategy for the diagnosis management, and prevention of chronic

obstructive pulmonary disease. Updated 2003. Available at: *http://www.goldcopd.com.* Accessed November 1, 2004.

3. (A) Dry mouth is a side effect.

Ref: Global Initiative for Chronic Obstructive Lung Disease. Global strategy for the diagnosis management, and prevention of chronic obstructive pulmonary disease. Updated 2003. Available at: *http://www.goldcopd.com.* Accessed November 1, 2004.

4. (C) An anticholinergic.

Ref: Global Initiative for Chronic Obstructive Lung Disease. Global strategy for the diagnosis management, and prevention of chronic obstructive pulmonary disease. Updated 2003. Available at: *http://www.goldcopd.com*. Accessed November 1, 2004.

5. (C) Dosage form and duration of action. Tiotropium is dosed once daily and is available in a dry powder inhaler, whereas Ipratropium is dosed three to four times a day and is available as a meter dose inhaler and solution for nebulization.

Ref: Global Initiative for Chronic Obstructive Lung Disease. Global strategy for the diagnosis management, and prevention of chronic obstructive pulmonary disease. Updated 2003. Available at: *http://www.goldcopd.com*. Accessed November 1, 2004.

6. (A) One inhalation once a day.

Ref: Global Initiative for Chronic Obstructive Lung Disease. Global strategy for the diagnosis management, and prevention of chronic obstructive pulmonary disease. Updated 2003. Available at: *http://www.goldcopd.com*. Accessed November 1, 2004.

7. (C) One tablet twice a day when being used for smoking cessation.

Ref: Global Initiative for Chronic Obstructive Lung Disease. Global strategy for the diagnosis management, and prevention of chronic

obstructive pulmonary disease. Updated 2003. Available at: *http://www.goldcopd.com*. Accessed November 1, 2004.

8. (B) It should be initiated 1 week before the patient stops smoking. This provides the greatest chance of success.

Ref: Global Initiative for Chronic Obstructive Lung Disease. Global strategy for the diagnosis management, and prevention of chronic obstructive pulmonary disease. Updated 2003. Available at: *http://www.goldcopd.com*. Accessed November 1, 2004.

9. (B) Stage I mild COPD because of her FEV_1 being 80% and having minimal daily symptoms.

Ref: Global Initiative for Chronic Obstructive Lung Disease. Global strategy for the diagnosis management, and prevention of chronic obstructive pulmonary disease. Updated 2003. Available at: *http://www.goldcopd.com*. Accessed November 1, 2004.

10. (B) Prednisone tablets. This product should only be used in a short-term manner because of the risk of adverse effects.

Ref: Global Initiative for Chronic Obstructive Lung Disease. Global strategy for the diagnosis management, and prevention of chronic obstructive pulmonary disease. Updated 2003. Available at: *http://www.goldcopd.com*. Accessed November 1, 2004.

PATIENT PROFILE 240
^{18}F-FDG

ANSWERS

1. (A)

Ref: Saha GB. *Fundamentals of Nuclear Pharmacy*, 4th edition. New York: Springer-Verlag, 1997:244.

2. (C)

Ref: Saha GB. *Fundamentals of Nuclear Pharmacy*, 4th edition. New York: Springer-Verlag, 1997:14.

3. (E)

Ref: Saha GB. *Fundamentals of Nuclear Pharmacy*, 4th edition. New York: Springer-Verlag, 1997:243.

4. (B)

Ref: Saha GB. *Fundamentals of Nuclear Pharmacy*, 4th edition. New York: Springer-Verlag, 1997:243.

5. (C)

Ref: Saha GB. *Fundamentals of Nuclear Pharmacy*, 4th edition. New York: Springer-Verlag, 1997:308.

6. (D)

Ref: Saha GB. *Fundamentals of Nuclear Pharmacy*, 4th edition. New York: Springer-Verlag, 1997:14.

7. (D)

Ref: Zatz J. *Pharmaceutical Calculations*, 3rd edition. New York: Wiley-Interscience, 1995:308.

8. (E)

Ref: Zatz J. *Pharmaceutical Calculations*, 3rd edition. New York: Wiley-Interscience, 1995:308.

9. (B)

Ref: Saha GB. *Fundamentals of Nuclear Pharmacy*, 4th edition. New York: Springer-Verlag, 1997:21.

10. (A)

Ref: Saha GB. *Fundamentals of Nuclear Pharmacy*, 4th edition. New York: Springer-Verlag, 1997:52–53.

PATIENT PROFILE 241
SMOKING CESSATION

ANSWERS

1. (D) The Fagerstrom Test for Nicotine Dependence (FTND) is a six-item instrument that can be completed by the patient or administered in an interview with the patient. An individual's FTND scale score can range from 0 to 10 and is computed as a sum of the responses to the six questions. Scores higher than 5 are indicative of substantial nicotine dependence.

   The DSM-IV is the Diagnostic and Statistical Manual of Mental Disorders.
   The PANSS is the Positive and Negative Symptom Scale for Schizophrenia.
   The BPRS is the Brief Psychiatric Rating Scale.
   The CAGE is an assessment tool for screening alcohol abuse disorders.

   Ref: Corelli RL, Hudmon KS. Tobacco use and dependence. In: Koda-Kimble MA, Young LY, Kradjan WA, et al., eds. *Applied Therapeutics: The Clinical Use of Drugs,* 8th edition. Baltimore, MD: Lippincott Williams & Wilkins 2005:1–29.

2. (B) Polycyclic aromatic hydrocarbons are products of incomplete combustion of tobacco. Polycyclic aromatic hydrocarbons are potent inducers of the cytochrome P450 microsomal enzymes CYP1A1 and CYP1A2, and possibly CYP2E1. Most drug interactions with tobacco smoke result from the induction of CYP1A2.

   Ref: Corelli RL, Hudmon KS. Tobacco use and dependence. In: Koda-Kimble MA, Young LY, Kradjan WA, et al., eds. *Applied Therapeutics: The Clinical Use of Drugs,* 8th edition. Baltimore, MD: Lippincott Williams & Wilkins 2005:1–29.

3. (D) Smoking can increase the metabolism of theophylline via induction of CYP1A2. Theophylline levels should be monitored if cigarette smoking is initiated, discontinued, or changed.

   Ref: Corelli RL, Hudmon KS. Tobacco use and dependence. In: Koda-Kimble MA, Young LY, Kradjan WA, et al., eds. *Applied Therapeutics: The Clinical Use of Drugs,* 8th edition. Baltimore, MD: Lippincott Williams & Wilkins 2005:1–29.

4. (C) Smoking cessation is a process that might take months or even years to achieve. Clinicians should discuss pharmacotherapeutic options for smoking cessation and should educate patients that medications, when taken correctly, can substantially increase the likelihood of quitting. Furthermore, arranging follow-up counseling is important because a patient's ability to quit increases with multiple counseling interactions.

Ref: Corelli RL, Hudmon KS. Tobacco use and dependence. In: Koda-Kimble MA, Young LY, Kradjan WA, et al., eds. *Applied Therapeutics: The Clinical Use of Drugs,* 8th edition. Baltimore, MD: Lippincott Williams & Wilkins 2005:1–29.

5. (B) Patients who abruptly stop smoking may experience constipation (intestinal movement decreases for a brief period), difficulty concentrating (time needed to adjust to not having constant stimulation from nicotine), hunger (cravings for cigarettes can be confused with hunger pangs; oral cravings are common), insomnia (nicotine affects brain wave function and influences sleep patterns). Palpitations are uncommon. Other common nicotine withdrawal symptoms include dry cough and nasal drip (as the body rids itself of mucus), craving for a cigarette, dizziness (the body is getting extra oxygen), fatigue (nicotine is a stimulant), and irritability.

   Ref: Corelli RL, Hudmon KS. Tobacco use and dependence. In: Koda-Kimble MA, Young LY, Kradjan WA, et al., eds. *Applied Therapeutics: The Clinical Use of Drugs,* 8th edition. Baltimore, MD: Lippincott Williams & Wilkins 2005:1–29.

6. (E) The nicotine gum, lozenge, and oral inhaler have similar concentration curves. The nicotine nasal spray reaches its peak plasma concentration most rapidly. The nicotine transdermal patch has the slowest onset, but provides more consistent blood levels of nicotine over a longer period of time. Nicotine is categorized by the FDA as pregnancy risk category D, indicating that there is evidence of risk to the human fetus.

   Ref: Corelli RL, Hudmon KS. Tobacco use and dependence. In: Koda-Kimble MA, Young LY, Kradjan WA, et al., eds. *Applied Therapeutics: The Clinical Use of Drugs,* 8th edition. Baltimore, MD: Lippincott Williams & Wilkins 2005:1–29.

7. (C) The most common side effects associated with the nicotine patch are erythema, burning, and pruritus at the skin application site. To minimize the potential for local skin reactions, it is important to counsel patients to rotate the patch application site daily. The same area should not be used again for at least 1 week. The patient should ensure that the patch adheres well to the skin, especially around the edges. Exposure to water and exercise do not reduce the effectiveness of the nicotine patch if it is applied correctly. Nicotine transdermal patch products are available over the counter and via prescription. The 24-hour nicotine transdermal patches theoretically offer the advantage of continuous nicotine delivery over a 24-hour period and provide coverage for early morning cravings.

The 16-hour patch offers the advantage of less sleep interference, insomnia, and vivid dreams.

Ref: Corelli RL, Hudmon KS. Tobacco use and dependence. In: Koda-Kimble MA, Young LY, Kradjan WA, et al., eds. *Applied Therapeutics: The Clinical Use of Drugs,* 8th edition. Baltimore, MD: Lippincott Williams & Wilkins 2005:1–29.

8. (D) Zyban (bupropion SR) is a nonnicotine agent. It inhibits the neuronal reuptake of dopamine and norepinephrine in the central nervous system. The exact mechanism of action in smoking cessation is unknown, but clinical trials confirm that bupropion SR can reduce cravings for tobacco and nicotine withdrawal symptoms. Approximately 1 week of bupropion SR dosing is required to reach steady-state blood levels and treatment should be initiated while the patient is still smoking. Bupropion SR can be used safely in conjunction with NRT, and data suggest that the combination may be more effective than monotherapy with either agent.

Ref: Corelli RL, Hudmon KS. Tobacco use and dependence. In: Koda-Kimble MA, Young LY, Kradjan WA, et al., eds. *Applied Ther-*

apeutics: The Clinical Use of Drugs, 8th edition. Baltimore, MD: Lippincott Williams & Wilkins 2005:1–29.

9. (A) The nicotine polacrilex gum is more viscous than ordinary chewing gum and is more likely to adhere to fillings, bridges, dentures, crowns, and braces. TS should not use nicotine polacrilex gum because she wears dentures.

Ref: Corelli RL, Hudmon KS. Tobacco use and dependence. In: Koda-Kimble MA, Young LY, Kradjan WA, et al., eds. *Applied Therapeutics: The Clinical Use of Drugs,* 8th edition. Baltimore, MD: Lippincott Williams & Wilkins 2005:1–29.

10. (B) Although not FDA approved specifically for smoking cessation, the prescription medications clonidine and nortriptyline are recommended as second-line agents for smoking cessation. Bupropion SR is FDA approved for smoking cessation and is considered a first-line agent.

Ref: Corelli RL, Hudmon KS. Tobacco use and dependence. In: Koda-Kimble MA, Young LY, Kradjan WA, et al., eds. *Applied Therapeutics: The Clinical Use of Drugs,* 8th edition. Baltimore, MD: Lippincott Williams & Wilkins 2005:1–29.

PATIENT PROFILE 242

HYPERCHOLESTEROLEMIA

ANSWERS

1. (B) JW's four CHD risk factors that independent of an elevated LDL are; age (>55 years), smoking, hypertension, and a low HDL (<40 mg/dL).

Ref: Third Report of the National Cholesterol Education Program (NCEP) Expert Panel on Detection, Evaluation, and Treatment of High Blood Cholesterol in Adults (Adult Treatment Panel III) final report. *Circulation* 2002;106:3143–3421.

2. (C) The usual daily dose of colesevelam for the treatment of hypercholesterolemia is 2.6 to 3.8 g daily.

Ref: Third Report of the National Cholesterol Education Program (NCEP) Expert Panel on Detection, Evaluation, and Treatment of High Blood Cholesterol in Adults (Adult Treatment Panel III) final report. *Circulation* 2002;106:3143–3421.

3. (C) The recommend time interval for obtaining a lipid panel to assess the efficacy of lipid lowering therapy once a medication is initiated or there is a change in therapy is 6 weeks.

Ref: Third Report of the National Cholesterol Education Program (NCEP) Expert Panel on Detection, Evaluation, and Treatment of High Blood Cholesterol in Adults (Adult Treatment Panel III) final report. *Circulation* 2002;106:3143–3421.

4. (D) Bile acid sequestrants are contraindicated when serum triglycerides are >400 mg/dL.

Ref: Third Report of the National Cholesterol Education Program (NCEP) Expert Panel on Detection, Evaluation, and Treatment of High Blood Cholesterol in Adults (Adult Treatment Panel III) final report. *Circulation* 2002;106:3143–3421.

5. (A) Drug interactions with bile acid sequestrants can be avoided when concomitant medications are given 1 hour before or 4 hours after the sequestrant.

Ref: Third Report of the National Cholesterol Education Program (NCEP) Expert Panel on Detection, Evaluation, and Treatment of High Blood Cholesterol in Adults (Adult Treatment Panel III) final report. *Circulation* 2002;106:3143–3421.

6. (D) Bile acid sequestrants do not exhibit an elevation of liver function tests as a major adverse effect.

Ref: Third Report of the National Cholesterol Education Program (NCEP) Expert Panel on Detection, Evaluation, and Treatment of High Blood Cholesterol in Adults (Adult Treatment Panel III) final report. *Circulation* 2002;106:3143–3421.

7. (D) Bile acid sequestrants work by binding bile acids in the intestine using anionic exchange.

Ref: Third Report of the National Cholesterol Education Program (NCEP) Expert Panel on Detection, Evaluation, and Treatment of High Blood Cholesterol in Adults (Adult Treatment Panel III) final report. *Circulation* 2002;106:3143–3421.

8. (B) The initial starting dose of ezetimibe to treat hypercholesterolemia is 10 mg daily.

    Ref: Drug Information 2004. *American Hospital Formulary Service* 2004;1642–1643.

9. (E) Both ezetimibe and statins can elevate serum liver function tests; thus, when used in combination there is an increased risk of elevating serum liver function tests.

    Ref: Drug Information 2004. *American Hospital Formulary Service* 2004;1642–1643.

10. (C) Ezetimibe works by decreasing the absorption cholesterol in the intestine.

    Ref: Drug Information 2004. *American Hospital Formulary Service* 2004;1642–1643.

PATIENT PROFILE 243

BACTERIAL VAGINOSIS

ANSWERS

1. (B) *Gardnerella vaginalis*, an anaerobic bacteria, is associated with bacterial vaginosis. Other organisms, such as *Prevotella* sp., *Mobiluncus* sp., and *Mycoplasma hominis,* also are implicated.

    Ref: Sexually transmitted diseases treatment guidelines, 2002. Centers for Disease Control Website. Available at: *http//www.cdc.gov/STD/ treatment/5-2002TG.htm*. Accessed October 17, 2004.

2. (E) Bacterial vaginosis is associated with douching, lack of vaginal lactobacilli, and multiple sex partners. Bacterial vaginosis occurs from the replacement of H_2O_2-producing lactobacillus with high amounts of the organisms listed in the answer to Question 1.

    Ref: Sexually transmitted diseases treatment guidelines, 2002. Centers for Disease Control Website. Available at: *http//www.cdc.gov/STD/ treatment/5-2002TG.htm*. Accessed October 17, 2004.

3. (D) Goals of therapy include minimizing the risk for infectious complications after hysterectomy and abortion and relieving signs and symptoms such as white vaginal discharge and malodor. It is unclear if bacterial vaginosis results from a sexually transmitted pathogen; the treatment of a male sex partner does not prevent recurrence of bacterial vaginosis.

    Ref: Sexually transmitted diseases treatment guidelines, 2002. Centers for Disease Control Website. Available at: *http//www. cdc.gov/STD/treatment/5-2002TG.htm*. Accessed October 17, 2004.

4. (B) The alternate agent for the treatment of bacterial vaginosis, if an individual has an allergy to metronidazole, is clindamycin. Erythromycin, ofloxacin, and tetracycline are not effective treatments and changing the route of administration to intravaginal metronidazole would not be tolerated.

    Ref: Sexually transmitted diseases treatment guidelines, 2002. Centers for Disease Control Website. Available at. *http//www. cdc.gov/STD/treatment/5-2002TG.htm*. Accessed October 17, 2004.

5. (E) Metronidazole may cause adverse effects including but not limited to diarrhea, dizziness, headache, loss of appetite, metallic taste, and nausea.

    Ref: Metronidazole (Drug Monograph). In: Klasco RK, ed. DRUGDEX® System. Thomson MICROMEDEX®, Greenwood Village, CO (Edition expires 9/2004).

6. (B) A disulfiram reaction may occur if alcohol is ingested during metronidazole therapy. Metronidazole interferes with ethanol metabolism. An individual experiencing this reaction may develop severe facial flushing, headache, nausea and vomiting, weakness, confusion, hypotension, and blurred vision.

    Ref: Metronidazole (Drug Monograph). In: Klasco RK, ed. DRUGDEX® System. Thomson MICROMEDEX®, Greenwood Village, CO (Edition expires 9/2004).

7. (E) All statements are counseling points for patient education about metronidazole.

    Ref: Metronidazole (Drug Monograph). In: Klasco RK, ed. DRUGDEX® System. Thomson MICROMEDEX®, Greenwood Village, CO (Edition expires 9/2004).

8. (B) Treatment for the male sex partner is not routinely recommended because it does not help to decrease the recurrence of bacterial vaginosis.

    Ref: Sexually transmitted diseases treatment guidelines, 2002. Centers for Disease Control Website. Available at: *http//www.cdc. gov/STD/treatment/5-2002TG.htm*. Accessed October 17, 2004.

9. (D) Both clindamycin cream 2% and metronidazole gel 0.75% are alternatives to oral metronidazole in the

treatment of bacterial vaginosis. Both are used intravaginally once a day.

Ref: Sexually transmitted diseases treatment guidelines, 2002. Centers for Disease Control Website. Available at: *http//www. cdc.gov/STD/treatment/5-2002TG.htm*. Accessed October 17, 2004.

10. (B) The duration of therapy of metronidazole is 5 days for bacterial vaginosis. Clindamycin therapy is 7 days.

Ref: Sexually transmitted diseases treatment guidelines, 2002. Centers for Disease Control Website. Available at: *http//www. cdc.gov/STD/treatment/5-2002TG.htm*. Accessed October 17, 2004.

PATIENT PROFILE 244

ALZHEIMER'S DISEASE

ANSWERS

1. (D) All of the symptoms associated with JB's condition result from memory loss. This is the first noticeable symptom of AD. JB's memory loss is more significant than the typical memory loss associated with age since she is forgetting to eat, resulting in weight loss and forgetting to refill her prescriptions, a sign of nonadherence.

Ref: Difilippi JL, Crismon ML, Clark WR. Alzheimer's disease. In: DiPiro JT, Talbert RL, Yee GC, et al., eds. *Pharmacotherapy: A Pathophysiologic Approach,* 5th edition. New York: McGraw-Hill, 2002:1165–1182.

2. (A) Malnutrition is a complication associated with AD because patients such as JB will forget to eat. Other complications include falls, aspiration, infection, violent behavior, and dehydration.

Ref: Difilippi JL, Crismon ML, Clark WR. Alzheimer's disease. In: DiPiro JT, Talbert RL, Yee GC, et al., eds. *Pharmacotherapy: A Pathophysiologic Approach,* 5th edition. New York: McGraw-Hill, 2002:1165–1182.

3. (C) Galantamine is a nicotinic receptor agonist as well as a cholinesterase inhibitor. This action promotes the release of acetylcholine. The other cholinesterase inhibitors do not act at the nicotinic receptor.

Ref: Difilippi JL, Crismon ML, Clark WR. Alzheimer's disease. In: DiPiro JT, Talbert RL, Yee GC, et al., eds. *Pathophysiologic Approach,* 5th edition. New York: McGraw-Hill, 2002:1165–1182.

4. (D) The starting dose of galantamine is 4 mg po bid. The drug may be titrated up by 8 mg daily every 4 weeks to a maximum of 8 to 16 mg po bid.

Ref: Difilippi JL, Crismon ML, Clark WR. Alzheimer's disease. In: DiPiro JT, Talbert RL, Yee GC, et al., eds. *Pharmacotherapy: A Pathophysiologic Approach,* 5th edition. New York: McGraw-Hill, 2002:1165–1182.

5. (A) Nausea is the most reported adverse effect occurring in 24% of patients. Other common adverse effects include vomiting, diarrhea, dizziness, and headache.

Ref: Difilippi JL, Crismon ML, Clark WR. Alzheimer's disease. In: DiPiro JT, Talbert RL, Yee GC, et al., eds. *Pharmacotherapy: A Pathophysiologic Approach,* 5th edition. New York: McGraw-Hill, 2002:1165–1182.

6. (C) Even though olanzapine can cause anticholinergic side effects, it is preferred over the other therapies. The more recent atypical antipsychotics are ideal because they have fewer side effects than the other therapeutic modalities.

Ref: Difilippi JL, Crismon ML, Clark WR. Alzheimer's disease. In: DiPiro JT, Talbert RL, Yee GC, et al., eds. *Pharmacotherapy: A Pathophysiologic Approach,* 5th edition. New York: McGraw-Hill, 2002:1165–1182.

7. (B) Patients with AD often experience depression towing to the frustration caused by the memory loss. The recommended treatment is the selective serotonin reuptake inhibitor class because of the decreased incidence of cholinergic effects, OSHT, and drowsiness.

Ref: Difilippi JL, Crismon ML, Clark WR. Alzheimer's disease. In: DiPiro JT, Talbert RL, Yee GC, et al., eds. *Pharmacotherapy: A Pathophysiologic Approach,* 5th edition. New York: McGraw-Hill, 2002:1165–1182.

8. (B) Sundowning can occur late in the afternoon and is characterized by the magnification of symptoms because of a decrease in cognition. The severity of symptoms can change throughout the course of the disease, becoming worse with the advanced stages.

Ref: Difilippi JL, Crismon ML, Clark WR. Alzheimer's disease. In: DiPiro JT, Talbert RL, Yee GC, et al., eds. *Pharmacotherapy: A Pathophysiologic Approach,* 5th edition. New York: McGraw-Hill, 2002:1165–1182.

9. (C) It is important not to over stimulate AD patients by arguing with them or having them perform tasks that will cause frustration. Orientation cues become important during the disease progression because patients can become disoriented even in their own homes. These cues can be in the form of colored papers in doorways that will help the patient remain oriented.

Ref: Difilippi JL, Crismon ML, Clark WR. Alzheimer's disease. In: DiPiro JT, Talbert RL, Yee GC, et al., eds. *Pharmacotherapy: A Pathophysiologic Approach,* 5th edition. New York: McGraw-Hill, 2002:1165–1182.

10. (D) Vitamin E has been identified as an antioxidant and may be used by patients with AD. It is an over-the-counter preparation and is relatively inexpensive. JB may benefit from its use in terms of slowing the progression of the disease but it is important to note that it will not cure AD and should not be used as the only treatment modality.

Ref: Difilippi JL, Crismon ML, Clark WR. Alzheimer's disease. In: DiPiro JT, Talbert RL, Yee GC, et al., eds. *Pharmacotherapy: A Pathophysiologic Approach,* 5th edition. New York: McGraw-Hill, 2002:1165–1182.

PATIENT PROFILE 245
TYPE 2 DIABETES MELLITUS

ANSWERS

1. (C) The United Kingdom Prospective Diabetes Study (UKPDS) was a landmark report on the care of patients with type 2 diabetes mellitus, confirming the importance of glycemic control for reducing microvascular complications. The major portion of the study compared conventional therapy versus intensive therapy with either a sulfonylurea or insulin and found that microvascular complications are reduced by 25% when median HbA1C is 7% compared with 7.9%.

Ref: Oki JC, Isley WL. Diabetes mellitus. In: Dipiro JT, Talbert RL, Yee GC, et al., eds. *Pharmacotherapy: A Pathophysiologic Approach,* 5th edition. New York: McGraw-Hill, 2002: 1335–1358.

2. (C) The most common side effect of sulfonylureas is hypoglycemia.

Ref: Oki JC, Isley WL. Diabetes mellitus. In: Dipiro JT, Talbert RL, Yee GC, et al., eds. *Pharmacotherapy: A Pathophysiologic Approach,* 5th edition. New York: McGraw-Hill, 2002: 1335–1358.

3. (D) Sulfonylureas exert a hypoglycemic effect by stimulating pancreatic secretion of insulin by binding to the pancreatic β-cell plasma membrane associated with the ATP-dependent K^+ channel, resulting in closing of these channels, and opening of the voltage-dependent $Ca2^+$ channels. An increase in intracellular calcium leads to an increase in insulin secretion.

Ref: Oki JC, Isley WL. Diabetes mellitus. In: Dipiro JT, Talbert RL, Yee GC, et al., eds. *Pharmacotherapy: A Pathophysiologic Approach,* 5th edition. New York: McGraw-Hill, 2002: 1335–1358.

4. (B) Upon initiation of therapy with a thiazolidinedione such as rosiglitazone, baseline liver function tests (AST and ALT) should be obtained, then repeated every other month for the first 12 months, and then periodically thereafter. Thiazolidinediones should not be initiated if baseline AST or ALT exceeds 2.5 times the upper limit of normal and they should be discontinued if the AST or ALT exceeds three times the upper limit of normal or if signs and symptoms of liver injury are present.

Ref: Oki JC, Isley WL. Diabetes mellitus. In: Dipiro JT, Talbert RL, Yee GC, et al., eds. *Pharmacotherapy: A Pathophysiologic Approach,* 5th edition. New York: McGraw-Hill, 2002: 1335–1358.

5. (C) Metformin can be initiated with immediate release tablets at 500 mg bid with meals or 850 mg once a day.

Ref: Oki JC, Isley WL. Diabetes mellitus. In: Dipiro JT, Talbert RL, Yee GC, et al., eds. *Pharmacotherapy: A Pathophysiologic Approach,* 5th edition. New York: McGraw-Hill, 2002: 1335–1358.

6. (B) The onset of action of the thiazolidinediones, Actos® and Avandia® is slow, often taking 2 to 3 months to see a full effect.

Ref: Oki JC, Isley WL. Diabetes mellitus. In: Dipiro JT, Talbert RL, Yee GC, et al., eds. *Pharmacotherapy: A Pathophysiologic Approach,* 5th edition. New York: McGraw-Hill, 2002: 1335–1358.

7. (A) Metformin should be avoided in patients with renal insufficiency to reduce to incidence of lactic acidosis.

Ref: Oki JC, Isley WL. Diabetes mellitus. In: Dipiro JT, Talbert RL, Yee GC, et al., eds. *Pharmacotherapy: A Pathophysiologic Approach,* 5th edition. New York: McGraw-Hill, 2002: 1335–1358.

8. (D) β-Blockers may prolong and mask the symptoms of hypoglycemia.

Ref: Carlisle BA, Kroon LA, Koda-Kimble MA. Diabetes mellitus. In: Koda-Kimble MA, Young LY, Kradjan WA, et al., eds. *Applied Therapeutics: The Clinical Use of Drugs,* 8th edition. Baltimore: Lippincott Williams & Wilkins, 2005:1–86.

9. (D) Numerous studies have documented the effectiveness of ACE inhibitors and angiotensin-receptor blockers (ARBs) in retarding the development and progression of nephropathy; therefore, these agents are considered optimal first-line therapy for the management of hypertension in patients with diabetes.

Ref: Carlisle BA, Kroon LA, Koda-Kimble MA. Diabetes mellitus. In: Koda-Kimble MA, Young LY, Kradjan WA, et al., eds. *Applied Therapeutics: The Clinical Use of Drugs,* 8th edition. Baltimore: Lippincott Williams & Wilkins, 2005:1–86.

10. (B) The National Cholesterol Education Program (NCEP) Adult Treatment Panel III (ATP III) guidelines classify the presence of DM as a coronary heart disease risk equivalent, and therefore recommend that LDL-C be lowered to <100 mg/dL.

Ref: Oki JC, Isley WL. Diabetes mellitus. In: Dipiro JT, Talbert RL, Yee GC, et al., eds. *Pharmacotherapy: A Pathophysiologic Approach,* 5th edition. New York: McGraw-Hill, 2002:1335–1358.

PATIENT PROFILE 246

MIGRAINE

ANSWERS

1. (E) All three are considered headache triggers, and may be contributing factors in AL's migraines. Both excessive caffeine use and caffeine withdrawal may precipitate migraines. Alcohol in general is known to precipitate migraines. Red wine in particular contains tyramine, which also has been identified as a migraine trigger. Chocolate can precipitate migraines as well.

Ref: Alldredge BK. Neurologic disorders. In: Koda-Kimble MA, Young LY, Kradjan WA, et al., editors. *Applied Therapeutics: The Clinical Use of Drugs,* 8th edition. Baltimore: Lippincott Williams & Wilkins; 2005:1–27.

Ref: Wagner ML, Sotirhos MM, Sibersteine SD. Headache. In: Herfindal ET, Gourley DR, eds. *Textbook of Therapeutics,* 7th edition. Baltimore: Lippincott Williams & Wilkins, 2000: 1083–1105.

2. (A) Oral contraceptives with high-potency estrogen are associated with precipitating and exacerbating migraine headaches. Of the agents listed, Estrostep® has the lowest estrogenic activity. The other agents have high estrogenic activity.

Ref: Alldredge BK. Neurologic disorders. In: Koda-Kimble MA, Young LY, Kradjan WA, et al., editors. *Applied Therapeutics: The Clinical Use of Drugs,* 8th edition. Baltimore: Lippincott Williams & Wilkins; 2005:1–27.

3. (D) The triptans are 5-HT$_{1B/1D}$ receptor agonists. 5-HT$_3$ antagonists (e.g., ondansetron) are used in the treatment of emesis.

Ref: Alldredge BK. Neurologic disorders. In: Koda-Kimble MA, Young LY, Kradjan WA, et al., editors. *Applied Therapeutics: The Clinical Use of Drugs,* 8th edition. Baltimore: Lippincott Williams & Wilkins; 2005:1–27.

4. (D) Triptans have been linked to vascular events such as coronary vasospasm, angina, myocardial infarction, and stroke, but these events usually are associated with patients who have pre-existing coronary artery disease or significant cardiovascular risk factors. Chest tightness and pressure are potential side effects of triptan therapy. These symptoms do not correlate with cardiac ischemia and typically are mild and do not last more than 2 hours (not all day). Triptan therapy may cause vasoconstriction and should be avoided in patients with hypertension, peripheral or cerebral vascular disease, coronary artery disease, prior myocardial infarction, Prinzmetal's angina, or coronary vasospasm.

Ref: Alldredge BK. Neurologic disorders. In: Koda-Kimble MA, Young LY, Kradjan WA, et al., editors. *Applied Therapeutics: The Clinical Use of Drugs,* 8th edition. Baltimore: Lippincott Williams & Wilkins; 2005:1–27.

5. (E) This is the correct dosing for intranasal Zomig® (zolmitriptan); dosing for the oral formulation of zolmitriptan is 2.5 mg. Amerge® (naratriptan) and Maxalt® (rizatriptan) are not available in intranasal formulations. Frova® (frovatriptan) is not available in a parenteral formulation. Imitrex® (sumatriptan) is available as a subcutaneous injection, but the dose is excessive, appropriate dosing is 6 mg SQ or 25–50 mg po.

Ref: Alldredge BK. Neurologic disorders. In: Koda-Kimble MA, Young LY, Kradjan WA, et al., editors. *Applied Therapeutics: The Clinical Use of Drugs,* 8th edition. Baltimore: Lippincott Williams & Wilkins; 2005:1–27.

6. (C) β Blockers are effective in preventing migraines when taken daily. β Blockers with ISA (intrinsic sympathomimetic activity) are not effective for migraine prophylaxis.

Ref: Beckett BE, Herndon KC. Headache disorders. In: DiPiro JT, Talbert RL, Yee GC, et al., eds. *Pharmacotherapy: A*

Pathophysiologic Approach, 5th edition. New York: McGraw-Hill, 2002:1119–1133.

7. (E) DHE (dihydroergotamine) is an ergot derivative and should not be given within 24 hours of a triptan because of the potential to cause serotonin syndrome. Fluoxetine also may precipitate serotonin syndrome when combined with triptans. SSRIs are not contraindicated in patients taking triptans, but if these agents are combined the patient should be monitored for symptoms of serotonin syndrome (e.g., weakness, incoordination). Propranolol reduces the clearance of frovatriptan, zolmitriptan, rizatriptan, and eletriptan.

Ref: Alldredge BK. Neurologic disorders. In: Koda-Kimble MA, Young LY, Kradjan WA, et al., editors. *Applied Therapeutics: The Clinical Use of Drugs,* 8th edition. Baltimore: Lippincott Williams & Wilkins; 2005:1–27.

Ref: Beckett BE, Herndon KC. Headache disorders. In: DiPiro JT, Talbert RL, Yee GC, et al., eds. *Pharmacotherapy: A Pathophysiologic Approach,* 5th edition. New York: McGraw-Hill, 2002:1119–1133.

8. (E) All three statements are true. The correct regimen for butorphanol nasal spray is one spray in one nostril (1 mg) at the onset of migraine. The dose may be repeated in 1 hour if needed. Butorphanol is a narcotic analgesic and does have abuse potential.

Ref: Beckett BE, Herndon KC. Headache disorders. In: DiPiro JT, Talbert RL, Yee GC, et al., eds. *Pharmacotherapy: A Pathophysiologic Approach,* 5th edition. New York: McGraw-Hill, 2002:1119–1133.

9. (D) Migranal® is the brand name of DHE. This ergot derivative is available in an intranasal formulation. Cafergot® (ergotamine tartrate) is also an ergot derivative that is available as oral tablets and rectal suppositories. Axert® (almotriptan) and Relpax® (eletriptan) are both second-generation triptans. Fioricet® is a combination of butalbital, APAP, and caffeine.

Ref: Alldredge BK. Neurologic disorders. In: Koda-Kimble MA, Young LY, Kradjan WA, et al., editors. *Applied Therapeutics: The Clinical Use of Drugs,* 8th edition. Baltimore: Lippincott Williams & Wilkins; 2005:1–27.

Ref: Beckett BE, Herndon KC. Headache disorders. In: DiPiro JT, Talbert RL, Yee GC, et al., eds. *Pharmacotherapy: A Pathophysiologic Approach,* 5th edition. New York: McGraw-Hill, 2002: 1119–1133.

10. (E) Midrin contains all three ingredients: APAP (analgesic), isometheptene mucate (sympathomimetic amine), and dichloralphenazone (chloral hydrate derivative).

Ref: Beckett BE, Herndon KC. Headache disorders. In: DiPiro JT, Talbert RL, Yee GC, et al., eds. *Pharmacotherapy: A Pathophysiologic Approach,* 5th edition. New York: McGraw-Hill, 2002: 1119–1133.

PATIENT PROFILE 247

TULAREMIA

ANSWERS

1. (C) *Francisella tularensis* is a small aerobic gram-negative bacillus.

Ref: Dennis D, Inglesby T, Henderson D, et al. Tularemia as a biological weapon: medical and public health management. *JAMA* 2003;285(21):2763–2773.

Ref: Weinstein R, Alibek K. *Biological and Chemical Terrorism: A Guide for Healthcare Providers and First Responders.* New York: Thieme, 2003:106–107.

2. (D) The incubation period may range from 1 to 14 days, with most people experiencing symptoms in 3 to 5 days, depending on the amount of bacteria to which one is exposed.

Ref: Dennis D, Inglesby T, Henderson D, et al. Tularemia as a biological weapon: medical and public health management. *JAMA* 2003;285(21):2763–2773.

Ref: Weinstein R, Alibek K. *Biological and Chemical Terrorism: A Guide for Healthcare Providers and First Responders.* New York: Thieme, 2003:106–107.

3. (D) *F. tularensis* can be carried by many small mammals. A bite from a rabbit, rodent, woodchuck, muskrat, fox, coyote, or skunk could transmit the disease. The bacterium also is carried by arthropods such as mosquitoes, deerflies, or ticks.

Ref: Dennis D, Inglesby T, Henderson D, et al. Tularemia as a biological weapon: medical and public health management. *JAMA* 2003;285(21):2763–2773.

Ref: Weinstein R, Alibek K. *Biological and Chemical Terrorism: A Guide for Healthcare Providers and First Responders.* New York: Thieme, 2003:106–107.

4. (A) Streptomycin is the drug of choice per the CDC guidelines. Gentamicin is more readily available in the United States and is an acceptable alternative.

Ref: Dennis D, Inglesby T, Henderson D, et al. Tularemia as a biological weapon: medical and public health management. *JAMA* 2003;285(21):2763–2773.

Ref: Weinstein R, Alibek K. *Biological and Chemical Terrorism: A Guide for Healthcare Providers and First Responders.* New York: Thieme, 2003:106–107.

5. (B) The typical length of treatment for tularemia is 10 days.

Ref: Dennis D, Inglesby T, Henderson D, et al. Tularemia as a biological weapon: medical and public health management. *JAMA* 2003;285(21):2763–2773.

Ref: Weinstein R, Alibek K. *Biological and Chemical Terrorism: A Guide for Healthcare Providers and First Responders.* New York: Thieme, 2003:106–107.

6. (D) Blood urea nitrogen, blood drug concentrations, and creatinine clearance are all important monitoring parameters with aminoglycosides. Aminoglycosides are eliminated by the kidneys; those with renal dysfunction must have doses or frequency modified in response to these laboratory results.

Ref: *AHFS DI Bioterrorism Resource Manual.* Bethesda, MD: American Society of Health-System Pharmacists, 2002:313–318.

7. (B) In mass prophylaxis doxycycline or ciprofloxacin 500 mg po q 12 hours are the drugs of choice. Tetracycline 500 mg po qid is also recommended.

Ref: Dennis D, Inglesby T, Henderson D, et al. Tularemia as a biological weapon: medical and public health management. *JAMA* 2003;285(21):2763–2773.

Ref: Weinstein R, Alibek K. *Biological and Chemical Terrorism: A Guide for Healthcare Providers and First Responders.* New York: Thieme, 2003:106–107.

8. (A) Doxycycline is in the class of antibiotics called tetracyclines.

Ref: Thomson MICROMEDEX, *http://micromedex/Doxycyline/ overview.* MicroMedex® Healthcare Series Vol 121. Expires 12/2004.

9. (E) The patient needs to be counseled to finish the full course of therapy and take each dose with a full glass of water. Antacids and iron-containing products must be separated because they decrease the absorption of the antibiotic. Doxycycline may cause photosensitivity of the skin. Precautions such as wearing hats, long sleeves, and sunscreen need to be discussed with the patient.

Ref: *AHFS DI Bioterrorism Resource Manual.* Bethesda, MD: American Society of Health-System Pharmacists, 2002:82–91.

10. (E) Surveillance from data indicating a surge of unusual diseases or diseases that do not naturally occur in one geographic area should be reported to the local public health department. These are all indicators that a possible biological agent has been released.

Ref: Dennis D, Inglesby T, Henderson D, et al. Tularemia as a biological weapon: medical and public health management. *JAMA* 2003;285(21):2763–2773.

Ref: Weinstein R, Alibek K. *Biological and Chemical Terrorism: A Guide for Healthcare Providers and First Responders.* New York: Thieme, 2003:106–107.

PATIENT PROFILE 248

GERIATRIC MENTAL ILLNESS TREATMENT

ANSWERS

1. (B) Amitriptyline is very anticholinergic and blockade of central cholinergic receptors can lead to decreases in cognitive ability.

Ref: Jacobson S, Pies R, Greenblatt D, eds. *Handbook of Geriatric Psychopharmacology.* Washington, DC: American Psychiatric Publishing, 2002.

2. (D) Both amitriptyline and fluphenazine potently block cholinergic receptors.

Ref:Schatzberg AF, Nemeroff CB, eds. *Essentials of Clinical Psychopharmacology.* Washington, DC: American Psychiatric Publishing, 2001.

3. (A) Albuterol is a β-adrenergic receptor agonist. With overuse patients can feel anxiety, agitation, and jitteriness.

Ref:Micromedex, available at *http://www.micromedex.com.* Accessed 2004.

4. (C) Ziprasidone has virtually no affinity for the cholinergic receptor, whereas chlorpromazine, haloperidol, and perphenazine are moderate to potent blockers of cholinergic receptors. Blockade of cholinergic receptors can lead to decreases in cognitive function.

Ref: Jacobson S, Pies R, Greenblatt D, eds. *Handbook of Geriatric Psychopharmacology.* Washington, DC: American Psychiatric Publishing, 2002.

5. (A) Donepezil increases acetylcholine by slowing its metabolism by blocking acetylcholinesterase. However, the increase in acetylcholine will have little effect on the receptor because it is potently blocked by fluphenazine.

Ref: Jacobson S, Pies R, Greenblatt D, eds. *Handbook of Geriatric Psychopharmacology.* Washington, DC: American Psychiatric Publishing, 2002.

DIABETES

ANSWERS

1. (E) IV has glucose intolerance, low HDL, and high triglycerides. The presence of three or more of the following qualifies as metabolic syndrome: (a) abdominal obesity (>40 in. for men, >35 in for women), (b) glucose intolerance (fasting blood glucose ≥110 mg/dL), (c) blood pressure of at least 130/85, (d) high triglycerides (≥150 mg/dL), (e) low HDL (<40 mg/dL in men, and <50 mg/dL in women).

    Ref: The Seventh Report of the Joint National Committee. Prevention, detection, evaluation, and treatment of high blood pressure. *JAMA* 2003;289:2560–2572.

2. (B) ASA reduces incidence of myocardial infarction by inhibiting TxA_2-mediated platelet activation. The Early Treatment Diabetic Retinopathy Study (ETDRS) consisted of type 1 and 2 diabetic men and women, approximately half of whom had established cardiovascular disease. The relative risk for myocardial infarction in the first 5 years in those randomized to aspirin therapy was lowered significantly to 0.72 (CI 0.55 to 0.95). The Hypertension Optimal Treatment (HOT) Trial compared the outcomes of 18,790 patients receiving 75 mg/day of aspirin versus placebo. Aspirin significantly reduced myocardial infarction by 36%, and cardiovascular events by 15% in patients with diabetes who are treated for hypertension.

    Ref: The ETDRS Investigators. Aspirin effects on mortality and morbidity in patients with diabetes mellitus: Early Treatment Diabetic Retinopathy Study report 14. *JAMA* 1992;268:1292–1300.

    Ref: Hansson L, Zanchetti A, Carruthers SG, et al. Effects of intensive blood-pressure lowering and low dose aspirin on patients with hypertension: principal results of the Hypertension Optimal Treatment (HOT) randomized trial. *Lancet* 1998;351:1755–1762.

3. (E) The UKPDS studies have established the importance of intensive blood pressure and blood glucose control for reduction of diabetes-related morbidity and mortality. Glyburide and metformin are associated with improved glycemic control and the reduction of microvascular complications. Metformin is associated with reduction of diabetes-related mortality and all-cause mortality in obese patients. Aggressive blood pressure control strategies using ß-blockers or ACE-inhibitors have been associated with a reduction of microvascular and macrovascular complications.

    Ref: UK Prospective Diabetes Study (UKPDS) Group. Intensive blood-glucose control with sulfonylureas or insulin compared with conventional treatment and risk of complications in patients with type 2 diabetes. *Lancet* 1998;352:837–853.

    Ref: UK Prospective Diabetes Study Group. Effect of intensive blood-glucose control with metformin on complications in overweight patients with type 2 diabetes. *Lancet* 1998;352:854–865.

    Ref: UK Prospective Diabetes Study Group. Tight blood pressure control and risk of macrovascular and microvascular complications in type 2 diabetes. *BMJ* 1998;317:703–713.

    Ref: UK Prospective Diabetes Study Group. Efficacy of atenolol and captopril in reducing risk of macrovascular and microvascular complications in type 2 diabetes. *BMJ* 1998;317:713–720.

4. (A) Extensive analysis of data from patients with diabetes in the HOPE and MICRO-HOPE studies consistently show reduction of macrovascular endpoints of myocardial infarction, revascularization, and stroke along with reduction of cardiovascular death among patients treated with ACE-inhibitor therapy (ramipril). ACE-inhibitor therapy has not been able to conclusively demonstrate a reduction of unstable angina in the diabetic population. Other benefits from ACE-inhibitor therapy among patients with diabetes from the HOPE and MICRO-HOPE include reductions in microvascular complications of nephropathy, optical laser-photocoagulation, or dialysis. Data from the ALLHAT trial suggest that lisinopril and chlorthalidone have a similar relative risk reduction of cardiovascular death, all-cause mortality, stroke, and nonfatal myocardial infarction.

    Ref: The Heart Outcome Prevention Evaluation Study Investigators. Effects of an angiotensin-converting-enzyme inhibitor ramipril, on cardiovascular events in high-risk patients. *N Engl J Med* 2000; 342:145–153.

    Ref: Heart Outcomes Prevention Evaluation Study Investigators. Effects of ramipril on cardiovascular and microvascular outcomes in people with diabetes mellitus: results of the HOPE study and MICRO-HOPE substudy. *Lancet* 2000;355:253–259.

    Ref: The ALLHAT Officers and Coordinators for the ALLHAT Collaborative Research Group. Major outcomes in high-risk hypertensive patients randomized to angiotensin-converting enzyme inhibitor or calcium channel blocker vs diuretic: The Antihypertensive and Lipid-Lowering Treatment to Prevent Heart Attack Trial. *JAMA* 2002;288:2981–2997.

5. (D) Hypoglycemia triggers an adrenergic nervous system response, resulting in increased hepatic gluconeogenesis and common symptoms of tachycardia, tremor, and palpitations. Sweating is a common response to hypoglycemia but is triggered by the parasympathetic nervous system. Thirst is a common symptom of uncontrolled hyperglycemia in patients with type 1 and 2 diabetes. Usually, excessive thirst is accompanied by hunger and

frequent urination in the classic triad of symptoms: polyuria, polydipsia, and polyphagia.

Ref: Steil CF. Diabetes mellitus. In: DiPiro JT, Talbert RL, Yee GC, et al., eds. *Pharmacotherapy: A Pathophysiologic Approach,* 4th edition. Stamford, CT: Appleton & Lange, 1999:1219–1243.

6. (B) Sweating is a parasympathetic-mediated response to hypoglycemia not affected by β-blockers. Tachycardia, tremor, palpitations, and increases in systolic and diastolic blood pressure are sympathetic-mediated responses to hypoglycemia. β-Blockers frequently blunt the adrenergic response so common symptoms of hypoglycemia such as tachycardia, tremor, and palpitations are not experienced. Patients with diabetes who are receiving β-blockers may be counseled to be aware of sweating, confusion, and fatigue as key signs of hypoglycemia.

Ref: Steil CF. Diabetes mellitus. In: DiPiro JT, Talbert RL, Yee GC, et al., eds. *Pharmacotherapy: A Pathophysiologic Approach,* 4th edition. Stamford, CT: Appleton & Lange, 1999:1219–1243.

7. (D) The primary site of mechanism of action of HCTZ is the inhibition of the Na^+Cl^- transporter in the distal convoluted tubule. HCTZ also inhibits Na^+Cl^- transporters in the proximal convoluted tubule and the renal cortex as secondary and tertiary sites of action.

Ref: Jackson EK. Diuretics. In: Hardman JG, Limbird LE, Molinoff PB, Ruddon RW, Goodman-Gilman A, eds. *Goodman & Gilman's: The Pharmacological Basis of Therapeutics*, 9th edition. New York: McGraw-Hill, 1996:685–713.

8. (A) A double-blind placebo-controlled study of gabapentin titrated from 900 mg to goal 3600 mg daily in patients with diabetic neuropathy documents significant improvement in pain, global assessment, and quality of life.

Ref: Backonja M, Beydoun A, Edwards KR, et al. Gabapentin for the symptomatic treatment of painful neuropathy in patients with diabetes mellitus. *JAMA* 1998;280:1831–1836.

9. (E) IV is considered at high risk for developing coronary disease in the future. New updates to the ATP III issued in 2004 summarize and provide new evidence that LDL-C levels ≤70 mg/dL are the ideal therapeutic target in patients with diabetes.

Ref: Grundy SM, Cleeman JI, Merz CNB, et al. Implications of recent clinical trials for the National Cholesterol Education Program Adult Treatment Panel III Guidelines. *Circulation* 2004;110: 227–239.

10. (E) The mean LDL-C reduction observed using simvastatin 40 mg the Heart Protection Study was approximately 40 mg/dL. More importantly, 40 mg of simvastatin was associated with approximately 25% reduction in major coronary events, stroke, revascularization, and vascular events.

Ref: The Heart Protection Study Collaborative Group. MRC/BHF Heart Protection Study of cholesterol-lowering with simvastatin in 5963 people with diabetes: a randomized placebo-controlled trial. *Lancet* 2003;361:2005–2016.

PATIENT PROFILE 250

GASTROENTERITIS

ANSWERS

1. (B) When travelers from industrialized countries spend time in developing countries, they frequently experience a rapid and dramatic change in organisms that occupy their gastrointestinal tract. Some of these new organisms are potential enteric pathogens. Travelers who develop traveler's diarrhea have ingested a sufficient amount of pathogenic organisms to overcome their individual defense mechanisms. Enterotoxigenic *E. coli* are among the most common single causative agent of traveler's diarrhea in countries where such surveys have been conducted. Infections with *Shigella, Salmonella,* and *Campylobacter jejuni* are less frequent causes; they may be more common in specific traveled areas.

Ref: Bern C, Herwaldt B, Kozarsky P, et al. National Center for Infectious Diseases Traveler's Health. *The Yellow Book, Health Information for International Travel, 2003–2004.* Available from: *http://www.cdc.gov/travel/diarrhea.htm.*

2. (C) Fluoroquinolones can be used to treat traveler's diarrhea resulting from ETEC, *Shigella,* and *Salmonella.* Although fluoroquinolones have activity against *Campylobacter jejuni,* resistance has been increasing; macrolides remain the treatment of choice for gastroenteritis caused by this organism. TMP/SMX has been used in the past for traveler's diarrhea, but resistance has limited its utility.

Ref: Guerrant RL, Gilder TV, Steiner TS, et al. Practice guidelines for the management of infectious diarrhea. *Clin Infect Dis* 2001;32:331–350.

3. (A) Rifaximin is a poorly absorbed rifamycin derivative with activity against several enteric pathogens. Like other rifamycin antibiotics (e.g., rifampin, rifabutin), its

antibacterial activity results from it binding the bacterial DNA-dependent RNA polymerase. It is indicated for use in the treatment of traveler's diarrhea caused by noninvasive strains of *E. coli* (i.e., ETEC).

Ref: Steffen R. Rifaximin: a nonabsorbable antimicrobial as a new tool for treatment of traveler's diarrhea. *J Travel Med* 2001; 8(suppl 2):S34–39.

4. (B) The protective efficacy in clinical trials with fluoroquinolones is 80% to 100%; bismuth subsalicylate has a protective efficacy of 40% to 65%. Because of resistance among *E. coli* strains, TMP/SMX efficacy is limited to certain areas and seasons, such as when traveling to inland Mexico during the summer months. Loperamide may be used for treatment but does not have a role in prophylaxis.

Ref: Rendi-Wagner P, Kollaritsch H. Drug prophylaxis for traveler's diarrhea. *Clin Infect Dis* 2002;34:628–633.

5. (C) Gastric acidity and normal enteric flora are components of the enteric host defense against enteric infections. Most ingested bacterial pathogens do not reach the lower gastrointestinal tract because they do not survive the acidic pH of the stomach. In the lower gastrointestinal tract, normal bacterial floras prevent colonization by potentially pathogenic bacteria. Agents that raise the stomach pH (esomeprazole) or kill normal gastrointestinal flora (antibiotics) increase the likelihood that ingested potential pathogens will survive and cause gastroenteritis.

Ref: Richard I. Guerrant RL, Steiner TS. Principles and syndromes of enteric infection. In: Mandel GL, Bennett JE, Dolin R, eds. *Principles and Practice of Infectious Diseases,* 5th edition. Philadelphia: Churchill Livingstone, 2000:1076–1093.

6. (D) Because the etiologic organism is located in the colon, antimicrobial treatment of *C. difficile* diarrhea requires enteral delivery of metronidazole or vancomycin. Information in case reports suggest that IV metronidazole also may be effective because of this drug's fecal excretion. Although metronidazole and vancomycin are considered equally effective, concerns with promoting vancomycin resistance in enterococci have prompted many national guidelines to recommend oral metronidazole over oral vancomycin as first-line treatment.

Ref: Bartlett JB. Antibiotic-associated diarrhea. *N Engl J Med* 2002;346:334–339.

7. (A) Because metronidazole inhibits alcohol dehydrogenase, disulfiram-like reactions (flushing, headache, nausea, vomiting, abdominal cramps, sweating) may occur in patients who ingest alcohol while receiving metronidazole. Patients receiving metronidazole should be warned about the possibility of this reaction. The manufacturers recommend that alcohol not be consumed during therapy and for at least 1 day (or at least 3 days with the oral capsules or extended-release oral tablets) after completing metronidazole therapy.

Ref: McEnvoy GK, ed. *AHFS drug information.* Bethesda, MD: American Society of Health-System Pharmacists, 2004.

8. (B) Antimotility agents, alone or in combination with antimicrobial therapy, may be used for the treatment of gastroenteritis resulting from noninvasive enteric pathogens (i.e., ETEC). For enteric pathogens (e.g., *Salmonella typhi, Shigella, C. difficile*) that produce more invasive disease (e.g., fecal leukocytes, blood in stool, fever), it is prudent to avoid antimotility agents because of concerns with prolonging or worsening the enteric infection or increasing the risk for complications associated with infection by these organisms.

Ref: Ansdell VE, Ericsson CD. Prevention and empiric treatment of traveler's diarrhea. *Med Clin North Am* 1999;83:945–973.

9. (D) Although almost all antibiotics have been associated with *C. difficile* gastroenteritis, studies commonly implicate clindamycin, cephalosporins, and penicillins (especially aminopenicillins).

Ref: Thielman NM. Antibiotic-associated colitis. In: Mandel GL, Bennett JE, Dolin R, eds. *Principles and Practice of Infectious Diseases,* 5th edition. Philadelphia: Churchill Livingstone, 2000:1111–1126.

10. (B) Although relapse may be higher with antibiotic treatment of gastroenteritis produced by nontyphoidal *Salmonella* species, certain groups of patients should receive such therapy because of the risk for complications after the development of *Salmonella* bacteremia (observed in 2% to 4% of cases). Therapy should be initiated in patients at extremes of age (<2 or >50 years of age), patients who are immunodeficient, and patients at risk for metastatic seeding because of vascular grafts, artificial joints, or valvular heart disease.

Ref: Thielman NM. Antimicrobial therapy of infectious diarrhea. *J Infect Dis Pharmacother* 2000;4(suppl 2):29–42.

PATIENT PROFILE 1
FOOD AND DRUG ADMINISTRATION RECALLS

ANSWERS

1. (D) This is considered a Class III, Retail Level incident because the off-colored tablets do not have any medical or health risk and a retail level recall that will remove remaining product from retail shelves. In this case, the FDA did not deem it necessary to remove the product from consumer possession.

   Ref: 21 CFR 7.51

2. (A) A Class I recall is reserved for significant and major medical or health risks.

   Ref: 21 CFR 7.51

3. Pharmaceutical manufacturers may refuse to participate in recalls that are voluntary under statute and regulation. However, FDA may institute other punitive measures to persuade manufacturers to comply with their request for a product recall.

   Ref: 21 CFR 7.51

PATIENT PROFILE 2
CONTROLLED SUBSTANCES ACT

ANSWERS

1. (A) The Federal Controlled Substances Act permits pharmacists to fill prescriptions in an emergency situation provided that the patient's medical condition requires immediate treatment, that the prescription is for a CII controlled substance only, and that the prescriber is unable to give the patient a hard-copy prescription. Physicians have 7 days in which to mail a hard-copy prescription to the pharmacist who dispensed the emergency prescription.

   Ref: 21 CFR 1306.11(d)

2. (C) Correct DEA registration numbers are determined with a formula. Practitioners have the letter A or B in the first alpha position followed by the first letter of their last names. Wholesalers and other distributors have the first letter R. To verify whether a DEA registration number on a prescription is correct, the formula is as follows:

   1. Add digits 1, 3, and 5 and determine a sum.
   2. Add digits 2, 4, and 6, determine a sum, and multiply the sum by 2.
   3. Add the two sums; the second digit of this sum (called the check digit) equals the last digit of the DEA registration number.

   Ref: 21 CFR 1301

3. (C) For all oral prescription orders for controlled substances in Schedule II through V, a hard-copy prescription must be mailed or sent to the dispensing pharmacy within 7 days.

   Ref: 21 CFR 1306.21

4. (E) Pharmacies are permitted under federal regulation to accept prescription orders by facsimile and maintain the faxed copy as an original hard copy provided the patient has a medically diagnosed terminal illness, is in hospice care, or is in a long-term care facility. For faxed prescriptions for CII controlled substances, a written hard copy from the prescriber is required.

   Ref: 21 CFR 1306.11

5. (E) When pharmacists dispense any prescription, regardless of federal schedule, they must affix a child-resistant closure unless authorized by the patient to do otherwise or unless they are dispensing an exempt medication, such as nitroglycerine SL tablets. A federal transfer label also is required to be affixed to any prescription container in the dispensing of federally controlled substances in Schedules II through IV. All prescriptions for CII controlled substances must be kept in a file separate from other prescriptions for controlled substances.

   Ref: 16 CFR 1700.14(a)(10), 21 CFR 1308

6. (D) Pharmacists may call patients to offer counseling if the person receiving the prescription is not the patient, may give a toll-free telephone number, or may post a sign offering counseling.

   Ref: Pub L No. 101–508

7. (B) Federal OBRA 90 regulations require pharmacists to offer counseling to Medicaid patients only. States may impose their own requirements.

    Ref: Pub L No. 101–508

8. (C) Pharmacists are correspondingly responsible for prescriptions they fill that are not for a legitimate medical purpose and not in the usual course of professional practice.

    Ref: 21 CFR 1306.04

9. (C) For a prescription for a controlled substance to be complete, the DEA registration number of the prescriber must be placed on the prescription.

    Ref: 21 CFR 1306.05

10. (E) The federal CSA does not address the type of prescriptions that may be called in to pharmacies in emergency situations. The act does permit agents of prescribers to telephone all prescriptions into pharmacies.

    Ref: 21 CFR 1306.11(d)

PATIENT   PROFILE   3

ORPHAN DRUG APPROVAL

ANSWERS

1. (B) Technically, orphan drugs may only be orphan drugs and not have any other indications for use other than that for which they have been approved.

    Ref: PL 97-414

2. (E) All of the above are incentives for the manufacture of an orphan drug.

    Ref: PL 97-414

3. (A) If a company cannot produce enough product to meet demand, that company would lose its exclusive right to manufacture the product under the definition of the Orphan Drug Act.

    Ref: PL 97-414

PATIENT   PROFILE   4

CONTROLLED SUBSTANCES ACT

ANSWERS

1. (E) DEA Form-222 is used when a DEA registrant wants to order for stock controlled substances in schedules I and II.

    Ref: 21 CFR 1305

2. (B) The DEA permits registrants to take an inventory of federally controlled substances at any time with the two calendar years of the initial inventory.

    Ref: 21 CFR 1304

3. (D) A pharmacist granted power of attorney by a registrant is permitted by the DEA to sign DEA Form-222 to order for pharmacy stock controlled substances in Schedule II.

    Ref: 21 CFR 1305.07

4. (B) DEA Form-106 is used when a DEA registrant is required to report a theft or substantial loss of federally controlled substances.

    Ref: 21 CFR 1307

5. (D) DEA Form-41 is used when a DEA registrant wants to remove from inventory unused, expired, or damaged controlled substances.

    Ref: 21 CFR 1307

EXPIRATION DATING AND NATIONAL DRUG CODE (NDC)

ANSWERS

1. (D) OTC products for human use, considered to be used in a relatively short time, and medicated are exempt from FDA expiration dating regulations.

   Ref: 21 CFR 133

2. (A) National Drug Code numbers on product labels are not required by the FDA for use by manufacturers.

Use of NDC numbers is voluntary for product identification.

Ref: 21 CFR 207.35

3. (A) If a manufacturer chooses to use an NDC number of its product labels, the number is required to appear on the top third of the principal display panel of all drug product labels.

   Ref: 21 CFR 207.35

PRACTITIONERS AND PRESCRIPTIVE AUTHORITY

ANSWERS

1. (D) Ophthalmologists are medical doctors who specialize in the treatment of diseases and conditions of the human eye. This means that they were trained as physicians first and learned about all the body's organ systems and the diseases that may occur. However, in this case, even though the ophthalmologist has chosen to specialize, he still has the legal authority to treat diseases and conditions that may not be ophthalmic in nature.

2. (B) Chiropractors are not considered to be practitioners under federal law. They are not entitled to apply for DEA registration and may not write prescriptions for federally controlled substances.

3. (E) The answer to this question is both A and C. Physicians or medical doctors (MDs) can prescribe methadone in certain circumstances. It may be prescribed for pain, although there may very well be more effective treatments available, or, in the case of an opioid-addicted individual, methadone may be prescribed in a limited fashion until the patient enters a drug treatment program.

MIDLEVEL PRACTITIONERS

ANSWERS

1. (C) Correct DEA registration numbers are determined with a formula. Midlevel practitioners such as nurse practitioners and physcian assistants have the letter *M* in the first alpha position followed by the first letter of their last name. Pharmacists verify whether a DEA registration number on a prescription is correct by using the following formula:
   1. Add digits 1, 3, and 5 and determine the sum.
   2. Add digits 2, 4 and 6, determine the sum, and multiply this by 2.

3. Add the two sums. The second digit of this sum (called the *check-digit*) equals the last digit of the DEA registration number.

    Ref: 21 CFR 1301

2. (D) As with all regulations, federal regulations take precedence unless those of a state are more stringent. In this case, the DEA allows prescriptive privileges to midlevel prescribers as long as the state in which the person practices allows them as well.

    Ref: 21 CFR 1304

3. (E) Documentation is required of all midlevel prescribers who are given prescribing privileges by states. Practice guidelines, agreements, and protocols may be used and must be readily available for inspection by the DEA.

    Ref: 21 CFR 1301

PATIENT PROFILE 8

FOOD, DRUG, AND COSMETIC ACT

ANSWERS

1. (C) Misbranding can be most easily understood as a violation of a labeler, either the manufacturer or the dispenser, that misrepresents the product in the container.

    Ref: USP DI, Vol. III, FDCA. Sect. 505

2. (B) The Controlled Substances Act places certain products or ingredients into schedules according to potential for abuse.

    Ref: 21 CFR 1308

3. (C) The federal orange book, or *Therapeutic Drug Products with Therapeutic Equivalence Evaluations,* serves as a guide to practitioners regarding the therapeutic equivalence drug products.

    Ref: USP DI, Vol. III

4. (C) Drug products given an A rating in the FDA *Approved Drug Products with Therapeutic Equivalence Evaluations* would be characterized as therapeutically equivalent. Drug products given a B rating in the FDA Approved Drugs with Therapeutic Equivalence Evaluations would be characterized as not therapeutically equivalent.

    Ref: USP DI, Vol. III

5. (A) The National Drug Code consists of an 11-digit code in which the first four digits identify the labeler, the next four digits identify the product, and the two digits identify the package size. NDC numbers on product labels do not necessarily indicate that the product is a legend or prescription drug.

    Ref: 21 CFR 207

6. (C) The Prescription Drug Marketing Act prohibits pharmacies from storing, dispensing, or purchasing prescription drug samples and requires state boards of pharmacy to license drug wholesalers.

    Ref: 21 USC 1301

7. (D) The Kefauver-Harris Amendments to the federal Food, Drug and Cosmetic Act required examination of all prescription medications manufactured between 1938 and 1962 to determine drug effectiveness.

    Ref: 21 USC 1301

8. (C) Phase III is the largest human-testing phase in drug development. More data on safety and efficacy are gathered for a more diverse test population.

    Ref: 21 CFR 505

9. (D) Phase IV is the phase during which long-term safety, efficacy, and monitoring are established after marketing approval is granted.

   Ref: 21 CFR 505

10. (C) A product may be considered adulterated if it becomes contaminated after it is shipped to a retail outlet. A product may be considered misbranded if the label does not reflect the true contents of the container to which it is affixed.

    Ref: 21 CFR 50511

11. (D) An abbreviated new drug application (ANDA) is used by manufacturers of generic products to gain approval for an off-patent drug product.

    Ref: 21 CFR 505, 21 CFR 314

12. (A) The FDA drug monograph was a panel review of ingredients for OTC products to determine safety and efficacy as well as labeling, indications, instructions, and warnings.

    Ref: 21 CFR 310

PATIENT PROFILE 9

CONTROLLED SUBSTANCES ACT

ANSWERS

1. (E) U.S. postal regulations permit the mailing of any filled prescription with any controlled substance in any quantity.

   Ref: 18 USC 1716

2. (D) Although a seemingly difficult request in that the remaining refills may constitute a large quantity of tablets, federal law does not prohibit the dispensing of multiple prescription refills at one time. However, pharmacists may feel that this practice raises issues of professional liability. Pharmacists must rely on their own professional judgement in these situations.

   Ref: 21 CFR 1306, 18 USC 1716

3. (D) U.S. postal regulations permit the mailing of any filled prescription with any controlled substance in any quantity. The inner prescription container must be labeled in accordance with federal laws and regulations. The outer container or its packaging must not be labeled in any way that indicates the contents within.

   Ref: 18 USC 1716

4. (B) A psychologist has a doctorate and is specially trained to treat patients with mental illness by means of counseling. Psychologists are not eligible under federal law to obtain DEA registration and therefore are not considered practitioners. Some states may, however, depending on their laws, permit psychologists to have limited prescribing authority as midlevel prescribers. The other choices are considered practitioners under the CSA. A psychiatrist is a physician whose specialty is the medical treatment of mental illness. An allopathic physician is by general definition a person with a doctor of medicine degree who practices any specialty in conventional medicine, such as dermatology, internal medicine, oncology, or cardiology. A veterinarian is a specialist in the medical treatment of animals. A podiatrist is a specialist in the medical treatment of the feet.

   Ref: 21 CFR 1306

5. (A) Pharmacists may lawfully fill prescriptions written by medical interns or foreign physicians when these persons are assigned a suffix to be used with the institutional (e.g., hospital) DEA registration number. No cosignature is required.

   Ref: 21 CFR 1301

6. (E) According to federal law, a prescription for a controlled substance must be written in ink or indelible pencil or typewritten and signed by the prescriber in his or her own handwriting.

   Ref: 21 CFR 1306

7. (D) The federal Controlled Substances Act limits prescription refills of up to 5 times within 6 months for any CIII and CIV prescriptions with authorized refills.

PRESCRIPTION DRUG MARKETING ACT

ANSWERS

1. (C) One of the main intents of the PDMA was to prevent the diversion of prescription drug samples from a public health and a law enforcement standpoint. The FDA believed many of the samples being sold to pharmacies were expired, damaged or otherwise adulterated.

   Ref: 21 CFR 503

2. (E) The PDMA was implemented to prevent pharmacies from dispensing or storing samples. However, in many institutional settings, it may be more sensible for the pharmacy to store sample medications in an effort to better control them. The PDMA permits this activity under the conditions listed in the question.

   Ref: 21 CFR 503

3. (B) The PDMA requires drug wholesalers to register with states in which they operate to better monitor their activities and to prevent diversion.

   Ref: 21 CFR 503

STATUTORY AUTHORITY

ANSWERS

1. (C) The Federal Trade Commission (FTC) is responsible for truth in advertising in federal government. Consequently, it has jurisdiction and authority to regulate many medicinal and health-related products. However, the FDA has the authority to regulate prescription drugs. The FTC regulates medical devices and over-the-counter drugs, though; the agency may confer or defer decisions on advertising to the FDA.

   Ref: FDCA, 1938

2. (E) The FDA is well within its statutory rights to determine the accuracy of the claims made by pharmaceutical manufacturers about their prescription drug products. However, although the agency can request removal of the advertisement or commercial, they cannot remove the advertisement by themselves. In cases where a pharmaceutical company refuses to remove an advertisement that is considered inaccurate, the FDA may employ a number of remedies such as teaming up the FTC, the Department of Justice, and so on.

   Ref: FDCA, 1938

3. (B) The answer to this question is misbranded, or an inaccuracy in product labeling, which includes all written, spoken, and print advertisement. Therefore, a television or print ad that makes unsubstantiated medical claims about the efficacy of a drug product is considered misbranded under the FDCA. An adulterated product is one in which the integrity of the product is compromised; that is, contaminated, expired, and so on.

   Ref: FDCA, 1938

PATIENT PROFILE 12

POISON PREVENTION PACKAGING ACT

ANSWERS

1. (A) All prescription drugs for oral use, unless exempt by regulation, the patient, or the physician, must be dispensed in child-resistant containers.

   Ref: 16 CFR 1700.14

2. (E) The Poison Prevention Packaging Act permits certain medications, such as nitroglycerin, to be packaged in non–child-resistant containers. OTC products for elderly persons with arthritis also may be packaged in containers with non–child-resistant closures that are clearly marked as such and in only one package size.

   Ref: 16 CFR 1700.14

3. (D) Prescription refills must be dispensed in new containers if the original filling was dispensed in a plastic container because of the possibility that the locking mechanism may become worn after repeated opening. Prescriptions dispensed in glass containers need only replacement of child-resistant caps. Patients may orally request that prescriptions be dispensed to them in non–child resistant containers. However, the Consumer Product Safety Commission recommends that pharmacists obtain a written exemption statement before dispensing medication in non–child-resistant caps.

   Ref: 16 CFR 1700.15

PATIENT PROFILE 13

FOOD, DRUG, AND COSMETIC ACT

ANSWERS

1. (D) Recalls are not under the statutory authority of the FDA. However, the agency can recommend that a company recall a product from the market-place if the product is under FDA jurisdiction and if that product jeopardizes the health and safety of the public. Companies whose products are under FDA jurisdiction and are a danger to the health of the public may recall these products at any time. Class I recalls indicate grave danger or possible irreversible threat to public safety. That is, the product may cause death or grave bodily injury if ingested. Class II recalls indicate a public safety threat but one that is reversible or not life threatening. That is, the product may cause fever or vomiting if ingested. Class III recalls indicate no threat to public safety but that the product is defective, for example, leaving the butter out of buttered popcorn. A consumer-level recall indicates that the product in question must be removed from the consumer's home or elsewhere. A retail-level recall indicates that the product in question must be removed from pharmacy shelves and indicates that the product in question must be removed from pharmacy wholesalers or other sites of distribution.

   Ref: 21 CFR 3085

2. (E) There is no federal requirement regarding product expiration. Expiration is based on results of stability studies conducted by manufacturers that involve a number of conditions, such as packaging and storage.

   Ref: United States Pharmacopoeia. 22nd revision, 1990.

3. (E) The USP recommends that prescription labels used when a medication is dispensed from a community retail pharmacy bear an expiration date, which is the date on the manufacturer's stock bottle or 1 year from the date on which the product is dispensed to the patient, whichever is earlier.

   Ref: United States Pharmacopoeia. 22nd revision, 1990.

4. (D) The USP recommends that prescription labels used when a medication is dispensed in unit-dose from a hospital or institutional pharmacy bear an expiration date of 25% of the time remaining on the manufacturer's stock bottle or 6 months from the date repackaged, whichever is earlier.

   Ref: United States Pharmacopoeia. 22nd revision, 1990.

5. (D) The proper expiration date on insulin products is 2 years from the date manufactured.

   Ref: United States Pharmacopoeia. 20th revision, 1980.

OVER-THE-COUNTER DRUGS

ANSWERS

1. (A) OTC product labels must by written in understandable language and provide information necessary for safe and effective use by consumers who are expected to medicate themselves without intervention by a physician.

   Ref: 21 CFR 330

2. (E) The OTC drug review process ultimately gives companies a plan to consult when developing OTC products for market. It permits scientific and public comment about OTC product categories, ingredients, and combinations.

   Ref: 21 CFR 330

3. (B) The monograph process, a petition, or a supplemental NDA can be used to facilitate a prescription to OTC switch.

   Ref: 21 CFR 330

4. (E) The criteria used by the FDA to classify drugs as having prescription status include whether the product has been shown to be habit forming in clinical trials and whether the drugs require a physician's supervision for proper use.

   Ref: 21 CFR 330

CONTROLLED SUBSTANCES ACT

ANSWERS

1. (E) Obviously, Agent Biggs will wish to see all of these and more. DEA has the authority to audit when they wish. An agent will check and verify that your DEA registration is current and up to date. He or she will also check to see that a federal biennial inventory was conducted and signed by the registrant. He or she will check completed copies of DEA 222 forms, used in ordering drugs in Schedule I and II, which are required signed and dated by the person receiving the drugs and filed in the pharmacy. Also, the agent may check your current invoices that account for the ordering of federally controlled substances in Schedules III, IV, and V.

   Ref: 21 CFR 1305

2. (D) In order for a written prescriptions to be valid under the Controlled Substances Act (CSA), the prescription must contain the name and address of the practitioner, the name and address of the patient, the date the prescription was written, the practitioner's DEA registration number, name, strength, dosage form, quantity, directions for use, and the number of refills if authorized as well as the prescriber's signature.

   Ref: 21 CFR 1306

3. (A) The federal transfer label is required to be affixed or appear on prescription containers that are filled for drugs listed in Schedules II, III, and IV. A federal transfer label is not required to appear on containers filled with drugs listed in Schedule V.

   Ref: 21 CFR 1308

LABORATORY VALUES OF CLINICAL IMPORTANCE

INTRODUCTORY COMMENTS

All laboratory appendices should be interpreted with caution since normal values differ widely among clinical laboratories. The values given in this Appendix are meant primarily for use with this text. In preparing the Appendix, the editors have taken into account the fact that the system of international units (SI, système international d'unités) is now used in most countries and in most medical and scientific journals.[1] However, clinical laboratories in many countries continue to report values in traditional units. Therefore, both systems are used in the Appendix. Values in SI units appear first, and traditional units appear in parentheses after the SI units. The dual system is also used in the text except for (1) those instances in which the numbers remain the same but only the terminology is changed (mmol/L for meq/L or IU/L for mIU/mL), when only the SI units are given; and (2) most pressure measurements (e.g., blood and cerebrospinal fluid pressures), when the traditional units (mmHg, mmH$_2$O) are used. In all other instances in the text the SI unit is followed by the traditional unit in parentheses. The SI base units, SI derived units, other units of measure referred to in Appendix, and SI prefixes are listed in Tables A-1 to A-3 at the end of Appendix. Conversions from one system to another can be made as follows:

$$mmol/L = \frac{mg/dL \times 10}{\text{atomic weight}}$$

$$mg/dL = \frac{mmol/L \times \text{atomic weight}}{10}$$

BODY FLUIDS AND OTHER MASS DATA

Body fluid, total volume: 50 percent (in obese) to 70 percent (lean) of body weight
    Intracellular: 0.3–0.4 of body weight
    Extracellular: 0.2–0.3 of body weight

Blood
    Total volume:
        Males: 69 mL per kg body weight
        Females: 65 mL per kg body weight
    Plasma volume:
        Males: 39 mL per kg body weight
        Females: 40 mL per kg body weight
    Red blood cell volume:
        Males: 30 mL per kg body weight (1.15–1.21 L/m² of body surface area)
        Females: 25 mL per kg body weight (0.95–1.00 L/m² of body surface area)

CEREBROSPINAL FLUID[2]

		Conversion Factor (CF) $C \times CF = SI$
Osmolarity	292–297 mmol/kg water (292–297 mOsm/L)	—
Electrolytes:		
Sodium	137–145 mmol/L (137–145 meq/L)	—
Potassium	2.7–3.9 mmol/L (2.7–3.9 meq/L)	—
Calcium	1.0–1.5 mmol/L (2.1–3.0 meq/L)	0.5
Magnesium	1.0–1.2 mmol/L (2.0–2.5 meq/L)	0.5

[1] Young DS: Implementation of SI units for clinical laboratory data. Ann Intem Med 106:114,1987.

		Conversion Factor (CF) $C \times CF = SI$
Chloride	116–122 mmol/L (116–122 meq/L)	—
CO$_2$ content	20–24 mmol/L (20–24 meq/L)	—
P$_{co_2}$	6–7 kPa (45–49 mmHg)	0.1333
pH	7.31–7.34	—
Glucose	2.2–3.9 mmol/L (40–70 mg/dL	0.05551
Lactate	1–2 mmol/L (10–20 mg/dL)	0.1110
Total protein:	0.2–0.5 g/L (20–50 mg/dL)	0.01
Albumin	0.066–0.442 g/L (6.6–44.2 mg/dL)	0.01
IgG	0.009 –0.057 g/L (0.9–5.7 mg/dL)	0.01
IgG index[3]	0.29–0.59	
Oligoclonal bands (OGB)	<2 bands not present in matched serum sample	
Ammonia	15–47 μmol/L (25–80 μg/dL)	0.5872
Creatinine	44–168 μmol/L (0.5–1.9 mg/dL)	88.40
Myelin basic protein	<4 μg/L	—
CSF pressure	50–180 mmH$_2$O	—
CSF volume (adult)	~150 mL	—
Leukocytes		
Total	<5 per mL	—
Differential:		
Lymphocytes	60–70 percent	—
Monocytes	30–50 percent	—
Neutrophils	None	—

CHEMICAL CONSTITUENTS OF BLOOD

See also function tests, especially "Metabolic and Endocrine Tests."

	Conversion Factor (CF) $C \times CF = SI$
Acetoacetate, plasma: <100 μmol/L (<1 mg /dL)	97.95
Albumin, serum: 35–55 g/L (3.5–5.5 g/dL)	10.00
Aldolase: 0–100 nkat/L (0–6 U/L)	16.67
Alpha$_1$ antitrypsin, serum: 0.8–2.1 g/L (85–213 mg/dL)	0.01
Alpha fetoprotein (adult), serum: <30 μg/L (<30 ng/mL)	—
Aminotransferase, serum:	
Aspartate (AST,SGOT): 0–0.58 μkat/L (0–35 U/L)	0.01667
Alanine (ALT, SGPT): 0–0.58 μkat/L (0–35 U/L)	0.01667
Ammonia, as NH$_3$, plasma: 6–47 μmol/L (10–80 μg/dL)	0.5872
Amylase, serum: 0.8–3.2 μkat/L: 60–180 U/L	0.01667
Angiotensin-converting enzyme (ACE): <670 nkat/L (<40 U/L)	16.67
Arterial blood gases:	
[HCO$_3$$^-$]: 21–28 mmol/L (21–30 meq/L)	—
P$_{co_2}$: 4.7–5.9 kPa (35–45 mmHg)	0.1333
pH: 7.38–7.44	—
P$_{o_2}$: 11–13 kPa (80–100 mmHg)	0.1333
Ascorbic acid (vitamin C), serum: 23–57 μmol/L (0.4–1.0 mg/dL)	56.78

[2] Since cerebrospinal fluid concentrations are equilibrium values, measurements of the same parameters in blood plasma obtained at the same time are recommended. However, there is a time lag in attainment of equilibrium, and cerebrospinal levels of plasma constituents that can fluctuate rapidly (such as plasma glucose) may not achieve stable values until after a significant lag phase.

[3] igG index = $\dfrac{\text{CSF IgG(mg/dL)} \times \text{serum albumin(g/dL)}}{\text{Serum IgG(g/dL)} \times \text{CSF albumin(mg/dL)}}$

	Conversion Factor (CF) $C \times CF = SI$

Barbiturates, serum: normal, nondetectable

    Phenobarbital, "potentially fatal" level: approximately 390 μmol/L (9 mg/dL) — 43.06

    Most short-acting barbiturates, "potentially fatal" levels: approximately 150 μmol/L (35 mg/L) — 4.419

β-Hydroxybutyrate, plasma: <300 μmol/L (<3 mg/dL) — 96.05

Bilirubin, total, serum (Malloy-Evelyn): 5.1–17 μmol/L (0.3–10 mg/dL) — 17.10

    Direct, serum: 1.7–5.1 μmol/L (0.1–0.3 mg/dL) — 17.10

    Indirect, serum: 3.4–12 μmol/L (0.2–0.7 mg/dL) — 17.10

Calciferols (vitamin D), plasma:

    1,25-dihydroxyvitamin D [1,25(OH)$_2$D]: 40–160 pmol/L (16 to 65 pg/mL) — 2.4

    25-hydroxyvitamin D [25(OH)D]: 20–200 nmol/L (8–80 ng/mL) — 2.496

Calcium, ionized: 1.1–1.4 mmol/L (4.5–5.6 mg/dL) — 0.2495

Calcium, plasma: 2.2–2.6 mmol/L (9–10.5 mg/dL) — 0.2495

Carbon dioxide content, plasma (sea level): 21–30 mmol/L (21–30 meq/L) — —

Carbon dioxide tension (P$_{CO_2}$), arterial blood (sea level): 4.7–5.9 kPa (35–45 mmHg) — 0.1333

Carbon monoxide content, blood: symptoms with over 20 percent saturation of hemoglobin

Carotenoids, serum: 0.9–5.6 μmol/L (50–300 μg/dL) — 0.01863

Ceruloplasmin, serum: 270–370 mg/L (27–37 mg/dL) — 10.00

Chloride, serum (Cl$^-$): 98–1.6 mmol/L (98–106 meq/L) — —

Cholesterol: see Table A-4

Complement, serum:

    C3: 0.55–1.20 g/L (55–120 mg/dL) — 0.01

    C4: 0.20–0.50 g/L (20–50 mg/dL) — 0.01

Copper, serum: 11–22 μmol/L (70–140 μg/dL) — 0.1574

Creatine kinase, serum (total):

    Females: 0.17–1.17 μkat/L (10–70 U/L) — 0.01667

    Males: 0.42–1.50 μkat/L (25–90 U/L) — 0.01667

Creatine kinase-MB: 0–7 μg/L — —

Creatinine, serum: <133 μmol/L (<1.5 mg/dL) — 88.40

Digoxin serum:

    Therapeutic level: 0.6–2.8 nmol/L — 1.281

    Toxic level: >3.1 nmol/L (>2.4 ng/mL) — 1.281

Ethanol, blood:

    Behavioral changes: >4.3 mmol/L (>20 mg/dL) — 0.2171

    Legal intoxication: >17 mmol/L (>80 mg/dL) — 0.2171

    Coma and death: >65 mmol/L (>300 mg/dL) — 0.2171

Fatty acids, free (nonesterified), plasma: 180 mg/L (<18 mg/dL) — 10.00

Ferritin, serum: — —

    Women: 10–200 μg/L (10–200 ng/ml)

    Men: 15–400 μg/L (15–400 ng/ml)

Folic acid, red cell: 340–1020 nmol/L cells (150–450 ng/mL cells) — 2.266

Folic acid, serum: 7–36 nmol/L cells (3–16 ng/mL cells) — —

Gastrin, serum: 40–200 ng/L (40–200 pg/mL) — —

Glucose (fasting), plasma:

    Normal: 4.2–6.4 mmol/L (75–115 mg/dL) — 0.05551

    Diabetes mellitus: >7.8 mmol/L [>140 mg/dL (on more than one occasion)] — 0.05551

Glucose, 2 h postprandial, plasma:

    Normal: <7.8 mmol/L (<140 mg/dL) — 0.05551

    Impaired glucose tolerance: 7.8–11.1 mmol/L (140–200 mg/dL) — 0.05551

    Diabetes mellitus: >11.1 mmol/L on more than one occasion (>200 mg/dL) — 0.05551

Hemoglobin, blood (sea level):

    Male: 140–180 g/L (14–18 g/dL) — 10.00

    Female: 120–160 g/L (12–16 g/dL) — 10.00

    Hemoglobin A$_{1c}$: up to 6 percent of total hemoglobin — —

	Conversion Factor (CF) C × CF = SI
Immunoglobulins, serum:	
IgA: 0.9–3.2 g/L (90–325 mg/dL)	0.01
IgD: 0–0.08 g/L (0–8 mg/dL)	0.01
IgE: <0.00025 g/L (<0.025 mg/dL)	0.01
IgG: 8.0–15.0 g/L (800–1500 mg/dL)	0.01
IgM: 0.45–1.5 g/L (45–150 mg/dL)	0.01
Iron, serum: 9–27 μmol/L (50–150) μg/dL	0.1791
Iron-binding capacity, serum: 45–66 μmol/L (250–370 μg/dL)	0.1791
Saturation: 0.2–0.45 (20–45 percent)	
Lactate dehydrogenase, serum: 1.7–3.2 μkat/L (100–190 U/L)	0.01667
Lactate dehydrogenase isoenzymes, serum (agarose):	
Fraction 1 (of total): 0.14–0.25 (14–26 percent)	0.01
Fraction 2: 0.29–0.39 (29–39 percent)	0.01
Fraction 3: 0.20–0.25 (20–26 percent)	0.01
Fraction 4: 0.08–0.16 (8–16 percent)	0.01
Fraction 5: 0.06–0.16 (6–16 percent)	0.01
Lactate, venous plasma: 0.6–1.7 mmol/L (5–15 mg/dL)	0.1110
Lead, serum: <1.0 μmol/L (<20 μg/dL)	0.04826
Lipase, serum: 0–2.66 μkat/L (0–160 U/L)	0.01667
Lipids: see Table A-4	—
Lipids, triglyceride, serum: see "Triglycerides"	—
Lipoprotein: see Table A-4	—
Lithium, serum:	
Therapeutic level: 0.6–1.2 mmol/L (0.6–1.2 meq/L)	—
Toxic level: >2 mmol/L (2 meq/L)	—
Magnesium, serum: 0.8–1.2 mmol/L (1.8–3 mg/dL)	0.4114
Osmolality, plasma: 285–295 mmol/kg serum water (285–295 mosmol/kg serum water)	—
Oxygen content:	
Arterial blook (sea level): 17–21 volume percent	—
Venous blood, arm (sea level): 10 to 16 volume percent	—
Oxygen percent saturation (sea level):	
Arterial blood: 0.97 mol/mol (97 percent)	0.01
Venous blood, arm: 0.60–0.85 mol/mol (60–85 percent)	0.01
Oxygen tension (P_{o_2}) blood: 11–13 kPa (10–100 mmHg)	0.1333
pH, blood: 7.38–7.44	—
Phenytoin, plasma: See Harrison's Fig. 365–8*	
Phosphatase, acid, serum: 0.90 nkat/L (0–5.5 U/L)	—
Phosphatase, alkaline, serum: 0.5–2.0 nkat/L (30–120 U/L)	—
Phosphorus, inorganic, serum: 1.0–1.4 mmol/L (3–4.5 mg/dL)	0.3229
Potassium, serum: 3.5–5.0 mmol/L (3.5–5.0 meq/L)	
Protein, total, serum: 55–80 g/L (5.5–8.0 g/dL)	10.00
Protein fractions, serum:	
Albumin: 35–55 g/L [3.5–5.5 g/dL (50–60 percent)]	10.00
Globulin: 20–35 g/L [2.0–3.5 g/dL (40–50 percent)]	10.00
Alpha$_1$: 2–4 g/L [0.2–0.4 g/dL (4.2–7.2 percent)]	10.00
Alpha$_2$: 5–9 g/L [0.5–0.9 g/dL (6.8–12 percent)]	10.00
Beta: 6–11 g/L [0.6–1.1 g/dL (9.3–15 percent)]	10.00
Gamma: 7–17 g/L [0.7–1.7 g/dL (13–23 percent)]	10.00
Pyruvate, venous, plasma: 60–170 μmol/L (0.5–1.5 mg/dL)	113.6

*Fauci AS, Braunwald E. Isselbacher KJ. et al. *Harrison's Principles of Internal Medicine, 14th edition.* McGraw-Hill, New York 1998.

	Conversion Factor (CF) C × CF = SI

Quinidine, serum:

    Therapeutic range: 4.6–9.2 μmol/L (1.5–3 mg/L) — 3.082

    Toxic range: 15.4–18.5 μmol/L (5–6 mg/L) — 3.082

Salicylate, plasma: 0 mmol/L — —

    Therapeutic range: 1.4–1.8 mmol/L (20–25 mg/dL) — 0.07240

    Toxic range: >2.2 mmol/L (>30 mg/dL) — 0.07240

Sodium, serum: 136–145 mmol/L (136–145 meq/L) — —

Steroids: see "Metabolic and Endocrine Tests" — —

Transferrin, serum: 2.3–3.9 mg/L (230–390 μg/dL) — 10.00

Triglycerides: <1.8 mmol/L (<160 mg/dL) — 0.01129

Troponin l, serum: 0–0.4 μg/L (0–0.4 ng/mL) — —

Troponin T, serum: 0–0.1 μg/L (0–0.1 ng/mL) — —

Urea nitrogen, serum: 3.6–7.1 mmol/L (10–20 mg/dL) — 0.3570

Uric acid, serum:

    Men: 150–480 μmol/L (2.5–8.0 mg/dL) — 59.48

    Women: 90–360 μmol/L (1.5–6.0 mg/dL) — 59.48

Vitamin A, serum: 0.7–3.5 μmol/L (20–100 μg/dL) — 0.03491

Vitamin B$_{12}$, serum: 148–443 pmol/L (200–600 pg/mL) — 0.7378

Zinc, serum: 11.5–18.5 μmol/L (75–120 μg/dL) — 0.1530

CIRCULATORY FUNCTION TESTS

Arteriovenous oxygen difference: 30–50 mL/L

Cardiac output (Fick): 2.5–3.6 L/m^2 of body surface area per minute

Contractility indexes:

    Maximum left ventricular dp/dt: 1650 mmHg/s (range, 1320–1880, mmHg/s)

    $(dp/dt)/DP$ when DP = 40 mmHg: 37.6 ± 12.2 s^{-1} (DP, diastolic pressure)

    Mean normalized systolic ejection rate (angiography): 3.32 ± 0.84 end-diastolic volumes per second

    Mean velocity of circumferential fiber shortening (angiography) 1.66 ± 0.42 circumferences per second

Ejection fraction, stroke volume/end-diastolic volume (SV/EDV): normal range: 0.55–0.78; average: 0.67

End-diastolic volume: 75 mL/m^2 (range, 60–88 mL/m^2)

End-systolic volume: 25 mL/m^2 (range, 20–33 mL/m^2)

Left ventricular work:

    Stroke work index: 30–110 (g·m)/m^2

    Left ventricular minute work index: 1.8–6.6 [(kg·m)/m^2]/min

    Oxygen consumption index: 110–150 mL

Maximum oxygen uptake: normal range 20–60 mL/min; average: 35 mL/min

Pulmonary vascular esistance: 20–120 (dyn·s)/cm^5 (2–12 kPa·s/L)

Systemic vascular resistance: 770–1500 (dyn·s)/cm^5 (77–150 kPa·s/L)

GASTROINTESTINAL TESTS

See also "Stool Analysis."

Absorption tests:

    D-Xylose absorption test: After an overnight fast, 25 g xylose is given in aqueous solution by mouth.

        Urine collected for the following 5 h should contain 33–53 mmol (5–8 g) (or >20 percent of ingested dose). Serum xylose should be 1.7–2.7 mmol (25–40 mg/dL) l h after the oral dose.

    Vitamin A absorption test: A fasting blood specimen is obtained and 200,000 units of vitamin A in oil is given by mouth. Serum vitamin A levels should rise to twice fasting level in 3–5 h.

Bentiromide test (pancreatic function): 500 mg bentiromide (chymex) orally; p-aminobenzoic acid

    (PABA) measured in plasma and/or urine

        Plasma: >3.6 (± 1.1) μg/mL at 90 min

        Urine: >50 percent recovered as PABA in 6 h

Gastric juice:
  Volume:
    24 h: 2–3 L

      Nocturnal: 600–700 mL
      Basal, fasting: 30–70 mL/h
  Reaction:
    pH: 1.6–1.8
    Titratable acidity of fasting juice: 4–9 μmol/s (15–35 meq/h)   0.261
  Acid output:
    Basal:
      Females (mean ± 1 SD): 0.6 ± 0.5 ρmol/s (2.0 ± 1.8 meq/h)   0.2778
      Males (mean ± 1 SD): 0.8 ± 0.6 μmol/s (3.0 ± 2.0 meq/h)   0.2778
    Maximal (after subcutaneous histamine acid phosphate 0.004 mg/kg body weight
    and preceded by 50 mg promethazine or after betazole 1.7 mg/kg body wt or
    pentagastrin 6 μg/kg body wt):
      Females (mean ± 1 SD): 4.4 ± 1.4 μmol/s (16 ± 5 meq/h)   0.2778
      Males (mean± 1 SD): 6.4 ± 1.4 μmol/s (23 ± 5 meq/h)   0.2778
    Basal acid output/maximal acid output ratio: 0.6 or less
Gastrin, serum: 40–200 ng/L (40–200 pg/mL)   —
Secretin test (pancreatic exocrine function): 1 unit per kg body wt, Intravenously
  Volume (pancreatic juice): >2.0 mL/kg in 80 min   —
  Bicarbonate concentration: >80 mmol/L (>80 meq/L)   —
  Bicarbonate output: >10 mmol in 30 min (>10 meq in 30 min)   —

METABOLIC AND ENDOCRINE TESTS

Adrenocorticotropin (ACTH) plasma, 8 A.M.: 2–11 pmol/L (9–52 pg/mL)   0.2202
Adrenal cortex function tests: see Harrison's Chap. 322*   —
Adrenal medulla function tests: see Harrison's Chap. 333*   —
Adrenal steroids, plasma:
  Aldosterone, 8 A.M.: <220 pmol/L (patient supine, 100 meq Na and 60–100 meq K intake) (<8 ng/dL)   27.74
  Cortisol:
    8 A.M.: 140–690 nmol/L (5–25 μg/dL)   27.59
    4 P.M.: 80–330 nmol/L (3–12 μg/dL)   27.59
  Dehydroepiandrosterone (DHEA): 7–31 nmol/L (2–9 μg/L)   3.467
  Dehydroepiandrosterone sulfate (DHEA sulfate): 1.3–6.8 μmol/L (500–2500 μg/L)   0.002714
  11-Deoxycortisol (compound S): <30 nmol/L (<1 μg/dL)   28.86
  17-Hydroxyprogesterone:
    Women: follicular phase, 0.6–3 nmol/L (0.20–1 μg/L);   3.026
      luteal phase 1.5–10.6 nmol/L (0.5–3.5 μg/L)   3.026
    Men: 0.2–9 nmol/L (0.06)–3 μg/L)   3.026
Adrenal steroids, urinary excretion
  Aldosterone: 14–53 nmol/d (5–19 μg/d)   2.774
  Cortisol, free: 55–275 nmol/d (20–100 μg/d)   2.759
  17-Hydroxycorticosteroids: 5.5–28 μmol/d (2–10 mg/d)   2.759
  17-Ketosteroids:
    Men: 20–69 ρmol/d (6–20 mg/d)   3.467
    Women: 20–59 μmol/d (6–17 mg/d)   3.467
    Angiotensin II, plasma, 8 A.M.: 10–30 nmol/L (10–30 pg/mL)   —

*Fauci AS, Braunwald E, Isselbacher KJ, et al. *Harrison's Principles of Internal Medicine, 14th edition.* McGraw-Hill, New York 1998.

	Conversion Factor (CF) C × CF = SI

Arginine vasopressin (AVP), plasma:

    Random fluid intake: 1.5–5.6 pmol/L (1.5–6 ng/L) — 0.92

Calcitonin, plasma: <50 ng/L (<50 pg/mL) — —

Catecholamines, urinary excretion:

    Free catecholamines: <590 nmol/d (<100 μg/d) — 5.911

    Epinephrine: <275 nmol/d (<50 μg/d) — 5.458

    Metanephrines: <7 μmol/d (<1.3 mg/d) — 5.458

    Norepinephrine: 89–473 nmol/d (15–80) μg/d) — 5.91

    Vanillylmandelic acid (VMA): <40 μmol/d (<8 mg/d) — 5.046

Glucagon, plasma: 50–100 ng/L (50–100 pg/mL) — —

Gonadal function tests: see Harrison's Chaps. 336 and 337* — —

Gonadal steroids, plasma:

    Androstenedione:

        Women: 3.5–7.0 nmol/L (1–2 ng/mL) — 3.492

        Men: 3.0–5.0 nmol/L (0.8–1.3 ng/mL) — 3.492

    Estradiol:

        Women: 70–220 pmol/L (20–60 pg/mL), higher at ovulation — 3.671

        Men: <180 pmol/L (<50 pg/mL) — 3.671

    Progesterone:

        Men, prepubertal girls, preovulatory women, and postmenopausal women: <6 nmol/L (<2 ng/mL) — 3.180

        Women, luteal, peak: 6–60 nmol/L (2–20 ng/mL) — 3.180

    Testosterone:

        Women: <3.5 nmol/L (<1 ng/mL) — 3.467

        Men: 10–35 nmol/L (3–10 ng/mL) — 3.467

        Prepubertal boys and girls: 0.17–0.7 nmol/L (0.05–0.2 ng/mL) — 3.467

Gonadotropins, plasma:

    Women, mature, premenopausal, except at ovulation:

        FSH: 1.4–9.6 IU/L (1.4–9.6 mIU/mL) — —

        LH: 0.8–26 IU/L (0.8–26 mIU/mL) — —

    Ovulatory surge:

        FSH: 2.3–21 IU/L (2.3–21 mIU/mL) — —

        LH: 25–57 IU/L (25–57 mIU/mL) — —

    Postmenopausal women:

        FSH: 34–96 IU/L (34–96 mIU/mL) — —

        LH: 40–104 IU/L (40–104 mIU/mL) — —

    Men, mature:

        FSH: 0.9–15 IU/L (0.9–15 mIU/mL) — —

        LH: 1.3–13 IU/L (1.3–13 mIU/mL) — —

    Children of both sexes, prepubertal:

        LH: 1.0–5.9 IU/L (1.0–5.9 mIU/mL) — —

Growth hormone, after 100 g glucose by mouth: <2 μg/L (<2 ng/mL) — —

Human chorionic gonadotropin, β subunit (β-hCG), plasma:

    Men and nonpregnant women: <3 IU/L (<3 mIU/mL) — —

Insulin, serum or plasma, fasting: 43–186 pmol/L (6–26 μU/mL) — 7.175

Insulin-like growth factor I (somatomedin C, IGF-1/SM C): see Harrison's Chap. 329* — —

Oxytocin: random 1–4 pmol/L (1.25–5 ng/L) — 0.80

    Ovulatory peak in women 4–8 pmol/L (5–10 ng/L) — —

Pancreatic islet function tests: see Harrison's Chap. 334* — —

Parathyroid function tests: see Harrison's Chap. 354* — —

Pituitary function tests: see Harrison's Chaps. 328 to 330* — —

*Fauci AS, Braunwald E, Isselbacher KJ. et al. *Harrison's Principles of Internal Medicine, 14th edition.* McGraw-Hill, New York 1998.

	Conversion Factor (CF) $C \times CF = SI$
Pregnancy tests: *see* Harrison's Chap. 337*	—
Prolactin, serum: 2.15 µg/L (2–15 ng/mL)	—
Renin-angiotensin function tests: *see* Harrison's Chap. 332*	—
Semen analysis: *see* Harrison's Chap. 336*	—
Thyroid function tests:	
Dynamic tests of thyroid function: *see* Harrison's Chap. 331*	—
Radioactive iodine uptake, 24 h: 5–30 percent (range varies in different areas due to variations in iodine intake)	—
Resin T_3 uptake: 0.25–0.35 (25–35 percent) (varies among laboratories; for calculation of free T4 estimate, *see* Harrison's Chap. 331)*	0.01
Reverse triiodothyronine (rT_3), plasma: 0.15–0.61 nmol/L (10–40 ng/dL)	0.01536
Thyroid-stimulating hormone (TSH): 0.4–5 mU/L (0.4–5 µU/mL)	—
Thyroxine (T_4), serum radioimmunoassay: 64–154 nmol/L (5–12 µg/dL)	12.86
Triiodothyronine (T_3), plasma: 1.1–2.9 nmol/L (70–190 ng/dL)	0.01536

PULMONARY FUNCTION TESTS

See Table A-9

RENAL FUNCTION TESTS

	Conversion Factor (CF) $C \times CF = SI$
Clearances (corrected to 1.72 m² body surface area):	
Measures of glomerular filtration rate:	
Insulin clearance (C1):	
Males (mean ± 1 SD): 2.1 ± 0.4 mL/s (124 ± 25.8 mL/min)	0.01667
Females (mean ± 1 SD): 2.0 ± 0.2 mL/s (119 ± 12.8 mL/min)	0.01667
Endogenous creatinine clearance: 1.5–2.2 mL/s (91–130 mL/min)	0.01667
Urea: 1.0–1.7 mL/s (60–100 mL/min)	0.01667
Measures of *effective renal plasma flow* and *tubular function*:	
p-Aminohippuric acid clearance (Cl_{PAH}):	
Males (mean ± 1 SD):10.9 ± 2.7 mL/s (654 ± 163 mL/min)	0.01667
Females (mean ± 1 SD):9.9 ± 1.7 mL/s (594 ± 102 mL/min)	0.01667
Concentration and dilution test:	
Specific gravity of urine:	
After 12-h fluid restriction: 1.025 or more	—
After 12-h deliberate water intake: 1.003 or less	—
Protein excretion, urine: <0.15 g/d (150 mg/d)	0.01
Males: 0–0.06 g/d (0–60 mg/d)	0.01
Females: 0–0.09 g/d (0–90 mg/d)	0.01
Specific gravity, maximal range: 1.002–1.028	—
Tubular reabsorption, phosphorus: 79–94 percent of filtered load	—

*Fauci AS, Braunwald E, Isselbacher KJ. et al. *Harrison's Principles of Internal Medicine, 14th edition.* McGraw-Hill, New York 1998.

HEMATOLOGIC EVALUATIONS

See also "Chemical Constituents of Blood."

	Conversion Factor (CF) $C \times CF = SI$
Bone marrow: see Table A-6	—
Carboxyhemoglobin:	
Nonsmoker: 0–0.023 (0–2.3 percent)	0.01
Smoker: 0.021–0.042 (2.1–4.2 percent)	0.01
Erythrocyte:	
Count: $4.15–4.90 \times 10^{12}/L$ ($4.15–4.90 \times 10^{6}/mm^3$)	—
Distribution width: 0.13–0.15 (13–15 percent)	—
Glucose-6-phosphate dehydrogenase: 12.1 ± 2 IU/gHb (WHO)	—
Life span:	
Normal survival: 120 days	—
Chromium-labeled, half-life ($t_{1/2}$): 28 days	—
Mean corpuscular hemoglobin (MCH): 28–33 pg/cell (28–33 pg/cell)	—
Mean corpuscular hemoglobin concentration (MCHC): 320–360 g/L (32–36 g/dL)	10.00
Mean corpuscular volume (MCV): 86–98 fl (86–98 μm^3)	—
Ham's test (acid serum): negative	—
Haptoglobin, serum 0.5–2.2 g/L (50–220 mg/dL)	0.01
Hematocrit	
Males: 0.42–0.52 (42–52%)	—
Females: 0.37–0.48 (37–48%)	—
Hemoglobin:	
Plasma: 0.01–0.05 g/L (1–5 mg/dL)	0.01
Whole blood:	
Males: 8.1–11.2 mmol/L (13–18 g/dL)	—
Females: 7.4–9.9 mmol/L (12–16 g/dL)	—
Hemoglobin A_2 (HbA$_2$): 0.015–0.035 (1.5–3.5 percent)	0.01
Hemoglobin, fetal (HbF): <0.02 (<2 percent)	0.01
Leukocytes:	
Alkaline phosphatase (LAP): 0.2–1.6 μkat/L (13–100 μ/L)	—
Count: $4.3–10.8 \times 10^{9}/L$ ($4.3–10.8 \times 10^{3}/mm^3$)	
Differential:	
Neutrophils: 0.45–0.74 (45–74 percent)	
Bands: 0–0.04 (0–4 percent)	
Lymphocytes: 0.16–0.45 (16–45 percent)	
Monocytes: 0.04–0.10 (4–10 percent)	
Eosinophils: 0–0.07 (0–7 percent)	
Basophils: 0–0.02 (0–2 percent)	
Methemoglobin: <2 mg/L (<2 μg/mL)	—
Osmotic fragility:	
Slight hemolysis: 0.45–0.39 percent	—
Complete hemolysis: 0.33–0.30 percent	—
Platelets and coagulation parameters:	
Alpha$_2$ antiplasmin: 70–130 percent	
Antithrombin III: 80–120 percent	
Bleeding time:	
Simplate: <7 min	
Euglobulin lysis time: >2 h	
Factor II: 60–100 percent	
Factor V: 60–100 percent	
Factor VII: 60–100 percent	
Factor IX: 60–100 percent	

	Conversion Factor (CF) C × CF = SI

Factor X: 60–100 percent
Factor XI: 60–100 percent
Factor XII: 60–100 percent
Factor XIII: 60–100 percent
Fibrinogen: 200–400 mg/dL
Plasminogen: 2.4–4.4 CTA U/mL
Protein C (antigenic assay): 58–148 percent
Protein S (antigenic assay): 58–148 percent
Partial thromboplastin time (activated PTT): comparable to control
Prothrombin time (quick one-stage): control ± 1 s
Platelets: $130–400 \times 10^9$/L (130,000–400,000/mm^3)
Thrombin time: control ± 3 s
von Willebrand's antigen: 60–150 percent

Protoporphyrin, free erythrocyte (FEP): 0.28–0.64 μmol/L of red blood cells (16–36 μg/dL of red blood cells) — 0.0177

Red cells: (see "Erythrocytes")
Schilling test: 7–40 percent of orally administered vitamin B$_{12}$ excreted in urine
Sedimentation rate:
  Westergren, <50 years of age:
    Males: 0–15 mm/h
    Females: 0–20 mm/h
  Westergren, >50 years of age:
    Males: 0–20 mm/h
    Females: 0–30 mm/h
Sucrose hemolysis: negative
Viscosity
  Plasma: 1.7–2.1
  Serum: 1.4–1.8
White blood cells: (see "Leukocytes")

STOOL ANALYSIS

	Conversion Factor (CF) C × CF = SI
Bulk:	
Wet weight: <197.5 (115 ± 41) g/d	—
Dry weight: <66.4 (34 ± 15) g/d	—
Alpha$_1$ antitrypsin: 0.98 (± 0.17) mg/g dry weight stool	—
Coproporphyrin: 600–1500 nmol/d (400–1000 μg/d)	1.527
Fat (on diet containing at least 50 g fat): <6.0 (4.0 ± 1.5) g/d when measured on a 3-day (or longer) collection	
Percent of dry weight: 0.30 (<30.4 percent)	0.01
Coefficient of fat absorption: >0.95 (>95 percent)	0.01
Fatty acid:	
Free: 0.01–0.10 (1–10 percent of dry matter)	0.01
Combined as soap: 0.005–0.12 (0.5–12 percent of dry matter)	0.01
Nitrogen: <1.7 (1.4 ± 0.2) g/d	—
Protein content: minimal	—
Urobilinogen: 68–470 μmol/d (40–280) mg/d)	1.693
Water: 0.65 (approximately 65 percent)	0.01

URINE ANALYSIS

See also "Metabolic and Endocrine Tests"

	Conversion Factor (CF) $C \times CF = SI$
Acidity, titratable: 20–40 mmol/d (20–40 meq/d)	—
Ammonia: 30–50 mmol/d (30–50 meq/d)	—
Amylase: 35–260 Somogyi units/h	—
Amylase/creatinine clearance ratio [$(Cl_{am}/Cl_{cr}) \times 100$]: 1–5	—
Bentiromide (pancreatic function): 50 percent excreted in 6 h as p-amino benzoic acid (PABA) after 500 mg oral bentiromide	—
Calcium (10 meq/d or 200-mg/d calcium diet): <3.8 mmol/d (<7.5 meq/d)	0.5
Catecholamines: see under "Metabolic and Endocrine Tests"	—
Copper: 0–0.4 µmol/d (0–25 µg/d)	0.01574
Coproporphyrins (types I and III): 150–460 nmol/d (100–300 µg/d)	1.527
Creatine, as creatinine:	
Adult males: <380 µmol/d (<50 mg/d)	7.625
Adult females: <760 µmol/d (<100 mg/d)	7.625
Creatinine: 8.8–14 mmol/d (1.0–1.6 g/d)	8.840
Glucose, true (oxidase method): 0.3–1.7 mmol/d (50–300 mg/d)	0.5551
5-Hydroxyindoleacetic acid (5-HIAA): 10–47 µmol/d (2–9 mg/d)	5.230
Lead: <0.4 µmol/d (<80 µg/d)	0.004826
Protein: <0.15 g/d (<150 mg/d)	0.1
Porphobilinogen: none	—
Potassium: 25–100 mmol/d [25–100 meq/d (varies with intake)]	—
Sodium:100–260 mmol/d [100–260 meq/d (varies with intake)]	—
Urobilinogen: 1.7–5.9 µmol/d (1–3.5 mg/d)	1.693
D-Xylose excretion: 5 to 8 g within 5 h after oral dose of 25 g	—

Table A-1

SI and Other Units

Quantity	Name of Unit	Symbol for Unit	Derivation of Units
SI BASE UNITS			
Length	meter	m	
Mass	kilogram	kg	
Time	second	s	
Thermodynamic temperature	Kelvin	K	
Amount of substance	mole	mol	
SI DERIVED UNITS			
Area	square meter	m^2	
Force	newton	N	$(m \cdot kg)/s^2$
Pressure	pascal	Pa	$N \cdot m^2$
Work, energy	joule	J	$N \cdot m$
Celsius temperature	degree Celsius	°C	K
OTHER UNITS RETAINED FOR USE			
Time	minute	min	
	hour	h	
	day	d	
Volume	liter	L	

Table A-2

Radiation Derived Units

Quantity	Old Unit	SI Unit	Name for SI Unit (and Abbreviation)	Conversion
Activity	curie (Ci)	Disintegrations per second (dps)	becquerel (Bq)	$1 \text{ Ci} = 3.7 \times 10^{10} \text{ Bq}$ $1 \text{ mCi} = 37 \text{ mBq}$ $1 \text{ μCi} = 0.037 \text{ MBq or } 37 \text{ GBq}$ $1 \text{ Bq} = 2.703 \times 10^{-11} \text{ Ci}$
Absorbed dose	rad	joule per kilogram (J/kg)	gray (Gy)	$1 \text{ Gy} = 100 \text{ rad}$ $1 \text{ rad} = 0.01 \text{ Gy}$ $1 \text{ mrad} = 10^{-3} \text{ cGy}$
Exposure	roentgen (R)	coulomb per kilogram (C/kg)	—	$1 \text{ C/kg} = 3876 \text{ R}$ $1 \text{ R} = 2.58 \times 10^{-4} \text{ C/kg}$ $1 \text{ mR} = 258 \text{ pC/kg}$
Dose equivalent	rem	joule per kilogram (J/kg)	sievert (Sv)	$1 \text{ Sv} = 100 \text{ rem}$ $1 \text{ rem} = 0.01 \text{ Sv}$ $1 \text{ mrem} = 10 \text{ μSv}$

Table A-3

SI Prefixes and Their Symbols

Factor	Prefix	Symbol for Prefix
10^9	giga	G
10^6	mega	M
10^3	kilo	k
10^2	hecto	h
10^1	deka	da
10^{-1}	deci	d
10^{-2}	centi	c
10^{-3}	milli	m
10^{-6}	micro	μ
10^{-9}	nano	n
10^{-12}	pico	p
10^{-15}	femto	f
10^{-18}	alto	a

Table A-4

Classification of Total Cholesterol, LDL-Cholesterol, and HDL-Cholesterol Values

	Total Plasma Cholesterol	LDL-Cholesterol	HDL-Cholesterol	Conversion Factor (C to SI)
Desirable	<5.20 mmol/L (<200 mg/dL)	<3.36 mmol/L (<130 mg/dL)	>1.55 mmol/L (>60 mg/dL)	0.02586
Borderline	5.20–6.18 mmol/L (200–239 mg/dL)	3.36–4.11 mmol/L (130–159 mg/dL)	0.9–1.55 mmol/L (35–60 mg/dL)	0.02586
Undesirable	≥6.21 mmol/L (≥240 mg/dL)	≥4.14 mmol/L (≥160 mg/dL)	<0.9 mmol/L (<35 mg/dL)	0.02586

SOURCE: Modified from the report of the Expert Panel on Detection, Evaluation, and Treatment of High Blood Cholesterol in Adults: Second Report of the National Cholesterol Education Program (NCEP) expert panel on detection, evaluation, and treatment of high blood cholesterol (Adult Treatment Panel II). Circulation 89:1329, 1994.

Table A-5

Normal Values of Doppler Echocardiographic Measurements in Adults

	Range	*Mean*
RVD (cm)	0.9 to 2.6	1.7
LVID (cm)	3.5 to 5.7	4.7
Posterior LV wall thickness (cm)	0.6 to 1.1	0.9
IVS wall thickness (cm)	0.6 to 1.1	0.9
Left atrial dimension (cm)	1.9 to 4.0	2.9
Aortic root dimension (cm)	2.0 to 3.7	2.7
Aortic cusps separation (cm)	1.5 to 2.6	1.9
Percentage of fractional shortening	34 to 44%	36%
Mitral flow (m/sec)	0.6 to 1.3	0.9
Tricuspid flow (m/sec)	0.3 to 0.7	0.5
Pulmonary artery (m/sec)	0.6 to 0.9	0.75
Aorta (m/sec)	1.0 to 1.7	1.35

NOTE: RVD, right ventricular dimension; LVID, left ventricular internal dimension; LV, left ventricle; IVS, interventricular septum.

SOURCE: From H. Feigenbaum, *Echocardiography,* 5th ed, Philadelphia, Lea & Febiger, 1994

Table A-6

Differential Nucleated Cell Counts of Bone Marrow

	*Norma, Mean %**	*Range, %†*		*Normal, Mean %**	*Range, %†*
Myeloid	56.7		Erythroid	25.6	
Neutrophilic series	53.6		Pronormoblasts	0.6	0.2–1.3
Myeloblast	0.9	0.2–1.5	Basophilic normoblasts	1.4	0.5–2.4
Promyelocyte	3.3	2.1–4.1	Polychromatophilic	21.6	17.9–29.2
Myelocyte	12.7	8.2–15.7	normoblasts		
Metamyelocyte	15.9	9.6–24.6	Orthochromatic normoblasts	2.0	0.4–4.6
Band	12.4	9.5–15.3	Megakaryocytes	<0.1	
Segmented			Lymphoreticular	17.8	
Eosinophilic series	3.1	1.2–5.3	Lymphocytes	16.2	11.1–23.2
Basophilic series	<0.1	0–0.2	Plasma cells	2.3	0.4–3.9
			Reticulum cells	0.3	0–0.9

* From MM Wintrobe et al, *Clinical Hematology,* 8th ed. Philadelphia, Lea & Febiger, 1981.
† Range observed in 12 healthy men.

Table A-7

Erythrocytes and Hemoglobin: Normal Values at Various Ages

Age	Red Blood Cell Count,* 10^{12}/L	Hemoglobin,* g/L (g/dL)	Vol. Packed RBCs,* mL/dL	Corpuscular Values			
				MCV, fL	MCH, pg	MCHC, g/L (g/dL)	MCD, μm
Days 1–13	5.1 ± 1.0	195 ± 50 (19.5 ± 5)	54.0 ± 10.0	106–98	38–33	340–360 (36–34)	8.6
Days 14–60	4.7 ± 0.9	140 ± 33 (14 ± 3.3)	42.0 ± 7.0	90	30	330 (33)	8.1
3 months to 10 years	4.5 ± 0.7	122 ± 23 (12.2 ± 2.3)	36.0 ± 5.0	80	27	340 (34)	7.7
11–15 years	4.8	131 (13.14)	39.0	82	28	340 (34)	
Adults:							
Females	4.8 ± 0.6	140 ± 20 (14 ± 2)	42.0 ± 5.0	90 ± 7	29 ± 2	340 ± 20 (34 ± 2)	7.5 ± 0.3
Males	5.4 ± 0.9	160 ± 20 (16 ± 2)	47.0 ± 5.0	90 ± 7	29 ± 2	340 ± 20 (34 ± 2)	7.5 ± 0.3

* The range of values represents almost the extremes of observed variations (93 percent or more) at sea level. The blood values of healthy persons should fall well within these mean ± SD figures.

NOTE: MCV, mean corpuscular volume; MCH, mean corpuscular hemoglobin; MCHC, mean corpuscular hemoglobin concentration; MCD, mean corpuscular diameter.

SOURCE: MM Wintrobe et al, *Clinical Hematology,* 8th ed, Philadelphia, Lea & Febiger, 1981.

Table A-8

Normal Leukocyte Count, Differential Count, and Hemoglobin Concentration at Various Ages

Age	Leukocytes, Total	Neutrophils			Eosinophills	Basophils	Lymphocytes	Monocytes
		Total	Band	Segmented				
12 mo	11.4(6.0–17.5)	3.5(1.5–8.5) *31*	0.35 *3.1*	3.2 *28*	0.3(0.05–0.7) *0.4*	0.05(0–0.20) *0.4*	7.0(4.0–10.5) *61*	0.55(0.05–1.1) *4.8*
4 yr	9.1(5.5–15.5)	3.8(1.5–8.5) *42*	0.27(0–1.0) *3.0*	3.5(1.5–7.5) *39*	0.25(0.02–0.65) *2.8*	0.05(0–0.20) *0.6*	4.5(2.0–8.0) *50*	0.45(0–0.8) *5.0*
6 yr	4.3(1.5–8.0)	0.25(0–1.0) *51*	4.0(1.5–7.0) *3.0*	4.0(1.5–7.0) *48*	0.23(0–0.65) *2.7*	0.05(0–0.20) *0.6*	3.5(1.5–7.0) *42*	0.40(0–0.8) *4.7*
10 yr	8.1(4.5–13.5)	4.4(1.8–8.0) *54*	0.24(0–1.0) *3.0*	4.2(1.8–7.0) *51*	0.20(0–0.60) *2.4*	0.04(0–0.20) *0.5*	3.1(1.5–6.5) *38*	0.35(0–0.8) *4.3*
21 yr	7.4(4.5–11.0)	4.4(1.8–7.7) *59*	0.22(0–0.7) *3.0*	4.2(1.8–7.0) *56*	0.20(0–0.45) *2.7*	0.04(0–0.20) *0.5*	2.5(1.0–4.8) *34*	0.30(0–0.8) *4.0*

NOTE: Values are expressed as "cells × 10^9/L." The numbers in italic are percentages.

SOURCE: E Beutler et al (eds), *Williams Hematology,* 5th ed, New York, McGraw-Hill, 1995. By permission.

Table A-9

Summary of Values Useful in Pulmonary Physiology

	Symbol	Typical Values Man Aged 40, 75 kg, 175 cm Tall	Typical Values Woman Aged 40, 60 kg, 160 cm Tall
PULMONARY MECHANICS			
Spirometry—volume-time curves:			
Forced vital capacity	FVC	4.8 L	3.3 L
Forced expiratory volume in 1 s	FEV_1	3.8 L	2.8 L
FEV_1/FVC	$FEV_1\%$	76%	77%
Maximal midexpiratory flow	MMF (FEF 25–27)	4.8 L/s	3.6 L/s
Maximal expiratory flow rate	MEFR (FEF 200–1200)	9.4 L/s	6.1 L/s
Spirometry—flow-volume curves:			
Maximal expiratory flow at 50% of expired vital capacity	V_{max} 50 (FEF 50%)	6.1 L/s	4.6 L/s
Maximal expiratory flow at 75% of expired vital capacity	V_{max} 75 (FEF 75%)	3.1 L/s	2.5 L/s
Resistance to airflow:			
Pulmonary resistance	RL (R_L)	<3.0 (cmH$_2$O/s)/L	
Airway resistance	Raw	<2.5 (cmH$_2$O/s)/L	
Specific conductance	SGaw	>0.13 cmH$_2$O/s	
Pulmonary compliance:			
Static recoil pressure at total lung capacity	Pst TLC	25 ± 5 cmH$_2$O	
Compliance of lungs (static)	CL	0.2 L cmH$_2$O	
Compliance of lungs and thorax	C(L + T)	0.1 L cmH$_2$O	
Dynamic compliance of 20 breaths per minute	C dyn 20	0.25 ± 0.05 L/cmH$_2$O	
Maximal static respiratory pressures:			
Maximal inspiratory pressure	MIP	>90 cmH$_2$O	>50 cmH$_2$O
Maximal expiratory pressure	MEP	>150 cmH$_2$O	>120 cmH$_2$O
LUNG VOLUMES			
Total lung capacity	TLC	6.4 L	4.9 L
Functional residual capacity	FRC	2.2 L	2.6 L
Residual volume	RV	1.5 L	1.2 L
Inspiratory capacity	IC	4.8 L	3.7 L
Expiratory reserve volume	ERV	3.2 L	2.3 L
Vital capacity	VC	1.7 L	1.4 L
GAS EXCHANGE (SEA LEVEL)			
Arterial O$_2$ tension	Pa$_{O_2}$	12.7 ± 0.7 kPa (95 ± 5 mmHg)	
Arterial CO$_2$ tension	Pa$_{CO_2}$	5.3 ± 0.3 kPa (40 ± 2 mmHg)	
Arterial O$_2$ saturation	Sa$_{O_2}$	0.97 ± 0.02 (97 ± 2%)	
Arterial blood pH	pH	7.40 ± 0.02	
Arterial bicarbonate	HCO$_3^-$	24 + 2 meq/L	
Base excess	BE	0 ± 2 meq/L	
Diffusing capacity for carbon monoxide (single breath)	DL$_{CO}$	0.42 mLCO/s/mmHg (25 mL CO/min/mmHg)	
Dead space volume	V$_D$	2 ml/kg body wt	
Physiologic dead space; dead space-tidal volume ratio	V$_D$/V$_T$		
Rest		≤ 35% V$_T$	
Exercise		≤ 20% V$_T$	
Alveolar-arterial difference for O$_2$	P(A−a)$_{O_2}$	≤ 2.7 kPa ≤ 20 kPa (≤20 mmHg)	